The Attentive Brain

The Attentive Brain

edited by Raja Parasuraman

A Bradford Book
The MIT Press
Cambridge, Massachusetts
London, England

This book was set in Palatino on the Monotype "Prism Plus" PostScript Imagesetter by Asco Trade Typesetting Ltd., Hong Kong and was printed and bound in the United States of America.

Library of Congress Cataloging-in-Publication Data

The attentive brain / edited by Raja Parasuraman.
   p.   cm.
"A Bradford book."
Includes indexes.
ISBN 0-262-16172-9 (alk. paper)
1. Attention. 2. Cognitive neuroscience. I. Parasuraman, R.
[DNLM: 1. Attention. 2. Brain. 3. Neurosciences—methods. BF
321 A885 1998]
QP405.A876   1998
612.8′2—dc21
DNLM/DLC
for Library of Congress   97-22985
                                                            CIP

For Rashmi, Rachna, and Shanta

Contents

Preface   xi

I   Introduction   1

1   The Attentive Brain: Issues and Prospects   3
     Raja Parasuraman

II   Cognitive Neuroscience Methods   17

2   Neuroanatomy of Visual Attention   19
     Maree J. Webster and Leslie G. Ungerleider

3   Neurochemistry of Attention   35
     Richard T. Marrocco and Matthew C. Davidson

4   Neurophysiology of Visual Attention   51
     Brad C. Motter

5   Electrophysiological Approaches to the Study of Selective
     Attention in the Human Brain   71
     Steven J. Luck and Massimo Girelli

6   Functional Anatomy of Visual Attention in the Human Brain:
     Studies with Positron Emission Tomography   95
     Maurizio Corbetta

7   Functional Magnetic Resonance Imaging and the Study
     of Attention   123
     James V. Haxby, Susan M. Courtney, and Vincent P. Clark

8   Cortical Lesions and Attention   143
     Diane Swick and Robert T. Knight

9   Computational Architectures for Attention   163
Ernst Niebur and Christof Koch

III Varieties of Attention   187

10   Arousal and Attention: Psychopharmacological and
Neuropsychological Studies in Experimental Animals   189
Trevor W. Robbins

11   Brain Systems of Vigilance   221
Raja Parasuraman, Joel S. Warm, and Judi E. See

12   Visuospatial Attention and Parietal Function: Their Role
in Object Perception   257
Lynn C. Robertson

13   Attention, Pattern Recognition, and Pop-Out in Visual Search   279
Ken Nakayama and Julian S. Joseph

14   Attention and Visual Object Segmentation   299
Jon Driver and Gordon C. Baylis

15   Divided Attention: Narrowing the Gap between Brain and
Behavior   327
Jochen Braun

16   Spatial Working Memory and Spatial Selective Attention   353
Edward Awh and John Jonides

17   Attention and Language   381
Ira Fischler

18   Executive Attention: Conflict, Target Detection, and Cognitive
Control   401
Michael I. Posner and Gregory J. DiGirolamo

IV Development and Pathologies of Attention   425

19   Developing an Attentive Brain   427
Mark H. Johnson

20   Attention-Deficit/Hyperactivity Disorder: Symptom Domains,
Cognitive Processes, and Neural Networks   445
*James Swanson, Michael I. Posner, Dennis Cantwell, Sharon Wigal,
Francis Crinella, Pauline Filipek, Jane Emerson, Don Tucker, and
Orhan Nalcioglu*

21 Selective Attention in Aging and Dementia   461
    Raja Parasuraman and Pamela M. Greenwood

22 Neglect   489
    Robert D. Rafal

23 The Mind Adrift: Attentional Dysregulation in Schizophrenia   527
    Paul G. Nestor and Brian F. O'Donnell

    Contributors   547
    Author Index   551
    Subject Index   575

Preface

There is perhaps no more compelling discipline in the behavioral and brain sciences today than cognitive neuroscience. This book provides a systematic examination of the cognitive neuroscience of attention, taking as its thesis that attention is not a unitary function of the brain. To fully understand attention, therefore, requires examination of the components of attention, an undertaking first begun in my previous book *Varieties of Attention*, published in 1984. More than a decade later, the startling advances made in cognitive neuroscience now make possible an understanding of the neural events that are associated with the different forms of attentive behavior.

The Attentive Brain discusses the major cognitive neuroscience techniques used for examining attention, the mechanisms of the different varieties of attention, and the influence of development and pathology on attention. My attempt in the coverage of topics was to be as broad as possible and to discuss areas in which the most progress has been made in research. It is no longer possible for any book in cognition or neuroscience to be comprehensive, and this book is no exception. Nevertheless, several of the major areas of modern attention research are discussed.

This book had its origins two years ago in "brown bag" meetings, colloquia, lunches, and dinners with various colleagues and students. Discussions with members of the Cognitive Science Laboratory at The Catholic University of America, particularly with Pamela Greenwood, David Hardy, and Sangeeta Panicker, helped shape the initial ideas for the book. My research collaborations with Vince Clark, James Haxby, and Alex Martin at the Laboratory of Brain and Cognition at the National Institute of Mental Health, where I am a visiting scientist, also helped hone the form of this book.

I thank the contributors to this book for their excellent chapters. Their enthusiasm for this project helped it along considerably. Brad Motter deserves special mention for contributing a fine chapter at very short notice.

Over the years my research has been supported by the National Institutes of Health, the National Aeronautics and Space Administration, the U.S. Navy, and the Alzheimer's Association. Their financial support is gratefully acknowledged.

Jennifer Engle and Carol Cairns helped considerably in preparing the final manuscript, and David Hardy helped in copyediting and initial photocopying.

Thanks also to Jackie Duley for preparing the indexes and to Fiona Stevens, Amy Pierce, Michael Rutter, and Katherine Arnoldi of The MIT Press for their guidance during the preparation and production of this book.

Most of all, I thank my wife, Rashmi Sinha, and our children, Rachna and Shanta, for their continual love, encouragement, and support.

I   Introduction

1   The Attentive Brain: Issues and Prospects

Raja Parasuraman

ABSTRACT   Attention is not a single entity but the name given to a finite set of brain processes that can interact, mutually and with other brain processes, in the performance of different perceptual, cognitive, and motor tasks. Although there is no completely agreed-upon taxonomy of attention, a good case can be made for the relative independence of at least three components of attention: *selection*, *vigilance*, and *control*. At the most general level all three aspects of attention serve the purpose of allowing for and maintaining goal-directed behavior in the face of multiple, competing distractions. The contribution of cognitive neuroscience to the understanding of the functional characteristics and neural implementation of those varieties of attention is discussed.

How does the human brain attend? Of all the myriad tasks that the brain has to perform, perhaps none is as crucial to the performance of other tasks as attention. For when the brain attends, it also perceives. When the brain attends and perceives, it learns. What is learned is sometimes spontaneously recalled in the absence of attention, but voluntary recollection requires an attentive brain. To develop skill at a complex task, the brain must reduce the need for constant attention to components of the task, allowing them to be carried out automatically. Attention is thus important for many activities—perception, voluntary recall, and the development of skill. When the brain must carry out those or other activities concurrently, the coordination of their execution to minimize interference also involves attention. Finally, how the human brain produces conscious experience remains a mystery, but the brain mechanisms of attention may be closely related to those of consciousness.

When confronted with such a list of putative functions, at least two reactions are possible. The first is to recognize the multifaceted nature of attention and to attempt to meet the challenge of understanding the similarities and differences between the varieties of attention. The second is to question the very concept of attention. If attention participates in all those functions, is it separate from each or is it an integral part of them? Or is attention epiphenomenal? Alternatively, if attention is not a single entity with a single definition, is it not an ill-conceived concept?

Questions such as these have worried theorists and researchers for many years, as if the second of the two reactions to the diversity of attention were the stronger. For example, in a classic volume on attention published in the heyday of the "cognitive revolution" in psychology, Moray (1969) complained that he found more than a dozen meanings for the term *attention* in the literature. He therefore wondered whether a fully satisfactory theory of attention would ever emerge. [More recently, Moray, who has argued for the continued viability (1993) of Broadbent's filter theory of selective attention (1958) for practical design purposes, has withdrawn from the debate on the mechanisms of attention.] Some time thereafter, Neisser (1976), an early leader of the cognitive revolution, categorically stated that separate mechanisms of attention do not exist. A decade later, Johnston and Dark wondered whether "understanding the nature of selective attention is ultimately futile" (1986, p. 70). In a more recent, sweeping review of the literature, Allport (1993) similarly questioned whether attention is a coherent field of study and whether any theoretical progress had been made in 25 years of research. Finally, Johnston and Dark observed that William James (1890) anticipated many modern attentional phenomena and theories in his classic *Principles of Psychology* and closed their review by commenting that, following completion of his seminal work, James "abandoned psychology altogether" (Johnston and Dark, 1986, p. 70). The implication: that a satisfactory understanding of attention did not yield even to the prodigious intellect of James, and that little real progress had occurred in more than a century of research on attention.

The Attentive Brain can be taken as a potential antidote to these rather gloomy assessments of the state of research on attention. The central thesis is that attention is not a single entity but the name given to a finite set of brain processes that can interact, mutually and with other brain processes, in the performance of different perceptual, cognitive, and motor tasks. At the psychological level attention is not any one thing. Neither, certainly, is it everything, nor is it a chimera. Hence, there cannot be a single definition of, and probably not a single, overarching theory of, attention. Far from being abandoned, the study of attention should be continued vigorously, for significant strides in understanding have been made in recent years. A second thesis of this volume is that although the psychology of attention should not be abandoned, it can be considerably enriched by the methods and theories of cognitive neuroscience. Of course, the idea that attention is not unitary is not new and can be traced at least as far back as James (1890). However, in contrast to older approaches, which often have been based on limited empirical evidence or on intuition, the cognitive neuroscience approach provides detailed and testable hypotheses concerning different attentional processes. This introductory chapter provides a brief overview of the issues surrounding the diversity of attention, of the impact of cognitive neuroscience on those issues, and of the prospects for further advancement.

THE VARIETIES OF ATTENTION

The pessimistic assessment of attention research, even by those who have made important contributions to the field, is somewhat puzzling. Much of the criticism centers on the lack of a definition and a single theory that can accommodate all the data (e.g., Johnston and Dark, 1986). But why should there be a single definition or theory of attention? No one asks for *the* definition of memory or for *the* theory of memory. Knowing that an apple is a fruit or that lions are carnivorous, for example, would seem to involve cognitive processes distinct from those invoked while mentally rehearsing a 10-digit telephone number that must be immediately dialed. Yet both are referred to as memory phenomena, although usually with the qualifiers "semantic" and "working," respectively. Similar qualifiers are used in the study of attention—"selective" and "sustained," for example—to refer to different processes. The diversity of memory has also been explicitly recognized (Roediger and Craik, 1989; Schacter and Tulving, 1994). Memory processes have been distinguished on the basis of their spatiotemporal characteristics, their influence on other cognitive processes, and their representation in the brain (Tulving, 1995). The same would appear to be true of attention.

The diversity of attentional functions has been discussed since at least the time of James (1890). James distinguished between sensory attention driven by environmental events and voluntary attention to both external stimuli and to internal thoughts. A century later, the diversity of attentional processes was explicitly treated in the precursor to this volume, *Varieties of Attention* (Parasuraman and Davies, 1984), the title of which was taken from a chapter title in James's book.

James is widely recognized for his insights into attention, which were largely gained without the benefit of sophisticated behavioral experimentation. Now, more than 100 years later, what more do we know about attention? Ralph Waldo Emerson said that the "measure of a genius is success in bringing everyone around to his views 50 years later (Emerson, 1883, p. 171)." By that criterion, James is certainly a genius. It seems we have largely confirmed what James knew. But that may say more about James's foresight than it says, as some have suggested, about the sterility of empirical research in the intervening period. Progress has been made. James's views have been elaborated on in ways that were unavailable or unknown during his time. Recent neuroscience studies have forced the fractionation of attention into multiple operations, as discussed further in this volume. In general, whereas behavioral studies have been useful in identifying the functional characteristics of attention, neuroscience studies have enabled further examination of how and why those functions are implemented in the brain. That knowledge has prompted new types of behavioral studies, which in turn have stimulated new types of neuroscience research. Such reciprocity should prove highly beneficial in advancing the study of attention on all fronts.

Although the diversity of attention is recognized, it is also true that no completely satisfactory taxonomy of attention has been put forward. By the same token, however, taxonomies of memory continue to be debated, and no single one is universally accepted (Mishkin and Appenzeller, 1987; Squire et al., 1993; Tulving, 1995). Nevertheless, different major aspects of attention can and have been distinguished (Parasuraman and Davies, 1984; Posner and Boies, 1971). It would be remarkable (however unlikely) if each of those were carried out by a single center in the brain. Indeed, modern neuroscience research has confirmed that the many functions of attention are carried out by different, though interacting, neural systems in the brain.

What are the varieties of attention? First, many brain processes run automatically and are influenced by attention slightly or not at all (Shiffrin and Schneider, 1977). Automatic processes may summon attention, as in the case of the response to the sudden onset of a peripheral stimulus (Yantis and Jonides, 1990), but they can also operate outside awareness. With respect to attentive processes, a good case can be made for the relative independence and fundamental importance of at least three components: *selection, vigilance,* and *control.* Although Posner and Boies (1971) used somewhat different terms (selection, alertness, and capacity), they showed, on the basis of behavioral evidence, that those components of attention have different functional characteristics. The distinction has been reinforced by the results of more recent cognitive neuroscience investigations.

In a broad sense, all three components of attention can be thought of as serving the purpose of allowing for and maintaining goal-directed behavior in the face of multiple, competing distractions. LaBerge (1995) more specifically proposed that attention serves the goals of accurate and speedy perception and action and the maintenance of processing over time. Of course, an organism's goals are themselves determined not only by the environment but by the organism's internal dispositions, both temporary and enduring; that is presumably what links attention to motivation and to emotion. Given a goal, however, components of attention can help implement and maintain it.

Selection

A critically important component is selection, which is perhaps the most widely studied area of attention. Selectivity of processing is required because of the computational limitations imposed by fully parallel processing of all sources on any intelligent agent (animate or inanimate) (see Niebur and Koch, chapter 9, this volume). The physiological properties (e.g., large receptive field size) of neurons in higher perceptual processing areas of the primate brain are also consistent with such a computational limitation (Desimone and Duncan, 1995). The primate brain presumably evolved mechanisms of selective attention to cope with that limitation. Views differ on whether attention selection is facilitatory (LaBerge and Brown, 1989), inhibitory (Tipper, 1985), or both (Posner and Dehaene, 1994), and on whether selection is location-based (Cave and Pashler, 1995), object-based (Duncan, 1984), or object token–based (Kanwisher and Driver, 1992); the requirement for selectivity, however, is not disputed seriously. Without such selectivity, organisms would be ill-equipped to act coherently in the face of competing and distracting sources of stimulation in the environment.

Vigilance

If selective attention serves coherent, goal-directed behavior, *vigilance*—or sustained attention—ensures that goals are maintained over time. The need for sustained attention defines a component of attention that is distinct from selection. In fact, some evidence suggests that selective and sustained attention might be opponent processes that ensure a kind of attentional balance in the organism. For example, although a high rate of stimulus presentation increases selectivity and enhances focused attention (Posner, Cohen, Choate, Hockey, and Maylor, 1984) and associated brain electrical activity (Hillyard, Hink, Schwent, and Picton, 1973), it decreases vigilance (Parasuraman, 1979; See, Howe, Warm, and Dember, 1995). Conversely, a spatial cue that temporarily inhibits location-based selection (Posner, 1980) enhances vigilance (Bahri and Parasuraman, 1989). Irrespective of the correctness of this view, and without implying that selection cannot be maintained for long periods of time (i.e., that selective sustained attention is not possible), a large body of behavioral data points to a distinction between those two forms of attention. Recent cognitive neuroscience investigations have provided further support for the distinction (Parasuraman, Warm, and See, chapter 11 this volume; Posner and Petersen, 1990).

Control

The ability to sustain information-processing activity over time in the face of distraction is only one means of maintaining goal-directedness. The activity may need to be temporarily stopped (in order to respond to some other important information) and then resumed; there may be other concurrent activities; and the future course of all such activities must be coordinated. The term *attentional control* has been applied to that function of attention. Theories of working memory (Baddeley, 1986) and of planning (Norman and Shallice, 1986) prominently feature the concept of control.

In contrast to selection and vigilance, attention control is less well understood. The control function has often been associated with a so-called central executive that coordinates and manages all information-processing activities in the brain. Some of the dissatisfaction with the diversity of definitions of attention, which was discussed earlier, may stem from the many functions that are subsumed under the concept of a central executive (Allport, 1993). Another criticism is that such a conceptualization raises the specter of a homunculus in the brain, with the attendant loss of explanatory power because of infinite regress (e.g., what controls the executive, and so on).

Yet no one would deny the importance of control processes in the development of skill and in the maintenance of efficient task performance. Furthermore, one aspect of attentional control provides possibly the only support for the argument that attention involves a special function that is quite distinct from other functions such as perception and memory. For example, it has been argued that selective attention reflects the interaction of mechanisms of perception and working memory (Desimone and Duncan, 1995) and that sustained attention can be incorporated within theories of arousal and sleep (Kinomura, Larsson, Gulyas, and Roland, 1996), in which case the separate status of attention is put in jeopardy. There is one characteristic of attention, however, that cannot be easily accounted for in terms of other theories. In a now classic study, Duncan (1980) showed that people can effectively monitor many sources of information simultaneously without loss in efficiency, but only when critical targets do not occur simultaneously. The moment that attention is given to a source in order to detect a target, processing of targets at any other source is dramatically reduced. This fundamental limitation in attentional control cannot be explained by a sensory deficiency, by a deficit in working memory, or by a problem in motor control.

Processing multiple simultaneous targets is only one aspect of attentional control. The challenge is to develop similarly well-specified conceptualizations of other subcomponents of attentional control that can be tested rigorously. There are already movements in this direction, with cognitive neuroscience leading the way. Two examples are briefly noted here. Niebur and Koch (1994) have described a computational model of neurons in higher cortical areas that function as coincidence detectors and that therefore allow for differentiation of attended (synchronous) from unattended (asynchronous) stimuli. The detectors can, in principle, affect motor control systems, thereby allowing for attentional control without the need for a processing homunculus. In chapter 18 of this volume, Posner and DiGirilamo propose a model of attentional control that makes specific predictions for several subcomponents. They go on to provide empirical support for the predictions from behavioral, electrophysiological, and functional brain-imaging data. As discussed in the next section, the methods used in these two examples define the field of cognitive neuroscience.

COGNITIVE NEUROSCIENCE AND ATTENTION

What Is Cognitive Neuroscience?

Cognitive neuroscience represents the merger of cognitive psychology and neuroscience, which are both now mature fields of investigation. The aims of both disciplines are ostensibly the same: to gain an understanding of the workings of the human mind and brain. Until recently, however, the two disciplines had little productive interchange. Cognitive psychology emphasized theories of mental processes that often had little to do with known facts of brain function. Neuroscience took a lengthy detour from its original mission of studying brain *and* mind to focus solely on the details of neural structure, physiology, chemistry, and molecular biology. The need to relate the two disciplines was recognized for several years, and attempts at forging interrelationships were made. In a prescient and memorable phrase, the philosopher Mario Bunge (1980) characterized such interrelationships as requiring "progress beyond 'mindless neuroscience' and 'brainless psychology' to a true neuropsychology" (1980).

Cognitive neuroscience represents the rapprochement that became possible with the development of computational models of cognitive (Rumelhart and McClelland, 1986) and brain processes (Churchland and Sejnowski, 1992), the emergence of technologies for noninvasive imaging of human brain functions (Posner and Raichle, 1994), and other factors (see Kosslyn and Koenig, 1992). The three cornerstones of this field for the study of behavior are methods from cognitive psychology, neuroscience studies, and computational modeling (Gazzaniga, 1995). Figure 1.1 shows a general framework for cognitive neuroscience, taken from Klein (1996). The three major subdisciplines are indicated in the outer pathway of links. In addition, examining the effects of damage can provide valuable information that can constrain and test models of cognition and their instantiation in the brain: the effects of "lesions" to a computational model can be pitted against those associated with induced brain lesions in animals or acquired brain damage in humans, or both. Consistent with that approach, the present volume not only examines the major neuroscientific and computational methods available for studying attention, but also examines lesion studies in animals and in humans.

Cognitive neuroscience should ideally also proceed in parallel with perspectives from development and evolution. To paraphrase Diamond (1997), if psychology, neuroscience, and computer science can be used to discover the proximate causes of attentional phenomena, one must then turn to development and evolution for the ultimate causes. As Geschwind (1979) proposed, localization of function should never be the end point of explanation in neuropsychology. To take a simple example, it is well known that Broca's area lies adjacent to the area of motor cortex that controls the vocal musculature, and that Wernicke's area is situated close to the primary auditory cortex. Rather than simply note the localization of different language functions to those areas, Geschwind proposed the need for evolutionary explanations for such localization: for example, that language is based on adaptations of brain areas in early humans who were preliterate and for whom language was primarily spoken (Broca's area) and heard (Wernicke's area), rather than written and read. Similarly, as neural systems of attention are discovered, one needs to ask how they evolved from earlier neural systems, and how they develop in individuals. Although evolutionary perspectives are not explicitly treated in this volume (for a thorough discussion, see Tooby and Cosmides, 1995), the development of attention, both in infancy and in adulthood is discussed.

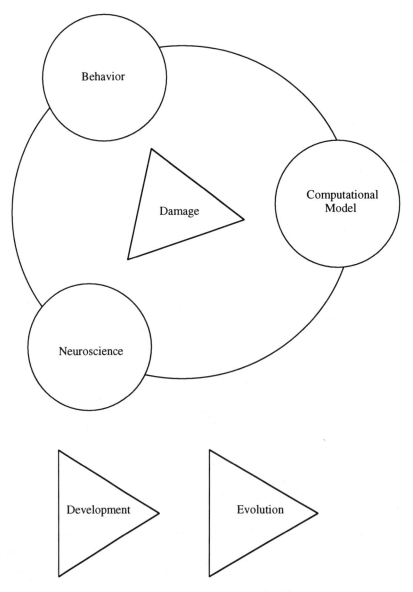

Figure 1.1 A framework for cognitive neuroscience. (After Klein, 1996.)

Cognitive Neuroscience and Attention

While the first thesis of this volume is that the different varieties of attention must be carefully distinguished, the second is that cognitive neuroscience can help considerably in that enterprise. There is already much evidence of such achievement, as discussed throughout this volume. At the same time, the prospects for further advancement look very good.

It is also possible that the optimism that always accompanies the birth of a new paradigm—in this case, cognitive neuroscience—is misplaced and will in time fall prey to the pessimism that has been noted previously. There are some reasons why this is less likely to occur now than in the past. Cognitive neuroscience is not just the addition of new dependent measures to study attention; that is, it is not just the use of neuroscience measures by cognitive psychologists and behavioral measures by neuroscientists. Instead, questions are being asked in a different way that represents a genuine interaction between disciplines. Two examples will suffice by way of illustration. Visual search tasks used in human cognitive studies have been adapted to examine issues relating to how neurons in the ventral temporal lobe of monkeys respond to objects that must be selectively attended (Chelazzi, Miller, Duncan, and Desimone, 1993). Conversely, primate single-unit and human functional brain-imaging studies have inspired new types of cognitive anatomical experiments that examine the behavioral consequences of a hypothesis concerning a particular brain area or circuit (Posner, Inhoff, Friedrich, and Cohen, 1987). Although those kinds of studies could have been done previously, they are both much more likely and much better motivated theoretically with the advent of cognitive neuroscience.

No claim is made that cognitive neuroscience will resolve all issues that have been debated by attention researchers. The explosion of cognitive neuroscience research on attention has led to a number of fundamental advances in knowledge. But many conceptual and methodological issues remain uncertain and controversial. This volume attempts to describe not only the advances but also the areas of disagreement or uncertainty, so as to serve as a springboard for further research.

At the same time, fundamental issues that have not yielded to cognitive analysis may benefit from the new paradigm. Many issues in attention research have been framed as dichotomies that have turned out to be simplifications. When dichotomies have been redefined, there has been theoretical progress. The early- versus late-selection debate on the temporal locus of selective attention represents one example. Clearly, both forms of selection can be used, but the challenge has been to provide reliable evidence of early selection and to identify the conditions under which it occurs. Although behavioral studies have been informative in this regard, studies using event-related brain potentials (ERPs) have clearly shown that selective attention modulates early-latency ERP components, both in the visual and in the auditory modality (Eason, Harter, and White, 1969; Hillyard et al., 1973; Näätänen, 1992; Parasuraman, 1978). More recent ERP studies have shown unequivocally that, under conditions of high perceptual load, early selection occurs as early as about 50 ms after stimulus onset and involves modulation of brain electrical activity in sensory-specific cortical areas in a manner consistent with a sensory gain-control mechanism (see Luck and Girelli, chapter 5 this volume). That conclusion is also supported by other functional brain-imaging studies (Corbetta, chapter 6 this volume). Thus, the early- versus late-selection debate can be redefined as the identification of the conditions under which selection occurs at multiple levels of representation in the brain (see also Johnston, McCann, and Remington, 1996).

Finally, some long-standing issues remain controversial. One issue that has stood since the time of James (1890) is whether attention represents a causal force that influences other activities such as perception (Treisman, 1996) or whether it is a by-product of other processes such as stimulus priming (Johnston and Dark, 1986) or competitive neural interactions (Desimone and Duncan, 1995). The issue of whether attention is a cause or an effect is closely related to the question of whether there exist attentional *systems* that are separate from other sensory and motor systems in the brain. Posner (Posner and Dehaene, 1994; Posner and Petersen, 1990) has been the most forceful proponent of the separate-system view, while others have suggested that attention represents an emergent property of other processing activities (Desimone and Duncan, 1995). Johnston and Dark (1986) favored "effect" theories over "cause" theories of attention (as did James). It is possible that this dichotomy, like others in cognitive theory, may also be redefined by cognitive neuroscience, so that evidence for both cause and for effect might be obtained. Functional brain-imaging studies have provided clear evidence for attentional effects in many parts of the brain (see Corbetta, chapter 6 this volume; Haxby, Courtney, and Clark, chapter 7 this volume). What has proven somewhat elusive is the identification of the causal source(s) of attentional effects, which would presumably implement the component of attentional control discussed earlier in this chapter. Posner (1995) has argued that the anterior cingulate gyrus of the frontal lobe plays a key role in attentional control and is therefore one of the brain areas that act as the causal source, but that is not a view that is held by all researchers (also, see Webster and Ungerleider, chapter 2 this volume). One reason why some researchers might be skeptical could be the feeling that postulating a specialized attentional control area in the brain creates a homunculus in the brain. However, as discussed earlier in this chapter, the notion of attentional control does not necessarily require a homunculus. Additional research should clarify whether the anterior cingulate or other higher cortical areas act as agents of attention, or whether all attentional phenomena can be explained without the need for such mechanisms. Whatever the outcome, the cognitive neuroscience paradigm has redefined the debate using more tractable questions that can be pursued empirically.

OVERVIEW OF THE BOOK

This volume comprises four sections, including a section containing this introductory chapter. The second section, Methods, describes the major neuroscience methods for studying attention, with chapters on methods used only in animals (anatomical tract tracing, single-unit electrophysiology, neurochemical manipulations); on noninvasive human brain-imaging techniques including ERPs, positron emission tomography (PET), and functional magnetic resonance imaging (fMRI); as well as chapters on studies with brain-damaged individuals. The second section also includes a chapter devoted to computational modeling.

The Methods section thus treats most of the techniques important for the cognitive neuroscience approach illustrated in figure 1.1. However, the focus of these chapters is not exclusively methodological. Their intent is to illustrate the unique contribution of each technique, in the spirit of converging operations, to the advancement of knowledge on specific varieties of attention.

The third section, Varieties of Attention, examines different attentional functions from the cognitive neuroscience perspective. Readers will find that the three major components of attention described earlier—selection, vigilance, and control—are well covered here, as are more specific issues within each of those domains.

The final section, Development and Pathologies, discusses the application of the findings developed in the previous sections to the analysis of normal and abnormal development and to pathologies of attention. The chapters in this section represent areas in which the use of the cognitive neuroscience framework has been particularly useful in understanding the development of attention and its breakdown with pathology.

CONCLUSIONS

Cognitive neuroscience research on attentional processes has led to a number of significant advances in knowledge. There are prospects for even greater progress in the future. Recognition and analysis of the varieties of attention and their associated brain mechanisms promises to significantly advance our understanding of attention in a manner that might well have impressed even William James.

ACKNOWLEDGMENT

Supported by National Institutes of Health grant AG05769.

REFERENCES

Allport, D. A. (1993) Attention and control: Have we been asking the wrong questions? A critical review of twenty-five years. In *Attention and Performance XIV*, edited by D. E. Meyer and S. Kornblum. Cambridge, MA: MIT Press.

Baddeley, A. D. (1986) *Working Memory*. Oxford: Oxford University Press.

Bahri, T. and Parasuraman, R. (1989) Covert shifts of attention enhance vigilance. *Bull. Psychon. Soc.* 27: 490.

Broadbent, D. E. (1958) *Perception and Communication*. London: Plenum Press.

Bunge, M. (1980, Jan.) From mindless neuroscience and brainless psychology to neuro-psychology. Paper presented at Annual Winter Conference for Brain Research, Keystone, CO.

Cave, K. R. and Pashler, H. (1995) Visual selection mediated by location: Selecting successive visual objects. *Percept. Psychophys.* 57: 421–432.

Chelazzi, L., Miller, E. K., Duncan, J., and Desimone, R. (1993) A neural basis for visual search in inferior temporal cortex. *Nature* 363: 345–347.

Churchland, P. and Sejnowski, T. (1992) *The Computational Brain.* Cambridge, MA: MIT Press.

Desimone, R. and Duncan, J. (1995) Neural mechanisms of selective attention. *Annu. Rev. Neurosci.* 18: 193–222.

Diamond, J. (1997) *Guns, Germs, and Steel: The Fate of Human Societies.* New York: W. W. Norton.

Duncan, J. (1980) The locus of interference in the perception of simultaneous stimuli. *Psychol. Rev.* 87: 272–300.

Duncan, J. (1984) Selective attention and the organisation of visual information. *J. Exp. Psychol. Gen.* 113: 501–517.

Eason, R. G., Harter, M. R., and White, C. T. (1969) Effects of attention and arousal on visually evoked cortical potentials and reaction time in man. *Physiol. Behav.* 4: 283–289.

Emerson, R. W. (1883) *Letters and Biographical Sketches.* Boston: Little Brown.

Gazzaniga, M. S. (1995) *The Cognitive Neurosciences.* Cambridge, MA: MIT Press.

Geschwind, N. (1979) Specializations of the human brain. *Sci. Am.,* June, 180–197.

Hillyard, S. A., Hink, R. F., Schwent, V. L., and Picton, T. W. (1973) Electrical signs of selective attention in the human brain. *Science* 182: 177–180.

James, W. (1890) *The Principles of Psychology.* New York: Dover Publications.

Johnston, J. C., McCann, R. S., and Remington, R. W. (1996) Selective attention operates at two processing loci. In *Converging Operations in the Study of Visual Selective Attention,* edited by A. F. Kramer, M. G. H. Coles, and G. D. Logan, pp. 439–458. Washington, DC: American Psychological Association.

Johnston, W. A. and Dark, V. J. (1986) Selective attention. *Annu. Rev. Psychol.* 37: 43–75.

Kanwisher, N. G. and Driver, J. (1992) Objects, attributes and visual attention: Which, what and where. *Curr. Dir. Psychol. Sci.* 1: 26–31.

Kinomura, S., Larsson, J., Gulyas, B., and Roland, P. E. (1996) Activation by attention of the human reticular formation and thalamic intralaminar nuclei. *Science* 271: 612–515.

Klein, R. (1996) Attention: Yesterday, today, and tomorrow. *Am. J. Psychol.* 109: 139–150.

Kosslyn, S. M. and Koenig, O. (1992) *Wet Mind.* New York: Free Press.

LaBerge, D. (1995) *Attentional Processing: The Brain's Art of Mindfulness.* Cambridge, MA: Harvard University Press.

LaBerge, D. and Brown, V. (1989) Theory of attentional operations in shape identification. *Psychol. Rev.* 96: 101–124.

Mishkin, M. and Appenzeller, T. (1987) The anatomy of memory. *Sci. Am.* 1–12.

Moray, N. (1969) *Attention: Selective Processes in Vision and Hearing.* London: Hutchinson Educational.

Moray, N. (1993) Designing for attention. In *Attention: Selection, Awareness and Control,* edited by A. D. Baddeley and L. Weiskrantz, pp. 111–134. New York: Oxford University Press.

Näätänen, R. (1992) *Attention and Brain Function.* Hillsdale, NJ: Lawrence Erlbaum.

Neisser, U. (1976) *Cognition and Reality.* San Francisco: W. H. Freeman.

Niebur, E. and Koch, C. (1994) A model for the neuronal implementation of selective visual attention based on temporal correlation. *J. Comput. Neurosci.* 1: 141–158.

Norman, D. A. and Shallice, T. (1986) Attention to action: Willed and automatic control of behavior. In *Consciousness and Self-Regulation*, edited by R. J. Davidson, G. E. Schwartz, and D. Shapiro, pp. 1–18. New York: Plenum Press.

Parasuraman, R. (1978) Auditory evoked potentials and divided attention. *Psychophysiology* 15: 460–465.

Parasuraman, R. (1979) Memory load and event rate control sensitivity decrements in sustained attention. *Science* 205: 924–927.

Parasuraman, R. and Davies, D. R. (1984) *Varieties of Attention*. San Diego, CA: Academic Press.

Posner, M. I. (1980) Orienting of attention. *Q. J. Exp. Psychol.* 32: 3–25.

Posner, M. I. (1995) Attention in cognitive neuroscience: An overview. In *The Cognitive Neurosciences*, edited by M. S. Gazzaniga, pp. 615–624. Cambridge, MA: MIT Press.

Posner, M. I. and Boies, S. J. (1971) Components of attention. *Psychol. Rev.* 78: 391–408.

Posner, M. I., Cohen, Y., Choate, L. S., Hockey, R., and Maylor, E. (1984) Sustained concentration: Passive filtering or active orienting? In *Preparatory States and Processes*, edited by S. Kornblum and J. Requin, pp. 49–65. Hillsdale, NJ: Lawrence Erlbaum.

Posner, M. I. and Dehaene, S. (1994) Attentional networks. *Trends Neurosci.* 17: 75–79.

Posner, M. I., Inhoff, A., Friedrich, F. J., and Cohen, A. (1987) Isolating attentional systems: A cognitive-anatomical analysis. *Psychobiol.* 15: 107–121.

Posner, M. I. and Petersen, S. E. (1990) The attention system of the human brain. *Annu. Rev. Neurosci.* 13: 25–42.

Posner, M. I. and Raichle, M. (1994) *Images of Mind*. New York: W. H. Freeman.

Roediger, H. L. and Craik, F. I. M. (1989) *Varieties of Memory and Consciousness*. Hillsdale, NJ: Lawrence Erlbaum.

Rumelhart, D. E. and McClelland, J. E. (1986) *Parallel Distributed Processing* (Vol. 1). Cambridge, MA: MIT Press.

Schacter, D. L. and Tulving, E. (1994) *Memory Systems*. Cambridge, MA: MIT Press.

See, J. E., Howe, S. R., Warm, J. S., and Dember, W. N. (1995) Meta-analysis of the sensitivity decrement in vigilance. *Psychol. Bull.* 117: 230–249.

Shiffrin, R. M. and Schneider, W. (1977) Controlled and automatic human information processing: II. Perceptual learning automatic attending, and a general theory. *Psychol. Rev.* 84: 127–190.

Squire, L. R., Knowlton, B., and Musen, G. (1993) The structure and organization of memory. *Annu. Rev. Psychol.* 44: 453–495.

Tipper, S. P. (1985) The negative priming effect: Inhibitory priming by ignored objects. *Q. J. Exp. Psychol.* 37A: 571–590.

Tooby, J. and Cosmides, L. (1995) Mapping the evolved functional organization of mind and brain. In *The Cognitive Neurosciences*, edited by M. S. Gazzaniga, pp. 1185–1197. Cambridge, MA: MIT Press.

Treisman, A. (1996) The binding problem. *Curr. Opin. Neurobiol.* 6: 171–178.

Tulving, E. (1995) Memory: Quo vadis? In *The Cognitive Neurosciences*, edited by M. S. Gazzaniga, pp. 839–847. Cambridge, MA: MIT Press.

Yantis, S. and Jonides, J. (1990) Abrubt visual onsets and selective attention. *J. Exp. Psychol.: Hum. Percept. Perf.* 16: 121–134.

II Cognitive Neuroscience Methods

2 Neuroanatomy of Visual Attention

Maree J. Webster and Leslie G. Ungerleider

ABSTRACT Neuroanatomical tract tracing methods used in studies with nonhuman primates have led to an explosion of information regarding connectivity in the central nervous system. This information is relevant for understanding the brain wiring that underlies such complex cognitive functions as visual attention and for providing constraints on neural network models of attention in the human brain.

Neuroanatomical tract tracing studies in nonhuman primates have provided detailed information about the precise brain wiring that underlies such complex functions as perception, attention, and memory. Initial neuroanatomical insights into attention were suggested by clinical studies of brain-damaged patients with the neglect syndrome, who exhibit deficits in attending to a particular location in space. Many studies implicated the parietal and frontal cortices and several subcortical structures, including the pulvinar nucleus of the thalamus and the superior colliculus, as critical regions involved in the syndrome (Mesulam, 1981; Bisiach and Vallar, 1988). Although lesion and electrophysiological studies in nonhuman primates have indicated that those discrete brain regions contribute uniquely to the completion of the attentive process, anatomical tracing studies point to intricate interconnections between those regions that form a complex neural network. As the pattern of interconnections has become better understood, several investigators have proposed neural network models of attention that are constrained by the anatomical structures involved (Mesulam, 1981, 1990; Posner and Petersen, 1990).

This chapter provides an overview of the methods used for anatomical tracing studies, of the principles of organization used to describe and understand cortical circuitry, and of the neural network models that attempt to incorporate anatomical organization into theories of visual selective attention. Because most of the investigations into attention have focused on attention in the visual modality, and because the visual system has been extremely well studied using anatomical, electrophysiological, behavioral, and psychophysical paradigms, the discussion here will be concerned primarily with the visual system.

A

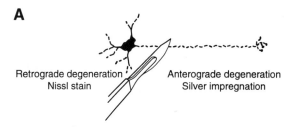

Retrograde degeneration
Nissl stain

Anterograde degeneration
Silver impregnation

B

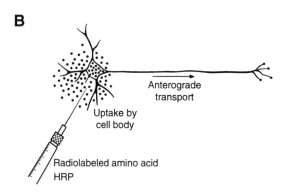

Anterograde
transport

Uptake by
cell body

Radiolabeled amino acid
HRP

C

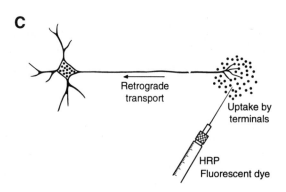

Retrograde
transport

Uptake by
terminals

HRP
Fluorescent dye

Figure 2.1 Different types of tract tracing methods. (A) Retrograde and anterograde degeneration following axotomy. (B) Anterograde transport of tracers. (C) Retrograde transport of tracers. (Adapted from Blackstad et al., 1981.)

NEUROANATOMICAL TRACT TRACING METHODS

The earliest neuroanatomical tracing studies ascertained interconnections in the brain by cutting axons (figure 2.1A). Following such a procedure, the cell bodies giving rise to those axons undergo retrograde degeneration, which is clearly visible in a Nissl stain. Likewise, the axonal terminals distal to the lesion undergo anterograde degeneration, which can be revealed by appropriate histochemical staining procedures, such as the silver impregnation method (Nauta and Gygax, 1951). Although such methods yielded, for the first time, information regarding intracerebral connectivity, the techniques themselves were often unreliable and the interpretation of the results could be questioned due to the frequent involvement of axons of passage at the site of the lesion (for a discussion of those early techniques, including their advantages and limitations, see Heimer and RoBards, 1981).

Neuroanatomy was revolutionized with the experimental application of fast axonal transport. By making use of intra-axonal anterograde transport, the neuroanatomist can inject substances into the brain that are then taken up by the cell body and by the dendrites of neurons within the injected area and are transported to the axonal terminals, where they may be examined in histologically processed brain slices (figure 2.1B). The most commonly used anterograde tracers are radiolabeled amino acids, such as proline and leucine, and the enzyme horseradish peroxidase (HRP). In the case of the former, sections of the brain are coated with a photographic emulsion that is sensitive to the radioactive emissions from the structures labeled by the tracers. When that emulsion is developed and viewed microscopically, labeled axons and terminals appear as black grains when viewed with normal bright-field optics, or as silver grains when viewed using dark-field optics (Cowan, Gottleib, Hendrickson, Price, and Woolsey, 1972; Hendrickson, Moe, and Nobel, 1972).

Tracing of neural pathways using HRP is a major technique in neuroanatomy. In this method the process of histochemical visualization is achieved by incubating the tissue in a medium that contains hydrogen peroxide (H_2O_2) and a chromogenic aromatic amine (e.g., tetramethylbenzidine). The chromogens polymerize and assume a more intense color when oxidized. Hence, at sites of HRP activity, the HRP-H_2O_2 complex oxidizes the chromogen and results in the precipitation of a colored reaction-product, which can be viewed in the light microscope and which acts as a marker for HRP activity (LaVail and LaVail, 1972; Mesulam, 1978, Gibson, Hansma, Houk, and Robinson, 1984).

The neuroanatomist can make use of intra-axonal retrograde transport by injecting substances into the brain that are taken up by the axonal terminals within the injected area and are then transported to the cell body, where they may be examined in processed sections (figure 2.1C). In addition to the histochemical technique described above for use with HRP, retrograde labeling can also be detected by injecting fluorescent dyes and viewing brain sections under specified wavelengths of illumination. Moreover, multiple pathways may be examined in the same animal by using dyes that fluoresce at different wavelengths and that are differentially compartmentalized in the nucleus and in the cytoplasm of the cell body (Bentivoglio, Kuypers, Catsman-Berrevoets, Loewe, and Dann, 1979; Bentivoglio, Van Der Kooy, and Kuypers, 1980). All of the anatomical tracers described here, anterograde and retrograde, have typically been used to examine long corticocortical projections and connections between cortical and subcortical structures.

PRINCIPLES OF ANATOMICAL ORGANIZATION IN THE BRAIN

Since the introduction of tract tracing methods there has been an explosion in the amount of information collected on the connectivity of the brain, particularly with respect to sensory and perceptual areas underlying vision. This information, together with electrophysiological recording, has led to the identification of at least 30 visual areas in the macaque monkey brain (Felleman and Van Essen, 1991). The myriad connections would be overwhelmingly incomprehensible if it were not for the development of two principles of organization that have been applied to the anatomical organization of the brain and in particular to the visual system. The first principle is that multiple cortical areas can be organized within parallel processing systems, and the second is that cortical areas of the same modality can be placed in hierarchical order.

Cortical Processing Streams for Object Vision and Spatial Vision

The first principle of cortical organization states that the visual areas appear to be divided into two major corticocortical processing pathways, each of which begins with the primary visual cortex. The ventral, or occipitotemporal, pathway is directed into the inferior temporal cortex and is important for visual object recognition, or what an object is. The dorsal, or occipitoparietal, pathway is directed into the posterior parietal cortex and is important for spatial perception, or where an object is (Desimone and Ungerleider, 1989).

The original evidence for separate processing pathways for object vision and spatial vision was the contrasting effects of inferior temporal and posterior parietal lesions in monkeys (Ungerleider and Mishkin, 1982). Inferior temporal cortex lesions severely impair performance on tasks requiring discrimination of visual object forms or patterns, but leave intact performance on tasks requiring visuospatial judgments. Conversely, lesions of posterior parietal cortex do not impair object discrimination performance but do produce marked visuospatial deficits (for a review, see Ungerleider and Mishkin, 1982).

Subsequent anatomical and physiological studies have supported the distinction between visual processing streams (Ungerleider, 1985). Using multidimensional scaling of anatomical data, Young (1992) confirmed the functional segregation of visual areas into dorsal and ventral processing streams with limited cross-talk between streams. Physiological studies have shown that neurons in areas along the occipitotemporal pathway (areas V1, V2, V4, TEO, and TE) respond selectively to visual features relevant to object identification, such as color and shape. On the other hand, neurons in areas along the occipitoparietal pathway (areas V1, V2, V3, MT, and MST) respond selectively to spatial aspects of stimuli, such as direction of motion, as well as to tracking eye movements (for reviews, see Maunsell and Newsome, 1987; Desimone and Ungerleider, 1989). Boussaoud, Ungerleider, and Desimone, (1990) have proposed a third visual processing pathway, directed to the cortex of the rostral superior temporal sulcus, that plays a role in either complex motion perception, the integration of object and spatial perception, or both. Moreover, there is now evidence that the dorsal and ventral pathways extend into the frontal lobes, such that the inferior prefrontal convexity, which receives information from the inferior temporal cortex, is important for keeping in mind what an object is, whereas the dorsolateral prefrontal cortex, which receives information from the parietal cortex, is important for keeping in mind where an object is (Wilson, O'Scalaidhe, and Goldman-Rakic, 1993).

Hierarchical Organization of Visual Cortical Areas

The second principle of cortical organization is that cortical areas within a pathway are organized hierarchically, such that projections from lower-order areas to higher-order areas originate mainly in layer III of cortex and terminate predominantly in layer IV, whereas projections from higher-order areas to lower-order areas originate mainly in layers V and VI of cortex and terminate both above and below layer IV but not in layer IV (Rockland and Pandya, 1979; Maunsell and Van Essen, 1983; also, see figure 2.2). The former type of projection has been termed "feedforward" and the latter type has been termed "feedback." Maunsell and Van Essen (1983) also described a third laminar pattern that was not clearly feedforward or feedback, in that the terminals varied their laminar pattern from one patch to another, or in that the terminals were homogeneously distributed across all layers, including layer IV. They termed this type of projection "intermediate" and suggested that it characterizes connections between areas at the same hierarchical level. Thus, by injecting either anterograde or retrograde tracers or both into

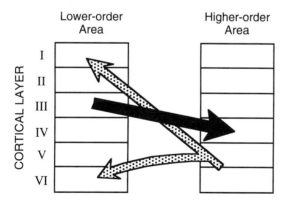

Figure 2.2 Interconnections of sensory cortical areas. Black arrow indicates feedforward projections form lower-order to higher-order areas, and stippled arrows indicate feedback projections from higher-order to lower-order areas.

known visual areas and observing the laminar distribution of labeled cells and terminals, one can establish the hierarchical organization among the multiple visual cortical areas.

Physiological studies have also supported the idea that much of the processing within the visual system is hierarchical (for a review, see Desimone and Ungerleider, 1989). For example, the earliest neuronal response latencies found in physiological recordings increase steadily as one proceeds from the primary visual cortex toward the temporal and parietal lobes. Likewise, the average receptive field size (that is, the portion of the visual field from which a stimulus evokes a neuronal response) also increases as one moves along the visual pathways, consistent with the idea that receptive fields of cells in later areas are built up from those in earlier areas.

Whereas the feedforward projection is obligatory for the functioning of a higher-order area, in that deactivation or removal of a lower-order cortical area (in vision or somesthesis) renders higher-order areas unresponsive (Schiller and Malpeli, 1977; Pons, Garraghty, Friedman, and Mishkin, 1987; Girard and Bullier, 1989), the feedback projection is thought to be modulatory, in that deactivation or removal of a higher-order area does not prevent activation of lower-order areas to which the higher-order area is connected (Sandell and Schiller, 1982). Although the precise function of feedback projections is still unclear, they are thought to play a top-down role in perceptual processing, as with the influence of selective attention in vision.

The two principles of cortical organization, parallel processing pathways and hierarchical organization, are illustrated in a current wiring diagram of the visual system, which is shown in figure 2.3 (and its color version, plate 1). Although the schematic is a representation of visual areas in the monkey brain, similar general principles of cortical organization may also apply to the human brain, although the details of the neural architecture and connectivity patterns undoubtedly differ. Visual areas appear to be similarly organized into dorsal and ventral streams in both Old World and New World monkeys (Weller, 1988), suggesting a common primate plan that probably extends to the organization of human visual cortex as well. Moreover, recent positron emission tomography studies have shown that the human brain also possesses separate cortical visual streams for object and spatial vision (Haxby, Grady, et al., 1991; Haxby, Horowitz, et al., 1994; Ungerleider and Haxby, 1994).

Those principles of organization are essential, not only to our understanding of the cortical circuitry underlying such processes as perception and attention, but also to our understanding of the effects of attention on other cognitive processes, such as learning and memory (see Desimone, Wessinger, Thomas, and Schneider, 1990; Colby, 1991; Posner and Dehaene, 1994; Desimone and Duncan, 1995). In addition, the role of subcortical structures and their connectivity must be included in any analysis of anatomical organization of cognitive function. The next section discusses these organizational principles in relation to anatomical models of attention.

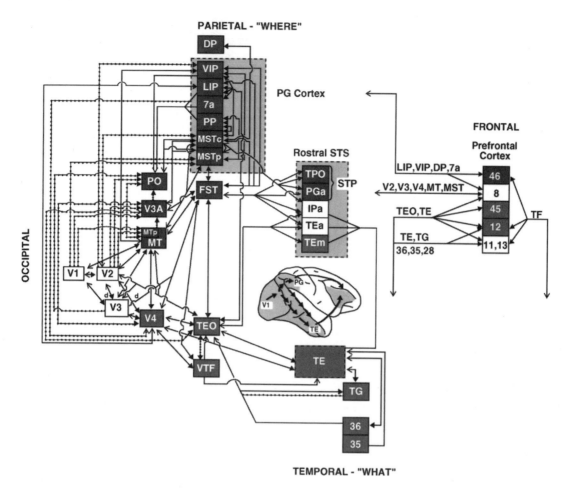

Figure 2.3 Visual processing pathways in monkeys derived from anatomical tract tracing methods. Heavy arrowheads indicate feedforward projections; open arrowheads indicate feedback projections. Solid lines indicate connections arising from both central and peripheral visual field representations; dotted lines indicate connections restricted to peripheral field representations. As shown in color plate 1, red boxes indicate ventral pathway areas related primarily to object vision, green boxes indicate dorsal pathway areas related primarily to spatial vision, and white boxes indicate areas not clearly allied with either pathway. Shaded region on the lateral view of the brain indicates the extent of the cortex included in the diagram. (Adapted from Ungerleider, 1995.) See table 2.1 for a key to abbreviations of visual areas.

ANATOMICAL MODELS OF ATTENTION

At any given time, the visual system can process only a limited amount of information and use that information for action. The filtering of irrelevant visual information is accomplished via selective attention mechanisms. Such mechanisms are thought to involve inputs to visual cortical areas from brain regions both within and outside of the visual system itself. Those brain regions might exert attentional control by filtering irrelevant information in either a bottom-up or top-down manner.

Table 2.1 Abbreviations for Visual Cortical Areas

DP	dorsal prelunate area
FEF	frontal eye fields
FST	fundus of superior temporal area
LIP	lateral intraparietal area
MSTc	medial superior temporal area, central visual field representation
MSTp	medial superior temporal area, peripheral visual field representation
MT	middle temporal area
PG	posterior parietal cortex
PO	parieto-occipital area
PP	posterior parietal sulcal zone
STP	superior temporal polysensory area
TE	anterior inferior temporal cortex
TEO	posterior inferior temporal cortex
TG	temporal pole area
V1	primary visual cortex
V2	visual area 2
V3	visual area 3
V3A	visual area 3, part A
V4	visual area 4
VIP	ventral intraparietal area

Anatomical models of attention have incorporated brain structures in which lesions produce varying degrees of neglect syndrome, that is, a deficit in attending to a particular location in space. Such structures include the parietal cortex (Bisiach and Vallar, 1988), the frontal cortex (Heilman and Valenstein, 1972), the cingulate gyrus (Watson, Heilman, Cauthen, and King, 1973), the basal ganglia (Hier, Davis, Richardson, and Mohr, 1977), the thalamus (Rafal and Posner, 1987; Watson and Heilman, 1979), and the midbrain and superior colliculus (Posner, Cohen, and Rafal, 1982). In general, those areas are considered to exert attentional effects via their inputs to perceptual processing areas.

Two models of attention that attempt to incorporate neuroanatomical connectivity of brain regions thought to be involved in the attentive process are those of Mesulam (1981, 1990) and of Posner and colleagues (Posner, 1990, 1995; Posner and Petersen, 1990; Posner and Rothbart, 1991; Posner and Driver, 1992). Both models include networks of similar brain structures, but the details of the two models differ. Whereas Mesulam's model provides greater anatomical specificity within the network, Posner's model gives greater weight to the cognitive functions performed by the different components of the network. Both models, however, are based on the standard view

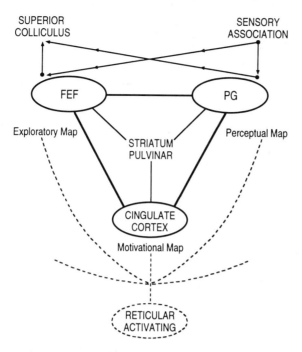

Figure 2.4 A neural network model for directed attention. (Adapted from Mesulam, 1990.) See table 2.1 for a key to abbreviations.

of attention, in which attention functions as a mental spotlight, enhancing the processing of the illuminated item.

Based on data from brain-damaged patients and from neuroanatomical studies of nonhuman primates, Mesulam proposed a network model of attention in which several distinct cortical regions interact. Those regions include the posterior parietal cortex (centered around area PG), the cingulate cortex, and the frontal cortex (centered around the frontal eye fields, or FEF), all of which are influenced by the reticular activating system (figure 2.4). According to this model, a separate spatial coordinate system is represented within each of those brain regions. The parietal component provides an internal perceptual map of the external world; the cingulate component regulates the spatial distribution of motivational valence; the frontal component coordinates the motor programs for exploration, scanning, reaching, and fixating; and the reticular component (including noradrenergic, dopaminergic, and cholinergic ascending systems) provides the underlying level of arousal (Marrocco, Witte, and Davidson, 1994; Robbins and Everett, 1995; Marrocco and Davidson, chapter 3 this volume).

Not only are the cortical components within this network modeled heavily and reciprocally interconnected (Pandya and Kuypers, 1969; Jones and Powell, 1970; Mesulam, Van Hoesen, Pandya, and Geschwind, 1977; Baleydier and Mauguière, 1980; Pandya, Van Hoesen, and Mesulam, 1981; Schwartz and Goldman-Rakic, 1982; Petrides and Pandya, 1984; Barbas and Mesulam,

1985; Huerta, Krubitzer, and Kaas, 1987; Vogt and Pandya, 1987; Cavada and Goldman-Rakic, 1989; Huerta and Kaas, 1990; Baizer, Ungerleider, and Desimone, 1991), but they are also connected with subcortical structures that are known to cause neglect syndrome when damaged in patients (Mesulam, 1990). Those structures include the superior colliculus, which is connected both to the frontal eye fields and to the parietal cortex (Fries, 1984; Colby and Olsen, 1985; Lynch, Graybiel, and Lobeck, 1985; Huerta, Krubitzer, and Kaas, 1986), and the pulvinar and striatum, which are connected to all three cortical regions in the network (Yeterian and Van Hoesen, 1978; Selemon and Goldman-Rakic, 1988; Alexander, DeLong, and Strick, 1986; Saint-Cyr, Ungerleider, and Desimone, 1990).

Finally, the cortical areas in this model are reciprocally interconnected not only with each other, but also with the same set of additional cortical areas, including the inferior temporal and orbitofrontal cortex (see Morecraft et al., 1993). This arrangement thus provides an anatomical substrate for parallel processing of information. However, only the parietal, cingulate, and frontal areas appear to be critical for the organization of directed attention, as neglect is specifically produced by damage to those and not to other areas. Moreover, the afferent inputs to those areas of cortex arise from separate populations of neurons rather than from axon collaterals of the same neurons (Baleydier and Mauguière, 1987; Morecraft, Geula, and Mesulam, 1993). Similarly, the outputs from those areas to target structures are virtually nonoverlapping (Selemon and Goldman-Rakic, 1988). Thus, the model provides both extensive interconnectivity and the capability for integration as well as parallel circuitry and the capacity for flexibility.

The model of attention proposed by Posner and his colleagues incorporates the same brain regions as that of Mesulam, but the regions are organized into somewhat different functional networks that perform presumably different cognitive computations. Thus, the model consists of a posterior attention network, an anterior attention network, and a vigilance network (figure 2.5). The posterior network involves the parietal cortex, the pulvinar, and the superior colliculus. Those areas cooperate in performing the operations needed to bring attention to, or to orient to, a location in space. Specifically, it is proposed that the parietal cortex disengages attention from the locus of the present target, the superior colliculus acts to move the spotlight of attention to the intended target, and the pulvinar is involved in the engagement of attention at the intended target (Posner and Petersen, 1990). The anterior attention network involves the anterior cingulate cortex and supplementary motor areas in the frontal cortex, which together appear to be active in a wide variety of situations involving the detection of events and the preparation of appropriate responses. It is the anterior attention network that is proposed to exercise executive control over voluntary behavior and thought processes. Finally, the vigilance network involves the locus coeruleus noradrenergic input to the cortex (Harley, 1987), which is crucial for maintaining a state of alertness.

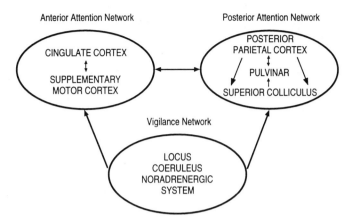

Figure 2.5 A diagrammatic representation of the neural network model of attention described by Posner and colleagues (Posner, 1990, 1995; Posner and Petersen, 1990; Posner and Rothbart, 1991).

Posner and Rothbart (1991) have proposed that the functions of orienting associated with the posterior network are dissociated from conscious processing, whereas the output of the anterior network provides the content of awareness. The vigilance network influences both the posterior and anterior networks by increasing the efficiency of orienting by the posterior system and by suppressing ongoing activity in the anterior system. This leads to a subjective state of readiness that is both alert and free of conscious content, a state that Posner and Rothbart (1991) refer to as the "clearing of consciousness."

In the two models of attention described here, attention focuses on one region of the visual field at a time. According to that view, attention is subserved by a system of spatially mapped structures that are revealed by the neglect syndrome following brain damage. The system operates to enhance perceptual processing at attended locations and reduce perceptual processing at unattended locations. These two models do not, however, specify the neuronal mechanisms that might mediate such effects. Nor do these models confront a fundamental problem posed by the existence of extremely large neuronal receptive fields at the highest levels of the processing pathways. It is known, for example, that single neurons within the inferior temporal cortex, which is the last station of the ventral pathway, have a receptive field size of about 25 degrees, or virtually the entire visual field. Although large receptive fields enable a global description of object features that is invariant over changes in retinal location, they also work against the problem that attentional mechanisms are supposed to solve; namely, to limit the amount of information that is processed by the visual system. Desimone and Duncan (1995) have recently proposed a model of attention based on neural competition that deals with this central problem.

According to the Desimone and Duncan (1995) model, at several points between input and response objects in the visual field compete for limited processing capacity and control of behavior. This competition can be biased by both bottom-up neural mechanisms that separate figures from their backgrounds as well as by top-down mechanisms that bias competition in favor of objects relevant to current behavior. Such bias can be controlled not only by selection of spatial location but also by selection of object features. The presumed mechanism for these selective attention effects is thought to operate at the level of an individual neuron's receptive field. Thus, neurons respond to an attended stimulus as if their receptive fields had contracted around it (Desimone et al., 1990). This would then allow neurons to communicate information with high spatial resolution despite their large receptive fields.

Desimone and Duncan (1995) have argued that, because many spatially mapped structures contribute to competition, the fact that damage to those structures produces neglect syndromes does not mean that they have a specific role in attentional control. For their model, attention is not a high-speed spotlight that scans each item in the visual field; rather, attention is an emergent property of slow competitive interactions that work in parallel across the visual field. Because these interactions are presumed to take place at the level of an individual neuron's receptive field, local anatomical network models may be more relevant to this alternative view than are large-scale network models.

CONCLUSIONS

Neuroanatomical tract tracing methods have provided detailed information on connectivity patterns underlying vision in nonhuman primates. These findings have led to two unifying principles of organization: segregation of visual cortical areas into dorsal and ventral processing streams, and hierarchical organization of cortical areas. Application of these principles can guide the investigation of cortical connectivity underlying vision in the human brain, and can inform neural network models that incorporate anatomical circuitry into theories of visual attention. Additional neuroanatomical information obtained from the use of these methods will be important in providing further constraints on such network models. Refinement of attentional network models will be required both at the macro level of interactions between cortical areas and at the micro level of local synaptic interactions.

REFERENCES

Alexander, G. E., DeLong, M. R., and Strick, P. L. (1986) Parallel organization of functionally segregated circuits linking basal ganglia and cortex. *Annu. Rev. Neurosci.* 9: 357–381.

Baizer, J. S., Ungerleider, L. G., and Desimone, R. (1991) Organization of visual inputs to the inferior temporal and posterior parietal cortex in macaques. *J. Neurosci.* 11: 168–190.

Baleydier, C. and Mauguière, F. (1980) The duality of the cingulate gyrus in rhesus monkey: Neuroanatomical study and functional hypothesis. *Brain Res.* 103: 525–554.

Baleydier, C. and Mauguière, F. (1987) Network organization of the connectivity between parietal area 7, posterior cingulate cortex and medial pulvinar nucleus: A double fluorescent tracer study in monkey. *Exp. Brain Res.* 66: 385–393.

Barbas, H. and Mesulam, M. (1985) Cortical afferent input to the principalis region in rhesus monkey. *Neurosci.* 15: 619–637.

Bentivoglio, M., Kuypers, H. G. J. M., Catsman-Berrevoets, C. E., Loewe, H., and Dann, O. (1980) Two new fluorescent retrograde neuronal tracers which are transported over long distances. *Neurosci. Lett.* 18: 25–30.

Bentivoglio, M., Van Der Kooy, D., and Kuypers, H. G. J. M. (1979) The organization of the efferent projections of the substantia nigra in the rat. A retrograde fluorescent double labeling study. *Brain Res.* 174: 1–17.

Bisiach, E. and Vallar, G. (1988) Hemineglect in humans. In *Handbook of Neuropsychology*, edited by F. Boller and J. Graffman, pp. 195–222. Amsterdam: Elsevier.

Blackstad, T. W., Heimer, L., and Mugnaini, E. (1981) Experimental anatomy: General approaches and laboratory procedures. In *Neuroanatomical Tract-Tracing Methods*, edited by L. Heimer and M. J. RoBards, pp. 1–53. New York: Plenum Press.

Boussaoud, D., Ungerleider, L. G., and Desimone, R. (1990) Pathways for motion analysis: Cortical connections of the medial superior temporal and fundus of the superior temporal visual areas in the macaque. *J. Comp. Neurol.* 296: 462–495.

Cavada, C. and Goldman-Rakic, P. S. (1989) Posterior parietal cortex in rhesus monkey, I: Parcellation of areas based on distinctive limbic and sensory corticocortical connections. *J. Comp. Neurol.* 287: 393–421.

Colby, C. L. (1991) The neuroanatomy and neurophysiology of attention. *J. Child Neurol.* 6: S90–S118.

Colby C. L. and Olsen, C. R. (1985) Visual topography of cortical projections to monkey superior colliculus. *Soc. Neurosci. Abstr.* 11: 1244.

Cowan, W. M., Gottlieb, D. I., Hendrickson, A. E., Price, J. L., and Woolsey, T. A. (1972) The autoradiographic demonstration of axonal connections in the central nervous system. *Brain Res.* 37: 21–51.

Desimone, R. and Duncan, J. (1995) Neural mechanisms of selective visual attention. *Annu. Rev. Neurosci.* 18: 193–222.

Desimone, R. and Ungerleider, L. G. (1989) Neural mechanisms of visual processing in monkeys. In *Handbook of Neuropsychology* (Vol. 2), edited by F. Boller and J. Grafman, pp. 267–299. New York: Elsevier.

Desimone, R., Wessinger, M., Thomas, L., and Schneider, W. (1990) Attentional control of visual perception: Cortical and subcortical mechanisms. *Cold Spring Harb. Symp. Quant. Biol.* 60: 963–971.

Felleman, D. J. and Van Essen, D. C. (1991) Distributed hierarchical processing in primate cerebral cortex. *Cereb. Cortex* 1: 1–47.

Fries, W. (1984) Cortical projections to the superior colliculus in the macaque monkey: A retrograde study using horseradish peroxidase. *J. Comp. Neurol.* 230: 55–76.

Gibson, A. R., Hansma, D. I., Houk, J. C., and Robinson, F. R. (1984) A sensitive low artifact TMB procedure for the demonstration of WGA-HRP in the CNS. *Brain Res.* 298: 235–241.

Girard, P. and Bullier, J. (1989) Visual acuity in area V2 during reversible inactivation of area 17 in the macaque monkey. *J. Neurophysiol.* 62: 1287–1302.

Harley, C. W. (1987) A role for norepinephrine in arousal, emotion and learning: Limbic modulation by norepinephrine and the key hypothesis. *Prog. Neuro-Pharm. Biol. Psychiatr.* 11: 419–458.

Haxby, J. V., Grady, C. L., Horwitz, B., Ungerleider, L. G., Mishkin, M., Carson, R. E., Herscovitch, P., Schapiro, M. B., and Rapoport, S. I. (1991) Dissociation of spatial and object visual processing pathways in human extrastriate cortex. *Proc. Natl. Acad. Sci. USA* 88: 1621–1625.

Haxby, J. V., Horwitz, B., Ungerleider, L. G., Maisog, J. M., Pietrini, P., and Grady, C. L. (1994) The functional organization of human extrastriate cortex: A PET-rCBF study of selective attention to faces and locations. *J. Neurosci.* 14: 6336–6353.

Heilman, K. M. and E. Valenstein. (1972) Frontal lobe neglect in man. *Neurology* 22: 660–664.

Heimer, L. and RoBards, M. J. (1981) *Neuroanatomical Tract-Tracing Methods.* New York: Plenum Press.

Hendrickson, A., Moe, L. and Nobel, B. (1972) Staining for autoradiography of the central nervous system. *Stain Technol.* 47: 283–290.

Hier, D. B., Davis, K. R., Richardson, E. P., and Mohr, J. P. (1977) Hypertensive putaminal hemorrhage. *Ann. Neurol.* 1: 152–159.

Huerta, M. F. and Kaas, J. H. (1990) Supplementary eye field as defined by intracortical microstimulation: Connections in macaques. *J. Comp. Neurol.* 293: 299–330.

Huerta, M. F., Krubitzer, L. A., and Kaas, J. H. (1986) Frontal eye fields as defined by intracortical microstimulation in squirrel monkeys, owl monkeys, and macaque monkeys, I: Subcortical connections. *J. Comp. Neurol.* 253: 415–439.

Huerta, M. F., Krubitzer, L. A. and Kaas, J. H. (1987) Frontal eye fields as defined by intracortical microstimulation in squirrel monkeys, owl monkeys, and macaque monkeys, II: Cortical connections. *J. Comp. Neurol.* 265: 332–361.

Jones, E. G. and Powell, T. P. S. (1970) An anatomical study of converging sensory pathways within the cerebral cortex of the monkey. *Brain* 93: 793–820.

LaVail, J. H. and LaVail, M. M. (1972) Retrograde axonal transport in the central nervous system. *Science* 176: 1416–1417.

Lynch, J. C., Graybiel, A. M., and Lobeck, L. J. (1985) The differential projection of two cytoarchitectonic subregions of the inferior parietal lobule of macaque upon the deep layers of the superior colliculus. *J. Comp. Neurol.* 235: 241–254.

Marrocco, R. T., Witte, E. A., and Davidson, M. C. (1994) Arousal systems. *Curr. Opin. Neurobiol.* 4: 166–170.

Maunsell, J. H. R. and Newsome, W. T. (1987) Visual processing in monkey extrastriate cortex. *Annu. Rev. Neurosci.* 10: 363–401.

Maunsell, J. H. R. and Van Essen, D. C. (1983) The connections of the middle temporal visual area (MT) and their relationship to a cortical hierarchy in the macaque monkey. *J. Neurosci.* 3: 2563–2586.

Mesulam, M.-M. (1978) Tetramethyl benzidine for horseradish peroxidase neurohistochemistry: A non-carcinogenic blue reaction product with superior sensitivity for visualizing neural afferents and efferents. *J. Histochem. Cytochem.* 26: 106–117.

Mesulam, M.-M. (1981) A cortical network for directed attention and unilateral neglect. *Ann. Neurol.* 10: 309–325.

Mesulam, M.-M. (1990) Large-scale neurocognitive networks and distributed processing for attention, language, and memory. *Ann Neurol.* 28: 597–613.

Mesulam, M.-M., Van Hoesen, G. W., Pandya, D. N., and Geschwind, N. (1977) Limbic and sensory connections of the inferior parietal lobule (area PG) in the rhesus monkey: A study with a new method for horseradish peroxidase histochemistry. *Brain Res.* 136: 393–414.

Morecraft, R. J., Geula, C., and Mesulam, M. (1993) Architecture of connectivity within a cingulo-fronto-parietal neurocognitive network for directed attention. *Arch. Neurol.* 50: 279–284.

Nauta, W. J. H. and Gygax, P. A. (1951) Silver impregnation of degenerating axon terminals in the central nervous system. (1) Technique. (2) Chemical notes. *Stain Technol.* 26: 5–11.

Pandya, D. N. and Kuypers, H. G. J. M. (1969) Cortico-cortical connections in the rhesus monkey. *Brain Res.* 13: 13–36.

Pandya, D. N., Van Hoesen, G. W., and Mesulam, M. M. (1981) Efferent connections of the cingulate gyrus in the rhesus monkey. *Exp. Brain Res.* 42: 319–330.

Petrides, M. and Pandya, D. N. (1984) Projections to the frontal cortex from the parietal region in the rhesus monkey. *J. Comp. Neurol.* 228: 105–116.

Pons, T. P., Garraghty, P. E., Friedman, D. P., and Mishkin, M. (1987) Physiological evidence for serial processing in somatosensory cortex. *Science* 237: 417–420.

Posner, M. I. (1990) Hierarchical distributed networks in the neuropsychology of selective attention. In *Cognitive Neuropsychology and Neurolinguistics*, edited by A. Caramazza, pp. 187–210. Hillsdale, NJ: Lawrence Erlbaum.

Posner, M. I. (1995) Attention in cognitive neuroscience: An overview. In *Handbook of Cognitive Neuroscience*, edited by M. S. Gazzaniga, pp. 615–624. Cambridge, MA: MIT Press.

Posner, M. I., Cohen, Y., and Rafal, R. D. (1982) Neural systems control of spatial orienting. *Philos. Trans. R. Soc. London Ser. B.* 298: 187–198.

Posner, M. I. and Dehaene, S. (1994) Attentional networks. *Trends Neurosci.* 17: 75–79.

Posner, M. I. and Driver, J. (1992) The neurobiology of selective attention. *Curr. Opin. Neurobiol.* 2: 165–169.

Posner, M. I. and Petersen, S. E. (1990) The attention system of the human brain. *Annu. Rev. Neurosci.* 13: 25–42.

Posner, M. I. and Rothbart, M. K. (1991) Attentional mechanisms and conscious experience. In *The Neuropsychology of Consciousness*, edited by A. D. Milner, and M. D. Rugg, pp. 91–112. London: Academic Press.

Rafal, R. D. and Posner, M. I. (1987) Deficits in human visual spatial attention following thalamic lesions. *Proc. Natl. Acad. Sci. U S A.* 84: 7349–7353.

Robbins, T. W. and Everett, B. J. (1995) Arousal systems and attention. In *Handbook of Cognitive Neuroscience*, edited by M. S. Gazzaniga, pp. 703–720. Cambridge, MA: MIT Press.

Rockland, K. S. and Pandya, D. N. (1979) Laminar origins and terminations of cortical connections of the occipital lobe in the rhesus monkey. *Brain Res.* 179: 3–20.

Saint-Cyr, J. A., Ungerleider, L. G., and Desimone, R. (1990) Organization of visual cortical inputs to the striatum and subsequent outputs to the pallido-nigral complex in the monkey. *J. Comp. Neurol.* 298: 129–156.

Sandell, J. H. and Schiller, P. H. (1982) Effect of cooling area 18 on striate cortex cells in the squirrel monkey. *J. Neurophysiol.* 48: 38–48.

Schiller, P. H. and Malpeli, J. G. (1977) The Properties and tectal projections of monkey retinal ganglion cells. *J. Neurophysiol.* 40: 428–445.

Schwartz, M. L. and Goldman-Rakic, P. S. (1982) Single cortical neurons have axon collaterals to ipsilateral and contralateral cortex in fetal and adult primates. *Nature* 299: 154–156.

Selemon, L. D. and Goldman-Rakic, P. S. (1988) Common cortical and subcortical targets of the dorsolateral prefrontal and posterior parietal cortices in the rhesus monkey: Evidence for a distributed neural network subserving spatially guided behavior. *J. Neurosci.* 8: 4049–4068.

Ungerleider, L. G. (1985) The corticocortical pathways for object recognition and spatial perception. In *Pattern Recognition Mechanisms*, edited by C. Chagas, R. Gattass, and C. G. Gross, pp. 21–37. Vatican City: Pontifical Academy of Sciences.

Ungerleider, L. G. (1995) Functional brain imaging studies of cortical mechanisms for memory. *Science* 270: 769–775.

Ungerleider, L. G. and J. V. Haxby. (1994) "What" and "where" in the human brain. *Curr. Opin. Neurobiol.* 4: 157–165.

Ungerleider, L. G. and Mishkin, M. (1982) Two cortical visual systems. In *Analysis of Visual Behavior*, edited by D. J. Ingle, M. A. Goodale, and R. J. W. Mansfield, pp. 549–586. Cambridge, MA: MIT Press.

Vogt, B. A. and Pandya, D. N. (1987) Cingulate cortex of the rhesus monkey, II: Cortical afferents. *J. Comp. Neurol.* 262: 271–289.

Watson, R. T. and Heilman, K. M. (1979) Thalamic neglect. *Neurology* 29: 690–694.

Watson, R. T., Heilman, K. M., Cauthen, J. C., and King, F. A. (1973) Neglect after cingulectomy. *Neurology* 23: 1003–1007.

Weller, R. E. (1988) Two cortical visual systems in Old World and New World primates. In *Progress in Brain Research* (Vol. 75), edited by T. P. Hicks and G. Benedek, pp. 293–306. Amsterdam: Elsevier.

Wilson, F. A. W., O'Scalaidhe, S. P., and Goldman-Rakic, P. S. (1993) Dissociation of object and spatial processing domains in primate prefrontal cortex. *Science* 260: 1955–1958.

Yeterian, E. H. and Van Hoesen, G. W. (1978) Cortico-striate projections in the rhesus monkey: The organization of certain cortico-caudate connections. *Brain Res.* 139: 43–63.

Young, M. P. (1992) Objective analysis of the topological organization of the primate cortical visual system. *Nature* 358: 152–154.

3 Neurochemistry of Attention

Richard T. Marrocco and Matthew C. Davidson

ABSTRACT The strengths and weaknesses of neurochemical (neuropharmacological and excitotoxic lesioning) methods in the study of attention are evaluated. Because attention is labile the need for simple, well-controlled attentional and mnemonic paradigms is stressed. The most frequent approaches are (1) systemic alteration of neurotransmitter function with receptor-specific drugs, and (2) neurochemically specific excitotoxic lesions. Results from those approaches have provided ample evidence that norepinephrine and acetylcholine play key roles in purely attentional tasks and in tasks with attentional components that are largely free of concomitant changes in arousal or in perceptual processing. The transmitters facilitate shifts of attention, the utilization of cues, and the maintenance of attention during arousing environmental conditions.

What is the neurochemistry of attention? It is the understanding of the functions and dysfunctions of the brain's attentional systems at the cellular and molecular levels. Neuropharmacological, biochemical, and molecular methods are used to manipulate neuron function and its effect on behavior. The pharmacological approach has yielded the most useful information about attention. Molecular methods such as genetic mutational analysis have yet to be employed and may be inappropriate at present because the key attentional operations (e.g., filtering, selecting, or enhancing neural activity) are organized at the single-cell, neural network, and systems levels, rather than at the subcellular level. The "level gap" may narrow, however, with increased understanding of the molecular specificity of individual cells and with the development of methods for highly selective manipulation of cell systems.

A number of different cell systems may be responsible for the filtering and selection of information. Attentional operations appear to be distributed across several networks of structures (Posner and Petersen, 1990; Morecraft, Geula, and Mesulam, 1993; also, see Webster and Ungerleider, chapter 2, this volume). The anterior network, which includes the frontal and cingulate cortex and the basal ganglia, is active during target detection and sustained attention (Pardo et al., 1991; Morecraft et al., 1993; Jackson and Houghton, 1994). The posterior network, which includes the parietal and inferotemporal cortices, the superior colliculus, and the medial pulvinar, becomes active during visuospatial attention tasks and during the selection of objects in the visual field (Corbetta, Miesin, Shulman, and Petersen, 1993; LaBerge and

Buchsbaum, 1990). In addition, network activity may be modified by input from the brainstem projection systems (BPSs). Each BPS may have a different impact on the attentional networks by virtue of its unique neurotransmitter actions on target neurons.

What are the general effects of manipulating neurotransmitter activity on neuronal activity? Systemic manipulations of the brain environment can cause quite extensive changes in brain chemistry; the sheer complexity of the cellular systems affected may be appreciated as follows. Each synaptic bouton contains one or more neuroactive substances that affects postsynaptic membranes as well as affecting the parent terminal. In addition, the boutons may release membrane-diffusible gases (e.g., nitric oxide) that influence postsynaptic neurons within a wide area. Postsynaptic membranes contain many receptor types and subtypes, each of which may be coupled directly to ionophores or may act through a half dozen different second messenger–linked, intracellular reactions that eventually alter ion channel activity and the membrane potential. The presynaptic influences also include modulatory substances that affect the long-term excitability of the postsynaptic cell. The synaptic potentials produced by these inputs are then weighted spatially and temporally to determine whether a change in impulse activity will occur.

Several challenges must be met in order to develop a systematic neurochemistry of attention. First, the gap between chemical manipulation and overt behavior must be narrowed, both by the use of methods that affect neuronal communication within and between structures and by analysis of the simplest possible attentional behaviors. Second, methods must be used initially that provide maximum isolation of the neural system of interest. There is little hope for understanding the network if the unique contribution of its components is unclear. Third, neurochemical methods should be used in conjunction with other, convergent methods to achieve a broad understanding of attentional processes. Important beginnings have already been made in each of these areas.

SCOPE OF THE CHAPTER

Recent reviews (Clark, Geffen, and Geffen, 1987; Colby, 1991; Posner and Petersen, 1990; Robbins and Everett, 1995) have described the anatomy and physiology of visuospatial and sustained attention in rats and in monkeys. Some of the basic behavioral results in rats are consistent in a general way with results of human studies using somewhat similar tasks, but many of the basic phenomena from neurochemical manipulations have not been demonstrated in other species, and their generality remains to be proven. For example, the mechanisms underlying visuospatial attention in the afoveate rat, including BPS anatomy and neurotransmitter distribution, are different than those of the Old World monkey. A broad neurobiological understanding of attention can be best acquired with parallel studies of primate and human attentional behavior and their underlying neural systems. The rhesus monkey is the ideal subject for such studies because its visual attentional capacities studied to date appear to be virtually identical to those of humans (Witte, 1994).

Behavioral tasks of attention must be designed and analyzed appropriately. Attending to an object may involve several closely related behaviors, including attention shifting, sustained attention, and arousal shifts. Both spatial attention and arousal can dynamically change in direction or intensity, thus confounding the dependent variable of interest. It is therefore important to choose paradigms that engage specific aspects of attention and that allow for the independent evaluation of attentional and arousal effects on behavior.

NEUROTRANSMITTER SYSTEMS IMPLICATED IN ATTENTION

The BPSs innervating the cortex originate primarily in the magnocellular basal forebrain (MBF) nuclei, the ventral tegmental area (VTA), the nucleus locus coeruleus (LC), the dorsal raphe nucleus (DR), and the tuberomammillary region of the hypothalamus (TMH). Additional projections originate in the glutamatergic intralaminar and midline thalamocortical projections, but their roles are less well understood. Many of the BPSs contain colocalized substances (peptides, adrenaline, excitatory amino acids) whose functions in attention are as yet unknown.

The Cholinergic System

The majority of acetylcholine (ACh) is supplied to the cortex by the nuclei of the MBF. ACh binds to nicotinic and muscarinic receptors, each of which has several subtypes. (These and other transmitter subtypes have only recently been discovered and their role, if any, in attention is unknown). Nicotinic receptors are found on presynaptic cholinergic and non-cholinergic terminals (for a recent review, see Wonnacott, Drasdo, Sanderson, and Rowell, 1990) but postsynaptic sites are also present. Muscarinic receptors tend to be located postsynaptically on target neurons. Muscarinic and nicotinic postsynaptic receptors are distributed differentially in cortical areas and across laminae.

The action of ACh on nicotinic receptors is mediated by direct receptor–ionophore coupling, whereas the postsynaptic responses mediated by muscarinic receptors are linked to second messenger systems. Nicotinic responses are usually excitatory and fast. Muscarinic responses are relatively slow and may be excitatory or inhibitory, depending on the properties of the second messenger system activated.

The Noradrenergic System

Noradrenaline (NA) is supplied to the cerebral cortex principally by the LC, whose axons travel in the dorsal tegmental bundle. In rats, monkeys, and humans, the vast majority of LC cells contain NA (but, see Chan-Palay and

Asan, 1989). NA is released onto alpha-1, alpha-2, and beta receptors, each of which has three subtypes with differential distributions in cortical laminae. Alpha-2 receptors are found at pre- and postsynaptic sites and, at least in the cortex, are more numerous than the postsynaptic alpha-1 receptors.

The effects of NA on target cells are complex. There are multiple actions on cell membrane currents presumably mediated by multiple receptor types or subtypes. As a result, the effects of NA on spontaneous and evoked activity may vary for different cells and for different recording locations (McCormick, Wang and Huguenard, 1993).

The Dopaminergic System

Dopamine (DA) is supplied to the cerebral cortex by the A8 and A10 groups of pontomedullary nuclei, which contain cells whose axons travel in the median forebrain bundle and which bifurcate widely to innervate the hemispheres. DA is released onto D-1, D-2, D-3, and D-4 receptors, each of which has two or more subtypes that are distributed differentially across cortical laminae. On cortical neurons, D-1 and D-2 receptors appear to be postsynaptic and presynaptic, respectively. The effects of DA on neurons may be excitatory or inhibitory, depending on the direction of changes produced in adenylyl cyclase activity.

The Histaminergic System

The TMH is the sole source of cortical histamine. Histamine binds to three types of receptors and its effects on postsynaptic neurons are similar to those of ACh and NA in that it produces a mixture of excitatory and inhibitory effects and a shift in firing patterns. Unlike other systems, there appears to be little tendency for selective innervation of cortical laminae.

The Serotonergic System

The main source of cerebral serotonin (5-HT) arises from the DR nucleus of the pons. 5-HT neurons impinge on three major receptors, each with two minor subtypes. Most 5-HT receptors are located postsynaptically, although iontophoretic application of 5-HT onto cells in DR produces an inhibition of spontaneous activity. 5-HT receptors mediate either purely inhibitory effects or mixed excitatory and inhibitory effects via second messenger systems. 5-HT receptor subtypes are differentially distributed across cortical laminae.

It is important to remember that the target cells of the BPSs are not only the intrinsic neurons of cortical (and subcortical) structures but are also the cells of other projection systems. For example, brainstem cholinergic neurons make contact with noradrenergic LC neurons (Reader and Jasper, 1984), and DA neurons in nucleus accumbens modulate GABAergic inhibition of structures within the MBF. This suggests that attentional computations may be modified by patterned inputs from a network of neuromodulatory structures.

PHARMACOLOGICAL ALTERATION OF BRAIN NEUROTRANSMITTER ACTIVITY

There are potentially many approaches to the neurochemical study of attention. The two most frequently used methods to manipulate the intact attentional system are pharmacological alteration and cytotoxic ablation. These methods are considered in turn.

Each of the ten or so stages in the life cycle of a neurotransmitter molecule represents an opportunity for pharmacological alteration of transmitter function. An important strategy is to augment or suppress receptor action by agonists or antagonists. The objective of this approach is to maximize action at the receptor of interest while minimizing nonspecific action at the receptors of other systems.

Local injections of drugs into brain tissues via iontophoresis, pressure, or microdialytic probes affect neural elements only near the injection site. Nonspecific effects are relatively infrequent and are limited primarily by diffusion. Promising new immunohistochemical methods may restrict the site of action even further to specific proteins within cells (see altering Brain activity by cytotoxic Lesions, below). These methods, however, are technically demanding, subject to placement errors, and impractical for injections into more than a single site. In contrast, systemic injections of a drug are easy to give, and such injections increase or decrease activity in many locations almost simultaneously. Unfortunately, there is little control over spatial distribution of the drug within the brain or within the peripheral nervous system, and nonspecific effects may be present. Deductions can be made about the site of action based on the known locations of the target receptors, but there is no guarantee that the receptors at a particular location are involved in the behavior of interest.

Nonspecific effects may include actions in the peripheral nervous system. In attentional tasks, such effects may include general metabolic effects (e.g., sympathetic stimulation) that may reduce alertness or motivation and nonspecific sensory (e.g., pupillary or accommodational changes) or motor effects (ataxia, tremor). One method to combat such effects is to test forms of the drug that do not cross the blood-brain barrier. However, because peripherally acting forms of the drugs may not be available, and because many studies use highly specific target behaviors and internal controls, that strategy is seldom used. Systemic injections have been used to study two types of attentional tasks: visuospatial and sustained attention.

Visuospatial Attention

The method of choice for studying visuospatial attention is the cued-target detection (CTD) task (Posner and Cohen, 1984). Central (cues at the fixation point) and peripheral (cues in the peripheral visual field) versions of this task have been used to measure reaction times (RTs) to target stimuli. Four types of cues are used in the most recent, peripheral version of this task (Witte, Davidson, and Marrocco, 1997). A valid cue accurately predicts the spatial location on most trials. However, to prevent the subject from attending to the target location continuously, the target occasionally appears at the opposite spatial location. The frequency of those invalid trials may be varied to alter cue predictability. The difference between valid and invalid RTs is the validity effect, an index of the benefits of spatial orienting.

The target typically follows the cue by some predetermined time interval. Therefore, the cue provides spatial and temporal information, but the relative contributions of the two types of cues to RT are not clear. To separate the temporal information from the spatial, a third trial type, the double cue (sometimes called a neutral cue) is added. For this cue, both left and right cues are presented simultaneously and the target occurs near one of them. Any decrease in RT must be due to increases in readiness or arousal provided by the increased temporal certainty of target onset. Finally, a no-cue condition omits all cues and serves to measure RTs without spatial or temporal information. Subtracting the no-cue trial averages from the double cue averages gives an index of the alerting effect, which is the increased arousal in anticipation of the impending target. In this regard, the CTD is one of the few methods that achieves the desired separation of arousal from spatial orienting effects.

Results using this paradigm are shown in figure 3.1. In both humans and in rhesus monkeys the valid cue mean RT is about 25 ms faster than the invalid cue mean RT, and the double-cue mean RT is about the same number of ms faster than the RT mean of the no-cue trials. Thus, the combined effects on

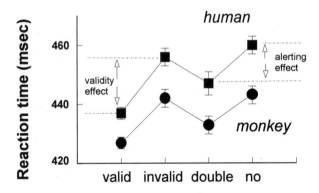

Cue type

Figure 3.1 Behavioral reaction times for monkeys and humans to different cue types in the attention shifting task. The difference between valid and invalid trials is the validity effect; the difference between double-cue and no-cue trials is the alerting effect. Rhesus monkeys are faster overall than humans but both produce the same pattern of reaction times. (Adapted from Davidson et al., 1994.)

RT of spatial and temporal information confer about 50 ms of processing advantage over the no-cue trials alone. These results suggest that attentional allocation has an evanescent effect on sensory and motor processing, and that measurement of that effect must take place within a narrow temporal window. The results also suggest that the visuospatial attention shifting systems of the primate and the human are virtually identical.

Noradrenaline The consequences of altering levels of brain noradrenergic, dopaminergic, or cholinergic neurotransmitters on the RTs of rhesus monkeys trained to perform the CTD task have been recently examined (Witte, Lickey, and Marrocco, 1992; Witte and Marrocco, 1997; Davidson, Villareal, and Marrocco, 1994; Witte et al., 1997). Results typical for drugs that bind to the alpha-2 adrenoceptor are shown in figure 3.2, which shows the effects of the alpha-2 agonist clonidine on alerting and validity. With doses that produce little if any sedation, clonidine had no effect on validity scores, but

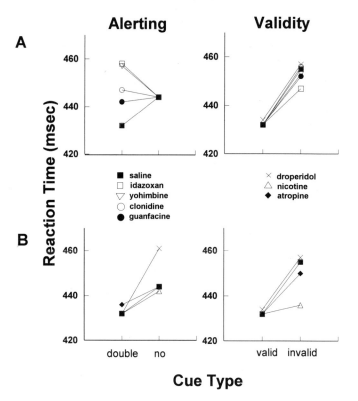

Figure 3.2 The effects of drugs on alerting and validity reaction times in primates. The data were computed by subtracting the main effect of each drug (i.e., overall reaction time) from the mean reaction times for each trial type. The resulting effects may be seen by comparing drug conditions with the saline control condition. Yohimbine HCl, 0.10mg/kg; idazoxan HCl, 0.10 mg/kg; clonidine HCl, 0.001 mg/kg; guanfacine HCl, 0.0001 mg/kg; nicotine ditartrate, 0.006 mg/kg; droperidol, 0.01 mg/kg; atropine sulfate, 0.01 mg/kg; saline, 0.9%.

it significantly reduced alerting scores by slowing the RTs to double cues. Similar effects were found for guanfacine, which acts at the same class of receptor sites.

Yohimbine and idazoxan normally act in the opposite fashion as clonidine, by blocking alpha-2 adrenoceptors. When administered with clonidine or guanfacine, they blocked clonidine's reduction of the alerting effect (Witte and Marrocco, 1997). By themselves, however, they reduced the alerting effect in a dose-dependent manner (Davidson et al., 1994). Because alpha-2 receptors are found both pre- and postjunctionally our results could be explained by assuming that clonidine and yohimbine are acting at presynaptic and postsynaptic sites, respectively. An alternative explanation, supported by recent work with aged primates (Arnsten, Cai, and Goldman-Rakic, 1988; Arnsten and Cai, 1993), is that yohimbine and guanfacine may act either pre- or postsynaptically, depending on the dose. Recent work with very low doses of yohimbine (50 μg/kg) suggests that it may act at different synaptic sites, and further explorations of these observations are in progress.

Somewhat different findings have been reported for visuospatial attention in humans (Clark, Geffen, and Geffen, 1989). Clonidine or a placebo was administered intravenously, and trial type (valid, invalid, and neutral) was indicated by central, symbolic cues. Clonidine decreased response cost (invalid RTs − neutral RTs) but did not change response benefit (neutral RTs − valid RTs). Comparable results can be shown for the data of Witte et al. (1992). However, because the humans and monkeys performed central and peripheral cue tasks, respectively, further comparisons are difficult.

Dopamine In primates, the dopaminergic antagonist droperidol altered alerting scores but had little effect on validity scores (Witte, 1994). The principal effect on alerting was an increase in RTs to no-cue trials, the opposite of the effect of the noradrenergic drugs. No impairment in double trials was seen. These effects were interpreted as reflecting impairment of tonic arousal, even though sedation ratings were not significantly elevated. Phasic arousal was thought to be unaffected, because cued trials had normal RTs. Recent work in our laboratory has also found enhanced alerting for the D-2 antagonist eticlopride, and the opposite result for the D-2 agonist quinpirole.

The effect of intravenous dopamine on human visuospatial attention was also tested in the Clark et al. study (1989). In contrast to the monkey data, the human data showed a decreased response cost and an unchanged response benefit. Because of the aforementioned task differences, a closer comparison with the monkey work is of limited use.

Acetylcholine Studies of the involvement of ACh in purely attentional tasks with subhuman primates are scarce. However, there is an extensive, although conflicting, attentional literature on the effects of scopolamine-induced reduction in ACh activity in rats and humans (e.g., see Meador et al.,

1993; Wesnes and Warburton, 1984) that is not discussed here. In primates nicotine reduces validity scores in the CTD task but has no effect on alerting scores (see figure 3.2). Nicotine decreases RTs overall and specifically reduces RTs for invalid trials, thus decreasing the validity effect (Witte, Davidson and Marrocco, 1997). The muscarinic cholinergic drug atropine appears to have little effect on either validity or alerting scores.

Additional support for the involvement of the cholinergic system has been obtained from studies of human tobacco smokers. Heavy smokers (those who smoke more than 20 cigarettes per day) demonstrated a reduction in overall RTs and a statistically significant reduction in the validity effect but not in the alerting effect (Witte et al., 1997), results similar to those obtained in monkeys. Witte et al. (1995) have recently replicated the human results on a different sample of smokers and, further, have shown that salivary nicotine levels were inversely proportional to the size of the validity effect. Curiously, whereas single injections of nicotine shortened invalid RTs in the monkeys, smoking a single cigarette caused no effect in human nonsmokers (Witte et al., 1997). Of course, the plasma and brain levels of nicotine achieved from inhaling may be quite different from those produced by a single intramuscular injection. Moreover, given that nicotine is but one component of tobacco smoke, successful replications using nicotine patches would firmly establish the specificity of the results. To summarize, these results and the noradrenergic manipulations strongly suggest a double dissociation between task and neurotransmitter system: catecholamines influence alerting but not orienting, whereas cholinergics alter orienting but not alerting.

What is the mechanism of nicotinic enhancement of invalid RTs? A decrease in invalid-cue RTs suggests a facilitation of attentional reorientation because the time taken to disengage from the invalid location and move to and engage at another location is much more rapid during invalid-cue trials than during control trials (Posner and Petersen, 1990). Which of those three operations is speeded? Because valid-cue RTs are unchanged, attentional disengagement from fixation, movement to the cue, and engagement on it must be minimally affected by nicotine. However, reorienting the attention requires a second disengagement from the invalid location, and nicotine may accelerate disengagement. One possible mechanism of nicotine enhancement is through presynaptic facilitation of glutamatergic neurotransmission in the parietal cortex, where disengagement is thought to occur (Posner and Peterson, 1990; Lena, Changeux, and Mulle, 1993). That interpretation is consistent with the rapid action of nicotinic synapses and with the finding that nicotinic receptors in frontal cortex may be located presynaptically on glutamatergic terminals (see Wonnacott et al., 1990).

Sustained Attention

Attention shifting is among the fastest known cognitive events. At the opposite end of the temporal continuum is sustained attention, in which subjects may maintain an attentive state for minutes or longer. Sustained attention is typically measured in vigilance tasks, in which a subject attempts to acquire infrequent information from the environment (Broadbent, 1971; Parasuraman, 1979; also, see Parasuraman, Warm, and See, chapter 11 this volume). The vigilant state is made up of several components: first, a passive arousal perhaps linked to the circadian cycle; second, an effortful arousal linked to the task and to cognitive factors (Eysenck, 1982); third, spatial attention as manifested by attention shifting or attentional breadth. A substantial case has been made for noradrenergic mediation of vigilant behavior, and there is recent work implicating GABA and ACh as well (McGaughy and Sarter, 1995).

Noradrenaline   NA agonists, as well as many other stimulants, increase sustained attention (Koelega, 1993), although there have been no controlled pharmacological studies in primates. However, cells of the monkey LC are activated by novel sensory stimuli but are quiescent during behaviors that turn the animal away from the external environment (reviewed by Aston-Jones, Chiang, and Alexinsky, 1991). The magnitude of the sensory response and the rate of LC background activity vary directly with arousal level (Aston-Jones and Bloom, 1981). However, LC background activity varies inversely with attentional effort (Rajkowski, Kubiak, and Aston-Jones, 1994). At first glance, that finding is unexpected. After all, a great number of studies tell us that vigilance and attentive effort are positively correlated (e.g., Broadbent, 1971), at least over part of the continuum of cognitive activation. However, the LC activity seems to be proportional to attentional lability rather than to attentional effort. Thus, LC activity is low when attention is turned inward during sleep or grooming and during effortful attention, and moderate or high when attention is turned outward in anticipation of sensory inputs. States of high arousal would presumably be like intense attentional effort and would therefore cause lowered LC activity. This suggests that organisms are less distractible by external events when highly aroused. A similar conclusion was reached by Carli, Robbins, Evenden, and Everitt, (1983), who suggested that the role of NA is to reduce distractability during states of high arousal (see Altering Brain Activity by Cytotoxic Lesions, below). Although the specific attentional component or components affected by the lesion remain unidentified, these results suggest that NA plays a role in sustained attention in both rats and in monkeys.

Attention and Working Memory

Attention is an integral part of the mnemonic process. It determines which information in the sensory store passes into working memory and it facilitates retrieval. A widely used memory task is the delayed response task, which requires a subject to remember the location of an object it has just seen. Spatial attention is probably required to facilitate the retrieval of information about a remembered location, and attention to the particular feature would minimize responses to incorrect objects. Because the delays between exposure and response may last tens of seconds, sustained attention during the trial is also required.

Noradrenaline   During normal senescence monkeys and humans show a loss of LC cell bodies and a decline in brain NA, resulting in increased distractibility, poorer short-term storage, and retrieval difficulties (Bartus and Dean, 1979). To understand these changes Arnsten et al. (1988) tested the effects of clonidine or guanfacine on performance deficits in object retrieval following delay periods. At low doses clonidine impaired performance whereas guanfacine improved it; the reverse pattern was observed at higher doses. The authors concluded that clonidine improved performance by increasing brain NA to non-aged levels, although basal NA levels were not actually measured. However, normal levels of NA are associated with efficient utilization of external cues. Thus, it is not clear whether the behavioral improvement was due to improved memory or to decreased distractability.

Arnsten and Contant (1992) tested whether alpha-2 agonists could reverse the performance deficits produced by distractors presented during the delay period. Error rates grew as the time increased between the distractor presentation and response time, but the errors were reduced by clonidine and guanfacine. In further work, the reduction was reversed by idazoxan or by the "specific" postsynaptic antagonist SKF 104078 (Arnsten and Cai, 1993). The authors interpreted the results as demonstrating that the agonists increase levels of NA in the prefrontal cortex, which enhances frontal inhibition of distractor responses in the primary sensory areas. However, other studies show that clonidine reduces brain NA (Brun, Suaud-Chagny, Gonon, and Buda, 1993; Heyn, 1994), which is suggestive of presynaptic action. In addition, SKF 104078 has been shown to antagonize clonidine presynaptically in some locations (Oriowo et al., 1991). Thus, an alternate hypothesis, supported by the findings of Witte et al. (1992), might be that distractors, like cues, are stimuli whose information is poorly processed following alpha-2 agonists because these drugs decrease the availability of NA in distractor (sensory) circuits. Further work is needed to decide between these alternatives hypotheses.

ALTERING BRAIN ACTIVITY BY CYTOTOXIC LESIONS

Current methods for producing brain lesions produce damage only at specific cell recognition sites. These sites, usually at neurotransmitter receptors, are often found on the somatodendritic surface, which accounts for cell-body damage. Axons of passage usually lack these receptors and are usually undamaged. In some areas, however, the terminal regions may contain receptors for the neurotoxic substance and could be damaged by the injection. One drawback of this method is that it may spare neighboring neurons that participate in the targeted behavior despite having a different neurochemical signature. Another drawback is that compensatory changes in receptor sensitivity may occur that mitigate the effects of the lesion on behavior.

The key issue with this method is the selectivity of the chemical lesion (for a comparison of several toxins, see Muir, Everitt, and Robbins, 1994). Toxins specific for noradrenergic, dopaminergic, serotonergic, and cholinergic neurons (Wenk, Stoehr, Quintana, Mobley, and Riley, 1994) are available. Diffusion from the injection site may be problematic, and the ideal control for nonspecific effects is to measure neurotransmitter content with high-performance liquid chromatography in the target area of interest.

Cholinergic Lesions

Studies of cognitive deficits with Alzheimer's disease, which results in severe depletion of cortical ACh, have suggested that the basal forebrain is involved in attentional computations (Parasuraman and Haxby, 1993; also, see Parasuraman and Greenwood, chapter 21 this volume). Experimental investigations with rats and monkeys have led to similar conclusions. For example, Voytko et al. (1994) found that MBF lesions produced significant increases in validity effects in the CTD task. Although no means to assess phasic alerting were included in the attentional task of this study, the results are generally complementary with a study by Witte et al. (1997) and with the nicotinic enhancement hypothesis mentioned previously. The lesions did not alter performance in several working memory tasks. In general, these results support the view that cholinergic activity may play a greater role in attention than in memory (Dunnett, Everitt, and Robbins, 1991).

Recent results using other behavioral tasks have yielded similar conclusions. In the serial RT task, a rat must attend to one section of a chamber and make a behavioral response to a brief target at a random location. This task, unlike the CTD task, involves overt orienting (eye, head, and perhaps body movements) as well as attention shifting to the targets. Using the serial RT task, Muir et al. (1994) have shown that MBF lesions in rats impaired several measures of attentional performance, a result that could be reversed by decreasing the attentional load. In those lesioned groups that showed behavioral recovery, deficits could be reinstated by increasing the attentional load. The most likely interpretation is that the intact basal forebrain is required for normal attentional function. Which particular attentional component requires the intact basal forebrain is not clear from these results, but both visuospatial attention and sustained attention are probably involved.

Noradrenergic Lesions

Carli et al. (1983) assessed the effects of lesions of the rat dorsal noradrenergic bundle on the serial RT task. They found that lesioned rats showed more errors, more impulsive and perseverative responses, and decreased response latencies for incorrect trials than controls when distractors were present during choice periods. The results suggest that the noradrenergic system normally makes attention more stable during conditions of heightened arousal. In general, the pattern of deficits found with NA lesions is distinct from the pattern found with DA and ACh lesions, supporting the idea that each BPS may be involved in different aspects of attentional performance.

In summary, neurochemical studies suggest that visuospatial attention may be modulated by both cholinergic and noradrenergic inputs. The results of these studies, taken together with the results of positron emission tomography (PET) scan experiments (see Corbetta, chapter 6, this volume) and with data on the impairment of directed attention that occurs with clinical neglect, suggest that the most likely site of modulation is the posterior system. Sustained attention clearly has a noradrenergic component, but it is also operational during delayed responses that are modified by cholinergic blockade. That data, along with PET data that point to activity in the frontal area (Pardo et al., 1991), suggest that sustained attention may be controlled by cholinergic and noradrenergic influences on the anterior attention system.

CONCLUSIONS

What impact has neurochemistry made on the major theoretical issues in attention? First, the neuropharmacological approach has contributed to our understanding of the components of attentional processes. The dissociation of the mechanisms underlying alerting and orienting components has been documented in primates and to a lesser extent in humans. Similarly, the cellular recordings in the LC strongly point to both phasic and tonic components of vigilant behavior. Lastly, the behavioral disruptions following NA lesions suggest that the capacity of attentional "bottlenecks" may be determined by neuromodulatory systems. Areas for future work include studies of the histaminergic and serotonergic systems and investigations into the roles of receptor subtypes or colocalized neurotransmitters in attention.

ACKNOWLEDGMENTS

Preparation of this manuscript was supported by National Institutes Health grant NS 32973 and by a grant from the McDonnell-Pew Foundations to the Center for the Cognitive Neuroscience of Attention at the University of Oregon.

REFERENCES

Arnsten, A. F. T. and Cai, J. X. (1993) Postsynaptic alpha-2 receptors stimulation improved memory in aged monkeys: Indirect effects of yohimbine versus direct effects of clonidine. *Neurobiol. Aging* 14: 597–603.

Arnsten, A. F. T., Cai, J. X., and Goldman-Rakic, P. S. (1988) The alpha-2 adrenergic agonist guanfacine improves memory in aged monkeys without sedative or hypotensive side-effects: Evidence for alpha-2 receptor subtypes. *J. Neurosci.* 8: 4287–4298.

Arnsten, A. F. T. and Contant, T. A. (1992) Alpha-2 agonists decrease distractibility in aged monkeys performing the delayed response task. *Psychopharmacology* 108: 159–169.

Aston-Jones, G. and Bloom, F. E. (1981) Activity of norepinephrine-containing locus coeruleus neurons in behaving rats anticipates fluctuations in the sleep-waking cycle. *J. Neurosci.* 1: 887–900.

Aston-Jones, G., Chiang, C., and Alexinsky, T. (1991) Discharge of noradrenergic locus coeruleus neurons in behaving rats and monkeys suggests a role in vigilance. *Prog. Brain Res.* 88: 501–520.

Aston-Jones, G., Rajkowski, J., Kubiak, P., and Alexinsky, T. (1994) Locus coeruleus neurons in monkey are selectively activated by attended cues in a vigilance task. *J. Neurosci.* 14: 4467–4480.

Bartus, R. T. and Dean, R. L. (1979) Recent memory in aged non-human primates: Hypersensitivity to visual interference during retention. *Exp. Aging Res.* 5: 385–400.

Broadbent, D. E. (1971) *Decision and Stress.* New York: Academic Press.

Brun, P., Suaud-Chagny, M. F., Gonon, F., and Buda, M. (1993) In vivo noradrenaline release evoked in the anteroventral thalamic nucleus by locus coeruleus activation: An electrochemical study. *Neuroscience,* 52: 961–972

Carli, M., Robbins, T. W., Evenden, J. L., and Everitt, B. J. (1983) Effects of lesions to ascending noradrenergic neurons of performance of a 5-choice serial reaction task in rats: Implications for theories of dorsal noradrenergic bundle function based on selective attention and arousal. *Behav. Brain Res.* 9: 361–380.

Chan-Palay, V. and Asan, E. (1989) Quantitation of catecholamine neurons in the locus coeruleus in human brains of normal young and older adults and in depression. *J. Comp. Neurol.* 287: 357–372.

Clark, C. R., Geffen, G. M., and Geffen, L. B. (1987) Catecholamines and attention. I. Animal and clinical studies. *Neurosci. Biobehav. Rev.* 11: 341–352.

Clark, C. R., Geffen, G. M. and Geffen, L. B. (1989) Catecholamines and the covert orienting of attention. *Neuropsychologia,* 27: 131–139

Colby, C. (1991) The neuroanatomy and neurophysiology of attention. *J. Child. Neurol.* 6: S90–S118.

Corbetta, M., Miesen, F. M., Shulman, G. L., and Petersen, S. E. (1993) A PET study of visuospatial attention. *J. Neurosci.* 13: 1202–1226.

Davidson, M. C., Villareal, M., and Marrocco, R. T. (1994) Pharmacological manipulation of noradrenaline activity influences covert orienting in rhesus monkey. *Neurosci. Abstr.* 21: 829.

Dunnett, S. B., Everitt, B. J., and Robbins, T. W. (1991) The basal forebrain-cortical cholinergic system: Interpreting the functional consequences of excitotoxic lesions. *Trends Neurosci.* 14: 494–500.

Eysenck, M. W. (1982) *Attention and Arousal.* Berlin: Springer.

Heyn, S. N. (1994) *The effect of clonidine on norepinephrine levels in the rat prefrontal cortex.* Unpublished honors thesis, University of Oregon, Eugene.

Jackson, S. and Houghton, G. (1994) Sensorimotor selection and the basal ganglia: A neural network model. In *Models of Information Processing in the Basal Ganglia,* edited by J. C. Houk, J. L. Davis, and D. G. Beiser, pp. 337–367. Cambridge, MA: MIT Press.

Koelega, H. S. (1993) Stimulant drugs and vigilance performance: A review. *Psychopharmacology* 111: 1–16.

LaBerge, D. and Buchsbaum, M. S. (1990) Positron emission tomographic measurements of pulvinar activity during an attention task. *J. Neurosci.* 10: 613–619.

Lena, C., Changeux, J. P., and Mulle, C. (1993) Evidence for "preterminal" nicotinic receptors on GABAergic axons in the rat interpeduncular nucleus. *J. Neurosci.* 13: 2680–2688.

Marrocco, R. T. and Witte, E. A. (1993) Systemic nicotine from cigarette smoking modifies covert orienting in human subjects. *Soc. Neurosci. Abstr.* 19: 561.

Marrocco, R. T., Witte, E., and Davidson, M. C. (1994) Arousal systems. *Curr. Opin. Neurobiol.* 7: 166–170.

McCormick, D. A., Wang, Z., and Huguenard, J. (1993) Neurotransmitter control of neocortical neuronal activity and excitability. *Cereb. Cortex* 3: 387–398.

McGaughy, J. and Sarter, M. (1995) Effects of chlordiazepoxide and scopolamine, but not aging, on the detection and identification of conditional visual stimuli. *J. Gerontol. A Biol. Sci. Med. Sci.* 50: 90–96.

Meador, K. J., Moore, E. E., Nichols, M. E., Abney, O. L., Taylor, H. S., Zamrini, E. Y., and Loring, D. W. (1993) The role of cholinergic systems in visuospatial processing and memory. *J. Clin. Exp. Neuropsychol.* 15: 832–842.

Morecraft, R. J., Geula, C., and Mesulam, M. M. (1993) Architecture of connectivity within a cingulo-fronto-parietal neurocognitive network for directed attention. *Arch. Neurol.* 50: 279–284.

Muir, J. L., Everitt, B. J., and Robbins, T. W. (1994) AMPA-induced excitotoxic lesions of the basal forebrain: A significant role for the cortical cholinergic system in attentional function. *J. Neurosci.* 14: 2313–2326.

Oriowo, M. A., Hieble, J. P., and Ruffolo, R. R., Jr. (1991) Evidence for heterogeneity of prejunctional alpha-2-adrenoceptors. *Pharmacology* 43: 1–13.

Parasuraman, R. (1979) Memory load and event rate control sensitivity decrements in sustained attention. *Science* 205: 924–927.

Parasuraman, R. and Haxby, J. V. (1993) Attention and brain function in Alzheimer's disease: A review. *Neuropsychology* 7: 242–272.

Pardo, J., Fox, P. T., and Raichle, M. (1991) Localization of a human system for sustained attention by positron emission tomography. *Nature* 349: 61–64.

Posner, M. I. and Cohen, Y. (1984) Components of performance. In *Attention and Performance X*, edited by H. Bouma and D. Bowhuis, pp. 531–556. Hillsdale, NJ: Lawrence Erlbaum.

Posner, M. I. and Petersen, S. E. (1990) The attention system of the human brain. *Annu. Rev. Neurosci.* 13: 25–42.

Rajkowski, J., Kubiak, P., and Aston-Jones, G. (1994) Locus coeruleus activity in monkey: Phasic and tonic changes are associated with altered vigilance. *Brain Res. Bull.* 35: 607–616.

Reader, T. A. and Jasper, H. H. (1984) Interactions between monoamines and other neurotransmitters in cerebral cortex. In *Monoamine Innervation of Cerebral Cortex*, edited by L. Descarriers, T. Reader, and H. Jasper, pp. 195–225. New York: Liss.

Robbins, T. W. and Everett, B. J. (1995) Arousal systems and attention. In *The Cognitive Neurosciences*, edited by M. S. Gazzaniga, pp. 703–720. Cambridge, MA: MIT Press.

Voytko, M. L., Olton, D. S., Richardson, R. T., Gorman, L. K., Tobin, J. R., and Price, D. L. (1994) Basal forebrain lesions in monkeys disrupt attention but not learning and memory. *J. Neurosci.* 14: 167–186.

Wenk, G. L., Stoehr, J. D., Quintana, G., Mobley, S., and Riley, R. G. (1994) Behavioral, biochemical, histological, and electrophysiological effects of 192 IgG-saporin injections into the basal forebrain of rats. *J. Neurosci.* 14: 5986–5995.

Wesnes, K. and Warburton, D. M. (1984) Effects of scopolamine and nicotine on human rapid information processing performance. *Psychopharmacology* 82: 147–150.

Witte, E. A. (1994) *The effects of pharmacological changes in the catecholaminergic and cholinergic systems on arousal and covert orienting.* Unpublished doctoral dissertation, University of Oregon, Eugene.

Witte, E. A., Lickey, M. E., and Marrocco, R. T. (1992) Pharmacological depletion of catecholamines modifies covert orienting in rhesus monkey. *Soc. Neurosci. Abstr.* 18: 537.

Witte, E. A., Davidson, M. C., and Marrocco, R. T. (1997) Effects of altering brain cholinergic activity on pharmacological manipulation of brain covert orienting of attention: Comparison of monkey and human performance. *Psychopharmacology* 132: 324–334.

Witte, E. A., and Marrocco, R. T. (1997) Alteration of brain noradrenergic activity in rhesus monkeys affects the alerting component of covert orienting. *Psychopharmacology* 132: 315–323.

Witte, E. A., McCracken, J. T., and Holmes, P. (1995) Attentional orienting altered by nicotine from tobacco smoke. *Soc. Neurosci. abstr.* 21: 939.

Wonnacott, S., Drasdo, A., Sanderson, E., and Rowell, P. (1990) Presynaptic nicotinic receptors and the modulation of transmitter release. In *The Biology of Nicotine Dependence.* Ciba Foundation symposium, pp. 87–105. Chichester, UK: Wiley.

4 Neurophysiology of Visual Attention

Brad C. Motter

ABSTRACT   The single-cell physiological method provides a unique view of the spatial and temporal components of information processing in the brain, and is therefore well suited to the investigation of the neural correlates of attention. With this method the stages of attentive selection can also be localized to populations of cells, and the mechanisms of selective limitations can be inferred from observed changes in processing. The constraints of this approach and the general methods and techniques employed are described. Studies using these methods to examine the neural correlates of focal visual attention in detection, discrimination, and search tasks are discussed.

The single-cell physiological method, or the recording of the electrical activity of individual neurons, provides a unique view of the spatial and temporal components of information processing in the brain. When combined with the use of appropriate tasks in the behaving animal, single-cell physiology provides information that cannot be obtained by other means. As discussed in other chapters in this volume, electrophysiological methods such as event-related potentials (ERPs) and functional brain-imaging techniques such as positron emission tomography (PET) can yield information on integrated brain activity underlying cognition in humans. However, only the single-cell physiological method possesses the requisite spatial and temporal resolution to disclose aspects of information processing at the neuronal level. Of course, unlike ERPs and PET, cellular recording is invasive. Each class of methods has its relative merits and costs.

With the use of the single-cell physiological method the flow of information through the circuitry of the nervous system can be directly examined in relation to behavior. The method is therefore well suited to the investigation of the neural correlates of attention. Furthermore, the stages of attentive selection can be localized to populations of cells and the mechanisms of selective limitations can be inferred from observed changes in processing.

In order to examine the neural mechanisms of attention, cellular recording must be carried out in conjunction with well-designed and carefully controlled behavioral tasks. The challenge is to design experimental paradigms so that principles of cognitive functions that arise from the concerted activity of millions of neurons can be deduced from a sampling of several hundred. This chapter outlines several of the constraints of the single-cell physiological approach, discusses some of the general methods and techniques employed, and summarizes a sampling of recent paradigms and results using these methods in the investigation of visual attention.

THE SINGLE-CELL PHYSIOLOGICAL METHOD

Discharge Activity of Neurons

The activity of individual neurons in awake and behaving animals is measured by placing a small metal electrical probe (a microelectrode) close enough to a neuron's cell body to observe the changes in the extracellular electrical field produced when the neuron generates an action potential. The voltages observed are typically on the order of 50–500 microvolts. With care and luck, the position of the electrode in relation to a given neuron can be maintained—without injuring the neuron or drifting out of range—for a period of time sufficient to characterize the neuron's activity in relation to several experimental variables. The extracellular electrode does not measure the neuron's membrane potential but rather the changes in extracellular field currents associated with intracellular and transmembrane ionic movements.

The field gradients generated by the fast transient discharge of action potentials (spikes) are sufficiently large and steep enough to discriminate the spikes generated by a single neuron from those of other nearby neurons. The discrimination is made by comparing the shapes of the temporal profiles of the voltage changes associated with each spike. Discharges associated with a single neuron often produce a rather consistent spike-like shape that differs significantly in its waveform from other nearby neurons. Differences in waveform are in part due to the exact positioning of the electrode with respect to the neuron but are also due to differences in the extracellular field structure resulting from different generator geometries. Usually only the time of occurrence of spikes from a discriminated neuron is measured and recorded.

Integration and Coding of Information

The significant result of synaptic integration is the generation of axonally propagated spikes. The set of intervals between spikes defines a time series of events that contains all of the information relayed from one neuron to the next set of neurons in the network. Although an interval code (a "Morse code") could be carried within spike trains, attempts to identify such codes have not produced clear examples of information coding. In fact, the variability in interspike intervals observed for many neurons in various locations in the nervous system is consistent with the presence of a random Poisson process (Perkel, Gerstein, and Moore, 1967). Given such variability, information appears to be coded within single neurons only by the average rate of firing and not by the precise composition of the intervals between spikes.

In fact, recent debate regarding interval coding is centered on explaining how synaptic integration can result in such a highly variable process. Cortical neurons receive around 5,000–10,000 synapses, of which about 85% are excitatory. If inputs actually arrived in a random fashion, their integration would result in a fairly regular output train (Softky and Koch, 1993). It has been argued that the large variability observed in interspike intervals arises both from a more contentious interaction between excitatory and inhibitory synaptic processes than was previously considered to be the case and from a more synchronous (coincident) arrival of input (Softky and Koch, 1993; Shadlen and Newsome, 1994). It has become increasingly clear that the role played by inhibition in cortical circuits is not simply an antagonistic balancing act versus excitation, but rather is a role in which inhibition acts as a trimming damper on the explosive growth of the positive feedback gain of excitatory cortical circuits. Relatively small amounts of inhibition provided at the correct time can shape the amplification of information (Douglas and Martin, 1991). Recent modeling studies emphasize these control structures and demonstrate the necessity of considering the collective action of groups of neurons in information processing (Somers, Nelson, and Sur, 1995). Furthermore, synaptic integration at most cortical synapses can be regulated by slow and long-acting neuromodulators, yet relatively little is understood about how these subsystems normally affect information transmission. Many of these widespread neuromodulator systems originate in areas of the basal forebrain and brainstem, areas that exert major state controls over waking and attentive behavior (see Marrocco and Davidson, chapter 3, this volume).

The recognition that selective response properties emerge within groups of neurons and that the emergent properties are manifest from the beginning of the response rather than arising in time from a more undifferentiated activity such as orientation sensitivity (Vogels and Orban, 1990; Somers et al., 1995) emphasizes the parallel and distributed processing aspects of neural function. The conveyance of parallel sets of information from one node in the neural net to the next emphasizes, in turn, the spatial aspects of synaptic integration of relatively coincident inputs. Within the context of small populations of neurons that provide information in a relatively instantaneous parallel manner, the lack of a temporal interval code for stimulus properties is perhaps more acceptable. That rationale appears to corroborate a long-held working assumption of neurophysiologists; namely, that the reconstruction of the temporal response profile of a single neuron, which is accomplished by averaging the results of repeated presentations of stimuli, provides a reasonable representation of the temporal profile of the response across a set of neurons. The strength of activity within the temporal profile (and its variability) are further taken to be reasonable indices of the validity of the information coded across the small group of participating neurons.

As it happens, one of earliest tools developed to summarize neural activity is still the most common and accepted analytic method—the peri-event time histogram (figure 4.1). The histogram depicts the temporal response profile

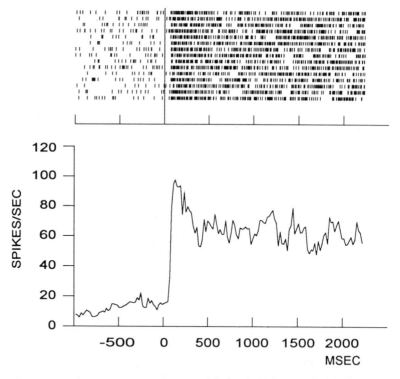

Figure 4.1 The peri-event time histogram shown at the bottom displays the average rate of neuronal firing occurring during a repeated series of behavioral trials. Here the activity of an extrastriate (V2) cortical neuron is shown synchronized to the onset (time 0.0) of a stimulus within its receptive field. Activity was averaged in 20 ms bins across the trials to produce the histogram. At the top of the figure is a spike raster for the same data that the histogram shows. Each row of tics is a temporal segment of a behavioral trial synchronized to the stimulus onset. Each tic represents the time of occurrence of a spike during the trial. The stimulus remained on for 3 s.

simply by averaging the activity per unit time relative to a particular event, for example a stimulus presentation or a motor act. The averaging occurs across stimulus repetitions spaced over a long enough period of time to insure independence of events. Histograms that combine information across sets of neurons usually normalize each neuron's response to some arbitrary scale value prior to averaging, in order to prevent a weighting bias within small samples of neurons. Histograms are often accompanied by examples of single-neuron activity displayed in a raster format that shows the actual timing of spikes during repeated trials. In such a display, trials are stacked one above the other and are synchronized in time to the relevant trial event (see figure 4.1). To an accustomed eye, at least, trial-to-trial variability in the neuronal response is easier to appreciate in such graphic displays.

Recording Techniques

Single-neuron recordings provide the highest available level of temporal and spatial resolution of functional brain activity, at the cost of measuring the simultaneous action of very small sets of neurons and of using invasive techniques. Single-neuron investigations into the role of attention in visual processing are carried out using animal models with appropriate levels of behavioral sophistication and visual performance necessary to probe fundamental processes underlying visual cognitive functions. In many cases non-human primates, usually macaque monkeys, are used as subjects.

The primary technical problem is the controlled placement of the recording microelectrode, which has a tip diameter of about a micron, near a cell body while the subject performs a behavioral task. In most cases it is necessary to be able to move the microelectrode to allow sampling of different neurons. In the case of recording from cortex, sampling is from a sheet of tissue about 2 mm thick with a typical targeted surface area of one to a few square centimeters that is often folded in several directions following the contours of the cortical sulcal patterns. The varied spatial sampling is accomplished with a lightweight drive unit that is usually attached, on a daily basis, to a chamber surgically affixed to the head. The chamber is positioned to provide access to the target area. The key to achieving stable recording is maintaining a hydraulic seal between the recording chamber, microdrive unit, and cranium that minimizes tissue movement relative to the electrode (Davies, 1956). In the absence of the seal, movement is produced by inter-cerebral pressure changes resulting from changes in posture, respiration and cardiac output. The electrode is slowly advanced into the brain until the target area is encountered. In recent years, improved waveform sorting techniques made possible by dramatic increases in computational capacity have made it possible to record from arrays of chronically implanted electrodes (usually small, 10–25 micron wires) mounted on much smaller, but far less precise, drive units. Such assemblies offer the potential of simultaneous recording from hundreds of neurons (Wilson and McNaughton, 1993).

Experimental Paradigms: Issues of Decision and Selection at the Neural Level

A critical methodological issue is the choice of experimental paradigm. Although paradigms from human studies of visual selective attention can be directly implemented behaviorally, many are not practical for single-neuron investigations. Neuronal studies have several major constraints related to the restricted information available to individual neurons and to the nature of decisions observed at the single-neuron level. Investigations must be tailored to accommodate the vantage point of a single neuron. Perhaps the simplest constraint is the issue of the neuron's receptive field. Stimuli must be presented in that restricted space for at least two conditions, usually one in which attention is somehow directed toward stimuli inside the receptive field and another in which attention is diverted to stimuli outside the receptive field. Because of the limited time available to study any given neuron, paradigms often have a limited characterization of the neuron's preferences and some spatial bias in the positioning of stimuli.

Behavioral measures of performance summarize information processing across both space and time domains. Attentive processes affect behavioral outcomes as the consequence of the modulation of networks of neurons. What can be observed in single neurons is only a small slice of the visual attentive process. What evidence, then, is an acceptable indication of a neural correlate of visual attentive processing? Single neurons have only a limited potential access to all information. Visually responsive neurons, for example, exhibit tuning sensitivities to various stimulus attributes—location, orientation, color, depth, motion, and so forth. Such sensitivities are realizable as the end products of arrangements of photo cells—intricately connected but nevertheless specialized collections that extract certain bits of information. Attention mechanisms may alter the gain of those sensitivities. In fact, altered responsiveness of neurons as a consequence of "directing attention to stimuli" has been used as evidence of attention in many studies. However, selective attention often implies a stage of cognition during which something more than a gain change occurs; selective attention implies that decisions are made about the sensory information. What evidence of decisions occurs at the level of neuronal activity? Decisions imply choices between alternatives (i.e., acceptance or preservation of certain lines of information) and active rejection or loss of other information. Evidence for selective attention processes can therefore be obtained under conditions in which preservation and elimination of information occur without gain changes.

Capturing evidence for the occurrence of decisions in the actions of a neuron at a given level is heavily constrained by the restricted sensitivities and the fleeting nature of information passage through the nervous system. Visually responsive neurons only have direct access to restricted portions of the visual field as defined by their receptive fields and are often sensitive only to certain attributes of the visual stimuli. Single-neuron experimental paradigms are thus constrained by the requirements to construct and place stimuli according to the preferences of the neuron under study. Such criteria create formidable barriers for multineuronal recording techniques in which overlapping receptive fields and different visual sensitivities make it difficult or impossible to simultaneously tailor stimuli for each neuron being studied.

Measures of the activity of a neuron do not have the advantage of behavioral measures that summarize outcomes of information processing. Single neurons participate in a small temporal slice of the visual attention process, a slice that may be nearly instantaneously thin, given the arguments for parallel processing mentioned in the previous section. Experimental paradigms are therefore constrained to obtain measurements of neural activity during very limited temporal periods. This problem is further exacerbated by the fact that networks governed by feedback systems settle as a function of time. When observations occur shortly after the onset of visual stimuli, the interpretation of results must take into account the non-stationarity of neuronal processing. Some neurobehavioral paradigms have deliberately attempted to extend the observation periods by providing information in stages (Motter, 1994a).

To summarize, the single-cell recording technique offers a potentially powerful means of investigating the mechanisms of attention at the neuronal level when the method is combined judiciously with appropriate behavioral paradigms. In the next section, the modern use of these methods to investigate visual attention is discussed. To provide pertinent background, earlier studies of sensory and attentive processes associated with neuronal activity in parietal and temporal association areas are described first.

ATTENTIVE PROCESSES IN PARIETAL AND TEMPORAL VISUAL ASSOCIATION AREAS

The initial neurobehavioral studies of visual cortical association areas were usually cast in terms of the exploration of correlations between the physical parameters of the stimulus, its form or position in space, and the discharge activity of neurons. Those studies depicted a variety of complex sensory correlations that often related the intensity of neural activity to the general attentive interest shown by the subject with regard to the set of stimuli being used. The observed correlations also supported the propositions that parietal and temporal visual cortical areas represented two distinct sensory hierarchies. The parietal visual association areas emphasized the visuospatial relationships between self and surrounding objects and represented a stage where sensory processes merged with systems directly associated with the organization and direction of behavior in the environment (Lynch Mountcastle, Talbot, and Yin, 1977; Mountcastle, Lynch, Georgopoulous, Sakata, and Acuna, 1975). In contrast, the emphasis of temporal association areas was clearly on object form and recognition and represented a stage where sensory processes became entwined with systems associated with object recognition and memory (Desimone and Gross, 1979; Rolls, Judge, and Sanghera, 1977; also, see Webster and Ungerleider, chapter 2, this volume).

As behavioral paradigms progressed beyond simple control of fixation to manipulation of the intent of the fixation act, it became clear that the neuronal processing observed in temporal and parietal association areas was as powerfully affected by the factors associated with the attentive viewing conditions as it was by the attributes of the physical stimuli themselves. The different information processing emphasis in the parietal and temporal areas was apparent even with respect to the attentional influences. Both sensitivity to visual stimuli and effective receptive field size were increased by a factor of three or more for parietal neurons during a focal attention fixation task (Mountcastle, Anderson, and Motter, 1981; Mountcastle, Motter, Steinmetz, and Sestokas, 1987), whereas under essentially the same conditions the receptive fields of inferior temporal cortical neurons were observed to collapse around a visible fixation target (Richmond, Wurtz, and Sato, 1983).

Understanding of the differential nature of attentive influences within parietal and temporal cortical areas was further refined with the introduction of paradigms that diverted attention, but not the eyes, away from the fixation target to other locations. Directing attention to a particular location suppression the responsiveness at that location of parietal visual neurons and increased sensitivity to surrounding regions of visual space (Mountcastle, Motter, Steinmetz, and Duffy, 1984; Steinmetz Connor, Constantinidis, and McLavghlin, 1993). In clear contrast, directing focal attention to a particular object or location results in an increased visual responsiveness in inferior temporal neurons (Richmond and Sato, 1987) that appears to be graded by the level of the attentive requirement (Spitzer and Richmond, 1991). These studies clearly demonstrated that selective attention is not a unitary event in the nervous system but instead occurs in different systems and places different limitations on processing in different parts of the visual field all at the same time.

NEUROPHYSIOLOGICAL STUDIES OF VISUAL ATTENTION

Selective Attention as a Focal Spatial Process

Attention is normally focused where one looks—usually where the eyes are fixating. Visual orienting and attention processes most often work together to bring objects into the central foveal region of vision where they can be scrutinized. Evidence from both cueing and task loading studies suggests that focal attention is directed at a single locus (object) at a time and cannot be subdivided (Posner, 1980; Duncan, 1984; Braun and Sagi, 1991). A number of theories, following Broadbent (1958), have depicted focal attention as a selective filter that passes information within a restricted dimension and actively depresses information outside that dimension. The dimension that has dominated consideration is spatial location. The designation of location, rather than a stimulus feature (such as the set of red objects), as the framework within which attention operates, produces a critical distinction. It implies a bottleneck for detection and recognition that is principally a spatial factor, resulting in a limited capacity sampling zone that must be shifted around the scene.

Current biological models utilize the retinotopic organization of the early visual system and the progressive enlargement of receptive field size within the hierarchy of the visual system as the framework for a selective filter based on spatial location. Focal attention is modeled as operating through a selection or highlighting of a dynamically determined subset of interconnected cortical (and subcortical) areas that are related in terms of retinotopic location. The mechanisms of the current models emphasize both the gating of information within the zone to higher levels of analysis and the suppression of information outside the zone of focused attention (Desimone,

1992; Koch and Ullman, 1985; Olshausen, Anderson, and Van Essen, 1993; Tsotsos et al., 1995). Correspondingly, neurophysiological investigations have concentrated on correlations with the shift of attention from one location to another and with the differential processing of information within attended versus nonattended locations.

Focal Attentive Processes in Visual Orienting

The close bond between the definition of focal attentive processes and the issues of spatial selectivity have played a major role in the development of studies of selective processing associated with visual orienting (for a review, see Colby, 1991). Goldberg and Wurtz (1972) were the first to note an enhanced discharge activity when a visual onset stimulus was the target for a saccade (see figure 4.2). The enhanced activation preceded the eye movement and was shown to be selective for the specific target of the impending saccadic eye movement and not for other potential targets presented at the

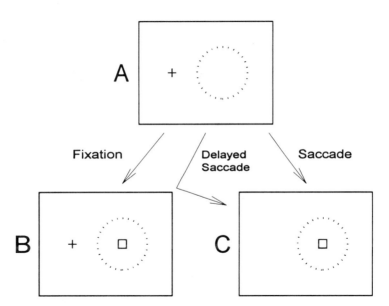

Figure 4.2 Initial studies of the role played by attention in visual orienting were based on variations of the fixation and saccade paradigms. (A) Each paradigm started with the requirement of steady fixation of a small target (+) that provided a fixed positioning of the receptive field (dashed circle) from trial to trial. Receptive field position and size were determined separately for each neuron. (B) The fixation paradigm required continuous fixation of the target (+) despite presentation of test stimuli (square). (C) In the saccade paradigm the target disappeared as the test stimulus appeared and the subject was required to saccade to and fixate on the test stimulus. A variation, the delayed saccade paradigm, combined the two by delaying the offset of the target until after the initial response to the test stimulus had occurred. Differences in the neural activity evoked by the test stimulus in different paradigms, either at onset or just prior to saccades, could reveal underlying focal attention shifts.

same time (Wurtz and Mohler, 1976b). Those observations in the superior colliculus were the first to demonstrate a process operating at the level of individual neurons that resulted in a preferential selection of information from a discrete spatial location, a process resembling attentive selection of a visual target. Similar enhanced (as well as suppressed) activity prior to a saccade has been observed in posterior parietal cortex (Yin and Mountcastle, 1977; Bushnell, Goldberg, and Robinson, 1981), frontal cortex (Goldberg and Bushnell, 1981), and extrastriate area V4 (Fischer and Boch, 1981), but not in striate cortex or in extrastriate area V2 (Wurtz and Mohler, 1976a; Baizer Robinson, and Dow, 1977). The lack of either enhancement or suppression of responses in early visual cortical areas (V1 and V2) was important because it suggested that the locus of attentive selection lay beyond striate cortex. As discussed later, however, more recent studies suggest a revision of this view.

Changes in activity associated with shifts in attention without concomitant eye movements have also been reported for neurons in posterior parietal cortex (Bushnell et al., 1981; Mountcastle et al., 1984; Steinmetz et al., 1994). In general, the results of those studies of visual orienting have been interpreted as indicating a lack of attentional influence on target selection in early visual cortical areas, suggesting an immutable encoding of basic visual features (but see later). In contrast, an active role for attentive processes in anatomically later visual areas, especially parietal cortex, appears to be in agreement with behavioral deficits resulting from damage to those areas, as in the neglect syndrome (Mesulam, 1981).

The sudden appearance of objects usually generates an involuntary shift of focal attention to the object (Yantis and Jonides, 1984). Such automatic attentional capture mechanisms may play a major role in the effects seen in many saccade paradigms. Most eye movements during visual search or reading, however, are not made to newly appearing stimuli. Fischer and Boch (1985) used a delayed saccade paradigm and reported that neurons in extrastriate area V4 that produced an initial transient response to the onset of a potential target stimulus became reactivated later in the behavioral trial when that stimulus became the target of a saccade. Fischer and Boch suggested that the reactivation could represent a shift in directed focal attention but also could be due to a change in visual sensitivity related to the active state of fixation. Later studies by Boch (1986) reported similar observations in striate cortex, again with a task requiring release of fixation and production of saccadic eye movements. Responses similar to reactivation also have been observed in a peripheral attention task that involved neither saccadic eye movements nor release of fixation (Motter, 1989). An increment in activity in neurons in areas V1, V2, and V4 was observed when a small cue that was placed inside the receptive field and used to guide focal attention to peripheral sites became the relevant cue during the trial. Together, these studies suggest that shifts in focal attention can be observed early in the cortical processing of visual information.

Focal Attention Processes in Discrimination Tasks

The most direct evidence that focal attention influences sensory processing in early visual cortical areas comes from two studies in which the subjects were required to discriminate the orientation of bars presented at an attended location (Motter, 1993; Press, Knierim, and Van Essen, 1994). Both studies demonstrated that focal attentive processes can modulate the response of cortical neurons as early as striate cortex (area V1). The two studies differed from previous investigations in two important ways. Both studies required orientation discrimination of a small bar as opposed to simple detection, as was required in previous studies. The importance of that difference lies in the observation that detection of the presence of oriented bars can be accomplished by a parallel prefocal attention process, but discrimination of the orientation of bars requires a serial focal attention process (Sagi and Julesz, 1985). Secondly, in both studies target stimuli were presented in the presence of competing stimuli, a condition in which a correct response clearly benefits from focal attention; focal attention provides no clear benefit, however, when isolated stimuli are presented against homogenous backgrounds (Engel, 1971; Grindley and Townsend, 1968). In both tasks focal attention, directed to the target location by spatial cueing procedures, produced response differences between stimuli at attended and nonattended locations, but typically only when multiple competing stimuli were present. Responses that were diminished by the presence of competing stimuli in the nonattended condition were, in the attended condition, returned to the activation levels observed for single isolated stimuli, suggesting that focused attention acts to isolate a target from surrounding competition. Similar observations for neurons in area V2 have been reported (Motter, 1993; Reynolds, Chelazzi, Luck, and Desimone, 1994). It remains to be established whether those effects are present under more natural scene conditions. In summary, and in contrast to visual orienting paradigms, the results from visual discrimination paradigms have demonstrated that focal attentive processes can act in the first cortical stages of visual processing to alter sensitivity to stimuli in select areas of the visual field.

Rather than explicitly cueing focal attention to a specific location, several neurophysiological studies have used a sustained monitoring task in which the subjects must detect the occurrence of a change in a sequential pattern of stimulus presentations (Moran and Desimone, 1985; Haenny and Schiller, 1988) or the occurrence of a cued target in a temporal sequence of stimuli (Haenny, Maunsell, and Schiller, 1988; Maunsell, Sclar, Nealey, and DePriest, 1991). The relevant stimulus attributes are usually orientation or color. Changes in neuronal sensitivity were measured between conditions in which a given stimulus was relevant to the correct completion of the task versus when it was not. When the task required reporting on a particular attribute (e.g., orientation) the sensitivities of the related receptive field characteristics were sharpened in striate and extrastriate V4 neurons (Haenny and Schiller,

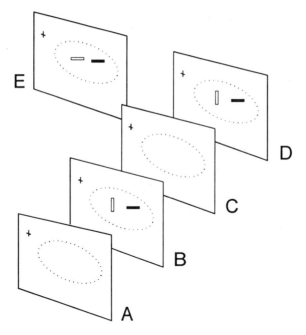

Figure 4.3 Sequential presentation paradigms require either the detection of a particular object (usually the repetition of the first object in a sequence) or a change in the sequence of objects. Moran and Desimone (1985) used a variation in which the subject had to detect a change in a particular object (one of the two bars), ignoring changes at other locations. The sequences A, B, C, D and A, B, C, E either differed or did not, depending upon whether the subject was to attend solely to the stimulus bar on the right or left. Object pairs were chosen so that one object was effective in activating the neuron and the other was not. Differences in the neuronal response to the pair of stimuli were found to be correlated with whether the subject was attending to the effective stimulus or not.

1988). The degree of observed sharpening (higher response rates and narrower orientation bandwidths) was positively correlated with the overall sensitivity of the neuron for that particular stimulus attribute. The lack of separate competing stimuli in these paradigms makes it difficult to distinguish between potentially feature- and focal-sensitive attentional mechanisms.

Moran and Desimone (1985) used a sequential presentation paradigm in which a set of two stimuli was repeatedly presented, with an interstimulus interval of 500 ms. The task was to detect a change from one presentation to the next in one of the two simultaneously presented stimuli while ignoring changes in the other stimulus (figure 4.3). During a block of trials the locations of the relevant and irrelevant stimuli were constant. Moran and Desimone reported that focal attention suppressed the response to the irrelevant, nonattended stimulus placed within the receptive fields of V4 neurons. In contrast, the relevant, attended stimulus produced a response that was essentially unaffected by the presence or absence of the irrelevant stimulus within the receptive field. Differential effects were observed only when both stimuli were within the receptive field. When either the relevant or irrelevant stimulus was placed outside the receptive field, the response to the stimulus remaining within the field was unchanged. Moran and Desimone concluded that their results supported a filter model of focal attention, in which information at the locus of focal attention was passed on and surrounding information within the receptive field was suppressed.

An alternate view of their results is that focal attention isolates the attended object from surrounding competition (Motter, 1993; Press et al., 1994; Reynolds et al., 1994), thereby returning response strengths closer to those observed in the absence of surrounding stimuli. That interpretation emphasizes the active processing of objects within the focus of attention and attributes the observed suppressive filtering to stimulus competition rather than to an active suppressive filtering of unattended objects that is limited to the receptive field. Changes in the sensitivity of the receptive fields of area V4 neurons as a function of the location of focal attention (Connor, Gallant, Preddie, and Van Essen, 1996) lends some support to this view. In Connor and colleagues' study, directing attention to locations at or near the edge of the receptive field tended to heighten sensitivity to probe stimuli delivered nearby within the receptive field, suggesting that the objects themselves and not the receptive field per se were the significant spatial determinants. Focal attention may be the key not only to how feature information is bound together for any one object, but also to how information from different objects is kept separate.

Directing of Attention: Dimensions Other Than Spatial Location

Other studies have concentrated on the influence of attention on the sensitivity of neurons to relevant stimulus dimensions other than location. Those observations suggest that early-stage analytic mechanisms for perceptual features are subject to top-down control that is more specific than simply a gain control. Haenny et al. (1988) demonstrated that such control could be achieved within extrastriate area V4 even with information from another sensory modality. They reported that the responses of V4 neurons to visual stimuli in a delayed match to sample task could be modulated by either visual or somatosensory sample cues. Their task required the detection of a particular grating orientation in a sequence of grating presentations.

The animal subjects were presented with the cued grating orientation before each trial. The cue was presented either visually or in the form of a raised pattern that could be felt with the hand. Across the population of neurons reported, various correlations were observed: potentiation of the stimulus response sometimes to all stimuli paired with a particular cue orientation, or sometimes to particular pairs of cue and stimulus though often not matching pairs. Maunsell et al. (1991) further demonstrated that the particular form of the modulation that occurs is not dependent upon the sensory modality of the cue, either visual or somatosensory. Although no consistent correlation between cue and stimulus response was found across neurons, the responses of individual neurons to specific stimuli were clearly altered by the cue information. These studies established a strong case for top-down control early in visual processing, adding significantly to the debate about whether early versus late selection has any clear meaning when a system can be dominated by feedback.

Attentional Processes in Visual Search

A large portion of the recent work in selective attention has employed a visual search paradigm to investigate visual attentive processes. Simple versions of these paradigms require the subject to make a decision about the presence of a specified target object in an array of simultaneously presented objects. The search can be structured by providing information about the search goal. Several neurobehavioral paradigms have been developed to examine the selective processes underlying shifts in focal attention.

By presenting multiple stimuli within the receptive fields of inferior temporal neurons, Chelazzi, Miller, Duncan, and Desimone (1993) were able to demonstrate that target recognition and selection reduces or truncates the processing of the other objects in the neuron's receptive field. Their paradigm used a match to sample task in which the target was first shown at fixation and then later reappeared at one of two (or more) peripheral locations. The required behavioral response was to capture the target with a single eye movement (figure 4.4). For arrays of two stimuli, changes in the neuronal response profile that indicated recognition and selection of the target occurred about 200 ms after onset of the array and preceded the actual eye movement by 90–120 ms.

A different approach has been to examine physiological processing for evidence of top-down control processes that can guide focal attentive search by manipulating the processing of features; that is, by biasing the search for a particular feature (Egeth, Virzi, and Garbart, 1984; Wolfe, Cave, and Franzel, 1989). Such correlates have been found in area V4 where simple objects can be attentionally segregated on the basis of color or luminance (Motter, 1994a, 1994b). These studies used a two-stage conditional discrimination task that required the subjects to select an elongated bar target on the basis of color and then report its orientation. In the initial stage, an array of stimuli and a color cue that identified a subset of the stimuli containing the target were presented. The presence of multiple stimuli of the correct color, however, required the subject to await a second stage in which the array was reduced to two stimuli, thereby revealing a single stimulus having the matching color (see figure 4.5). During the first stage, V4 neurons whose receptive fields included stimuli of the correct color were found to have a maintained activity, whereas V4 neurons whose fields contained incorrect color matches had depressed activity. When the cue was changed after the array was presented, the neural activity changed (without any change in the

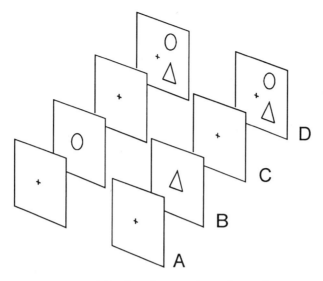

Figure 4.4 In a delayed match-to-sample paradigm, subjects are (A) trained to fixate a target (+) and maintain fixation centrally during (B) a brief presentation of the sample. Then, with the appearance of the choice array (D), subjects are required to make a single eye movement to fixate the stimulus presented initially as the sample. Object pairs were chosen so that one object was effective in activating the neuron and the other was not. Comparisons of the responses evoked by the different choice array conditions were used by Chelazzi et al. (1993) to demonstrate that the neural response in inferior temporal cortical neurons was truncated when the subjects' attention was directed away from the effective stimulus in the interval just before the eye movement was made.

receptive field stimulus) to reflect the correct match, with a latency of about 150–250 ms. This study provides the first clear physiological evidence of spatially parallel attentional processing of stimulus features that highlight potential targets for possible further scrutiny by focal attentive processes. These results fit a model of feature-based attention that can, in parallel, prioritize the stimuli in the scene for the purposes of guiding a focal attention search (Moore and Egeth, 1996).

CONCLUSIONS

Investigations into the actions of attention processes on the transmission of information through single neurons in the visual system have provided two new basic themes that must be incorporated into the development of our understanding of cognitive processes. First, information processing does not progress through a singular hierarchically staged system. Rather, it spreads in parallel through a divergent structure with numerous opportunities for feedback control, making early and late strategies metaphors for selection rather than for implementation. Second, selective processing appears along each branch of the network, often with quite different computational modes of implementation of the selective process. These physiologically based

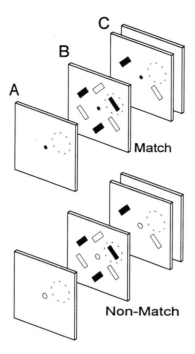

Figure 4.5 Staged conditional orientation discrimination paradigm used to study feature selection processes. The task was to report the orientation of a bar of a particular color. Subjects initially fixated a central dot (A) that provided the conditional color cue for the eventual orientation discrimination (C). During the presentation of an intervening array of stimuli (B), the cue color permitted a selection of a subset of stimuli based on the color feature, but the discrimination had to await the revelation of a clear choice at stage C. The response to the same physical stimulus in the receptive field during the array presentation was compared between conditions in which the stimulus either matches the cue color or does not (nonmatch). Neurons in area V4 were strongly activated during the array period (B) when their receptive fields contained a stimulus matching the cue color (Motter, 1994a).

themes require a redress of many ideas about attentional functions and place an emphasis on feedback control structures in coherent theories of attention.

ACKNOWLEDGMENTS

This work was supported by a grant from the Veterans Affairs Medical Research Program. I wish to thank my colleagues, in particular Denis Pelli, for discussions about decision making at the neuronal level.

REFERENCES

Baizer, J. S., Robinson, D. L., and Dow, B. M. (1977) Visual responses of area 18 neurons in awake, behaving monkey. *J. Neurophysiol.* 40: 1024–1037.

Boch, R. (1986) Behavioral modulation of neuronal activity in monkey striate cortex: Excitation in the absence of active central fixation. *Exp. Brain Res.* 64: 610–614.

Braun, J. and Sagi, D. (1991) Texture-based tasks are little affected by second tasks requiring peripheral or central attentive fixation. *Perception* 20: 483–500.

Broadbent, D. E. (1958) *Perception and Communication*. London: Pergamon Press.

Bushnell, M. C., Goldberg, M. E., and Robinson, D. L. (1981) Behavioral enhancement of visual responses in monkey cerebral cortex. I. Modulation in posterior parietal cortex related to selective visual attention. *J. Neurophysiol.* 46: 755–772.

Chelazzi, L., Miller, E. K., Duncan, J., and Desimone, R. (1993) A neural basis for visual search in inferior temporal cortex. *Nature* 363: 345–347.

Colby, C. L. (1991) The neuroanatomy and neurophysiology of attention. *J. Child Neurol.* 6: 90–118

Connor, C. E., Gallant, J. L., Preddie, D. C., and Van Essen, D. C. (1996) Responses in area V4 depend on the spatial relationship between stimulus and attention. *J. Neurophysiol.* 75: 1306–1308.

Davies, P. W. (1956) Chamber for microelectrode studies in the cerebral cortex. *Science* 124: 179–180.

Desimone, R. (1992) Neural circuits for visual attention in the primate brain. In *Neural Networks for Vision and Image Processing*, edited by G. A. Carpenter, and S. Grossberg, Cambridge, MA: MIT Press.

Desimone, R. and Gross, C. G. (1979) Visual areas in the temporal cortex of the macaque. *Brain Res.* 178: 363–380.

Douglas, R. and Martin, K. (1991) A functional microcircuit for cat visual cortex. *J. Physiol. (Lond.)* 440: 735–769.

Duncan, J. (1984) Selective attention and the organization of visual information. *J. Exp. Psychol. Gen.* 113: 501–517.

Egeth, H. E., Virzi, R. A., and Garbart, H. (1984) Searching for conjunctively defined targets. *J. Exp. Psychol. Hum. Percept. Perf.* 10: 32–39.

Engel, F. L. (1971) Visual conspicuity, directed attention and retinal locus. *Vis. Res.* 11: 563–576.

Fischer, B. and Boch, R. (1981) Enhanced activation of neurons in prelunate cortex before visually guided saccades of trained rhesus monkey. *Exp. Brain. Res.* 44: 129–137.

Fischer, B. and Boch, R. (1985) Peripheral attention versus central fixation: Modulation of the visual activity of prelunate cortical cells of the rhesus monkey. *Exp. Brain. Res.* 345: 111–123.

Goldberg, M. E. and Bushnell, M. C. (1981) Behavioral enhancement of visual responses in monkey cerebral cortex. II. Modulation in frontal eye fields specifically related to saccades *J. Neurophysiol.* 46: 773–787.

Goldberg, M. E. and Wurtz, R. H. (1972) Activity of superior colliculus in behaving monkey. II. Effect of attention on neuronal responses. *J. Neurophysiol.* 35: 560–574.

Grindley, G. C. and Townsend, V. (1968) Voluntary attention in peripheral vision and its effects on acuity and differential thresholds. *Q. J. Exp. Psychol.* 20: 11–19.

Haenny, P. E., Maunsell, J. H. R., and Schiller, P. H. (1988) State dependent activity in monkey visual cortex. II. Retinal and extraretinal factors in V4. *Exp. Brain. Res.* 69: 245–259.

Haenny, P. E. and Schiller, P. H. (1988) State dependent activity in monkey visual cortex. I. Single cell activity in V1 and V4 on visual tasks. *Exp. Brain. Res.* 69: 225–244.

Koch, C. and Ullman, S. (1985) Shifts in selective visual attention: Towards the underlying neural circuitry. *Hum. Neurobiol.* 4: 219–227.

Lynch, J. C., Mountcastle, V. B., Talbot, W. H., and Yin, T. C. T. (1977) Parietal lobe mechanisms for directed attention. *J. Neurophysiol.* 40: 362–389.

Maunsell, J. H. R., Sclar, G., Nealey, T. A., and DePriest, D. D. (1991) Extraretinal representations in area V4 in the macaque monkey. *Vis. Neuroscience* 7: 561–573.

Mesulum, M. M. (1981) A cortical network for directed attention and unilateral neglect. *Ann. Neurol.* 10: 309–325.

Moore, C. M. and Egeth, H. (1996) Attending to stimulus features: Contrasting results from reaction time and masked accuracy [Abstract]. *Invest. Ophthalmol. Vis. Sci.* 37: S299.

Moran, J. and Desimone, R. (1985) Selective attention gates visual processing in the extrastriate cortex. *Science* 229: 782–784.

Motter, B. C. (1989) Reactivation responses in striate and extrastriate visual cortex during a peripheral attention task. *Soc. Neurosci. Abstr.* 15: 119.

Motter, B. C. (1993) Focal attention produces spatially selective processing in visual cortical areas V1, V2 and V4 in the presence of competing stimuli. *J. Neurophysiol.* 70: 909–919.

Motter, B. C. (1994a) Neural correlates of attentive selection for color or luminance in extrastriate area V4. *J. Neurosci.* 14: 2178–2189.

Motter, B. C. (1994b) Neural correlates of feature selective memory and pop-out in extrastriate area V4. *J. Neurosci.* 14: 2190–2199.

Mountcastle, V. B., Andersen, R. A., and Motter, B. C. (1981) The influence of attentive fixation upon the excitability of the light-sensitive neurons of the posterior parietal cortex. *J. Neurosci.* 1: 1218–1235.

Mountcastle, V. B., Lynch, J. C., Georgopoulous, A., Sakata, H., and Acuna, C. (1975) Posterior parietal association cortex of the monkey: Command functions for operations within extrapersonal space. *J. Neurophysiol.* 38: 871–908.

Mountcastle, V. B., Motter, B. C., Steinmetz, M. A., and Duffy, C. J. (1984) Looking and seeing: Visual functions of the parietal lobe. In *Dynamic Aspects of Neocortical Function*, edited by G. M. Edelman, W. E. Gall, and W. M. Cowan, New York: Wiley.

Mountcastle, V. B., Motter, B. C., Steinmetz, M. A., and Sestokas, A. K. (1987) Common and differential effects of attentive fixation on the excitability of parietal and prestriate (V4) cortical visual neurons in the macaque monkey. *J. Neurosci.* 7: 2239–2255.

Olshausen, B., Anderson, C., and Van Essen, D. C. (1993) A neurobiological model of visual attention and invariant pattern recognition based on dynamic routing of information. *J. Neurosci.* 13: 4700–4719.

Perkel, D. H., Gerstein, G., and Moore, G. (1967) Neuronal spike trains and stochastic point processes. *Biophys. J.* 7: 391–418.

Posner, M. I. (1980) Orienting of attention. *Q. J. Exp. Psychol.* 32: 3–25.

Press, W. A., Knierim, J. J., and Van Essen, D. C. (1994) Neuronal correlates of attention to texture patterns in macaque striate cortex. *Soc. Neurosci. Abstr.* 20: 838.

Reynolds, J., Chelazzi, L., Luck, S., and Desimone, R. (1994) Sensory interactions and effects of selective spatial attention in macaque area V2. *Soc. Neurosci. Abstr.* 20: 1054.

Richmond, B. J. and Sato, T. (1987) Enhancement of inferior temporal neuronal response during visual discrimination. *J. Neurophysiol.* 58: 1292–1306.

Richmond, B. J., Wurtz, R. H., and Sato, T. (1983) Visual responses of inferior temporal neurons in awake rhesus monkeys. *J. Neurophysiol.* 50: 1415–1432.

Rolls, E. T., Judge, S. J., and Sanghera, M. K. (1977) Activity of neurons in the inferotemporal cortex of the alert monkey. *Brain Res.* 130: 229–238.

Sagi, D. and Julesz, B. (1985) Detection versus discrimination of visual orientation. *Perception* 14: 619–628.

Shadlen, M. N. and Newsome, W. T. (1994) Noise, neural codes and cortical organization. *Curr. Opin. Neurobiol.* 4: 5569–5579.

Softky, W. R. and Koch, C. (1993) The highly irregular firing of cortical cells is inconsistent with temporal integration of random EPSPs. *J. Neurosci.* 13: 334–350.

Somers, D. C., Nelson, S. B., and Sur, M. (1995) An emergent model of orientation selectivity in cat visual cortical simple cells. *J. Neurosci.* 15: 5448–5465.

Spitzer, H. and Richmond, B. J. (1991) Task difficulty: Ignoring, attending to, and discriminating a visual stimulus yield progressively more activity in inferior temporal neurons. *Exp. Brain. Res.* 83: 340–348.

Steinmetz, M. E., Connor, C. E., Constantinidis, C., and McLaughlin, J. R. (1994) Covert attention suppresses neuronal responses in area 7a of the posterior parietal cortex. *J. Neurophysiol.* 72: 1020–1023.

Treisman, A. and Gelade, G. (1980) A feature integration theory of attention. *Cognit. Psychol.* 12: 97–136.

Tsotsos, J. K., Culhane, S. M., Wai, W. Y. K., Lai, Y., Davis, N., and Nuflo, F. (1995) Modeling visual attention via selective tuning. *Artif. Intell.* 78: 507–545.

Vogels, R. and Orban, G. A. (1990) How well do response changes of striate neurons signal differences in orientation: A study in the discriminating monkey. *J. Neurosci.* 10: 3543–3558.

Wilson, M. A. and McNaughton, B. L. (1993) Dynamics of the hippocampal code for space. *Science* 261: 1055–1058.

Wolfe, J. M., Cave, K. R., and Franzel, S. L. (1989) Guided search: An alternative to the feature integration model for visual search. *J. Exp. Psychol. Hum. Percept. Perform.* 15: 419–433.

Wurtz, R. H. and Mohler, C. W. (1976a) Enhancement of visual responses in monkey striate cortex and frontal eye fields. *J. Neurophysiol.* 39: 766–772.

Wurtz, R. H. and Mohler, C. W. (1976b) Organization of monkey superior colliculus: Enhanced visual response of superficial layer cells. *J. Neurophysiol.* 39: 745–765.

Yantis, S. and Jonides, J. (1984) Abrupt visual onsets and selective attention: Evidence from visual search. *J. Exp. Psychol. Hum. Percept. Perform.* 10: 601–621.

Yin, T. C. T. and Mountcastle, V. B. (1977) Visual input to the visuomotor mechanisms of the monkey's parietal lobe. *Science* 197: 1381–1383.

5 Electrophysiological Approaches to the Study of Selective Attention in the Human Brain

Steven J. Luck and Massimo Girelli

ABSTRACT   Event-related potentials (ERPs) are electrophysiological responses that arise during sensory, cognitive, and motor processing and can be recorded noninvasively from normal human subjects. These potentials provide more precise information about the time course of information processing than is currently available from other noninvasive techniques and also yield coarse information about the neural substrates of cognitive processes. Because of these properties, the ERP technique has been used for more than 20 years in the study of selective attention. This chapter outlines the application of the ERP technique to the domain of attention research, including a description of the neural events that underlie the generation of ERPs and a discussion of some of the specific issues that have been addressed with ERP recordings.

There are now several techniques for studying the neural substrates of attention both in humans and in nonhuman primates. Other chapters in this volume describe some of these methods, including single-unit recordings in animals and human brain-imaging techniques such as positron emission tomography (PET) and magnetic resonance imaging (MRI). Each of these techniques has advantages and disadvantages, and so each tends to complement the others. This chapter describes the event-related potential (ERP) technique, which has certain unique advantages in the study of attentional processes in humans.

The principles underlying ERP recordings, the relationship between ERPs and other cognitive neuroscience techniques, and some of the contributions of ERP studies to attentional theory are examined. In particular, two issues that have been successfully addressed with the ERP technique are analyzed in some detail: (1) the stage of processing at which attention begins to select some inputs and suppress others (the locus-of-selection issue); and (2) the question of whether the same attentional mechanisms are used across different experimental paradigms (e.g., spatial cueing and visual search) and across different target stimuli (e.g., targets defined by color versus motion).

THE EVENT-RELATED POTENTIAL TECHNIQUE

When an electrode is placed on the scalp and the resulting signals are amplified and displayed on an oscilloscope, it is possible to observe voltage fluctuations that change according to factors such as arousal and activity

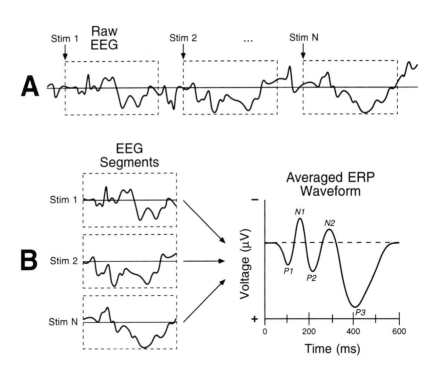

Figure 5.1 Example of the ERP averaging process. When stimuli are presented, it is very difficult to observe any clear response in (A) the raw EEG. However, if many stimuli are presented, it is possible to (B) extract the EEG segment following each stimulus, align those segments with respect to stimulus onset, and average them together. In most experiments, different stimulus types are randomly intermixed, and separate averages can be constructed for each stimulus type. Note that positive voltages are plotted downwards and that time zero represents the onset of the time-locking stimulus.

level. These fluctuations are commonly known as the electroencephalogram (EEG) and are widely used as markers for various global brain states. The EEG reflects the sum of a large number of simultaneously active neural systems; as a result, the specific neural activity underlying a particular cognitive process makes only a small contribution to the overall EEG. It is therefore difficult to measure specific neural processes in raw EEG data. However, specific neural processes that are tied to some particular event, such as the onset of a stimulus or a movement, can be extracted from the overall EEG by a simple averaging process, as is shown in figure 5.1. Typically, a stimulus is used to provide a time-locking point, and the EEG segments from multiple trials are first aligned with the onset of the stimulus and then are averaged. Any activity that is consistently time-locked to the stimulus will be present in every EEG segment and will therefore remain in the average, whereas any activity that is unrelated to the stimulus will become progressively attenuated as more trials are averaged. It should be noted that any measurable event can be used as the time-locking point, and ERP averages can therefore be synchronized with events such as button presses or the onset of electromyographic activity.

The resulting averaged ERP waveform consists of a set of positive and negative voltage deflections, which are referred to as peaks, waves, or components. Each peak is given a label, usually a *P* or *N* to indicate whether the peak is positive-going or negative-going, followed by a number to indicate the temporal position of the peak within the waveform. The number is sometimes given as a precise latency (e.g., P105 for a positive peak at 105 ms post stimulus) and is sometimes given as a single digit to indicate the ordinal position of the peak within the waveform (e.g., N2 for the second major negative peak). Because peak latencies may vary dramatically as a function of the stimuli and task, the use of exact latencies in component labels can be misleading; the P300 component, for example, may peak as late as 1000 ms under some conditions. We will therefore use ordinal positions to name ERP components in this chapter (see figure 5.1). It should also be noted that, following convention, ERP waveforms are plotted with negative voltages upward and positive voltages downward.

The sequence of ERP peaks that follows a stimulus is usually thought to reflect the sequence of neural and cognitive processes that is triggered by the onset of the stimulus. The amplitude and latency of each peak can therefore be used as a measure of the magnitude and timing of a given process. In addition, if multiple electrodes are used to measure activity at many scalp sites, the distribution of voltage over the scalp can be used as an index of the neuroanatomical loci of those neural and cognitive processes. Because of these attributes ERPs can be used to assess the effects of attention on sensory and cognitive processing, providing a precise index of the timing of attentional processes and a somewhat less precise index of the neural structures in which attentional processes operate. Before considering the use of ERPs in attention research, however, the cellular and biophysical events that give rise to ERPs are briefly examined, and the possibility of localizing the neural structures that generate a particular ERP component is considered.

ERP Generation and Localization

In contrast to single- and multiple-unit recordings of neuronal activity, which measure action potentials (see Motter, chapter 4, this volume), ERPs typically arise as a result of the postsynaptic potentials that are created when neurotransmitters bind with receptors on postsynaptic neurons (figure 5.2). Specifically, when an excitatory neurotransmitter binds with receptors on the apical dendrite of a pyramidal cell, positive ions enter into the neuron, creating a net negativity outside the cell in the region of the activated synapses. To maintain a complete circuit, the inward current is balanced by a passive outflow of current in the remainder of the cell, causing a net positivity in the region of the cell body and basal dendrites (figure 5.2A). Together, the positive and negative voltages create a small current dipole. If many similarly oriented cells are activated in this manner (an event that occurs primarily with cortical pyramidal cells), their dipoles will summate, and the summed

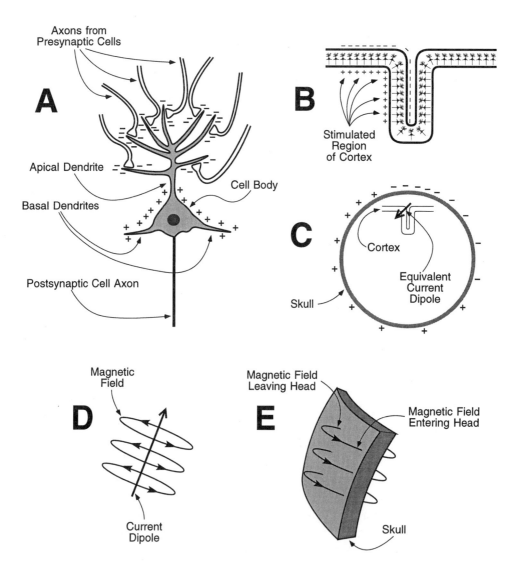

Figure 5.2 (A) Schematic pyramidal cell during neurotransmission. An excitatory neurotransmitter is released from the presynaptic terminals, causing positive ions to flow into the postsynaptic neuron. That activity creates a net negative extracellular voltage (−) in the area of the activated synapses and a net positive extracellular voltage (+) in other parts of the neuron, yielding a small dipole. (B) Folded sheet of cortex containing many pyramidal cells. When a region of the sheet is stimulated, the dipoles from the individual neurons summate. (C) The summated dipoles from the individual neurons can be approximated by a single equivalent current dipole, shown here as an arrow. The position and orientation of the dipole determine the distribution of positive and negative voltages recorded at the surface of the head. (D) Example of a current dipole with a magnetic field traveling around it. (E) Example of the magnetic field generated by a dipole that lies just inside the surface of the skull. If the dipole is roughly parallel to the surface, then the magnetic field can be recorded as it exits and enters the head; no field can be recorded if the dipole is oriented radially.

dipoles can be represented as a single, equivalent current dipole (figures 5.2B and 5.2C). This large dipole will then cause a passive volume conduction of voltage through the conductive medium of the brain. The meninges and skull have fairly high electrical resistance, which attenuates the voltage and causes it to spread widely, but some voltage can be recorded at the scalp. The recorded voltage will vary in amplitude over the scalp, with a distribution that depends on the position and orientation of the current dipole, which in turn depends on the position and orientation of the active neural tissue with respect to the surface of the skull (figure 5.2C). This simplified description of a complex set of biophysical events may be supplemented by the more complete accounts of Nunez (1981), Vaughan and Arezzo (1988), and Goff, Allison, and Vaughan (1978).

Although the scalp distribution of an ERP component is determined in a relatively straightforward manner by the position and orientation of the neural generator source, there are three factors that make it difficult or even impossible to localize a source based solely on scalp distribution information. The first difficulty arises from the fact that multiple brain areas usually contribute to the ERP waveform at any given time. It is relatively simple to solve the "forward problem" of computing the distribution of voltage that would be created at the scalp by one or more known generator dipoles, and it is even relatively simple to solve the "inverse problem" of determining the location of a single unknown generator dipole based on the observed distribution of voltage over the scalp. However, there is no unique solution to the inverse problem for the general case, in which one wishes to determine the locations of an unknown and potentially large number of sources that are all active at the same time. ERP generators cannot, therefore, be localized solely on the basis of scalp distribution data in the general case. However, the difficulties posed by multiple generator locations can be mitigated by making certain assumptions that limit either the number of generators or their positions or both. For example, Dale and Sereno (1993) have developed a technique in which MRI scans are used to divide each subject's cortical surface into an array of small patches; one dipole is then assumed for each patch, with an orientation that is perpendicular to the surface of the patch. Given those constraints, which are quite reasonable, the inverse problem can be solved by estimating the magnitude of activity for each of the finite number of patches at each time point. Cast in this manner, the inverse problem can be solved in a relatively straightforward manner using standard linear algebra techniques, assuming that the number of degrees of freedom in the observed scalp distribution is greater than the number of cortical patches.

The issue of degrees of freedom leads to the second difficulty in ERP localization, which is the spreading of voltage that is caused by the high resistance of the skull. Because of the spread of voltage, the signals recorded at nearby electrodes are highly correlated, so that each electrode site does not constitute an independent measurement. As a result, one cannot obtain an additional degree of freedom by adding a single electrode site, and even with an infinite number of electrodes the total possible number of degrees of freedom is too small to permit a unique solution of the inverse problem without additional constraints. This second difficulty does not make ERP localization impossible, but a reliable solution usually requires converging evidence from other techniques.

The problem of voltage spreading can be mitigated to a large extent by recording magnetic rather than electrical responses, because the skull is largely transparent to magnetic fields. Whenever an electrical dipole exists, a magnetic field is created that travels around the dipole in the perpendicular plane, as shown in figure 5.2D. As a result, when an ERP-generating dipole lies parallel to the surface of the skull, a magnetic field will flow out of and then back into the head, as shown in figure 5.2E. By placing an array of high-sensitivity magnetic sensors around the head, it is possible to measure these magnetic fields just as one can measure the EEG with an array of electrodes (Nunez, 1981; Williamson and Kaufman, 1987; Williamson, Lu, Karron, and Kaufman, 1991). In parallel with the nomenclature for electrical recordings, the overall magnetic signal is called the magnetoencephalogram (MEG) and the magnetic responses elicited by specific events are called event-related fields (ERFs). It is possible to estimate the location of an ERF generator by assessing the distribution of the magnetic field over the array of sensors, just as with ERPs, but two factors make this localization process more robust. First, as mentioned previously, the skull is essentially transparent to magnetic fields and does not cause them to spread laterally like the electrical potentials; as a result, more degrees of freedom are possible with ERF recordings than with ERP recordings. Second, a strong ERF signal can be recorded only for dipoles that are relatively near the surface of the brain and that are oriented roughly parallel to the surface of the skull. Although this limits the number of brain areas that can be measured with the ERF technique, it provides an important advantage for the localization process because it reduces the number of simultaneously recorded dipoles. Thus, ERFs provide a much better means of localization than do ERPs. It should be noted, however, that the ERF technique is orders of magnitude more expensive than the ERP technique because of the need for superconducting magnetic sensors and a magnetically shielded recording chamber.

There is a third factor that limits the effectiveness of both ERP and ERF localization techniques, namely noise. Of course, other imaging techniques such as PET and functional MRI (fMRI) are also influenced by noise, but the effects of noise are more problematic in ERP and ERF recordings, in which the relationship between the amount of noise and the size of the localization errors is often extremely complex. The complexity of the effects of noise occurs because very different sets of hypothetical generator locations can often lead to very similar voltage distributions at the surface; the noise level must be small relative to the difference in the voltage distributions in order for one to distinguish between the different hypothetical generator configurations. For example, a component that is broadly distributed across the scalp could arise from the activation of a large area of cortex near the surface or from a small area of cortex relatively deep in the brain; distinguishing between those alternatives can be an extremely difficult computational problem (see Dale and Sereno, 1993). Unfortunately, the signal-to-noise ratio in ERP averages is a function of the square root of the number of trials; doubling the signal-to-noise ratio, therefore, requires a fourfold increase in the number of trials. Reducing noise levels beyond a certain point is therefore difficult, because one can quadruple the number of trials only so many times without creating an unreasonably long experiment.

Given these difficulties, one might doubt that ERPs could ever be localized with a reasonable degree of accuracy. Such a conclusion would be unwarranted, however, because the difficulties just described apply primarily to the general case of ERP localization (i.e., attempts to determine the set of generator locations solely by examining the observed distribution of voltage over the scalp). As discussed previously, these difficulties can be mitigated to some extent by combining ERP recordings with structural MRI information and with ERF recordings. In addition, localization is much less problematic when the number of simultaneously active generators is small (see, e.g., Jewett and Zhang, 1995). This can be achieved by applying localization techniques to difference waveforms, in which the ERP waveforms recorded under one set of experimental conditions are subtracted from the ERP waveforms recorded under a slightly different set of conditions. When appropriate conditions are used, most of the generators will be equally active in both conditions and the difference waveform will therefore consist primarily of activity from the small set of generators that were differently active in the two conditions. It is also possible to use the known anatomy and physiology of the brain to generate specific hypotheses about the generator of a given component, which can then be tested by means of experimental manipulations rather than (or in addition to) mathematical analyses. For example, the upper and lower visual fields are represented in primary visual cortex by cortical patches that are at nearby locations but that differ in orientation by 180 degrees; several studies have examined the hypothesis that the C1 component is generated in primary visual cortex by testing whether the polarity of that component is inverted for stimuli in the upper visual field versus the lower visual field (Clark, Fan, and Hillyard, 1995; Jeffreys and Axford, 1972; Mangun, Hillyard, and Luck, 1993). This approach largely avoids the mathematical difficulties involved in ERP localization and can lead to a high degree of certainty.

Comparison with Other Techniques

Like any other widely used technique ERPs have certain unique advantages, especially in the context of attention research. Compared to behavioral measurements, for example, ERPs have the advantage of providing a continuous measure of processing between the stimulus and the response, allowing precise measurement of the time course of attentional processes. In addition, ERPs provide a means of covertly measuring information processing without requiring overt responses, which is particularly useful for assessing the processing of ignored stimuli. Compared to techniques such as PET and fMRI, which typically measure relatively slow changes in blood flow, ERPs have the advantage of millisecond temporal resolution. Although that advantage of the ERP technique has been widely discussed, there is a less well appreciated side effect of the temporal resolution, namely the ability to compare the processing of different stimuli presented within a single trial block. With PET, each image represents the average activity over a relatively long period of time (typically 40 s or longer), which makes it difficult to compare responses elicited by different stimulus classes such as attended and ignored stimuli. Functional MRI studies appear to be able to overcome this limitation, however, and may allow comparisons between stimuli presented at rates of up to one stimulus every two seconds. It should be noted that the poor temporal resolution of the PET and fMRI techniques is not due to intrinsically slow scanning, but instead reflects the fact that changes in blood flow develop over periods of several seconds. As a result, the PET and fMRI techniques will never attain high temporal resolution so long as they are used to measure relatively slow processes such as changes in blood flow.

In contrast to PET and fMRI, single-unit recordings, which are typically obtained from behaving animals, provide high temporal resolution in combination with high spatial resolution. However, the ERP technique maintains one obvious advantage over the single-unit recording technique; namely, ERPs can be recorded noninvasively from normal human subjects, which is an important factor in studies of cognitive processes such as attention. In addition, ERP recordings allow simultaneous measurement of many brain areas and neural processes, whereas single-unit recordings are typically restricted to one brain area at a given time.

Of course, the ERP technique has some disadvantages as well, two of which are particularly noteworthy. First, as discussed previously, it is difficult to determine the neural generator source of an ERP component, which is clearly an important limitation for a so-called brain-imaging technique. Second, most ERP components are quite small, and a very large number of trials must be averaged together in most experiments in order to obtain an adequate signal-to-noise ratio. The small component size makes the ERP technique inappropriate for some experimental paradigms, especially those for which single trials must be examined. With regard to practical signal-to-noise limitations, ERP recordings are certainly no worse than PET scans, but the signal-to-noise ratio of single-unit recordings and most behavioral measures is substantially better. Initial studies also suggest that the fMRI technique has a superior signal-to-noise ratio, but more research is necessary to make that determination with certainty.

ERPs and Eye Movements

Many studies of visuospatial attention are concerned with covert shifts of attention rather than with overt shifts in eye position, but the possible contribution of eye movements can be a vexing problem, no matter which behavioral or physiological technique is used. For example, faster and more accurate target detection at a cued than at an uncued location is not surprising when subjects fixate the cued location; similarly, it would not be surprising to find that a neurophysiological measure of processing differed as a function of the position of the eliciting stimulus on the retina. Most ERP studies of visuospatial attention, therefore, either use stimulus durations that are too short to permit saccadic eye movements (which is the usual strategy in behavioral experiments) or else record eye position and exclude trials during which there were eye movements from the averaged ERP waveforms (which is the more common strategy in electrophysiological recordings). In this respect, ERP research is no different from any other method used in studies of visual attention. However, eye movements cause an additional problem in ERP recordings that must be considered. Specifically, the eye movements can themselves generate ERPs that may overlap and confound the ERP waveforms that the experimenter intends to record.

Eye movements can generate spurious ERPs in two ways. First, the eyes contain fairly strong current dipoles that change in orientation when the eyes rotate, and those orientation changes result in potentials that can be recorded across the entire scalp. Fortunately, computational procedures are available to estimate and remove those potentials (Berg and Scherg, 1994; Gratton, Coles, and Donchin, 1983). However, there is a second and less widely appreciated consequence of eye movements. Specifically, as the eyes move across space any stimuli that strike the eyes (including the edges of the video monitor) will move across the retina, creating a great deal of motion-related neural activity even though such motion signals are suppressed before they reach awareness. The resulting ERPs are difficult to eliminate computationally, and it is therefore usually necessary to ensure that subjects maintain fixation during the recording period. This is not always possible, and in such cases one must be extremely careful that any ERP effects observed are not confounded by eye movement–related potentials. It should be noted, however, that eye movements produce analogous effects in other types of physiological recordings as well, and caution should therefore be used in interpreting any physiological data in which eye movements were not controlled.

THE LOCUS OF ATTENTIONAL SELECTION

Although almost all researchers agree that attention serves to select some sources of information and reject others, there has been a long-standing debate concerning the fundamental nature of the selection process. Many researchers assume that the perceptual processing capacity of the human brain is finite and argue that attention operates at an early stage to direct perceptual processing resources toward relevant stimuli so that they can be perceived faster and more accurately (e.g., Hawkins et al., 1990; Reinitz, 1990; Treisman and Gelade, 1980). Other researchers propose that the major limitations in processing capacity arise in postperceptual processes and argue that attention operates at a late stage to avoid overloading memory or response output systems (e.g., Duncan, 1980; Palmer, Ames, and Lindsey, 1993). This locus-of-selection issue has been very difficult to resolve on the basis of behavioral experiments, largely because behavioral responses reflect the sum of both early and late processes and do not provide a direct means of observing the sequence of processes interposed between a stimulus and a response. The ERP technique, in contrast, provides a relatively direct means of assessing the time course of information processing, and has been used for more than 20 years to address the locus-of-selection issue. This section summarizes some of the most recent locus-of-selection studies, which provide extremely clear evidence for the proposal that attention operates at an early stage, at least under certain conditions. Before discussing that evidence, however, it is necessary to clarify a few aspects of the early- versus late-selection debate.

There is little doubt that attention can operate at a late stage, after perceptual processing has been completed. For example, imagine an experiment in which letters are presented individually at the point of fixation for a duration of 1 s each, with some letters presented in red and some in blue. If an observer is asked to name the red letters and ignore the blue letters, he or she should have no difficulty selecting and naming only the red letters, even though both the red and blue letters would almost certainly be identified. This would be an example of selectivity at the very late stage of response selection, and there is little doubt that attention operates in this manner under some conditions. The real issue is whether attention might also— under some circumstances—operate at an early stage. Thus, the locus-of-selection issue cannot be resolved by providing cases in which selective processing occurs after perceptual processes are complete; rather, the burden of proof rests on proponents of early selection, who must demonstrate the existence of cases in which perceptual processes are degraded for ignored stimuli or enhanced for attended stimuli.

Early Selection in the Auditory Modality

Most of the early psychological and ERP studies of the locus of selection examined the auditory modality and used variants of the dichotic listening paradigm, in which different messages are presented in each ear and subjects are asked to attend to one ear and ignore the other. Behavioral experiments have shown that subjects are poor at reporting messages presented in the ignored ear, but it has been difficult to determine whether this is caused by early gating of sensory information from the ignored ear or by a late-stage selection process that prevents ignored information from being encoded into memory (for example, see Wood and Cowan, 1995a, 1995b). To distinguish between those alternatives, Hillyard and his colleagues conducted a number of studies in which they compared the ERPs elicited by stimuli presented in the attended and ignored ears (e.g., Hansen and Hillyard, 1980; Hillyard, Hink, Schwent, and Picton, 1973; Woldorff and Hillyard, 1991). They assumed that if attention operates at an early stage, then the early sensory ERP components should be enhanced for attended stimuli compared to ignored stimuli; if attention operates at a late stage, however, then the initial sensory responses should be identical and only the later ERP components should be affected by attention. In many studies, these researchers have obtained strong evidence for the proposal that attention influences the early sensory components, consistent with an early locus of selection. Specifically, the N1 component, which typically begins earlier than 100 ms post stimulus, is larger for attended than for ignored stimuli. In addition, under conditions of high perceptual load, attention begins to influence processing at an even earlier stage, beginning only 20 ms after stimulus onset (Woldorff, Hansen, and Hillyard, 1987; Woldorff and Hillyard, 1991)

The timing of those effects clearly indicates that attention operates at an early stage of processing. To determine the neuroanatomical source of the effects and thereby to provide additional evidence for early selection, Woldorff et al. (1993) recorded magnetic responses as well as ERPs during a dichotic listening paradigm. They found that the magnetic analog of the electrical N1 component (called the M1 wave) is modulated by attention just as the electrical N1 component is, and they localized the effect to the supra-temporal plane, which is the location of primary auditory cortex. Their results are shown in figure 5.3, which shows the ERP and ERF waveforms from their experiment, averaged over a group of seven subjects; figure 5.3 also shows the estimated location of the M1 wave for a single subject, super-imposed on top of that subject's MRI scan. The results of Woldorff et al. provide further evidence that attention begins to influence processing at an early stage, both temporally and neuroanatomically.

Early Selection in the Visual Modality

The locus-of-selection issue has also been addressed in the visual modality with the ERP technique, and many of those experiments have used a visual version of the paradigm developed by Hillyard and his colleagues for studying auditory attention. In the visual paradigm, which is illustrated in figure 5.4A, subjects fixate a central point and direct attention either to the left visual field (LVF) or to the right visual field (RVF). Streams of bars are then flashed at predefined locations in the LVF and RVF and subjects are required to press a button whenever a slightly smaller than normal bar is presented in

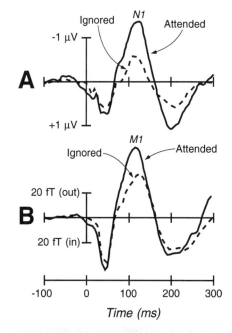

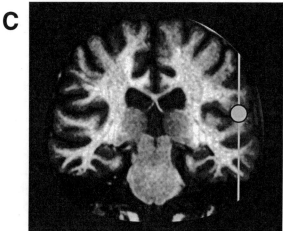

Figure 5.3 Data from the magnetoencephalographic study of Woldorff et al. (1993). (A) The electrical N1 component; (B) the magnetic counterpart, the M1; (C) the estimated generator site of the M1 for a single subject. The estimated generator site is shown as a circle centered in the cortex of the left supratemporal plane in the subject's MRI scan (the scan is oriented as if the subject were facing out from the page).

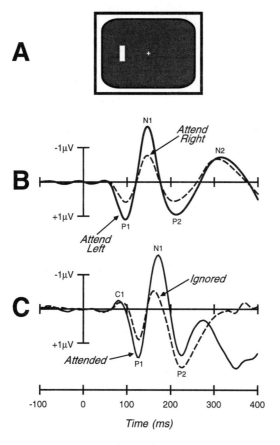

Figure 5.4 (A) Stimulus configuration commonly used in ERP studies of visual attention. White bars are flashed in random order to the left and right visual fields, and subjects attend to one location and ignore the other. (B) Idealized ERP waveforms that would be elicited by a stimulus in the left visual field. The P1 and N1 components are larger for this stimulus when it is attended than when attention is directed to the right visual field (the complementary pattern is observed for stimuli presented in the right visual field). (C) ERP waveforms from a study by Gomez Gonzales et al. (1994). In that experiment, the C1 component could be observed prior to the P1 and N1 components, but the C1 component was not affected by whether the stimulus was presented at the attended location or at the ignored location.

the attended visual field. Because these experiments are intended to examine the effects of covert shifts of attention rather than overt shifts in eye position, subjects are required to fixate a central point at all times, and trials contaminated by eye movements are rejected during the calculation of the averaged ERP waveforms.

Many experiments of this type have been conducted in the Hillyard laboratory (e.g., Mangun and Hillyard, 1988, 1990; Mangun et al., 1993; Van Voorhis and Hillyard, 1977) and also in other laboratories (e.g., Eason, Harter, and White, 1969; Neville and Lawson, 1987; Rugg, Milner, Lines, and Phalp, 1987). As shown in figure 5.4B, the initial P1 and N1 components are typically larger for stimuli presented at the attended location than at the ignored location, and the effects typically begin between 60 and 100 ms post-stimulus. Such effects provide clear evidence for an early locus of selection.

Although the P1 and N1 waves are the first ERP components that can usually be recorded following a visual stimulus, they do not appear to arise from the initial cortical visual area, which is called striate cortex. Instead, those components appear to arise from somewhat higher-level extrastriate areas of visual cortex, and the finding that attention modulates the amplitude of those components does not indicate whether or not attention also operates in striate cortex. Under certain conditions, however, it is possible to record an ERP component that precedes the P1 and N1 waves and is generated in striate cortex. The effects of attention on that striate cortex component, which is called the C1 wave, have been examined in three recent studies (Clark and Hillyard, 1996; Gomez Gonzales, Clark, Fan, Luck, and Hillyard, 1994; Mangun et al., 1993). As shown in figure 5.4C, the amplitude of the C1 component is the same for attended and ignored stimuli, whereas the P1 and N1 components are substantially larger for attended stimuli than for ignored stimuli. Such results indicate that attention does not influence visual processing until after striate cortex, a result that has been confirmed by single-unit experiments (Luck, Chelazzi, Hillyard, and Desimone, 1997; Moran and Desimone, 1985). These results contrast with the auditory experiments described in the previous section, in which the initial attention effects appear to arise in primary auditory cortex.

Although several investigators have recorded the magnetic responses elicited by visual stimuli, it has been much more difficult to localize ERP and ERF components in the visual modality than in the auditory modality, probably because a large number of visual areas are concurrently activated during visual processing. However, a recent study has provided a preliminary localization of the P1 attention effect by means of combined PET and ERP recordings (Heinze et al., 1994). Using a paradigm similar to that shown in figure 5.4A, Heinze and his collaborators found that blood flow was modulated by attention in a manner similar to P1 amplitude in a region of cortex on the ventral surface of the occipital lobe. In addition, modeling procedures indicated that a dipole located in the region of the PET attention effect could adequately account for the scalp distribution of the P1 attention effect. Thus, this study suggests that the P1 attention effect, which typically begins within 100 ms of stimulus onset, is generated in the visual cortical areas of the inferior occipital lobe, a result that provides additional evidence for an early locus of selection. It should be noted, however, that the PET and ERP techniques measure very different physiological processes, and it is very difficult to determine whether a PET effect and an ERP effect reflect the same underlying neural processes (for additional discussion, see Luck et al., 1997).

COMMON ATTENTIONAL MECHANISMS ACROSS EXPERIMENTAL PARADIGMS

During the past 20 years a large proportion of behavioral studies of visual attention have used two main paradigms, namely spatial cueing and visual search. In the spatial cueing paradigm a cue stimulus is presented at the beginning of each trial and is followed by a target stimulus that is presented either at the cued location (called a valid trial) or at an uncued location (called an invalid trial). In most experiments the target is more likely to appear at the cued location than at the uncued location, which is intended to motivate subjects to attend to the cued location in anticipation of the target's occurrence there. If attention is directed toward the cued location, then target detection and discrimination might be expected to be better on valid trials than on invalid trials, which is exactly the pattern that is observed in the majority of studies (Cheal, Lyon, and Gottlob, 1994; Jonides, 1981; Luck et al., 1994; Posner, 1980).

Attention has also frequently been studied with visual search tasks, which provide a less artificial means of assessing attention. In this paradigm the stimuli are arrays containing multiple objects, and the subjects are typically required to press one button if a predefined target object is present in the array and to press a different button if the target is absent. If attention must be focused on each individual item to determine whether or not it is the target, then the amount of time required to find the target should increase as the number of objects in the array increases. That pattern is observed under some conditions and not under others (Duncan and Humphreys, 1989; Treisman, 1985; Wolfe, Cave, and Franzel, 1989); such results have led to the proposal that certain types of stimuli can be detected without the serial application of attention, whereas other types of stimuli require focused attention in order to be detected (Braun and Sagi, 1990; Treisman and Gelade, 1980).

Although spatial cueing and visual search tasks ostensibly measure the same attentional mechanisms, the paradigms are sufficiently different that it is possible that they reflect entirely different psychological processes. However, almost all theories of attention assume that the same mechanisms of attention are manipulated by both tasks, and a great deal of theory revision would be necessary if this assumption were found to be incorrect. A few behavioral experiments have addressed that possibility and have generally concluded that the same attentional mechanisms are used in both paradigms (Briand and Klein, 1987; Prinzmetal, Presti, and Posner, 1986; Treisman, 1985), but the evidence has been relatively indirect. ERPs may provide a more direct means of addressing the issue, by indicating whether or not the same neural systems are modulated across the two paradigms. For example, finding that the P1 and N1 components are larger for stimuli presented at attended than at ignored locations in both paradigms would be fairly direct evidence that the same attentional mechanisms are involved

The first step in using ERPs to determine whether the same attentional mechanisms are used in both paradigms was to measure the effects of attention in the spatial cueing paradigm, which was accomplished by Mangun and Hillyard (1991) in an experiment illustrated in figure 5.5A. On each trial, an arrow appeared at fixation and indicated whether a subsequent target bar was likely to appear in the LVF or the RVF. When the target appeared, subjects made a speeded response, indicating whether the target was a tall bar or a short bar. As shown in figure 5.5B, reaction times were faster and the P1 and N1 components were larger on valid trials than on invalid trials, which indicates that sensory processing was facilitated at the cued location compared to the uncued location.

In the visual search task there are no explicit cues indicating that the subject should direct attention to a specific location; however, once the subject has located a potential target item, attention will typically be focused onto that item. Consequently, if subjects are given adequate time to locate the target, then stimuli subsequently presented at the location of the target item should be analogous to stimuli presented at a cued location, and stimuli presented at the location of a nontarget item should be analogous to stimuli presented at an uncued location. If the same mechanisms of attention are used in both the cueing and search paradigms, then the same P1 and N1 attention effects observed in the comparison of valid and invalid trials in the cueing paradigm should be found in a comparison of stimuli presented at target and nontarget locations during visual search. Luck, Fan, and Hillyard (1993) used this logic in a study of attentional mechanisms during visual search.

The task used by Luck et al. (1993) is illustrated in figure 5.5C. The stimulus arrays consisted of 1 red item, 1 green item, and 14 gray items; the items were randomly distributed across the display with the constraint that the red and green items were always in opposite hemifields. The arrays were presented for a duration of 700 ms, and trials in which there were eye movements were excluded from the ERP averages. At the beginning of each trial block subjects were told that one of the two colors would define the target stimulus for that block; for each array, they were required to indicate whether the item drawn in that color (i.e., the target) was an upright T or an inverted T. The design of the experiment had two main goals: (1) to allow subjects to locate the target item in a relatively short and consistent amount of time, which was possible because of the target's distinctive color; and (2) to ensure that attention was strongly focused onto the target item, which was achieved by requiring subjects to discriminate its form.

The ERP waveform elicited by a multiple-element stimulus array reflects the processing of the entire array, and it is not usually possible to measure the separate contribution of each individual stimulus to the overall ERP waveform. To measure sensory processing at specific locations, therefore, a probe technique was used. On each trial, a task-irrelevant probe square was presented either at the location of the target item or at the location of the

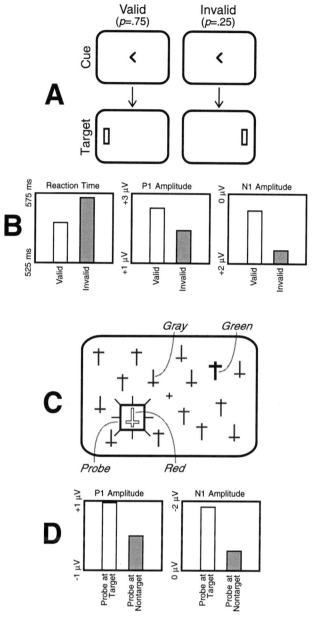

Figure 5.5 (A) Example of cue and target stimuli from the spatial cuing study of Mangun and Hillyard (1991). (B) Reaction times, P1 amplitudes, and N1 amplitudes for valid and invalid trials in that experiment. Note that the P1 and N1 amplitudes are displayed with larger bars representing greater amplitude (i.e., more positive for P1 and more negative for N1). (C) Stimulus configuration from the visual search study of Luck et al. (1993). The search array was presented for 700 ms, and the probe stimulus (the square) was flashed for 100 ms, beginning 250 ms after the onset of the search array. (D) P1 and N1 amplitudes from trials on which the probe was presented at the location of the target item, which are analogous to valid trials, and from trials on which the probe was presented at the location of a nontarget item, which are analogous to invalid trials.

colored nontarget item in the opposite hemifield, and the ERP elicited by this probe stimulus was used as a measure of sensory processing at the probed location. According to the logic outlined previously, the P1 and N1 components would be expected to be larger for probes presented at the location of a particular colored item when it was the target, and presumably attended, than when it was a nontarget, and presumably ignored. As is shown in figure 5.5D, this result was indeed obtained, indicating that the same attentional mechanisms are used in both the spatial cueing and visual search paradigms. It should be noted, however, that there were also some subtle differences between the results of this experiment and the P1 and N1 effects observed in cueing tasks, which indicates that there may be differences as well as similarities in the attentional mechanisms used in the two paradigms (see Luck et al., 1993).

Two attributes of the design are particularly noteworthy from a methodological perspective. First, it may seem strange that two colored items were used in each stimulus array instead of just one. However, this was necessary because it would be inappropriate to compare the ERP elicited by a probe presented at the location of a colored item with the ERP elicited by a probe presented at the location of one of the gray items. ERPs can be very sensitive to small differences in stimulus configurations such as this, and it is important to ensure that attentional manipulations are not confounded with stimulus differences. In this experiment, the ERP elicited by a probe presented at the location of a particular colored item could be measured when that item was the target and when the same item was a nontarget, ensuring that any ERP effects were due to attention rather than to physical stimulus differences. A second important attribute of the design is that the probe stimuli did not require a response and were completely irrelevant to the task. If subjects had been required to respond to the probe stimuli, it is likely that faster reaction times would have been observed for probes presented at the location of the target (such results have been obtained by Kim and Cave, 1995); however, such a response requirement may have changed the way in which the task was performed, making it difficult to be certain that the results reflect processes that are normally present during visual search. This is an example of the use of ERPs in the covert monitoring of information processing.

COMMON ATTENTIONAL MECHANISMS ACROSS STIMULUS TYPES

The majority of visual search studies have used target stimuli that are defined by attributes of color and form, features that are primarily processed by the so-called parvo pathway that passes through the parvocellular layers of the lateral geniculate nucleus (LGN) and feeds into relatively ventral areas of the occipital and temporal lobes. There is a parallel, magno pathway that remains somewhat segregated from the parvo pathway, passing through the magnocellular layers of the LGN and feeding primarily into relatively dorsal areas of the occipital and parietal lobes; the magno pathway appears to be specialized for processing features such as motion and depth (Livingstone and Hubel, 1987, 1988). Given the anatomical segregation of the two pathways and their different feature sensitivities, it seems plausible that different attentional mechanisms might be used for detecting visual search targets defined by different feature types, with one mechanism for the color and form features favored by the parvo pathway and another for the motion and depth features favored by the magno pathway. Indeed, when magno features have been used as visual search targets, the results have been somewhat different from those obtained with targets defined by parvo features (e.g., McLeod, Driver, and Crisp, 1988; Nakayama and Silverman, 1986). However, there is a substantial convergence between the two pathways in the extrastriate areas where attention appears to operate (Felleman and Van Essen, 1991; Maunsell, 1992), and so it is also possible that the same attentional mechanisms would be used independent of the features that define the target.

Just as the ERP technique can be used to assess whether the same attentional mechanisms are used across different tasks, it can also be used to determine whether the same mechanisms are used across different target types; a recent study used ERPs to determine whether the same mechanisms are involved in the detection of visual search targets defined by color, orientation, and motion (Girelli and Luck, 1997). Rather than using probe stimuli and looking for P1 and N1 attention effects, however, this study examined the ERPs elicited by the visual search arrays themselves, specifically an attention-related component called the N2pc wave. The N2pc wave is typically observed for visual search arrays containing targets, and is a negative deflection in the N2 latency range (200–300 ms post stimulus) that is primarily observed at posterior scalp sites contralateral to the position of the target item (N2pc is an abbreviation of N2-posterior-contralateral). Previous experiments have shown that the N2pc component reflects the focusing of attention onto a potential target item in order to suppress competing information from the surrounding distractor items (Luck and Hillyard, 1994a, 1994b). However, all of the experiments in which this component has been examined have used targets defined by parvo features such as color and orientation. If the same mechanisms of attention are used across different target types, then we would expect the N2pc component to be present for motion-defined targets as well as for color- and orientation-defined targets. As is shown in figure 5.6, that result was obtained. Thus, at least one neurophysiologically defined attentional mechanism is shared across parvo and magno targets in visual search.

CONCLUSIONS

The examples given in this chapter of the application of the ERP technique to issues in selective attention illustrate two main points. First, the main advantage of the ERP technique is its ability to provide a continuous measure

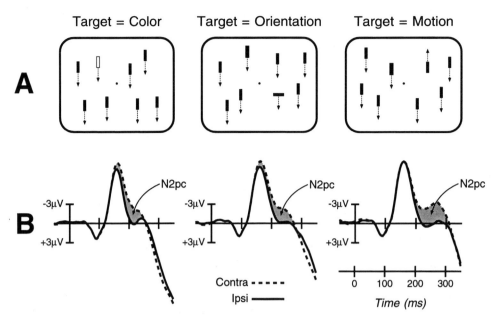

Figure 5.6 (A) Examples of the stimulus arrays that were used in the study of Girelli and Luck (1997). Each array consisted of eight bars. The bars were usually green, vertical, and downward moving, but some arrays contained a singleton item that differed in color, orientation, or direction of motion. Each of the three singleton types was the target in different trial blocks, and subjects were required to press one button when the target was present and another button when the target was absent. (B) ERP waveforms recorded at lateral occipital scalp sites for each of the three target types. The solid and broken lines reflect the responses recorded at electrode sites ipsilateral and contralateral to the position of the target, respectively. The shaded area is the difference between the ipsilateral and contralateral waveforms, and that difference defines the N2pc component.

of information processing, with different components corresponding to different neurocognitive processes. That attribute allows the time course of attention to be assessed and also makes it possible to determine whether the same processes are influenced by attention in different experimental situations. Second, although ERPs do not directly permit accurate localization of function, localization may be possible by combining ERP recordings with other sources of information. There have been relatively few studies of this nature, but multimethodological experiments are becoming increasingly common. It is important to note, however, that accurate localization is not always necessary in order to answer important theoretical questions, and the ERP technique will continue to provide a useful tool for studying attention even without improvements in its spatial resolution.

ACKNOWLEDGMENTS

Most of the research described in this chapter was conducted in the laboratory of Steve Hillyard, funded by grants and fellowships from the National Institutes of Health, the Office of Naval Research, the Human Frontier Science Program, the McDonnell-Pew Center for Cognitive Neuroscience at the University of California at San Diego, and the National Science Foundation. Preparation of this chapter was supported by a grant from the McDonnell-Pew Program in Cognitive Neuroscience. We would also like to acknowledge the important contributions of Jon Hansen, who developed most of the software used in these experiments.

REFERENCES

Berg, P. and Scherg, M. (1994) A multiple source approach to the correction of eye artifacts. *Electroencephalogr. Clin. Neurophysiol.* 90: 229–241.

Braun, J. and Sagi, D. (1990) Vision outside the focus of attention. *Percept. Psychophys.* 48: 45–58.

Briand, K. A. and Klein, R. M. (1987) Is Posner's "beam" the same as Treisman's "glue"?: On the relation between visual orienting and feature integration theory. *J. Exp. Psychol. Hum. Percept. Perform.* 13: 228–241.

Cheal, M. L., Lyon, D. R., and Gottlob, L. R. (1994) A framework for understanding the allocation of attention in location-precued discrimination. *Q. J. Exp. Psychol.* 47A: 699–739.

Clark, V. P., Fan, S., and Hillyard, S. A. (1995) Identification of early visually evoked potential generators by retinotopic and topographic analyses. *Hum. Brain Map* 2: 170–187.

Clark, V. P. and Hillyard, S. A. (1996) Spatial selective attention affects early extrastriate but not striate components of the visual evoked potential. *J. Cog. Neurosci.* 8: 387–402.

Dale, A. M. and Sereno, M. I. (1993) Improved localization of cortical activity by combining EEG and MEG with MRI cortical surface reconstruction: A linear approach. *J. Cog. Neurosci.* 5: 162–176.

Duncan, J. (1980) The locus of interference in the perception of simultaneous stimuli. *Psychol. Rev.* 87: 272–300.

Duncan, J. and Humphreys, G. (1989) Visual search and stimulus similarity. *Psychol. Rev.* 96: 433–458.

Eason, R., Harter, M., and White, C. (1969) Effects of attention and arousal on visually evoked cortical potentials and reaction time in man. *Physiol. Behav.* 4: 283–289.

Felleman, D. J. and Van Essen, D. C. (1991) Distributed hierarchical processing in the primate cerebral cortex. *Cereb. Cortex* 1: 1–47.

Girelli, M. and Luck, S. J. (1997) Are the same attentional mechanisms used to detect visual search targets defined by color, orientation, and motion? *J. Cog. Neurosci.* 9: 238–253.

Goff, W. R., Allison, T., and Vaughan, H. G., Jr. (1978) The functional neuroanatomy of event-related potentials. In *Event Related Brain Potentials in Man*, edited by P. Tueting, S. Koslow, and E. Callaway, pp. 1–92 New York: Academic Press.

Gomez Gonzales, C. M., Clark, V. P., Fan, S., Luck, S. J., and Hillyard, S. A. (1994) Sources of attention-sensitive visual event-related potentials. *Brain Topog.* 7: 41–51.

Gratton, G., Coles, M. G. H., and Donchin, E. (1983) A new method for off-line removal of ocular artifact. *Electroencephalogr. Clin. Neurophysiol.* 55: 468–484.

Hansen, J. C. and Hillyard, S. A. (1980) Endogenous brain potentials associated with selective auditory attention. *Electroencephalogr. Clin. Neurophysiol.* 49: 277–290.

Hawkins, H. L., Hillyard, S. A., Luck, S. J., Mouloua, M., Downing, C. J., and Woodward, D. P. (1990) Visual attention modulates signal detectability. *J. Exp. Psychol. Hum. Percept. Perform.* 16: 802–811.

Heinze, H. J., Mangun, G. R., Burchert, W., Hinrichs, H., Scholz, M., Münte, T. F., Gös, A., Scherg, M., Johannes, S., Hundeshagen, H., Gazzaniga, M. S., and Hillyard, S. A. (1994) Combined spatial and temporal imaging of brain activity during visual selective attention in humans. *Nature* 372: 543–546.

Hillyard, S. A., Hink, R. F., Schwent, V. L., and Picton, T. W. (1973) Electrical signs of selective attention in the human brain. *Science* 182: 177–179.

Jeffreys, D. A. and Axford, J. G. (1972) Source locations of pattern-specific components of human visual evoked potentials. I: Components of striate cortical origin. *Exp. Brain Res.* 16: 1–21.

Jewett, D. L. and Zhang, Z. (1995) Multiple-generator errors are unavoidable under model misspecification. *Electroencephalogr. Clin. Neurophysiol.* 95: 135–142.

Jonides, J. (1981) Voluntary versus automatic control over the mind's eye's movement. In *Attention and Performance IX*, edited by J. B. Long and A. D. Baddeley, pp. 187–203. Hillsdale, NJ: Lawrence Erlbaum.

Kim, M. S. and Cave, K. R. (1995) Spatial attention in visual search for features and feature conjunctions. *Psychol. Sci.* 6: 376–380.

Livingstone, M. S. and Hubel, D. H. (1987) Psychophysical evidence for separate channels for the perception of form, color, movement, and depth. *J. Neurosci.* 7: 3416–3468.

Livingstone, M. S. and Hubel, D. H. (1988) Segregation of form, color, movement, and depth: Anatomy, physiology, and perception. *Science* 240: 740–749.

Luck, S. J., Chelazzi, L., Hillyard, S. A., and Desimone, R. (1997) Neural mechanisms of spatial selective attention in areas V1, V2, and V4 of macaque visual cortex. *J. Neurophysiol.* 77: 24–42.

Luck, S. J., Fan, S., and Hillyard, S. A. (1993) Attention-related modulation of sensory-evoked brain activity in a visual search task. *J. Cog. Neurosci.* 5: 188–195.

Luck, S. J. and Hillyard, S. A. (1994a) Electrophysiological correlates of feature analysis during visual search. *Psychophysiology* 31: 291–308.

———. (1994b) Spatial filtering during visual search: Evidence from human electrophysiology. *J. Exp. Psychol. Hum. Percept. Perform.* 20: 1000–1014.

Luck, S. J., Hillyard, S. A., Mouloua, M., Woldorff, M. G., Clark, V. P., and Hawkins, H. L. (1994) Effects of spatial cuing on luminance detectability: Psychophysical and electrophysiological evidence for early selection. *J. Exp. Psychol. Hum. Percept. Perform.* 20: 887–904.

Mangun, G. R. and Hillyard, S. A. (1988) Spatial gradients of visual attention: Behavioral and electrophysiological evidence. *Electroencephalogr. Clin. Neurophysiol.* 70: 417–428.

Mangun, G. R., and Hillyard, S. A. (1990) Allocation of visual attention to spatial location: Event-related brain potentials and detection performance. *Percept. Psychophys.* 47: 532–550.

Mangun, G. R. and Hillyard, S. A. (1991) Modulations of sensory-evoked brain potentials indicate changes in perceptual processing during visual-spatial priming. *J. Exp. Psychol. Hum. Percept. Perform.* 17: 1057–1074.

Mangun, G. R., Hillyard, S. A., and Luck, S. J. (1993) Electrocortical substrates of visual selective attention. In *Attention and Performance XIV*, edited by D. Meyer and S. Kornblum, pp. 219–243. Cambridge, MA: MIT Press.

Maunsell, J. H. R. (1992) Functional visual streams. *Curr. Opin. Neurobiol.* 2: 506–510.

McLeod, P., Driver, J., and Crisp, J. (1988) Visual search for a conjunction of movement and form is parallel. *Nature* 332: 154–155.

Moran, J. and Desimone, R. (1985) Selective attention gates visual processing in the extrastriate cortex. *Science* 229: 782–784.

Nakayama, K. and Silverman, G. H. (1986) Serial and parallel processing of visual feature conjunctions. *Nature* 320: 264–265.

Neville, H. J. and Lawson, D. (1987) Attention to central and peripheral visual space in a movement detection task. I: Normal hearing adults. *Brain Res.* 405: 253–267.

Nunez, P. L. (1981) *Electric Fields of the Brain.* New York: Oxford University Press.

Palmer, J., Ames, C. T., and Lindsey, D. T. (1993) Measuring the effect of attention on simple visual search. *J. Exp. Psychol. Hum. Percept. Perform.* 19: 108–130.

Posner, M. I. (1980) Orienting of attention. *Q. J. Exp. Psychol.* 32: 3–25.

Prinzmetal, W., Presti, D. E., and Posner, M. I. (1986) Does attention affect visual feature integration? *J. Exp. Psychol. Hum. Percept. Perform* 12: 361–369.

Reinitz, M. T. (1990) Effects of spatially directed attention on visual encoding. *Percept. Psychophys.* 47: 497–505.

Rugg, M. D., Milner, A. D., Lines, C. R., and Phalp, R. (1987) Modulation of visual event-related potentials by spatial and non-spatial visual selective attention. *Neuropsychologia* 25: 85–96.

Treisman, A. M. (1985) Preattentive processing in vision. *Comp. Vis. Graphics Image Process.* 31: 156–177.

Treisman, A. M. and Gelade, G. (1980) A feature-integration theory of attention. *Cognit. Psychol.* 12: 97–136.

Van Voorhis, S. T. and Hillyard, S. A. (1997) Visual evoked potentials and selective attention to points in space. *Percept. Psychophys.* 22: 54–62.

Vaughan, H. G. and Arezzo, J. C. (1988) The neural basis of event-related potentials. In *Human Event-Related Potentials*, edited by T. W. Piction, pp. 45–96. Amsterdam: Elsevier.

Williamson, S. J. and Kaufman, L. (1987) Analysis of neuromagnetic signals. In *Methods of Analysis of Brain Electrical and Magnetic Signals*, edited by A. S. Gevins and A. Redmond, pp. 405–448. Amsterdam: Elsevier.

Williamson, S. J., Lu, Z. L., Karron, D., and Kaufman, L. (1991) Advantages and limitations of magnetic source imaging. *Brain Topogr.* 4: 169–180.

Woldorff, M. G., Hallen, C. C., Hampson, S. A., Hillyard, S. A., Pantev, C., Sobel, D., and Bloom, F. E. (1993) Modulation of early sensory processing in human auditory cortex during auditory selective attention. *Proc. Natl. Acad. Sci. USA* 90: 8722–8726.

Woldorff, M. G., Hansen, J. C., and Hillyard, S. A. (1987) Evidence for effects of selective attention to the midlatency range of the human auditory event related potential. In *Current Trends in Event-Related Brain Potential Research*, edited by R. Johnson, J. W. Rohrbaugh, and R. Parasuraman, pp. 146–154. London: Elsevier.

Woldorff, M. G. and Hillyard, S. A. (1991) Modulation of early auditory processing during selective listening to rapidly presented tones. *Electroencephalogr. Clin. Neurophysiol.* 79: 170–191.

Wolfe, J. M., Cave, K. R., and Franzel, S. L. (1989) Guided search: An alternative to the feature integration model for visual search. *J. Exp. Psychol. Hum. Percept. Perform.* 15: 419–433.

Wood, N. and Cowan, N. (1995a) The cocktail party phenomenon revisited: Attention and memory in the classic selective listening procedure of Cherry (1953). *J. Exp. Psychol. Gen.* 124: 243–262.

Wood, N. and Cowan, N. (1995b) The cocktail party phenomenon revisited: How frequent are attention shifts to one's name in an irrelevant auditory channel? *J. Exp. Psychol. Learn. Mem. Cogn.* 21: 255–260.

6

Functional Anatomy of Visual Attention in the Human Brain: Studies with Positron Emission Tomography

Maurizio Corbetta

ABSTRACT Positron emission tomography (PET) is a neuroimaging methodology that provides temporally integrated maps of regional cerebral blood flow (rCBF) across the whole brain. Maps of rCBF are indirectly related to neuronal activity and thus provide information about the functional anatomy of sensory, motor, and cognitive systems. Visual attention is conceptualized as a collection of neural mechanisms that generate and funnel cognitive biases (attentional templates) onto the visual system. PET studies indicate that these cognitive biases modulate activity in extrastriate visual cortex through a variety of selective and nonselective mechanisms. Parietal regions funnel spatial biases onto ventral extrastriate regions related to object analysis. Frontal regions may be involved in the generation and storage of attentional template signals.

The last decade has witnessed an explosion in the field of human brain imaging. New methodologies, most notably positron emission tomography (PET) and functional magnetic resonance imaging (fMRI), allow imaging of brain activity in vivo during sensory, motor, and cognitive behavior. The combination of brain imaging with task paradigms derived from cognitive psychology and psychophysics represent one of today's most effective ways to correlate in vivo cognition and brain activity (Raichle, 1994).

The current strategy for imaging human cognition is based on a set of assumptions regarding the use of metabolic measurements, such as blood flow in PET (Raichle, 1987) and deoxygenation signal in fMRI (Ogawa et al., 1992), to estimate neuronal activity and the underlying organization of the human brain. Metabolic measures represent an indirect but accurate way to measure neuronal activity but can image only a limited spatiotemporal bandwidth of neuronal activity. The brain is conceptualized as a modular system in which the neuronal activity necessary to execute a complex task is distributed across different brain modules (Posner, Petersen, Fox, and Raichle, 1988). The first part of this chapter describes the theory and practice at the base of PET imaging studies of cognition and critically discusses working assumptions and biological interpretations of the data. The second part discusses the contribution of PET toward understanding the neural basis of visual attention.

The problem of visual attention is central to theories of cognition and consciousness. Significant progress has been achieved in the last twenty years or so in elucidating the basic anatomical and physiological organization of the primate visual system (Felleman and Van Essen, 1991; Desimone and Ungerleider, 1989), but the means by which selection is achieved during vision are only beginning to be understood. The great challenge is to explain how internal states, including thought, memory, and emotions, interact with the visual system to create visual awareness. Brain-imaging methods can contribute to that effort by allowing researchers to monitor neural activity during attentional behavior across the whole brain.

POSITRON EMISSION TOMOGRAPHY MAPPING METHODOLOGY

History and Theory

PET defines an imaging methodology that employs a computerized tomograph to measure the concentration in the brain of positron-emitting compounds of natural molecules such as oxygen, nitrogen, or glucose. Several physiological metabolic parameters, including oxygen and glucose metabolism, blood flow, and blood volume, can be measured in vivo in the human brain (Raichle, 1987).

PET was originally developed by integrating the sophisticated mathematical algorithms for the reconstruction of the relative radiodensity of a body section in computerized tomography with the principles of tissue autoradiography. Tissue autoradiography quantitatively measures within slices of a tissue the accumulation of radioactively labeled compounds. Different compounds are used to measure different physiological variables, such as blood flow or glucose metabolism (Sokoloff et al., 1977). A PET scan can therefore be considered to be an in vivo autoradiogram, obtained with positron-emitting radioisotopes.

Positron-emitting radioisotopes were selected mostly because of their high energy, which allows their detection from outside the body through external detectors. Positrons are positively charged particles that are emitted by the nucleus during radioactive decay and that travel for a few millimeters before encountering an electron. The encounter results in a process called annihilation and produces two gamma rays traveling about 180 degrees apart from their origin, which may be located by external measurement of their temporal coincidence. The relative concentration of position-emitting radioisotopes, which reflects various physiological metabolic parameters, can therefore be estimated at different brain locations.

The first PET scanner for brain studies was built in the mid-1970s at Washington University (Ter-Pogossian, 1977). Initial attempts to correlate behavior with brain activity were based on measurements of glucose metabolism, which is directly correlated with neuronal activity (Reivich et al., 1979; Phelps, Kuhl, and Mazziotta, 1981). However, the long time needed for the accumulation of the relative glucose isotope in the brain (more than 40 minutes) and the long decay time prevented multiple measurements, making the method inefficient for studies of normal volunteers. By the mid-

1980s most groups had switched to measurements of regional cerebral blood flow (rCBF) with O^{15}-labeled water for physiological studies in vivo, primarily because its shorter half-life (123 s) allows multiple measurements in a single session.

Regional CBF Measurements and Neuronal Activity

In the normal brain, blood flow is indirectly related to neuronal activity. That relationship was first demonstrated in humans by Fulton (1926), who studied a patient who had been operated on for an arteriovenous malformation of the occipital lobe that proved not to be resectable. The patient was left with a craniotomy defect over which a bruit could be heard with a stethoscope. The patient reported that the noise in the back of his head intensified whenever he used his eyes. Fulton showed that the audible bruit over the occipital lobe increased selectively for visual stimulation but not for other types of stimuli. Several animal experiments later confirmed that cerebral blood flow represents an indirect but reliable indicator of neuronal activity in the brain (Schmidt and Hendrix, 1937; Serota and Gerard, 1938).

Teleologically, the local increment in blood flow provides an oversupply of metabolic substrates (oxygen and glucose) that is indispensable for the correct functioning of the neurons. However, the mechanisms coupling neuronal activity to vascular response are not well understood. Microcinematographic and optical imaging analyses document that vessels in the cortex increase their caliber within 400–1000 ms from the onset of changes in neuronal activity (Frostig, Lieke, Tso, and Grinvald, 1990; Cox, Woolsey, and Rovainen, 1993). This fast response suggests that the initial coupling is mediated by a direct neuronergic mechanism rather than by metabolic by-products of neuronal activity (e.g., increased pH or nitrous oxide; for a review, see Iadecola, 1993).

The vascular response is spatially blurred when compared to the underlying neuronal activity generating it, and optical imaging data indicate that this spatial mismatch may be within a few millimeters. Moreover, most metabolic (and blood flow) changes occur in the region of the neuropil (or synaptic region), which is the most active region metabolically, rather than at the level of the neuronal body (Schwartz et al., 1979).

The vascular response is also temporally blurred, as it takes several seconds for a vessel to return to baseline levels after being stimulated by neuronal activity, and its fidelity in the reproduction of neuronal signal is unclear. Some calculations indicate that most of the brain's metabolic demands are related to the maintenance of a correct ionic gradient across cellular membranes (neurons and glia), rather than to acute changes in neuronal activity (Creutzfeld, 1975). Measurements of glucose consumption in the superior cervical ganglion during stimulation of the rat cervical sympathetic trunk indicate that the relationship between stimulus rate and metabolism is not linear (Yarowsky, Kadekard, and Sokoloff, 1983). However, with PET a dependency has been observed in vivo between rate of stimulation and local blood flow in primary visual and somatosensory cortex (Fox and Raichle, 1985).

Finally, the neuronal sign of a vascular response is unknown. Blood flow increases locally both for excitatory and inhibitory neuronal activity, as both are equally demanding processes. These observations all carry important implications for the biological interpretation of PET data sets (for more information, see the section on Caveats of PET Activation Methodology).

PET measures blood flow by adapting the method originally developed by Seymour Kety for autoradiography in laboratory animals (Landau, Freygang, Roland, Sokoloff, and Kety, 1955; Raichle, Martin, Herscovitch, Mintun, and Markham, 1983). A small dose of O^{15}-labeled water is injected through an arm vein, and the dose distributes over several cardiac cycles to the brain in just longer than a minute. PET measures the accumulation of radioactive water in the brain, and the method computes an averaged distribution of rCBF over that time window. The corresponding image is an unknown combination of anatomical and physiological signals, due to the presence of baseline activity in gray and white matter, and of task-related neuronal signals proper. The half-life of O^{15}-labeled water is 123 seconds, and the whole injected dose decays within 10 minutes (5 half-lives) to baseline levels. The exposure to potentially dangerous effects of radiation is minimized, and multiple measurements can be performed in the same session.

In order to localize task-related activity changes, relative differences in rCBF between two behavioral states are measured by generating a subtraction image of the rCBF maps obtained in the two states. This approach eliminates most of the noise signal coming from the underlying brain anatomy. A typical PET subtraction image contains relative positive and negative rCBF regions of change that localize areas of difference between task and control condition. They do not provide, however, information about the absolute direction of change. For example, a positive rCBF change can represent an area of increased blood flow (activation) in the task condition, an area of decreased blood flow (deactivation) in the control condition, or any intermediate combination between activation and deactivation. The relationship between areas of activation and deactivation and underlying neuronal activity is governed by the previously discussed considerations regarding the sign of the vascular response.

The spatial resolution of this method—that is, the ability to resolve two nearby foci of rCBF change—is relatively low (typically 10–15 mm), but smaller differences in location (5–7 mm) can be resolved when single foci of activity are compared across different subtraction images. The spatial resolution is influenced by the distance travelled by the positron before annhilation, the sensitivity of the scanner, and the statistical noise in the image. The temporal resolution is about 40–60 s, and is limited by the time necessary to acquire images of good statistical quality.

Strategy for Brain-Mapping Studies

PET brain-mapping (or activation) studies are based on several assumptions concerning the organization of behavior in the brain. First, a complex behavior or task can be conceptualized as a series of simpler processing operations that can be analyzed through computational or task analysis (Marr, 1982). Second, a correspondence exists between a brain region and one or more of these processing operations; that is, the brain is conceptualized as a network of computational modules. Third, those operations—the brain regions—are recruited on task demands (Posner et al., 1988). Accordingly, any particular behavior (e.g., verbal fluency) does not map onto a single brain region but is the product of a processing interaction between a set of distributed brain modules.

PET activation experiments are designed to localize foci of brain activity that are related to specific processing operations. Two strategies have been employed. One strategy, directly derived from the work of Franciscus Donders on reaction time analysis (1869), compares pairs of tasks that are matched except for differences in a few stimuli or processes that are specifically of interest. For example, in a simple visual experiment, volunteers detect the onset of a grating stimulus in one scan and discriminate its orientation in the second scan. Subtraction between the two scans isolates regions specifically involved in discrimination, while subtracting away activity related to the sensory stimulus or processes related to detection. A second strategy, derived from the work of Sternberg (1969), uses similar control and experimental conditions but varies the relative processing time allocated to one processing component. For example, subjects hold in memory visual items for 500 ms in one scan and for 5 s in another scan. The corresponding subtraction will image processes related to visual short-term memory, which is the processing component differentially manipulated by the two conditions.

Data Averaging, Anatomical Localization, and Statistical Evaluation

Individual PET subtraction images are noisy, and several image-averaging techniques have been developed over the last 10 years to improve signal-to-noise ratios (Cox et al., 1993; Fox et al., 1988; Friston, Frith, Liddle, and Frackowiack, 1991; Silbersweig et al., 1993). Within-subject image averaging provides higher spatial resolution, as it removes the individual anatomical variability, but is limited by the low number of experimental conditions that can be studied in one subject. Across-subject averaging has a lower spatial resolution but allows more comparisons that are helpful during exploratory studies.

PET averaged subtraction images are transformed and standardized into a stereotactical anatomical atlas of the human brain (Talairach and Tournoux, 1988), which is the same for most imaging groups. Regional CBF regions of change are localized within this space using a three-dimensional coordinate system. More recently, the warping of PET images onto anatomical MRI images has allowed a finer correlation between rCBF responses and underlying brain anatomy (Cox et al., 1993; Woods, Maziotta, and Cherry, 1993). Finally, rCBF responses are evaluated for statistical significance with a variety of different methods (Fox and Mintun, 1989; Friston et al., 1991; Worsley, Evans, Marrett, and Neelin, 1992).

Caveats of PET Mapping Methodology

The ability of PET studies to image the true functional anatomy of a given task is limited by several factors. Most studies cannot rely on a precise computational model of the imaged behavior or task. Sometimes the putative processing operations are only broadly specified (e.g., detection versus discrimination); at other times the processing differences between task and control states are either too large to be informative or are not appropriately constrained by behavioral measures. Furthermore, the subtraction strategy in its simpler application assumes both additive recruitments of new modules without change to those modules previously engaged in the control state as well as a fixed correspondence between a brain module and one or more processing operations.

Those assumptions are challenged by new views that emphasize distributed processing across neuronal assemblies, time encoding, and flexibility in the operations performed by a particular module (Goldman-Rakic, 1994). Finally, small differences in the stimulus or timing parameters of a task produce major differences in the pattern of activations. For example, activity in a left temporal region during a verb generation task performed at a rate of one trial every 1.5 seconds (Raichle et al., 1994) is not significantly detected when the same task is performed at the rate of one trial per second (Petersen, Fox, Posner, Mintun, and Raichle, 1989). That difference, possibly related to a deeper encoding of verbal material at the slower rate of presentation, was difficult to predict in advance.

The problem of sensitivity to small methodological differences is common in psychology, but it is perhaps surprising in PET, a method that is intrinsically noisy and averaged. In terms of imaging, PET rCBF maps offer only a skewed representation of the true underlying functional anatomy of a given task. This is due both to the indirect relationship between rCBF and neuronal activity and to the spatiotemporal constraints of the instruments used to measure the vascular response. Issues of spatial localization, temporal integration and resolution, and sign of neuronal response are separately considered.

The accurate spatial localization of task-related neuronal activity is limited by the spatial blurring of the vascular response, by the resolution of the scanner (both conditions that were previously mentioned in this chapter), and by the concentration of task-related synaptic activity. As was discussed earlier, most metabolic (blood flow) changes occur at the level of the terminal synapses rather than at the level of the neuronal body (Schwartz et al., 1979). A task-related rCBF change, therefore, localizes nearby task-related neurons only when the concentration of task-related synapses is high; otherwise, it localizes near the terminal projection fields of the task-related neurons. There is very little data to support or contradict the assumption of spatial coincidence between rCBF and task-related neurons. The assumption is plausible in the cortex because of the high number of cortical interneurons, a reasonable correspondence between activations in primary sensory and motor areas, and known underlying physiology. However, the same assumption may be incorrect in the subcortical nuclei (caudate, putamen, thalamus), where autoradiographical metabolic changes make more sense when localized with the terminal projection fields of task-active neurons.

The temporal integration of the rCBF signal emphasizes operations that are phasically activated on each trial for a significant percentage of the total processing time (e.g., sensory and motor processes), as opposed to operations that are rapidly engaged and disengaged during a trial (e.g., putative switching control mechanisms proposed by computational models of visual attention; for example, see Olshausen, Anderson, and Van Essen, 1993) or that slowly change over time (e.g., long-term mechanisms of synaptic reorganization and facilitation; for example, see Gall and Lauterborn, 1991). Furthermore, the limited temporal resolution prevents any meaningful determinations about the temporal sequence of activations, that is, how information flows in the brain. PET rCBF maps therefore provide only an impoverished picture of a very dynamic pattern of neural activity, but serious attempts are under way to integrate metabolic imaging with electrical recording in order to improve their temporal resolution (for correlations between PET rCBF and scalp electrical activity, see Heintz et al., 1995; Snyder, Abdullaev, Posner, and Raichle, 1995).

Finally, the sign of a rCBF region of change can have multiple interpretations. Positive rCBF responses are thought to localize activity in brain regions participating in specific task operations, with the magnitude of the response related to the strength of participation. Therefore, most imaging studies covertly assume an excitatory neuronal sign and monotonicity between rCBF and neuronal activity. However, as was indicated earlier, the actual neuronal sign (excitation or inhibition) of a vascular response is unknown, and monotonicity between rCBF and neuronal activity has not been demonstrated. For example, more rCBF in one area may actually mean less participation in the task if the signal is mostly inhibitory. Moreover, other studies have related decrements in blood flow to presumably more efficient neuronal processing (Squire et al., 1992; Miller, Li, and Desimone, 1993).

Negative rCBF foci are affected by similar problems of interpretation. An additional issue, specific to negative responses, is the often quoted possibility that limitations in the "plumbing capacity" of the vascular supply might contribute to large regions of deactivation (Haxby et al., 1994). For example, large regions of deactivations in middle frontal and lateral hemispheric regions have been reported during visual tasks activating occipitotemporal regions (Haxby et al., 1994). Because the occipitotemporal region is supplied mostly by the posterior cerebral artery, it is possible that those deactivations merely represent relative flow decreases either in other branches of the same vascular distribution or in different vascular distributions (the anterior and middle cerebral arteries). Finally, brain regions that do not show any relative change are usually believed to be inactive, but an alternative possibility is that they are equally active in the control and in the task state. In conclusion, PET is a powerful tool for the investigation of human cognition, but it is important to realize its spatiotemporal limits and the various caveats affecting the biological interpretation of the data sets. The next section will consider how PET has been used to map the functional anatomy of visual attention in the human brain.

FUNCTIONAL ANATOMY OF VISUAL ATTENTION

Vision is an active process: the product of a dynamic interaction between visual signals entering the brain and a variety of internal biases that ensure the processing of behaviorally relevant over behaviorally irrelevant visual stimuli. Some biases are structural, hard-wired into the visual system, to facilitate the processing of certain stimulus configurations (e.g., a vertical bar in a field of horizontal bars) and likely reflect local interactions in the receptive field architecture. Other biases are related to information stored in long-term memory. For example, the familiarity of a stimulus modulates visual neurons in anterior inferotemporal cortex and area V4 of macaques, suggesting a general bias towards novelty (Miller et al., 1993). That habituation may reflect the dynamic selection in the population of responsive visual neurons of fewer units that are better tuned for the familiar stimuli. A final source of bias is the effect of cognitive expectations on visual processing.

Cognitive expectations are usually set up through a behavioral goal (e.g., look for the red apple), which can be either externally communicated via visual or verbal stimuli or triggered by such internal signals as memories, emotions, or homeostatic states (e.g., hunger). The neural signal (or set of signals) related to a particular behavioral goal, which biases neural activity at other brain sites (e.g., the visual system) to help achieve that goal, is defined as the attentional template (Duncan and Humphreys, 1989). Attentional templates can differ in complexity, consisting either of a single feature such as red or a complete object description involving multiple features (red, round, static). Attentional templates can be established in response to external visual or verbal information or triggered by internal states (e.g., hunger). Finally, they can be used to implement different goals, such as recognizing a target in a cluttered environment or reaching for it in three-dimensional space.

Consider a typical visual experiment on the effects of expectations on visual processing. The observer (monkey or human) is instructed to attend to a particular target object or feature (color, shape, motion) previous to the presentation of a test display containing multiple objects. It is easy to demonstrate that the advance instruction can improve target detection or discrimination, suggesting that a top-down signal has modulated visual processing. In this experiment it is important to distinguish between the activity related to the encoding of the behavioral goal (attentional template) and the activity related to the top-down effects of the attentional template on visual processing (selective visual modulations). The neural signals related to the attentional template can be considered the source of the attentional modulation, whereas the visual system is the site where the modulation occurs. The attentional template signal includes multiple operations, such as the encoding and storage of the instructions or their funneling into the visual system. Those operations may or may not be localized within the same brain regions.

One goal of current neuroimaging research is to understand the level of processing at which attentional templates can modulate visual activity. The locus of attentional selection has preoccupied the psychological literature on attention since the 1950s. Broadbent conceptualized attention as a bottleneck in the sensory transmission systems (1958). Early- and late-selection theorists have argued whether this bottleneck is located before or after recognition. Several PET and single-unit studies have demonstrated uneqivocally that attention can modulate visual processing and that attentional modulations occur at different levels of processing depending on task demands (see next section).

A second goal of interest is to define the type of attentional templates that can modulate visual activity. In primates, the visual system is organized in two hierarchical, functionally specialized processing pathways (Felleman and Van Essen, 1991; Desimone and Ungerleider, 1989; also, see Webster and Ungerleider, chapter 2, this volume). The occipitotemporal pathway, or ventral stream, which extends from primary visual cortex (area V1) into inferotemporal regions, is critical for the identification of objects. The occipitoparietal pathway, or dorsal stream, which extends from area V1 to posterior parietal regions, is critical for the analysis of spatial relations among objects and for guidance of eye and hand movements toward objects. Reciprocal connections (feedforward and feedback) exist between various processing stages in each pathway, supporting the idea that information can flow from lower to upper levels in the hierarchy (bottom-up), driven by the visual input, as well as from upper to lower levels (top-down), driven by cognitive signals (e.g., attentional biases). Psychological experiments over the course of the last decade have shown that attention can be independently allocated to regions of space, to objects, and to corresponding component features (color, shape, motion, location) (Kanwisher and Driver, 1992; Posner, 1980). Accordingly, early single-unit recording studies demonstrated selective modulations of visual activity related to the selection of a location (Bushnell, Goldberg, and Robinson, 1981; Wurtz, Goldberg, and Robinson, 1980; Moran and Desimone, 1985), and, more recently, both PET and single-unit studies have shown selective effects related to objects and features (Corbetta,

Miezen, Dobmeyer, Shulman, and Petersen, 1991; Haenny, Maunsell, and Schiller, 1988).

A third goal of current imaging research on attention is to localize the neural activity related to attentional templates, that is, the source of selective modulations in visual cortex. That neural activity is primarily unknown at the present time, but some working hypothesis have been proposed. One model identifies attentional template signals with short-term memory signals (Desimone and Duncan, 1995). Attentional templates for objects or features are encoded within a circuitry that includes ventrolateral prefrontal cortex, inferotemporal cortex, and their reciprocal connections. The object-related bias is funneled through inferotemporal cortex into other regions of the ventral object identity system. Similarly, spatial templates are generated in circuitries between dorsolateral prefrontal cortex and parietal areas, which are also reciprocally connected (Goldman-Rakic, 1994), and from there are transferred to other visual regions.

Another model (Posner and Petersen, 1990; Posner, 1994) postulates the existence of attentional brain systems independent from sensory, motor, or other cognitive networks (e.g., language or memory) that carry out various attentional operations. A vigilance system, identified with the noradrenergic projections from the locus coeruleus and various right hemisphere areas, maintains the alert state. A posterior orienting system, formed by posterior parietal cortex, superior colliculus, and the pulvinar nucleus of the thalamus, orients to sensory events. An anterior executive system, centered on the anterior cingulate region, acts as a central executive: it regulates the relative traffic between the lateral frontal region (language, working memory) and the posterior visual regions, and controls the access of relevant targets to premotor systems and focal awareness. Accordingly, attentional template signals for location, feature, or object originate in lateral prefrontal regions involved in working memory, and are funneled posteriorly (via the dorsal and ventral visual stream) through the anterior cingulate region. In summary, although both models postulate that working memory is somehow involved as a source of attentional template signals, only Posner's model regards the anterior cingulate to be a major node of processing interference and some brain regions such as anterior cingulate or posterior parietal cortex to be exclusively attentional in nature.

The next two sections will separately consider how attentional templates for objects, features of objects, or location modulate activity in the visual system; the third section will discuss the putative neural basis of attentional templates in relation to the two neurocognitive models of visual attention just presented.

Feature- or Object-Based Selective Visual Modulations

Visual objects can be described as the combination of simpler visual features (color, motion, orientation, texture, disparity, and location). Visual objects are encoded into object-centered neural representations, which are derived from earlier stages of processing related to feature analysis (Marr, 1982). One question is whether attention interacts with those representations to select behaviorally relevant visual objects. Earlier psychological reports failed to find consistent effects related to feature selection for suprathreshold discrimination, and suggested that spatial selection had prominence in vision (Allport, 1989). However, more recent data have shown convincing interference effects related to feature and object selection that are independent of location effects (Duncan, 1984; Vogel, Eekout, and Orban, 1988). Corbetta et al. (1991) demonstrated with PET that selective modulations related to visual feature processing systematically occur in human extrastriate visual cortex. In that study, participants were scanned during several match-to-sample visual discrimination tasks involving multiple colored moving objects. In three separate selective attention scans, observers reported a threshold change in either the color, shape, or speed of the objects. In a divided attention scan, participants reported a change in any of the three features. Both the selective and the divided condition require the creation of an attentional template of the relevant features and a comparison in memory (short-term memory) of the match and sample visual display. Passive viewing and fixation conditions, in which observers maintained fixation with and without presentation of the visual displays, respectively, were also included.

Two different types of modulation were observed in visual cortex. First, primary visual cortex and adjacent medial occipital areas were more active when subjects actively discriminated (selective and divided attention conditions) than when they passively viewed the same set of visual stimuli (active-passive modulation). Figure 6.1A (and its color version in plate 2) illustrates active-passive modulation in medial occipital cortex. Activity near the primary visual cortex is very high when fixation is subtracted from passive viewing, which reflects differences in sensory stimulation (figure 6.1A, left). However, visual cortex is still significantly more activated when any discrimination condition (motion, color, shape, divided) is compared to passive viewing (figure 6.1A, right). The active-passive modulation may or may not be selective, because no difference was observed within the spatial resolution of the method between selective and divided, or among selective conditions (not shown).

Active-passive differences have been reliably observed during some experiments involving active discrimination and passive viewing (Dupont et al., 1993; De Yoe, Schmit, and Neitz, 1995). Such differences are more robust in early visual regions such as primary visual cortex and in the lingual and fusiform gyri, than they are later in the visual system's inferotemporal cortex. Active-passive differences have been also observed in primary and secondary auditory cortex during auditory discrimination and passive listening tasks (Fiez et al., 1995). Nonselective task-dependent effects have been reported in primary visual cortex and extrastriate visual regions in primates (Wurtz et al., 1980; Mountcastle, Motter, Steinmatz, and Sestokas, 1987).

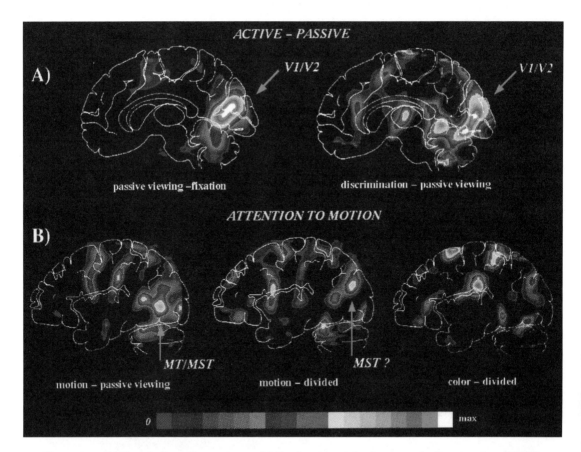

Figure 6.1 (A) Nonselective active-passive modulation in primary visual cortex and adjacent regions (V1/V2). Sagittal PET section 5 mm left off midline. (Left) V1/V2 activation for passive viewing of a colored moving array of objects minus viewing only a fixation point. (Right) V1/V2 modulation for discriminating threshold shape changes of the objects minus passive viewing. (B) Motion selective modulation in human homolog of middle temporal/middle superior temporal (MT/MST) area. Sagittal PET section 35 mm left off midline. (Left) MT/MST activity during threshold speed discrimination minus passive viewing. (Center) Activity when discriminating motion minus discriminating any attribute (color, shape, motion) in divided attention condition. (Right) Lack of activity during threshold color discrimination minus divided attention. See color plate 2.

Active-passive differences can be related to various mechanisms, including top-down attentional modulations, discriminatory processes, and differences in arousal. A recent large meta-analysis of nine visual processing experiments (involving more than 120 subjects) has demonstrated that active-passive blood flow increases in early visual areas are a robust phenomenon, and that those modulations are remarkably task selective in some experiments (Shulman et al., 1997a,b).

Second, extrastriate visual regions, specialized in processing a particular visual feature (e.g., motion processing regions), were more active above both a passive viewing and a divided attention baseline when subjects attended to that particular feature (e.g., motion). That type of modulation is known as feature selective modulation. Figure 6.1B illustrates the effects of attention to motion at the level of putative human MT, a region located laterally at the occipitotemporal junction specialized for motion analysis in humans (Tootell et al., 1995; Watson et al., 1993). The subtraction between attention to motion and passive viewing (figure 6.1B, left) isolates several foci of rCBF activity centered around MT/MST. Those responses can reflect a combination of signals, including discriminatory processes, arousal, and top-down modulations. The subtraction between attention to motion and divided attention (figure 6.1B, center) localizes additional activity, which is located more dorsally and posteriorly (about 17 mm in vector distance) and might represent later stations in the motion processing pathway (MST). This response reflects a selective modulation of visual activity (rCBF enhancement), because arousal and the discriminatory component are closely matched in this subtraction.

This modulation is motion selective because it is obtained when attention is focused on the speed of motion of the objects, but not when attention is focused on other features (e.g., color, as shown on the right side of figure 6.1B, or shape) or when it is divided across features. The modulation is also independent of location or space, because the random spatial distribution of the objects in the display discouraged spatial analysis, and there was no evidence of activation in parietal regions, which are related to spatial selection. The exact operation underlying the rCBF enhancement is not well specified and may include any combination of top-down activity related to the attentional template, to short-term memory, or to the matching signal for the attended feature or object. At the neuronal level, enhancement of visual activity has been reported in area MST for attending to moving objects (Maunsell, 1995), and both positive and negative modulatory effects have been reported in areas MT, MST, and 7a for attending to direction. The strength of the modulations increases for areas more "upstream" in the visual hierarchy (Ferrera, Rudolph, and Maunsell, 1994).

Figure 6.2 summarizes the location of other human extrastriate visual regions in which feature or object selective modulations have been reported. In all cases the modulation consists of an rCBF enhancement for the test task above that for the control tasks matched for visual stimulation and arousal. In an experiment by Corbetta et al. (1991), attention to color modulated a region in the collateral sulcus, between the fusiform and lingual gyri, and a more dorsal region in lateral occipital cortex. Attention to shape (size) bilaterally modulated the collateral sulcus, the fusiform and parahippocampal gyri, and the right inferior temporal cortex near the superior temporal sulcus (Corbetta et al., 1991). Those findings have been recently replicated with fMRI (Bush et al., 1995). Overlapping foci in ventral occipitotemporal cortex are activated by attention to face identity (Haxby et al., 1994; Sergent, Ohta, and MacDonald, 1992). A dorsolateral occipital region (about 1 cm more lateral than the dorsal focus for color) is active for attention to oriented gratings (Dupont et al., 1993). Finally, directing attention to visual words in a semantic monitoring task enhances rCBF above passive viewing of the same

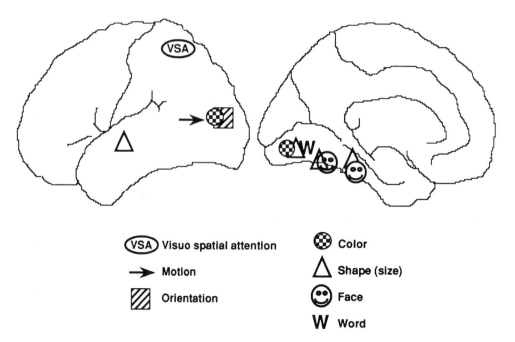

Figure 6.2 Selective feature and object modulations and visuospatial attention. Extrastriate visual regions showing feature selective modulations, and superior parietal region for visuospatial attention.

words in foci that are located near those that are active for color and shape (Petersen, Corbetta, Miezin, Shulman, and Raichle, 1993). Independent mapping and lesion studies demonstrate that those regions are specialized for processing the relevant visual attribute or object (e.g., color, motion, shape, faces, words) (see Haxby et al., 1994).

In summary, directing attention (under template conditions) toward features or objects independently of location significantly modulates activity in the visual system. Modulations in early visual areas may reflect nonselective processes like arousal in some cases, but are clearly task selective in other cases. Selective enhancements of blood flow occurs in extrastriate visual regions specialized in feature or object analysis when those feature or objects are in the focus of attention. In psychological terms, this modulation corresponds to an amplification of relevant information in the attended channel. In neural terms, enhancements of visual activity have been demonstrated in dorsal and ventral areas of the visual system (Maunsell, 1995) but it is unknown whether those modulations are restricted as in PET to task-relevant cortical processing areas (for an exception, see Ferrera et al., 1994).

Location-Based Selective Visual Modulations

Observers can attend to a location in an empty field, an example of space-based selection. Alternatively, an observer can attend to the location of an object; in that case, attention is distributed over the object and moves with the object, suggesting that the object, rather than an unrelated set of locations or a region of space, can be a unit of selection. The focus of attention typically changes every 200–300 ms, in conjunction with the execution of a saccadic eye movement, but covert shifts of attention can occur independently from such overt shifts. Finally, attention can be endogenously cued to a location or to an object location on the basis of spatial template information (e.g., "look to the left") can be or automatically attracted by a sensory event (e.g., a bright flash nearby) (Kanwisher and Driver, 1992; Posner, 1980).

Some PET experiments have studied the effects of directing attention to an object location. Heintz and colleagues reported that in a peripheral object discrimination task, in which the target object was presented to the upper visual field, the fusiform cortex was more strongly activated when attention was directed toward the object of interest than away from it (Heinze et al., 1994). Similar modulations occur in a more dorsolateral occipital region when objects are presented in the lower visual field (Woldorff et al., 1995). Petersen, Corbetta, Miezin, and Shulman (1994) also reported finding stronger activity in fusiform and dorsolateral occipital regions when attention was directed toward (rather than away from) a flashing checkerboard pattern, which stimulated both the upper and lower visual fields.

Across all these experiments the visual display contained objects in both visual fields during task and control conditions, and only the side of attention was manipulated. The instructed unit of selection (or attentional template) was the location of an object, and the resulting effect, therefore, likely reflects the presence of spatial selective modulations in task-relevant object-processing regions. At the neuronal level, about one-quarter to one-half of the neurons in ventral areas such as V4 and IT decrease their best visual response to an object (as assessed by previous sensory mapping) when attention is directed toward another object location within the cell's receptive field (Moran and Desimone, 1985). Therefore, spatial attention appears to restrict the focus of processing around the attended object to suppress activity coming from irrelevant objects. There is no contradiction between inhibition of neuronal activity and increases in rCBF, because inhibition is also a metabolically demanding process.

Interestingly, only one these studies (M. Woldorff, personal communication) localized activity in the parietal lobe, a region that has been classically associated with the control of spatial attention. In contrast, significant superior parietal activity (along with more ventral activations) has been reported in a different paradigm in which attention was peripherally allocated to detect a small difference in object orientation or to detect object onset. Activity was stronger in the discrimination condition, which may reflect focusing of attention onto the peripheral object (Vanderberghe et al., 1996, 1997). A possible difference across studies is the modality of stimulation, which involved a rapid continuous stream of peripheral stimuli (like in an evoked potential paradigm) in the former set of studies, and a discrete (trial-by-trial) stimulus presentation in the latter two experiments. The discrete modality of stimulation does not prevent covert shifts of attention in the intertrial interval, and they might be partly responsible for the superior parietal activation (see below). Alternatively, it is possible that some of the former experiments did not record activity from the dorsal parietal cortex because of the limited field view of some PET scanners.

Other PET studies have examined brain mechanisms related to directing attention to various spatial locations (as opposed to an object location) (Corbetta et al., 1993; Nobre et al., 1997). The distinction between attention to space or to object location is supported psychophysically, and there are no a priori reasons to believe that the two types of attention involve the same mechanisms. Varying the instructed locations while minimizing other type of processing (e.g., object analysis) also has the advantage of avoiding confounds between activations related to the source of the spatial bias and its effects on other task-related regions.

Corbetta et al. (1993) studied shifts of attention to various peripheral locations under conditions in which locations were either endogenously cued through instructions (template) or exogenously cued through sensory stimulation. In a third condition, attention was maintained centrally during the presentation of peripheral stimuli that were identical to the stimuli presented in the shifting conditions. The left panel of figure 6.3 shows a direct subtraction between conditions in which subjects endogenously shifted attention in the right visual field and conditions in which attention was maintained in the center (see also plate 3). The two conditions were matched in terms of peripheral visual stimulation, arousal, central fixation, and motor response (a

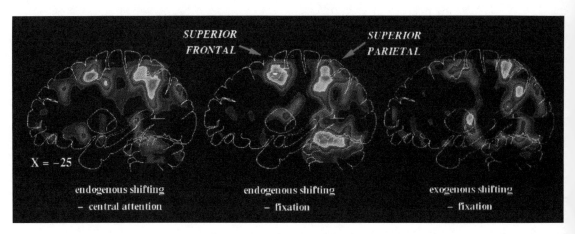

Figure 6.3 Shifts of visuospatial attention. PET sagittal section 25 mm left off midline. (Left) Superior frontal and parietal foci during endogenous shifts of attention in the right visual field (detect peripheral stimuli along a predictable series of location) minus central attention (detect dim central events). (Center) Endogenous shifts to the left visual field minus fixation (without detection). (Right) Exogenous shifts to left visual field (through passive presentation of peripheral stimuli) minus fixation. See color plate 3.

keypress). Two regions were more active in the shifting condition: one in the superior parietal lobule, near Brodmann's area 7, and one in the superior frontal cortex, near Brodmann's area 6. The center and right panels of figure 6.3 demonstrate that the superior parietal region was similarly active during both endogenous and exogenous shifts of attention independent of the execution of a motor response, which was required only in the endogenous condition. In contrast, the superior frontal region was more active for endogenous shifts of attention; its potential contribution to spatial selection is discussed in the attentional template section of this chapter. The dim visual stimulation prevented any extrastriate activity.

A working hypothesis to account for the results of Corbetta et al. is that the superior parietal cortex works as a spatial shifter mechanism to dynamically direct the focus of processing to peripheral locations or objects, independent of the mode of cueing (i.e., endogenous or exogenous), the requirements of a motor response, the response effector (i.e., eye versus hand), or the underlying task demands (i.e., detection versus discrimination). Accordingly, the superior parietal region is commonly active for attention to locations (as discussed previously) or for object location (Vandenberghe et al., 1994, 1995). That region is also active during visually and memory-guided saccadic eye movements to peripheral locations (Anderson et al., 1994; Petit et al., 1993; Petersen et al., 1994). Shifts of attention are common to both conditions but are endogenously cued in the memory task and exogenously cued in the visual task. Finally, superior parietal cortex is recruited during visual search tasks involving targets defined by color and orientation (Hunton, Corbetta, Shulman, Miezin, and Petersen, 1995) or by color and motion (Corbetta et al., 1995).

The putative link between shifts of spatial attention and superior parietal activity is particularly helpful because it provides some neurobiological constraints with which to test unresolved issues in psychology and vision. For example, a long-standing controversy in psychology is the one between parallel and serial models of visual search. The basic phenomenon is well known: the search time for a low-saliency target (e.g., a red triangle among red squares and green triangles) increases as the number of distractors increases, whereas the search time for a high-saliency target (e.g., a red square among green distractors) is independent of the number of distractors. The reasons for the difference are unclear. Some models, known as parallel search models, propose that visual analysis proceeds in parallel across the field in both cases, but that its efficiency declines in conditions of low target discriminability when more distractors are added to the system (Duncan and Humphreys, 1989). Others models propose that a spatial attention mechanism is additionally recruited in conditions of low discriminability to serially inspect each item in the field and discriminate between target and distractors (Treisman and Gelade, 1980).

Corbetta, Shulman, Miezin, and Petersen (1995) compared superior parietal activity during visual search tasks involving targets defined by color, by motion, or by the conjunction of color and motion. Psychophysically, the feature tasks yielded flat search functions, consistent with parallel search, whereas the conjunction task yielded the expected increasing search function. Across the entire brain, feature and conjunction tasks were best distinguished by activity in superior parietal cortex, which was significantly higher during the conjunction task, and which was colocalized in the regions previously activated by shifts of visuospatial attention. The common activation in superior parietal cortex for shifts of attention and conjunction targets is therefore consistent with serial models of search that uniquely predict the recruitment of a serial spatial attention mechanism in the conjunction task.

A different explanation is that the superior parietal activity reflects the binding of color and motion feature in the conjunction task. That explanation is consistent with recent findings showing that a patient with bilateral occipitoparietal lesions had severe difficulties in binding features of visually presented objects (Friedman-Hill, Robertson, and Treisman, 1995), and that blood flow in superior parietal cortex was higher when subjects had to report two (rather than one) features of the same object (Vanderberghe et al., 1997). Finally, recent findings indicate that TMS of parietal cortex disrupts the performance on a visual search task involving conjunction but not feature targets. The deficit disappears after extensive practice on the conjunction task (Ashbridge, Walsh, and Cowey, 1997). Practice may transform the conjunction task such that targets may begin to "pop out" in the display (Wolfe, Cave, and Franzel, 1989), therefore requiring fewer shifts of attention and/or less attentional binding of visual features. Explanations in terms of shifts of attention and feature binding are not necessarily exclusive if the superior parietal cortex contains a spatial map that is topographically connected (directly or indirectly through other structures, such as the pulvinar) to various feature maps (color, motion, or orientation). Parietal activity will therefore occur in tasks that emphasize processing at various locations, as does the shifting task, or in tasks that involve more than one feature at one location, as does the conjunction task.

It is important to emphasize at this point that the functional correspondence between superior parietal cortex and spatial selection operations does not make this area an attentional area, as some models suggest (Posner, 1994). In other words, spatial processing performed in this region can be used for other purposes, and it is possible that the same neurons could perform other operations within other behavioral contexts. For example, regions in posterior parietal cortex near the regions active for shifts of attention are also active during spatial analysis (Haxby et al., 1994), spatial working memory (Smith et al., 1993), and oculomotor behavior (Anderson et al., 1994; Petit et al., 1993). In some experiments, shifts of attention or spatial selection were controlled (Haxby et al., 1994). Correspondingly, anatomical and physiological data indicate that the parietal cortex is formed by several regions (LIP, VIP, 7a, 7B, MST), and that a combination of visual, attentional, memory, and planning neuronal signals can be recorded in those regions, sometimes within the same neuron (Andersen, 1989).

In summary, attention to object location produces selective increases of activity (rCBF enhancement) in specialized processing regions of the ventral, or object-oriented, visual system. That modulation is similar in terms of blood flow to the modulations obtained for attending to other features (i.e., color, motion, or shape), but the underlying neuronal mechanism may well differ in the two cases: neuronal enhancement for feature selection (Motter, 1994) and neuronal filtering of unattended objects for location selection (Moran and Desimone, 1985). The source of the spatial modulation is the superior parietal cortex, the activity of which is sensitive to location information and to integration across features and is independent of several other factors, including effector, presence of an overt response, and type of cueing.

Attentional Templates or Source Signals for Feature or Object and for Location

The neural activity underlying attentional templates is mostly unknown. Most imaging studies have concentrated on demonstrating the effect of attention on visual processing or selective modulations and have not systematically manipulated the template signal in terms of source of instruction (e.g., visual, verbal, or internal), content (e.g., feature, object, or location), or underlying behavioral goal (e.g., reaching or perceiving).

One theoretical proposal is that attentional template signals coincide with short-term memory signals located in prefrontal cortex (Desimone and Duncan, 1995). Single-unit recording in primates indicates that, although both prefrontal and visual areas contain neurons that fire in the delay period between a cue and a stimulus, only prefrontal neurons maintain delay activity across intervening nontarget stimuli (Chelazzi, Miller, Lueschow, and Desimone, 1993; Desimone and Duncan, 1995; Fuster, 1985). Several imaging studies have also demonstrated short-term memory activity in human prefrontal cortex (Smith et al., 1995; Courtney et al., in press). In one fMRI study of working memory for facial identity, activity in several right prefrontal regions preferentially covaried with working memory signal, while activity in several occipito-temporal regions preferentially covaried with selective and nonselective visual processing of face stimuli (Courtney, Ungerleider, Kell, and Haxby, 1997).

Some prefrontal regions that are active for short-term memory tasks are also recruited during attentional tasks involving templates. A superior frontal region, located near Brodmann's area 6, is commonly activated for locational working memory (Smith et al., 1995; Courtney et al., in press) and for endogenous shifts of spatial attention (figure 6.3). Endogenous shifts require a spatial template to direct attention to the relevant location. This region is not active during a conjunction visual search task for targets defined by color and motion (i.e., when the active template is nonspatial). The superior frontal region is a putative candidate for a region that encodes and holds spatial templates. In contrast, the superior parietal cortex, which is similarly active in the endogenous shifting and conjunction task, is better conceptualized as a "slave" spatial map, used to direct the focus of processing to relevant locations or objects under the guidance of both spatial and nonspatial templates.

A right middle prefrontal region, near Brodmann's areas 45 and 46, is commonly activated for object-oriented working memory (Smith et al., 1995; Courtney et al., in press) and when attention is divided across visual features (Corbetta et al., 1991). That region is not active when attention is focused on a single feature. As was previously discussed, the divided attention task places more demands on the attentional template and short-term memory. This region is also not active during the endogenous shifting task. The middle right dorsolateral prefrontal cortex is, therefore, a putative candidate for a region that encodes and holds feature and object templates.

The putative correspondence between short-term memory and attentional templates is speculative at this point. It is unknown whether short-term memory signals can produce the kind of psychophysical facilitation produced by template information (Wolfe, Cave, and Franzel, 1989), or whether short-term memory and template signals will still colocalize when template information is explicitly manipulated in terms of source, content, and behavioral goal.

The hypothesis that there are attentional networks in the brain (Posner and Petersen, 1990; Posner, 1994) is also relevant to the question of the neural activity associated with attentional templates. As discussed previously, the attentional network hypothesis postulates that attentional biases for location and for object identity are generated in lateral prefrontal regions that are related to working memory (as in Desimone and Duncan's model), but that the anterior cingulate region plays a major role in funneling such biases to posterior visual processing regions. The anterior cingulate, a central node in the so-called anterior executive system, is also critical for controlling the access of targets selected in visual regions to focal awareness and to premotor systems. These ideas are based on a variety of lesion, single-unit, and early imaging data, and have been recently reviewed (Posner, 1994; also, see Posner and DiGirolamo, chapter 18, this volume).

More recent PET imaging studies suggest that the anterior cingulate region is better conceptualized as a response selection region that is premotor in nature, rather than as a central executive that feeds top-down signals to posterior visual processing regions. First, several experiments have failed to consistently activate the anterior cingulate region during working memory tasks for location or object identity (Smith et al., 1995; Courtney, Ungerleider, Keil, and Haxby, 1996); consistent activation would be expected if attentional templates coincided with short-term memory and if the anterior cingulate region was feeding information to posterior regions. Moreover, in one experiment that correlated activity in frontal regions with length of the memory delay for face identity, the anterior cingulate was active only at longer delays (21 s) along with left prefrontal cortex, whereas right prefrontal cortex was active throughout (1–21 s) (Haxby et al., 1995). Those findings are consistent with a role for the right prefrontal cortex in visual encoding and storage, which presumably occurs throughout the delay, and for left prefrontal cortex and anterior cingulate in other processes, such as semantic encoding, that are recruited only later in the delay.

Second, other experiments have failed to generalize a role for the anterior cingulate in target detection across semantic and visual domains. Cognitive psychology experiments have indicated that target detection is a probe operation for conscious processing, and an earlier PET study has shown that anterior cingulate activity increased with the number of targets presented in a semantic monitoring task (Posner et al., 1988). More recently, several experiments have reevaluated the relationship between cingulate activity and target probability during visual discrimination tasks across a wide range of probabilities. Woldorff et al. (1995) had observers perform a peripheral object discrimination task with two different target rates (2% vs. 16%) and found no differential cingulate activation in the low vs. high probability condition. We have examined several visual search tasks using various combinations of features (e.g., color and orientation, color and motion) at different target probability levels (20% vs. 80%; 5% vs. 50%; 5% vs. 45%) (Corbetta et al., 1996). Target-probability effects were documented in visual regions, suggesting that a distinction between target and nontargets, at least for targets defined by the combination of simple features, does not necessarily involve anterior regions of the brain. Therefore, the anterior cingulate does not contain a general purpose mechanism for regulating the access of any target to conscious processing, although it may play a role in the detection of semantic targets.

Third, a recent large meta-analysis of PET experiments that compared brain activity during active visual processing versus passive viewing of the same stimuli failed to show any anterior cingulate activity that generalizes across tasks, which might have predicted if the cingulate works as a "central executive process" in different cognitive domains (Shulman et al., 1997a).

Fourth, anatomical, physiological, and imaging studies indicate that the anterior cingulate region is heterogeneous and includes multiple representations (Vogt et al., 1992). In monkeys, cingulate regions buried in the sulcus are predominantly motor-oriented, whereas regions on the gyrus have more connections with limbic structures. A recent meta-analysis of PET studies activating the cingulate region (Picard and Strick, 1996) distinguishes between three cingulate zones on the basis of task complexity and motor effector. The rostral cingulate zones are active during more complex internally generated and less deterministic responses, and as expected they co-localize with regions active during attentional paradigms (Corbetta et al., 1991; Pardo, Pardo, Janer, and Raichle, 1990; Petersen, Fox, Posner, Mintun, and Raichle,

1988). However, these zones also show somatotopy, which indicates a relationship with motor variables. Although the issue of whether attentional foci colocalize with foci obtained in more standard motor tasks will be resolved only through finer mapping experiments within the same subject, these data at least suggest that a premotor explanation of certain cingulate activity fits a large body of PET activation data and nicely fits current anatomo-physiological models.

In summary, the current PET evidence indicates that the anterior cingulate region (or the rostral cingulate zones, to use Picard and Strick's terms) is more involved in response selection than in central executive functions, including top-down funneling of cognitive biases in posterior visual regions. The type of response selection driving the cingulate region is not well specified, but appears to involve representational behavior. The prefrontal cortex, linked by various sources to representational internally guided behavior (Goldman-Rakic, 1994), is invariable activated along with the anterior cingulate cortex. Various flavors of representational behavior have been emphasized by different papers: inhibition of prepotent responses (Pardo et al., 1990), willed action (Frith, Friston, Liddle, and Frackowiack, 1991), integration across multiple channels (Corbetta et al., 1991), internally guided motor selection (Deiber et al., 1991), semantic associations (Petersen et al., 1989), and controlled speech or motor production (Raichle et al., 1994; Jenkins, Brooks, Nixon, Frackowiack, and Passingham, 1994).

CONCLUSIONS

PET has become a major tool for the exploration of human cognition. It allows researchers to monitor neuronal activity within a well-defined spatio-temporal bandwidth in the whole brain during cognitive processing. PET studies of human attention are providing new information about the functional anatomy of visual attention and awareness. Visual attention is not a unitary phenomenon, and multiple sites of selection have been localized in the brain as function of task demands. Visual responses can be clearly modulated by a combination of nonselective and selective signals as early as primary visual cortex and as late as frontal cortex. Attention to feature or to objects amplifies relevant information in specialized processing regions of extrastriate visual regions. Regions in the superior parietal cortex select locations and object locations for focal processing, biasing activity in ventral regions related to object processing. The neural basis of attentional templates is presently unknown, but may involve prefrontal regions related to working memory.

ACKNOWLEDGMENTS

I would like to thank Gordon Shulman and Steve Petersen for comments on an earlier draft. This work was supported by the Charles A. Dana Foundation, the McDonnell Center for Studies of Higher Brain Function, and by National Institutes of Health grants NS06833, NS2533, EY08775, and NS32979.

REFERENCES

Allport A. (1989) Visual attention. In *Foundations of Cognitive Science*, edited by M. I. Posner. Cambridge, MA: MIT Press.

Andersen, R. A. (1989) Visual eye movement functions of the posterior parietal cortex. *Annu. Rev. Neurosci.* 12: 377–403.

Anderson, T. J., Jenkins, I. H., Brooks, D. J., Hawken, M. B., Frackowiack, R. S. J., and Kennard, C. (1994) Cortical control of saccades and fixation in a man. A PET study. *Brain* 117: 1073–1084.

Broadbent, D. E. (1958) *Perception and Communication*. London: Pergamon Press.

Bush, G., Rosen, B., Belliveau, J., Reppas, J., Rauch, S. L., Kennedy, D., and Sutton, J. (1995) A functional magnetic resonance study of selective and divided attention during visual discrimination of shape, speed, and color. *Soc. Neurosci. Abstr.* 21: 936.

Bushnell, M. C., Goldberg, M. E., and Robinson, D. L. (1981) Behavioral enhancement of visual responses in monkey cerebral cortex. I. Modulation in posterior parietal cortex related to selective attention. *J. Neurophysiol.* 46: 755–772.

Chelazzi, L., Miller, E. K., Lueschow, A., and Desimone, R. (1993) Dual mechanisms of short-term memory: Ventral prefrontal cortex. *Soc. Neurosci. Abstr.* 19: 975.

Collins, D. L., Neelin, P., Peters, T. M., and Evans, A. C. (1994) Automatic 3D intersubject registration of MR volumetric data in standardized Talairach space. *J. Comp. Assist. Tomogr.* 18: 192–205.

Corbetta, M., Miezin, F. M., Dobmeyer, S., Shulman, G. L., and Petersen, S. E. (1991) Selective and divided attention during visual discrimination of shape, color, and speed: Functional anatomy by positron emission tomography. *J. Neurosci.* 11: 2383–2492.

Corbetta, M., Miezin, F. M., Shulman, G. L., and Petersen, S. E. (1993) A PET study of visuospatial attention. *J. Neurosci.* 13: 1202–1226.

Corbetta, M., Shulman, G. L., Miezin, F. M., and Petersen, S. E. (1995) Superior parietal cortex activation during spatial attention shifts and visual feature conjunction. *Science* 270: 802–805.

Courtney, S. M., Ungerleider, L. G., Keil, K., and Haxby, J. V. (1996) Object and spatial visual working memory activate separate neural systems in human cortex *Cereb. Cortex* 6: 39–49.

Courtney, S. M., Ungerleider, L. G., Kell, K., and Haxby J. V. (1997) Transient and sustained activity in a distributed neural system for human working memory. *Nature* 386: 608–611.

Cox, S. B., Woolsey, T. A., and Rovainen, C. M. (1993) Localized dymanic changes in cortical blood flow with whisker stimulation corresponds to matched vascular and neuronal architecture. *J. Cereb. Blood Flow Metab.* 13: 899–913.

Creutzfeld, O. D. (1975) Neurophysiological correlates of different functional states of the brain. In *Brain Work: The Coupling of Function, Metabolism and Blood Flow in the Brain*, edited by D. H. Ingvar and N. A. Lassen, pp. 22–47. Copenhagen: Munksgaard.

De Yoe, E. A., Schmit, P. W., and Neitz, J. (1995) Distinguishing cortical areas that are sensitive to task and stimulus variables with fMRI. *Soc. Neurosci. Abstr.* 21: 1760.

Deiber, M P., Passingham, R. E., Colebatch, J. G., Friston, K. J., Nixon, P. D., and Frackowiack, R. S. J. (1991) Cortical areas and the selection of movement: A study with positron emission tomography. *Exp. Brain Res.* 84: 393–402.

Desimone, R. and Duncan, J. (1995) Neural mechanisms of selective visual attention. *Annu. Rev. Neurosci.* 18: 193–222.

Desimone, R. and Ungerleider, L. E. (1989) Neural mechanisms of visual processing in monkeys. In *Handbook of Neuropsychology*, edited by H. Goodglass and A. R. Damasio, pp. 267–300. Amsterdam: Elsevier.

Donders, F. C. (1869) On the speed of mental processes. *Acta Psychol.* 30: 412–431.

Duncan, J. (1984) Selective attention and the organization of visual information. *J. Exp. Psychol. Gen.* 113: 501–517.

Duncan, J. and Humphreys, G. W. (1989) Visual search and stimulus similarity. *Psychol. Rev.* 96: 433–458.

Dupont, P., Orban, G. A., Vogels, R., Bormans, G., Nuyts, J., Schiepers, C., De Roo, M., and Mortelmans, L. (1993) Different perceptual tasks performed with the same visual stimulus attribute activate different regions of the human brain: A positron emission tomography study. *Proc. Natl. Acad. Sci.* 90: 10927–10931.

Felleman, D. J. and Van Essen, D. C. (1991) Distibuted hierarchical processing in the primate cerebral cortex. *Cereb. Cortex* 1: 1–47.

Ferrera, V. P., Rudolph, K. K., and Maunsell, J. H. R. (1994) Responses of neurons in the parietal and temporal visual pathways during a motion task. *J. Neurosci.* 14: 6171–6186.

Fiez, J. A., Raichle, M. E., Miezin, F. M., Petersen, S. E., Tallal, P., and Katz, W. F. (1995) PET studies of auditory and phonological processing: Effects of stimulus characteristics and task demands. *J. Cog. Neurosci.* 7: 357–375.

Fox, P. T. and Mintun, M. A. (1989) Noninvasive functional brain mapping by change-distribution analysis of averaged PET images of $H_2^{15}O$. *J. Nucl. Med.* 30: 141–149.

Fox, P. T., Mintun, M. A., Reiman, E. M., and Raichle, M. E. (1988) Enhanced detection of focal brain responses using intersubject averaging and change distribution analysis of subtracted PET images. *J. Cereb. Bloob Flow Metab.* 8: 642–653.

Fox, P. T. and Raichle, M. E. (1985) Stimulus rate determines regional blood flow in striate cortex. *Ann. Neurol.* 17: 303–305.

Fox, P. T. and Raichle, M. E. (1986) Focal physiological uncoupling of cerebral blood flow and oxidative metabolism during somatosensory stimulation in human subjects. *Proc. Natl. Acad. Sci. U S A* 83: 1140–1144.

Friedman-Hill, S. R., Robertson, L. C., and Treisman, A. (1995) Parietal contibutions to visual feature binding: Evidence from a patient with bilateral lesions. *Science* 269: 853–855.

Friston, K. J., Frith, C. D., Liddle, P. F., and Frackowiack, R. S. J. (1991) Comparing functional (PET) images: The assessment of significant change. *J. Cereb. Blood Flow Metab.* 11: 690–699.

Frith, C. D., Friston, K. J., Liddle, P. F., and Frackowiack, R. S. J. (1991) Willed action and the prefrontal cortex in man: A study with PET. *Proc. R. Soc. Lond. B. Biol. Sci.* 244: 241–246.

Frostig, R. D., Lieke, E. E., Tso, D. Y., and Grinvald, A. (1990) Cortical functional architecture and local coupling between neuronal activity and the microcirculation revealed by in-vivo high resolution optical imaging of intrinsic signals. *Proc. Natl. Acad. Sci. USA* 87: 6082–6086.

Fulton, J. F. (1926) Observations upon the vascularity of the human occipital lobe during visual activity. *Brain* 51: 310–328.

Fuster, J. M. (1985) The prefrontal cortex and temporal integration. In *Cerebral Cortex*, edited by E. G. Jones and A. Peters, pp. 151–177. New York: Plenum.

Gall, C. M. and Lauterborn, J. C. (1991) Activity-dependent neuronal gene expression: A potential memory mechanism? In *Memory: Organization and Locus of Change*, edited by L. R. Squire, N. M. Weinberger, G. Lynch, and G. L. McGaugh, pp. 301–329. New York: Oxford University Press.

Goldman-Rakic, P. S. (1994) The issue of memory in the study of prefrontal function. In *Motor and Cognitive Functions of the Prefrontal Cortex*, edited by A. M. Thierry, J. Glowinski, P. S. Goldman-Rakic, and Y. Christen, pp. 112–121. New York: Springer.

Haenny, P. E., Maunsell, J. H. R., and Schiller, P. H. (1988) State dependent activity in monkey visual cortex. II. Retinal and extraretinal factors in V4. *Exp. Brain Res.* 69: 245–259.

Haxby, J. V., Horwitz, B., Ungerleider, L. G., Maisog, J. M., Pietrini, P., and Grady, C. L. (1994) The functional organization of human extrastriate cortex: A PET-rCBF study of selective attention to faces and locations. *J. Neurosci.* 14: 6336–6353.

Haxby, J. V., Ungerleider, L. G., Horwitz, B., Rapoport, S. I., and Grady, C. L. (1995) Hemispheric differences in neural systems for face working memory: A PET-rCBF study. *Hum. Brain Map.* 3: 68–82.

Heintz, H. J., Mangun, G. R., Burchert, W., Hinrichs, H., Scholz, M., Munte, T. F., Gos, A., Scherg, M., Johannes, S., Hundeshagen, H., Gazzaniga, M. S., and Hillyard, S. A. (1995) Combined spatial and temporal imaging of brain activity during visual selective attention in humans. *Nature* 372: 543–546.

Hunton, D. L., Corbetta, M., Shulman, G. L., Miezin, F. M., and Petersen, S. E. (1995) common areas of parietal activation for shifts of spatial attention and tasks involving the conjunction of visual features. *Soc. Neurosci. Abstr.* 21: 937.

Iadecola, C. (1993) Regulation of the cerebral microcirculation during neural activity: Is nitric oxide the missing link? *Trends Neurosci* 16: 206–214.

Jenkins, I. H., Brooks, D. J., Nixon, P. D., Frackowiack, R. S. J., and Passingham, R. E. (1994) Motor sequence learning: A study with positron emission tomography. *J. Neurosci.* 14: 3775–3790.

Kanwisher, N. and Driver, J. (1992) Objects, attributes, and visual attention: Which, what, and where. *Psychol. Sci.* 1: 1–5.

Landau, W. M., Freygang, W. H. J., Roland, L. P., Sokoloff, L., and Kety, S. S. (1955) The local circulation of the living brain: Values in the unanestethized and anesthetized cat. *Trans. Am. Neurol. Assoc.* 80: 125–129.

Mangun, G. R., Hillyard, S. A., and Luck S. J. (1993) Electrocortical substrates of visual selective attention. In *Attention and Performance XIV*, edited by D. Meyer and S. Kornblum. Cambridge, MA: MIT Press.

Marr, D. E. (1982) *Vision*. San Francisco: W. H. Freeman.

Maunsell, J. H. R. (1995) The brain's visual world: Representation of visual targets in cerebral cortex. *Science* 270: 764–768.

Miller, E. K., Li, L., and Desimone, R. (1993) Activity of neurons in anterior inferior temporal cortex during a short-term memory task. *J. Neurosci.* 13: 1460–1478.

Moran, J. and Desimone, R. (1985) Selective attention gates visual processing in extrastriate cortex. *Science* 229: 782–784.

Motter, B. C. (1994) Neural correlates of attentive slection for color or luminance in extrastriate area V4. *J. Neurosci.* 14: 2178–2189.

Mountcastle, V. B., Motter, B. C., Steinmatz, M. A., and Sestokas, A. K. (1987) Common and differential effects of attentive fixation on the excitability of parietal and prestriate (V4) cortical visual neurons in the macaque monkey. *J. Neurosci.* 7: 2239–2255.

Nobre, A. C., Sebestyen, G. N., Gitelman, D. R., Mesulam, M. M., Frackoviack, R. S. J., and Frith, C. D. (1997) Functional localization of the system for visuospatial attention using positron emission tomography. *Brain* 120: 515–533.

Ogawa, S., Tank, D. W., Menon, R., Ellerman, J. M., Kim, S. G., Merkle, H., and Ugurbil, K. (1992) Intrinsic signal changes accompanying sensory stimulation: Functional brainmapping with magnetic resonance imaging. *Proc. Natl. Acad. Sci. U S A* 89: 5951–5955.

Olshausen, B. A., Anderson, C. H., and Van Essen, D. C. (1993) A neurobiological model of visual attention and invariant pattern recognition based on dynamic routing of information. *J. Neurosci.* 13: 4700–4719.

Pardo, J. V., Pardo, P. J., Janer, K.W., and Raichle, M. E. (1990) The anterior cingulate cortex mediates processing selection in the Stroop attentional conflict paradigm. *Proc. Natl. Acad. Sci. U.S.A.* 87: 256–259.

Petersen, S. E., Corbetta, M., Miezin, F. M., and Shulman, G. L. (1994) PET studies of parietal involvement in spatial attention: Comparison of different task types. *Can. J. Exp. Psych.* 48: 319–338.

Petersen, S. E., Corbetta, M., Miezin, F. M., shulman, G. L., and Raichle, M. E. (1993) The effects of selective attention on visual processing measured with performance and PET (positron emission tomography). In *Brain Mechanisms of Perception and Memory: From Neuron to Behavior*, edited by T. Ono, L. Squire, D. Perrett, and M. E. Raichle, pp. 413–425. New York: Oxford University Press.

Petersen, S. E., Fox, P. T., Posner, M. I., Mintun, M., and Raichle, M. E. (1989) Positron emission tomographic studies of the processing of single words. *J. Cog. Neurosci.* 1: 153–170.

Petit, L., Orssaud, C., Tzourio, N., Salamon, G., Mazoyer, B., and Berthoz, A. (1993) PET study of voluntary saccadic eye movements in humans: Basal ganglia-thalamocortical system and cingulate cortex involvement. *J. Neurophysiol.* 69: 1009–1017.

Phelps, M. E., Kuhl, D. E., and Mazziotta, J. C. (1981) Metabolic mapping of the brain's response to visual stimulation: Studies in humans. *Science* 211: 1445–1448.

Picard, N. and Strick, P. L. (1996) Motor areas of the medial wall: A review of their location and functional activation. *Cereb. Cortex* 6: 342–353.

Posner, M. I. (1980) Orienting of attention. *Q. J. Exp. Psychol.* 32: 3–25.

Posner, M. I. (1994) Attention: The mechanisms of consciousness. *Proc. Natl. Acad. Sci. U S A* 91: 7398–7403.

Posner, M. I. and Petersen, S. E. (1990) The attention system of the human brain. *Annu. Rev. Neurosci.* 13: 25–42.

Posner, M. I., Petersen, S. E., Fox, P. T., and Raichle, M. E. (1988) Localization of cognitive functions in the human brain. *Science* 240: 1627–1631.

Raichle, M. E. (1987) Circulatory and metabolic correlates of brain function in normal humans. In *Handbook of Physiology: Vol.5. The Nervous System*, edited by F. Plum, pp. 643–674. Bethesda, MD: American Physiological Society.

Raichle, M. E. (1994) Visualizing the mind. *Sci. Am.* 270: 36–42.

Raichle, M. E., Fiez, J. A., Videen, T. O., MacLeod, A. K., Pardo, J. V., Fox, P. T., and Petersen, S. E. (1994) Practice-related changes in human brain functional anatomy during non-motor learning. *Cereb. Cortex* 4: 8–26.

Raichle, M. E., Martin, W. R. W., Herscovitch, P., Mintun, M. A., and Markham J. (1983) Brain blood flow measured with intravenous $H_2{}^{15}O$. II. Implementation and validation. *J. Nucl. Med.* 24: 790–798.

Reivich, M., Kuhl, D., Wolf, A., Greenberg, J., Phelps, M. E., Ido, T., Casella, V., Fowler, J., Hofman E., Alavi, A., Som, P., and Sololoff, L. M. (1979) The [18F] fluorodeoxiglucose method for the measurment of local glucose utilization in man. *Circ. Res.* 44: 127–137.

Schmidt, C. F. and Hendrix, J. P. (1937) The action of chemical substances on cerebral blood vessels. *Res. Pub. Assoc. Res. Nerv. Ment. Dis.* 18: 229–276.

Schwartz, W. J., Smith, C. B., Davidsen, H., Savaki, L., Sokoloff, L., Mata, M., Fink, D. J., and Gainer, H. (1979) Metabolic mapping of functional activity in the hypothalamo-neurohypophysial system of the rat. *Science* 205: 723–725.

Sergent, J., Ohta, S., and MacDonald, B. (1992) Functional neuroanatomy of face and object processing: A positron emission tomography study. *Brain* 115: 15–36.

Serota, H. M. and Gerard, R. W. (1938) Localized thermal changes in the cat's brain. *J. Neurophysiol.* 1: 115–124.

Shulman, G. L., Corbetta, M., Buckner, R. L., Fiez, J. A., Miezin, M. E., and Petersen, S. E. (1997a) Common blood flow changes across visual tasks: I. Increases in subcortical structures and cerebellum, but not in non-visual cortexx. *J. Cog. Neurosci.*, in press.

Shulman, G. L., Fiez, J. A., Corbetta, M., Buckner, R. L., Miezin, F. M., Raichle, M. E., and Petersen, S. E. (1997b) Common blood flow changes across visual tasks: II. Decreases in cerebral cortex. *J. Cog. Neurosci.*, in press.

Silbersweig, D. A., Stern, E., Frith, C. D., Cahil, C., Schnorr, L., Grootoonk, S., Clark, J., Frackowiack, R. S. J., and Jones, T. (1993) Detection of thirty-second cognitive activations in single subjects with positron emission tomography: A new low dose $H_2^{15}O$ regional cerebral blood flow tridimensional imaging technique. *J. Cereb. Blood Flow Metab.* 1: 617–629.

Smith, E. E., Jonides, J., Koeppe, R. A., Awh, E., Schumacher, E. H., and Minoshima, S. (1995) Spatial versus object working memory: PET investigations. *J. Cog. Neurosci.* 7: 337–356.

Snyder, A. Z., Abdullaev, Y. G., Posner, M. I., and Raichle, M. E. (1995) Scalp electrical potentials reflect regional cerebral blood flow responses during processing of written words. *Proc. Natl. Acad. Sci. U S A* 92: 1689–1693.

Sokoloff, L. M., Reivich, M., Kennedy, C., Des Rosiers, M. H., Patlak, C. S., Pettigrew, K. D., Sakurada, O., and Shinohara, O. (1977) The [14C] deoxiglucose method for the measurement of local cerebral glucose utilization: Theory, procedure and normal values in the conscious nad anesthetized albino rat. *J. Neurochem.* 28: 897–916.

Squire, L. R., Ojemann, J. G., Miezin, F. M., Petersen, S. E., Videen, T. O., and Raichle, M. E. (1992) Activation of the hippocampus in normal humans: A functional anatomical study of memory. *Proc. Natl. Acad. Sci. U S A* 89: 1837–1841.

Sternberg, S. (1969) The discovery of processing stages: Extensions of Donder's method. *Acta Psychol.* 30: 276–315.

Talairach, J. and Tournoux, P. (1988) *Co-Planar Stereotaxic Atlas of the Human Brain.* New York: Thieme Medical.

Ter-Pogossian, M. M. (1977) Basic principles of computed axial tomography. *Semin. Nucl. Med.* 7: 109–127.

Tootell, R. B. H., Reppas, J. B., Kwong, K. K., Malach, R., Born, R. T., Brady, T. J., Rosen, B. R., and Belliveau, J. W. (1995) Functional analysis of hyman MT and related visual cortical areas using magnetic resonance imaging. *J. Neurosci.* 15: 3215–3230.

Treisman, A. M. and Gelade, G. (1980) A feature-integration of theory of attention. *Cognit. Psychol.* 12: 97–136.

Vanderberghe, R., Duncan, J., Dupont, P., Ward, R., Bormans, G., Mortemans, L., and Orban, G. A (1995) Superior parietal blood flow depends on the number of attended attributes. *Hum. Brain Map. Suppl.* 1: 269.

Vandenberghe, R., Dupont, P., Debruyn, B., Bormans, G., Michiels, J., Mortelmans, L., and Orban, G. A. (1996) The influence of stimulus location on the brain activation pattern in detection and orientation discrimination—A PET study of visual attention. *Brain* 119: 1263–1276.

Vanderberghe, R., Duncan, J., Dupont, P., Ward, R., Poline, J.-B., Bormans, G., Michiels, J., Mortelmans, L., and Orban, G. A. (1997) Attention to one or two features in left and right visual field: A positron emission tomography study. *J. Neurosci.* 17: 3739–3750.

Vanderberghe, R., Dupont, P., Rosier, A., Bruyn, B., Mortelmans, L., and Orban, G. A. (1994) Maintaining attention on an extrafoveal stimulus activates the contralateral parietal lobule in a feature discrimination task: A PET activation experiment. *Soc. Neurosci. Abstr.* 20: 1666.

Vogel, R., Eeckout, H., and Orban, G. (1988) The effect of feature uncertainty on spatial discriminations. *Perception* 17: 565–577.

Vogt, B. A., Finch, D. M., and Olson, C. R. (1992) Functional heterogeneity in cingulate cortex: The anterior executive and posterior evaluative regions. *Cereb. Cortex* 2: 435–443.

Watson, J. D., Myers, R., Frackowiak, R. S., Hajnal, J. V., Woods, R. P., Mazziotta, J. C., Shipp, S., and Zeki, S. (1993). Area V5 of the human brain: Evidence from a combined study using positron emission tomography and magnetic resonance imaging. *Cereb. Cortex* 3: 79–94.

Woldorff, M., Fox, T., Matzke, M., Veeraswamy, S., Jerabek, P., and Martin, C. (1995) Combined PET and ERP study of sustained visual spatial attention and visual target detection. *Hum. Brain Map. Suppl.* 1: 49.

Wolfe, J. M., Cave, K. R., and Franzel, S. L. (1989) Guided search: An alternative to the feature integration model for visual search. *J. Exp. Psychol. Hum. Percept. Perform.* 15: 419–433.

Woods, R. P., Mazziotta, J. C., and Cherry, S. R. (1993) MRI-PET registration with automated algorithm. *J. Comp. Ass. Tomogr.* 17: 536–546.

Worsley, K. J., Evans, A. C., Marret, S., and Neelin, P. (1992) A three-dimensional statistical analysis for CBF activation studies in human brain. *J. Cereb. Blood Flow Metabol.* 12: 900–918.

Wurtz, R. H., Goldberg, M. E., and Robinson, D. L. (1980) Behavioral modulation of visual responses in monkeys. *Prog. Psychobiol. Physiol. Psychol.* 9: 43–83.

Yarowsky, P., Kadekard, M., and Sokoloff, L. (1983) Frequency dependent activation of glucose utilization in the superior cervical ganglion by electrical stimulation of cervical sympathetic trunk. *Proc. Natl. Acad. Sci. U S A* 80: 4179–4183.

7 Functional Magnetic Resonance Imaging and the Study of Attention

James V. Haxby, Susan M. Courtney,
and Vincent P. Clark

ABSTRACT   Functional magnetic resonance imaging (fMRI) affords an unprecedented window onto function in the intact human brain. This chapter describes imaging methods using the blood oxygenation level dependent (BOLD) technique of fMRI. Experimental designs and image analysis methods for examining neural activity related to attention are discussed. Attention-related neural changes can reflect either (1) different modulatory effects on information processing, or (2) the activity of control systems that invoke and regulate those modulatory effects. At the current stage of fMRI research, only some effects in the former category have been reported. Although the latter category has not been studied with fMRI, appropriately designed fMRI studies may help to identify the components of attentional control systems.

In the early 1990s fortuitious insights and advances in the physics of magnetic resonance imaging (MRI) led to the discovery that MRI could be used to measure hemodynamic processes noninvasively in the human brain. Unlike positron emission tomography (PET), new methods for functional MRI (fMRI) required no exposure to ionizing radiation, no injections of tracers, and no sampling of blood. Technical difficulties imposed by working in a powerful ambient magnetic field were quickly overcome, and fMRI studies of the neural basis of human cognition have proliferated.

fMRI has the potential to be a powerful tool for investigating attention and other cognitive processes. At the time this review was written, numerous groups were already conducting fMRI studies of various types of attention. Because much of this work has been presented only at scientific meetings and has been published only in abstract form, this chapter focuses on a presentation of issues in imaging methods, experimental design, and image analysis that will influence the kind of information about attention that can be acquired using fMRI. Ongoing fMRI research on attention is referred to when relevant, but, aside from our own research, cannot yet be presented critically in detail.

THE PHYSICAL BASIS OF MRI

MRI uses the radio frequency (RF) electromagnetic waves emitted by the nuclei of hydrogen atoms with single-proton nuclei to construct detailed images of the brain and other organs. In an MRI scanner the magnetic dipoles of individual protons become aligned with the strong magnetic field of the scanner. The direction of the magnetic dipoles is perturbed by an RF pulse generated by gradient coils in the scanner. After the perturbation, the protons wobble, or precess, back to their original alignment. The precession has a frequency, called the Larmor or resonance frequency, that is specific to the type of nucleus, in this case single protons, and for the strength of the magnetic field. For example, single protons in a 1.5 tesla magnetic field, a strength typical of most scanners used for fMRI, has a resonance frequency of 63.84 MHz. A detectable radio signal at the resonance frequency is generated by protons that are precessing in phase with each other. The receiving coils in the scanner detect the radio signal emitted by the tiny senders. Spatial information about the location of the protons is afforded by slightly altering the strength of the magnetic field over the volume being imaged, and thereby altering the frequency and phase of signals emitted by protons at different locations.

Blood Oxygen Level Dependent fMRI

Broadly defined, fMRI refers to numerous methods for obtaining information about hemodynamic processes. This review focuses on the subset of those methods that is currently used for most fMRI studies of human cognition. This subset relies on blood oxygenation level dependent (BOLD) changes in the intensity of the magnetic resonance (MR) signal. MR imaging of BOLD changes is based on a difference in the magnetic property of oxygenated versus deoxygenated hemoglobin (Pauling and Coryell, 1936; Thulborn, Waterton, Matthews, and Radda, 1982). Whereas oxyhemoglobin is diamagnetic, or essentially nonmagnetic, deoxyhemoglobin is paramagnetic, meaning that it acquires a magnetic field of its own when placed in a magnetic field. In the magnetic field of a MRI scanner, deoxyhemoglobin molecules become magnetic. The presence of these small magnetic fields produces local inhomogeneities in the magnetic field that cause protons to precess out of phase with each other. The result is a decrease in the $T2^*$ component of the MR signal. A second, physiological phenomenon makes the change in MR signal useful for cognitive neuroscience studies. Changes in local neural activity cause a change in local blood flow (Roy and Sherrington, 1890). The change in blood flow is greater than the change in oxygen consumption (Fox and Raichle, 1986). The reason for the mismatch between blood flow and oxygen extraction changes is quite controversial. Whatever the physiological basis, the result is an increase in the level of blood oxygenation when blood flow increases, and, surprisingly, a decrease in blood oxygenation when blood flow decreases (Clark et al., 1996). The BOLD changes can be detected with $T2^*$-weighted MRI methods, affording indices of local hemodynamic changes that are induced by changes in neural activity (Kwong et al., 1992; Ogawa et al., 1992; Turner, LeBihan, Jezzard, Despres, and Taylor,

1992). A brightening of the image reflects an increase in blood oxygenation and indicates an increase in neural activity. A darkening of the image reflects a decrease in blood oxygenation and indicates a decrease in neural activity.

At the present time, those changes in image intensity cannot be translated into precise measures of the magnitude of change in blood oxygenation. Moreover, other hemodynamic factors, such as blood volume, also affect image intensity. The uncertainties about the physiological basis of the relationship between blood oxygenation, blood flow, and neural activity, and about the physiological basis of MR signal changes, are a matter of concern to everyone who uses fMRI. Nonetheless, these uncertainties need not inhibit cognitive neuroscience research using fMRI, because a strong link between the fMRI signal and changes in neural activity is beyond doubt, whatever its basis. Nevertheless, cognitive neuroscientists should be aware of progress in research on the physiological basis of fMRI and in MR imaging methods.

Fast Imaging Methods

The final advance in MRI physics that made modern fMRI possible was the development of fast imaging techniques (Turner and Jezzard, 1995). The most widely used fast imaging method is echo-planar imaging (EPI), which allows the acquisition of a complete cross-sectional image from one excitation pulse. A second rapid imaging method, spiral imaging, uses a more efficient search of frequency space than EPI and will probably be used more with improvements in gradient coil design, which are necessary to take full advantage of it. With those fast imaging methods and current standard echo-speed gradients, it is possible to obtain multiple cross-sectional images every second. A volume of cross-sectional images that contains most or all of the brain can be obtained every 2 to 6 seconds, depending on the spatial resolution of the images, the method being used, and the performance characteristics of the scanner system.

As was mentioned at the beginning of this section, other MRI methods are available that detect hemodynamic changes. Most promising among those are methods that directly measure blood flow, rather than the more indirect BOLD changes. At the present time, however, those blood flow measurement methods do not allow the rapid acquisition of volume images and are, therefore, not as useful for cognitive neuroscience studies.

The Hemodynamic Response Function

The signal change seen with fMRI typically lags behind the onset of stimulation or motor activity. The offset between sensory stimulation or motor activity and the associated change in neural activity is presumably on the order of tens or hundreds of milliseconds. The hemodynamic change measured by fMRI, on the other hand, does not reach its maximum for 4 to 8 seconds.

The function relating a change in neural activity to a hemodynamic change is called the hemodynamic response function (Boynton, Engel, Glover, and Heeger, 1996; Friston, Jezzard, and Turner, 1994). Most attempts to describe the transfer function have been atheoretical searches for mathematical functions that best fit the observed change in MR signal intensity. Those mathematical descriptions generally assume that the change in neural activity is a square wave, representing an essentially instantaneous change in neural activity to a new steady state that is coincident with the sensory, cognitive, or motor change. The delayed and smoothed hemodynamic change elicited by the change in neural activity has been modeled as a linear ramp or as a nonlinear curve with the shape of half of a Poisson or a Gaussian distribution.

A mathematical model of the hemodynamic response function is necessary for the analysis of fMRI data sets because it provides the basis for deriving the predicted fMRI time series so that the fit of the predicted response to the obtained response can be tested.

FMRI EXPERIMENTAL DESIGN AND DATA ANALYSIS

As compared to previous functional brain imaging methods, such as PET and other nuclear medicine procedures for measuring cerebral blood flow, fMRI offers the cognitive neuroscientist much greater freedom in experimental design. Unlike nuclear medicine procedures, which integrate activity over durations measured in tens of seconds, fMRI measures are virtually instantaneous, making the hemodynamic response the only factor that limits temporal resolution. A second advantage is the ability to obtain a virtually unlimited number of measures because fMRI is not limited by radiation dose restrictions. Consequently, enough data from one individual can be collected to perform massive signal averaging, increasing sensitivity and precision sufficiently to obtain detailed maps of responses in an individual brain. Removing the limit on data set size also allows the cognitive neuroscientist to test more experimental conditions in an individual subject and to test changes in neural response that occur over days, weeks, or months with various forms of learning.

Fundamentals of Experimental Design

An fMRI experiment consists of a series of images obtained over a period of time that typically lasts from one to 20 minutes. One such series of images shall be referred to as an fMRI time series. The length of the time series can be limited by scanner performance characteristics and scanner system memory capacity. Additional time series can be obtained, without removing the subject from the scanner, to increase the data set size and increase the signal-to-noise ratio. For every doubling of data set size, the standard error of the noise is reduced by $\sqrt{2}$. Consequently, obtaining four time series instead of one doubles the sensitivity of the experiment and affords detection of signal changes that are one half the magnitude of changes detected with a single series. Likewise, obtaining eight time series affords detection of signal changes that are 35% $(1/\sqrt{8})$ the size of changes detected with a single series.

Contrasts between conditions are best made within time series to minimize the confounding of BOLD changes with intensity changes due to head movement. Head movement is a major source of data degradation in fMRI experiments. A small head movement can cause a large change in signal intensity in an image volume element that is unrelated to blood oxygenation and neural activity. This signal intensity change is due to the change in the type of tissue or substance (gray matter, white matter, or cerebrospinal fluid) contained in that volume element. Signal intensities for those tissue types vary more than the differences caused by changes in blood oxygenation. Misalignment of scans caused by between-scan head movements can be partially corrected with software, but such corrections can be inadequate for correcting large movements.

Experimental Designs Based on Between-Task Contrasts: Subtraction and Parametric Variation

Most functional brain-imaging research is based on the assumption that the pattern of activity measured during the performance of a task reflects all of the sensory, cognitive, and motor components of that task. The functional image is seen as a measure of the total integrated neural activity associated with the complete task. That assumption makes sense for nuclear medicine procedures for measuring hemodynamics that integrate activity over periods measured in tens of seconds. It is not a necessary assumption for fMRI, however, as will be made clear in the next section. Under that assumption, the isolation of the activity related to a single cognitive component of a task requires the comparison of tasks that are matched on all other components except the one of interest. If the comparison is between a pair of tasks, then the comparison is a subtraction. If the comparison is across a series of tasks that systematically vary the component of interest in a graded fashion, then the comparison is a correlation.

Task subtraction is by far the most common experimental design in functional brain imaging research. In attention studies, tasks can be contrasted that involve attention to different stimulus locations (e.g., right or left field) or attributes (e.g., motion or color). Although used less often, parametric variation is a potentially more powerful experimental design because it has the potential to reveal the quantitative relationship between a cognitive parameter, such as attention or difficulty, and neural activity.

In a typical fMRI experiment using between-task contrasts, multiple scans are obtained over a period of 10 to 60 seconds while a subject performs each task. Each task block, therefore, has to consist of a homogeneous set of trials.

Haxby, Courtney, & Clark: Functional Magnetic Resonance Imaging

Experimental Designs That Examine Within-Task Changes in Activity

Experimental designs that contrast components between tasks preclude manipulations that can be critical for studies of attention. For example, if attention shifts between locations or attributes in a block of trials, then activity related to a specific location or attribute cannot be isolated. Sustained attention to a location or attribute can be studied, but any processes that are unique to transient focusing of attention cannot. Effects related to differences in expectation are also difficult or impossible to study with homogeneous blocks of trials. Responses to unexpected, infrequent, or sporadic events cannot be isolated. Moreover, with homogeneous blocks of trials, participants' ability to anticipate each successive trial can affect the nature of the cognitive and neural processes that are invoked.

The temporal resolution of fMRI, limited as it is only by the hemodynamic response function, makes it possible to use a different kind of experimental design that examines changes in activity that occur within a task (Courtney, Ungerleider, Keil, and Haxby, 1997). These changes can be between trials in a block or within a trial. The temporal blurring imposed by the hemodynamic response function necessarily imposes limits on the brevity of events that can be isolated in this type of experimental design, but the duration of those limits has not been clearly established.

In an early demonstration of the power of looking at within-task changes in activity, Engel et al. (1994) showed that moving a visual stimulus slowly over the visual field resulted in an observable movement of the peak of neural activity over retinotopically organized visual cortex, a result that made it possible to map the retinotopic organization and areal boundaries of early visual areas. More recently, Buckner et al. (1996) showed that the neural response to a single trial in a word generation task resulted in an observable increase in BOLD signal during a long resting interval that followed each trial.

We have conducted fMRI studies of working memory and visual recognition that demonstrate that within-task contrast designs can be devised that are more conducive for answering some cognitive questions (Courtney et al., 1997). In our studies of visual working memory, trials lasted 14–18 s and could be decomposed into epochs that reflected different cognitive processes. Each trial consisted of the presentation of stimuli to be held in memory, a delay interval, and the presentation of stimuli to test recognition memory. By analyzing the response to each epoch separately, responses related to perceptual encoding, working memory maintenance, and recognition could be distinguished. In these experiments, responses to events as short as 3 s could be distinguished from responses to events that immediately preceded and followed. The design and results from these studies are presented in more detail below.

Our study of visual recognition demonstrates even finer temporal resolution (Clark, Maisog, and Haxby, 1997). In that experiment, different types of visual stimuli (novel faces, a repeated target face, scrambled pictures, and blanks) were presented in a pseudorandom sequence at a rate of one every 2 s. Differentiating responses to the different types of stimuli could be reliably detected.

The temporal resolution of fMRI will probably never be adequate to distinguish responses separated by tens or hundreds of milliseconds. Investigation into the timing of neural events at that scale will probably always require different procedures, such as electrophysiological methods. Nonetheless, fMRI can be used to decompose tasks into events as brief as a couple of seconds and can be used to examine responses to trials that differ from others in a block.

FMRI Data Analysis

The data in an fMRI experiment consist of a series of scans. Each scan provides a single number, the MRI intensity, for each of a large number of locations in the brain, defined by each picture element (pixel) or volume element (voxel). Those MRI intensities mostly reflect brain anatomy, but the brightness is modulated over a small range, usually 0.5–3% at 1.5 tesla, by hemodynamic changes. Data analysis, therefore, is the analysis of the time series for each voxel or for groups of voxels defined as a regions of interest (ROI).

Time series analysis tests whether MRI intensities change significantly with changes in experimental conditions. Any parametric or nonparametric statistic that tests for differences between pairs or groups of conditions can be used. Fourier analysis has also been used to detect changes with frequencies that match the frequency of experimental condition changes. Because the hemodynamic response blurs the transition from one condition to the next over a 4–8 s period, statistics that test categorical contrasts must either discard data collected during that transition, resulting in a loss of sensitivity, or else must partition variance due to the slow change in BOLD signal to error variance, which also degrades sensitivity. Fourier analysis is also a suboptimal model of fMRI time series analysis because it assumes that the BOLD changes between conditions will have the shape of a sine wave. Any deviation from a sine wave, due to the shape of the hemodynamic response and to sustained levels of BOLD signal over longer task intervals, will result in a proportion of the signal being apportioned to other frequencies and a loss of power at the experimental frequency. Fourier analysis also requires that activations have a regular period, precluding the use of experimental designs with irregular time periods.

Regression analysis provides a method for testing the fit between an obtained and a predicted time series that can incorporate a better model of the hemodynamic response, and, therefore, optimize sensitivity to experimentally induced changes in MRI signal. For regression analysis, the predicted changes in neural activity, usually modeled as a square wave, are convolved with a model of the hemodynamic response function to incorporate the delay and dispersion of the hemodynamic change into the prediction, affording a better prediction of MRI intensities during the transition from one experimental condition to another.

The use of regression analysis for fMRI data was first proposed by Bandettini, Jesmanowicz, Wong, and Hyde, (1993), and was later refined by Friston, Jezzard, and Turner, (1994), to incorporate a better model of the hemodynamic response and to correct calculated probabilities for temporal autocorrelations. Because the hemodynamic response spreads out in time the change associated with a neural event, adjacent time points are influenced by the same neural events, resulting in temporal autocorrelations. Consequently, adjacent scans are not independent observations, and the degrees of freedom must be adjusted accordingly for all statistical tests.

The sophistication of regression analyses of fMRI data varies greatly. More complete models that use multiple regression can optimize sensitivity by factoring out variance related to factors of no interest (Friston et al., 1995) and by modeling more complex sets of between-task and within-task contrasts (Courtney et al., in 1997). Factors of no interest that can cause substantial changes in MRI intensities include shifts between repeated time series, which may be due to small head movements, and low-frequency changes within time series. Multiple regressors of interest can also be derived that test contrasts between several tasks or that test contrasts between different components of tasks.

FMRI SIGNAL CHANGES ASSOCIATED WITH ATTENTION

FMRI has the capability to detect changes in neural activity over intervals as brief as a few seconds in brain structures that are only a few millimeters across. Within those constraints, fMRI can be used to investigate a diverse array of neural effects related to attention, and, thereby, can shed light on the mechanisms by which attention can affect perceptual and cognitive processing.

Attention-related changes in neural activity can be divided into two broad classes, one reflecting the modulatory effects of attention on information processing and the other reflecting the control systems that invoke and regulate those modulatory effects. Modulatory effects refer to attention-driven changes in information processing, such as the amplification of attended information and the suppression of unattended information. Such effects have been amply demonstrated by single-cell recordings (e.g., Moran and Desimone, 1985), by event-related potentials (e.g., Mangun, Hillyard, and Luck, 1993) and by PET (Corbetta, Miezin, Dobmeyer, Shulman, and Petersen, 1991; Corbetta, Miezin, Shulman, and Petersen, 1993; Courtney, Ungerleider, Keil, and Haxby, 1996; Haxby et al., 1994; Kawashima, O'Sullivan, and Roland, 1995). FMRI can add to our understanding of modulatory effects by specifying the stages in information processing systems at which attention can exert influence, by demonstrating the circumstances under which that influence is enabled, and by elucidating the ways in which attention alters information processing.

Control systems, on the other hand, are a more elusive and hypothetical construct than are the modulatory effects they putatively invoke and regulate (also, see Parasuraman, chapter 1, this volume). Mechanisms must exist that cause the modulatory effects of attention, that translate the intention to attend to the act of attending. It is not clear, however, whether those systems have significant components that are purely supervisory with no direct role in the processing of attended and unattended information, or whether the information processing systems themselves also embody the mechanisms that control the influence of attention on their own activity. Studies that can discriminate between the modulatory effects of attention and the source or cause of the modulation have not yet been reported.

Modulatory Effects of Attention: Changes in Response Amplitude

All attention-related effects in functional brain-imaging studies are alterations in the amplitude of hemodynamic changes, but the characteristics of an amplitude change and the conditions under which it occurs can imply different mechanisms of attention-driven modulation.

The activity in a region that responds to a particular stimulus attribute can be altered depending on the focus of selective attention. Such an activity change implies that attention influences information processing by altering the firing rate of neurons that are sensitive to that attribute. For example, in a study of selective attention to the identity or the color of color-washed gray-scale pictures of faces, Clark, Parasuraman, et al. (1997) found that an area in the collateral sulcus, which has been found in PET-rCBF studies to respond to color during a passive viewing task, showed a larger change in MRI signal when attention was directed to the color of the stimuli than when attention was directed to face identity (figure 7.1 and color plate 4). Similarly, selective attention to moving stimuli modulated activity in the motion-sensitive extrastriate region, human MT/MST (hMT+), which has been found in both PET-rCBF and fMRI studies to respond to visual motion in passive viewing tasks (Tootell et al., 1995; Watson et al., 1993; Zeki et al., 1991). Attending selectively to moving dots that are interspersed with stationary dots further increased the amplitude of the response (O'Craven et al., 1995). Similarly, directing spatial attention to the sector of an array of dots in which the dots are moving increases the amplitude of the response in hMT+, even if attention is directed there in order to process a different attribute of the moving dots, namely color (Beauchamp et al., 1995). Directing both spatial attention and feature attention to the sector of moving dots, this time to detect changes in velocity, further increased the amplitude of response in hMT+, demonstrating that both spatial and feature attention can modulate the activity in this area.

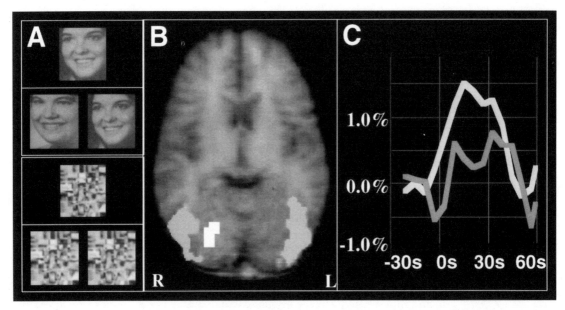

Figure 7.1 Selective attention to the color of color-washed faces resulted in a larger increase in fMRI BOLD signal in a region in the collateral sulcus. (A) A sample item from the delayed match-to-sample tests of attention to color and face identity and a sample control item. For the delayed match-to-sample tasks, subjects first saw a single color-washed face followed by two faces. For selective attention to color, subjects indicated which of the choice stimuli was closest in hue to the sample stimulus. For the control task, scrambled pictures were shown with the same timing and spatial configuration, and subjects responded to the pair of pictures by pressing both buttons. (B) The area indicated in yellow for this individual subject showed a greater response when attending to the color than to the identity of stimuli. The area shown in orange responded equally during both tasks, as compared to the control task. (C) Signal amplitude averaged over repeated cycles of control (−30 to 0 s), attention (0 to 30 s), and control (30 to 60 s) tasks during attention to color (yellow line) and attention to face identity (red line) for the region shown in yellow in (B) (From Clark et al., 1997.) See color plate 4.

Selective attention can also modulate activity in multiple areas that comprise a processing pathway. Directing attention to the identity or to the location of faces selectively activated several regions in ventral and dorsal extrastriate cortex, respectively, demonstrating a dissociation between the ventral object vision pathway and the dorsal spatial vision pathway (figure 7.2 and color plate 5) (Courtney et al., 1996a,b; Haxby, Clark, and Courtney, 1997).

Activation of cortical areas associated with one sensory modality is also associated with diminished activity in cortical areas associated with other sensory modalities, presumably reflecting suppression of processing of irrelevant and potentially distracting information from those modalities (Courtney, Ungerleider, et al., 1996; Haxby et al., 1994; Kawashima et al., 1995). In fMRI, those reductions of activity have been demonstrated as reduced BOLD signal (Clark et al., 1996), suggesting that reductions in blood flow are greater than the associated reductions in oxygen extraction.

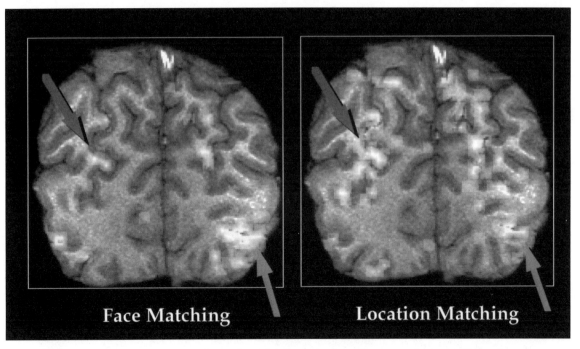

Figure 7.2 Differential activation of ventral and dorsal visual extrastriate areas in the occipital lobe when subjects selectively attend to the identity or location of faces. The results are from an fMRI study of an individual subject. Coronal sections are 3 cm from the occipital pole. Ventral lateral occipital areas that were more activated by face matching than by location matching are indicated with red arrows. Dorsal occipital areas that were more activated by location matching than by face matching are indicted with green arrows. (From Haxby et al., 1997.) See color plate 5.

Modulatory Effects of Attention: Changes in the Spatial Extent of an Activation

In addition to changes in the amplitude of activity in regions that are activated to some degree in both attended and unattended conditions, activation may be evident in some brain locations only when selective attention is directed towards relevant information. In practice, it is difficult to determine if a change in regional activity is an overall increase that raises the fringes of the activation above the statistical threshold for significance, or if the additional area of activation is showing a selectively greater increase in activity. The distinction may be important, as a change in the area of activated cortex may indicate the recruitment of additional columns or additional functional areas to represent attended information. The most convincing demonstration of attention-driven recruitment of additional cortex would be a demonstration that the upper confidence limit for activation in the unattended condition falls well below the magnitude of an increase that could be considered meaningful. An increase in the area of activation that is not merely an overall increase could also be indicated by a larger increase in activation, comparing unattended to attended conditions, in the voxels showing activation only in the attended condition as compared to the voxels showing significant activations during the unattended condition.

Demonstration of an increase in the area of activation is possible with fMRI but requires separate analysis of each individual subject. Group analyses tend to smooth the edges of areas of activation, making it more difficult to distinguish a change in area due to a threshold effect. The edges of activations in individual fMRI studies can be quite discrete. In an fMRI study of face perception, Clark et al. (1996) made a direct comparison between the size of activation in the voxels on the edge of an activated area and immediately adjacent voxels outside the activated area. Voxels contained within the activated area but at its outer edge demonstrated, on average, a 2% increase in BOLD signal. By contrast, the immediately adjacent voxels outside the activated area had a nonsignificant average increase in BOLD signal of less than 0.5%. At a distance of one voxel more distant from the activated area there was no tendency towards activation. Those results indicate that recruitment of adjacent cortical tissue by attention can be demonstrated with fMRI.

A change in the area of activation has been reported in a fMRI study of motor skill learning (Karni et al., 1995). Subjects practiced a finger opposition sequence over a period of several weeks. As they became more proficient at performing the learned sequence, the size of the cortical patch activated in motor cortex increased significantly, as compared to the activation associated with performing an unlearned sequence comprised of the same component movements. Those results suggest that, as learning occurred, the representation of the learned sequence included additional cortical columns in motor cortex.

Increases in the area of activated cortical regions are suggested by fMRI studies of attentional modulation, but none of those reports has attempted an analysis that could distinguish between a general increase in activity across an entire area that raises the fringe of activation above the threshold for statistical significance, and a selective increase in voxels that shows minimal or no activation in the unattended condition.

Modulatory Effects of Attention: Other Alterations of Response

In addition to changes in the amplitude and spatial extent of activation, attention may alter other aspects of the nature of a regional response that can be detected with fMRI. One such change is an alteration in the specificity of response to an aspect of a stimulus or to a component of a task. Changes of this type have been demonstrated in fMRI studies of visual working memory (Courtney, Maisog, Ungerleider, and Haxby, 1996). Another type of change involves a change in the functional connectivity between regions (Biswal, Yetkin, Haughton, and Hyde, 1995; Friston, Frith, Liddle, and Frackowiak, 1993; Horwitz, Grady, et al., 1992; Horwitz, Soncrant, and Haxby, 1992;

McIntosh et al., 1994). Such changes have been demonstrated in a PET-rCBF study of selective attention (McIntosh et al., 1994). FMRI has the potential to provide more powerful and compelling demonstrations of changes in functional connectivity, although to our knowledge no such demonstration has been reported yet.

In order to illustrate how fMRI can demonstrate a change in the specificity of a regional response to an attribute of a stimulus or to a component of a task, the design of our fMRI studies of working memory are presented in some detail. The working memory studies examined changes in activity that occurred within the task. Working memory is an ideal subject for studies that use this type of design, because each trial consists of components that last long enough to be distinguished with fMRI. In an initial study of working memory for face identity, subjects performed a task in which each trial began with the presentation of a single face to remember (Courtney et al., 1997)

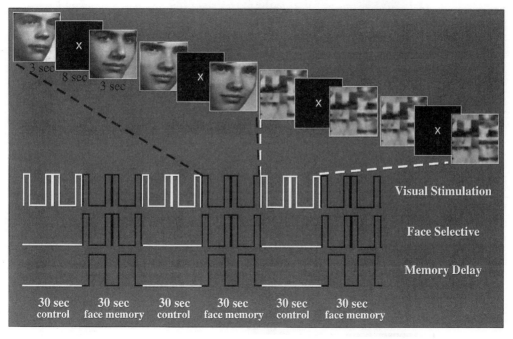

Figure 7.3 Experiment design for an fMRI study of working memory that used multiple regression to decompose the task into components that were segregated by time. Each memory task item began with the presentation of a single face for 3 s. A test face was presented after an 8 s delay, and subjects indicated whether the test face matched the face that began the item. For control items, scrambled pictures of faces were presented with the same timing, and subjects responded to the second picture in each item by pressing both buttons. For multiple regression analysis, the task was decomposed into three predicted responses, indicated by the square wave functions: a nonselective transient response to visual stimuli that was equal for faces and control stimuli; a selective transient response to faces; and a sustained response over memory delays. The square waves were convolved with a model of the hemodynamic response to produce the expected shape of a response in an fMRI time series. Multiple regression finds the optimal weights for a weighted sum of the regressors that best fits obtained fMRI time series. (From Courtney et al., 1997.)

(see figure 7.3). After an 8 s memory delay, a second test face was presented, and participants indicated whether it matched the face that began the trial. Two such working memory trials alternated with two control task trials that involved the presentation of scrambled pictures with the same timing that was used for the working memory task. The analysis of the results used multiple regression to obtain separate measures of activity that indicated (1) a nonselective response to either scrambled or intact pictures of faces; (2) a selectively greater response to faces than to scrambled pictures; and (3) a sustained response during the memory delay, indicating processing associated with the maintenance of an active representation in working memory. The results revealed six regions, three posterior extrastriate regions and three prefrontal regions, that demonstrated significant activation during the task. The multiple regression analysis showed that the relative strength of nonselective perceptual, selective perceptual, and memory-related activity varied systematically in the distributed neural system (figure. 7.4 and color plate 6). The response in early extrastriate regions was dominated by nonselective transient activation by the control and face stimuli. By contrast, the response in later extrastriate regions demonstrated a selective enhancement of the response to faces as compared to control stimuli. These later extrastriate areas also showed some sustained activity over memory delays, but even stronger sustained activity was seen in the prefrontal areas. Thus, all six areas were activated by the working memory task, but direct comparison of the relative strengths of activity during different components of the task in each area revealed that the functional role played by the six areas varied systematically.

A subsequent follow-up study, which contrasted working memory for face identity and for spatial location, suggested that both the selectivity of transient responses in later extrastriate cortex and the sustained activity during memory delays were modulated by selective attention (Courtney, Maisog, et al., 1996). When attention was directed away from face identity, the later ventral extrastriate areas demonstrated more equivalent responses to faces and to control stimuli. This result shows that selective attention did not operate simply by increasing activity in the areas that processed the attended information, but, rather, operated by selectively increasing the response in those areas to the relevant stimuli more than the response to irrelevant stimuli. When subjects selectively retained in working memory the spatial location rather than the identity of faces, the sustained response in ventral prefrontal areas was diminished and a different dorsal prefrontal area in the superior frontal sulcus demonstrated a sustained response that was smaller during facial identity working memory. This result shows that selective attention can modulate activity in cortical regions during a component of a task that is not related to the apprehension of a stimulus, but rather to a more purely cognitive operation, namely working memory maintenance.

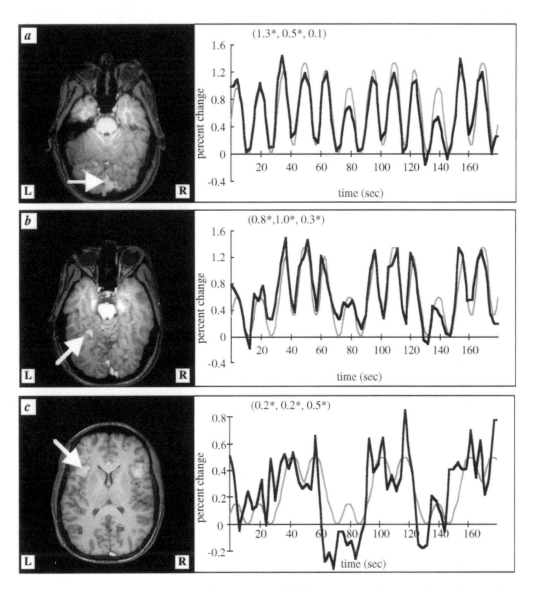

Figure 7.4 Two extrastriate and one prefrontal region with different patterns of response during a face working memory task. Data are from an individual subject. (a) A posterior ventral occipital area that demonstrated a mostly nonselective, transient response to visual stimuli. The weights calculated by multiple regression for the three regressors (figure 7.3) are shown in parentheses (*p < 0.05). The weighted sum of the regressors is shown in red (see color plate 6). The obtained fMRI time series, averaged over all voxels in the region and over repeated time series, is shown in black. (b) An anterior ventral temporal area that demonstrated a more selective, still mostly transient response to faces. The sustained activity over memory delays was small, but statistically significant. (c) A prefrontal region in the inferior frontal gyrus near the anterior end of the insula that demonstrated more sustained activity over memory delays. (Adapted from Courtney et al., 1997.)

Modulatory Effects of Attention: Altered Functional Connections Between Areas

Another way in which attention may modulate the activity of cortical regions that process attended and unattended information is to alter interactions between regions. In functional brain-imaging studies, changes in correlations between regions may indicate such alterations of functional connectivity (Friston et al., 1993; Horwitz, Grady, et al., 1992; Horwitz, Soncrant, and Haxby, 1992; McIntosh et al., 1994). Interregional covariance can be analyzed in a variety of ways, and the extent to which the different types of analysis reflect the same underlying connectivities is not clear.

Patterns of interregional correlations have been extensively investigated in PET-rCBF studies. Because of the limited number of scans that can be obtained in an individual subject with PET, analysis of interregional correlations are performed on group data. Two quite different types of group data analysis have been used. In the first, covariances in rCBF during a single task condition are examined (Horwitz, Grady, et al., 1992; Horwitz, Soncrant, and Haxby, 1992; McIntosh et al., 1994). These analyses examine the extent to which pairs of regions have higher or lower activity rates, in tandem, relative to whole brain activity. A positive correlation between two regions indicates that an individual subject with high rCBF in one region, relative to whole brain CBF, also has high rCBF in the other region, whereas another subject with relatively low rCBF in one region also has low rCBF in the other. Thus, these methods provide a very indirect index of whether the activity in one region has greater or lesser influence over the activity in another because no within-individual variation in regional activity is examined. Nonetheless, analyses of this type have indicated that selective attention increases the correlations between regions in distributed neural systems that process the attended information. For example, selective attention to face identity augmented interregional correlations in the ventral object vision pathway, whereas selective attention to the spatial location of faces augmented interregional correlations in the dorsal object vision pathway (McIntosh et al., 1994).

In the second type of covariance analysis used with PET-rCBF data, correlations between the extent to which regions change activity level between task conditions are analyzed (Friston et al., 1993). A positive correlation between two regions indicates that an individual subject who demonstrated a large activity increase in one region, comparing an activation and a baseline condition, also demonstrated a large increase in the second region, whereas a subject with a small activation in one region also had a small activation in the other. Thus, this method provides a somewhat more direct index of the extent to which two regions influence each other, but the index is still quite ambiguous. Two regions may be activated by different and relatively independent components of the task but nonetheless show greater or lesser activation in tandem because of interindividual variation in the extent to which subjects are engaged in the task or struggle with the task.

Because fMRI allows hundreds of scans to be obtained in one individual, potentially more powerful and convincing demonstrations of functional connectivity may be possible. FMRI methods examine the extent to which fluctuations in regional activity are correlated in an individual subject during a single task condition, or, better yet, during a component of a task. The fluctuations can be spontaneous and not under experimental control. Biswal et al. (1995) demonstrated that fMRI intensities in regions with known anatomical connections covaried during the resting state. In other words, when one region showed a spontaneous increase in BOLD signal, a connected region showed a similar increase. The fluctuations they examined had a temporal frequency that could not be explained by other physiological variables, such as the cardiac or respiratory cycles. Such correlated fluctations suggest that an increase in the neural activity in one region causes an increase in regions with which it is anatomically connected. The extent to which that index of the strength of a functional connection may change during the performance of a cognitive task has not been examined yet. Such an analysis, however, could determine whether and under what conditions attention can alter the efficacy of synaptic connections between regions.

Attention Control Systems: The Cause of Modulations

In theory, studies that vary the focus of selective attention also manipulate activity in systems that direct and maintain that focus. Consequently, areas that show greater activity during a selective attention condition may reflect a modulatory effect on information processing or a system that oversees that modulation or both. Such studies, therefore, confound the effect of attention and its cause. Although one may attempt to distinguish regions that are involved in perceptual processing from areas with executive functions based on a review of the neuroanatomical and neuropsychological literature, direct experimental demonstration of such a distinction is necessary. Such a demonstration would vary the activity of attention control operations while keeping the modulation of information processing, namely the focus or foci of attention and difficulty, constant. The power of the fMRI technique can be exploited to examine this vital issue in attention research.

CONCLUSIONS

Functional magnetic resonance imaging refers to a diverse set of methods for obtaining measures of physiological parameters. This review has focused on only a subset of these methods; namely, fMRI methods that measure changes in blood oxygenation and that use those changes as indices of changes in integrated regional neural activity. BOLD fMRI affords an unprecedented window onto function in the intact human brain, but a clear understanding of its capabilities and limitations is necessary to design fMRI experiments that can make the best use of this research tool. BOLD fMRI has a temporal resolution that is limited by the hemodynamic response, a transfer function that expresses the temporal course of a hemodynamic change elicited by a change in neural activity. Consequently, fMRI is capable of resolving events that are separated in time by a few seconds, and, under some conditions, can resolve events that are separated by less than a second. Resolving events on a millisecond time scale, however, requires other methods, like electrophysiology. With current scanning technology, the spatial resolution of BOLD fMRI is a few millimeters for most studies but can be pushed to submillimeter resolution. That level of resolution is sufficient for identifying functional cortical areas, for describing the functional topology within a cortical area (such as retinotopy in visual areas), and for delineating the borders between functional cortical areas.

Within these constraints, fMRI can detect a diverse array of neural events that reflect attentional processes. These effects include a variety of types of modulation of information processing, such as augmentation and suppression of processing, recruitment of additional cortical areas, altered specificity of response, and altered functional connectivity between regions. At this stage of fMRI research, only some of these effects have been demonstrated. A different and critical area for fMRI research concerns the neural systems that control, direct, and maintain attention. Again, no fMRI studies have been reported that clearly address these questions, but with an appropriate experimental design, fMRI may help to identify the components of these systems and characterize how they function.

REFERENCES

Bandettini, P. A., Jesmanowicz, A., Wong, E. C., and Hyde, J. S. (1993) Processing strategies for time-course data sets in functional MRI of the human brain. *Mag. Reson. Med.* 30: 161–173.

Beauchamp, M. S., Cox, R. W., and DeYoe, E. A. (1997) Graded effects of spatial and featural attention on human area MT and associated motion processing areas. *J. Neurophysiol.* 78: 516–520.

Biswal, B., Yetkin, F. Z., Haughton, V. M., and Hyde, J. S. (1995) Functional connectivity in the motor cortex of resting human brain using echo-planar MRI. *Mag. Reson. Med.* 34: 537–541.

Boynton, G. M., Engel, S. A., Glover, G. H., and Heeger, D. J. (1996) Linear systems analysis of functional magnetic resonance imaging in human V1. *J. Neurosci.* 16: 4207–4221.

Buckner, R. L., Bandettini, P. A., O'Craven, K. M., Savoy, R. L., Petersen, S. E., Raichle, M. E., and Rosen, B. R. (1996) Detection of cortical activation during averaged single trials of a cognitive task using functional magnetic resonance imaging. *Proc. Natl. Acad. Sci. U S A* 93: 14302–14303.

Clark, V. P., Keil, K., Maisog, J. M., Courtney, S., Ungerleider, L. G., and Haxby, J. V. (1996) Functional magnetic resonance imaging of human cortex during face matching: A comparison with positron emission tomography. *Neuroimage* 4: 1–15.

Clark, V. P., Maisog, J. M., and Haxby, J. V. (1997) FMRI Studies of face memory using random stimulus sequences. *NeuroImage* 5: S50.

Clark, V. P., Parasuraman, R., Keil, K., Kulanski, R., Fannon, S., Maisog, J. M., Ungerleider, L. G., and Haxby, J. V. (1997) Selective attention to face identity and color studied with fMRI. *Hum. Brain Map,* 5: 293–297.

Corbetta, M., Miezin, F. M., Dobmeyer, S., Shulman, G. L., and Petersen, S. E. (1991) Selective and divided attention during visual discriminations of shape, color, and speed: Functional anatomy by positron emission tomography. *J. Neurosci.* 11: 2383–2402.

Corbetta, M., Miezin, F. M., Shulman, G. L., and Petersen, S. E. (1993) A PET study of visuospatial attention. *J. Neurosci.* 13: 1202–1226.

Courtney S. M., Maisog, J. M., Ungerleider, L. G., and Haxby, J. V. (1996) Extrastriate and frontal contributions to face and location working memory. *Society for Neuroscience Abstracts* 22: 968.

Courtney, S. M., Ungerleider, L. G., Keil, K., and Haxby, J. V. (1996) Object and spatial working memory activate separate neural systems in human cortex. *Cereb. Cortex* 6: 39–49.

Courtney, S. M., Ungerleider, L. G., Keil, K. and Haxby, J. V. (1997) Transient and sustained activity in a distributed neural system for human working memory. *Nature* 386: 608–611

Engel, S. A., Rumelhart, D. E., Wandell, B. A., Lee, A. T., Glover, G. H., Chichilnisky, E. J., and Shadlen, M. N. (1994) fMRI of human visual cortex. *Nature* 370: 106.

Fox, P. T. and Raichle, M. E. (1986) Focal physiological uncoupling of cerebral blood flow and oxidative metabolism during somatosensory stimulation in human subjects. *Proc. Natl. Acad. Sci. U S A* 83: 1140–1144.

Friston, K. J., Frith, C. D., Liddle, P. F., and Frackowiak, R. S. J. (1993) Functional connectivity: The principal-component analysis of large (PET) data sets. *J. Cereb. Blood Flow Metab.* 13: 5–14.

Friston, K. J., Holmes, A. P., Polilne, J. B., Grasby, P. J., Williams, C. R., and Frackowiak, R. S. J. (1995) Analysis of fMRI time-series revisited. *NeuroImage* 2: 45–53.

Friston, K. J., Jezzard, P., and Turner, R. (1994) The analysis of functional MRI time series. *Hum. Brain Map.* 1: 153–171.

Haxby, J. V., Clark, V. P., and Courtney, S. M. (1997) Distributed hierarchical neural systems for visual memory in human cortex. In *Connections, Cognition, and Alzheimer's Disease,* edited by B. Hyman, C. Duyckaerts, and Y. Christen, pp. 167–180. New York: Springer.

Haxby, J. V., Horwitz, B., Ungerleider, L. G., Maisog, J. M., Pietrini, P., and Grady, C. L. (1994) The functional organization of human extrastriate cortex: A PET-rCBF study of selective attention to faces and locations. *J. Neurosci.* 14: 6336–6353.

Horwitz, B., Grady, C. L., Haxby, J. V., Ungerleider, L. G., Schapiro, M. B., Mishkin, M., and Rapoport, S. I. (1992) Functional associations among human posterior extrastriate brain regions during object and spatial vision. *J. Cog. Neurosci.* 4: 311–322.

Horwitz, B., Soncrant, T. T., and Haxby, J. V. (1992) Covariance analysis of functional interactions in the brain using metabolic and blood flow data. In *Advances in Metabolic Mapping Techniques for Brain Imaging of Behavioral and Learning Functions,* edited by F. Gonzalez-Lima, T. Finkenstaedt, and H. Scheich, pp. 189–217. Dordrecht, Netherlands: Kluwer Academic.

Karni, A., Meyer, G., Jezzard, P., Adams, M. M., Turner, R., and Ungerleider, L. G. (1995) Functional MRI evidence for adult motor cortex plasticity during motor skill learning. *Nature* 377: 155–158.

Kawashima, R., O'Sullivan, B. T., and Roland, P. E. (1995) Positron-emission tomography studies of cross-modality inhibition in selective attentional tasks: Closing the "mind's eye." *Proc. Natl. Acad. Sci. U S A* 92: 5969–5972.

Kwong, K. K., Belliveau, J. W., Chesler, D. A., Goldberg, I. E., Weisskoff, R. M., Poncelet, B. P., Kennedy, D. N., Hoppel, B. E., Cohen, M. S., and Turner, R. (1992) Dynamic magnetic resonance imaging of human brain activity during primary sensory stimulation. *Proc. Natl. Acad. Sci. U S A* 89: 5675–5679.

Mangun, G. R., Hillyard, S. A., and Luck, S. J. (1993) Electro-cortical substrates of visual selective attention. In *Attention and Performance XIV*, edited by D. E. Meyer and S. Kornblum, Cambridge, MA: MIT Press.

McIntosh, A. R., Grady, C. L., Ungerleider, L. G., Haxby, J. V., Rapoport, S. I., and Horwitz, B. (1994) Network analysis of cortical visual pathways. *J. Neurosci.* 14: 655–666.

Moran, J. and Desimone, R. (1985) Selective attention gates visual processing in the extrastriate cortex. *Science* 229: 782–784.

O'Craven, K. M., Rosen, B. R., Kwong, K. K., Treisman, A., and Savoy, R. L. (1997) Voluntary attention modulates fMRI activity in human MT-MST. *Neuron* 18: 591–598.

Ogawa, S., Tank, D. W., Menon, R., Ellermann, J. M., Kim, S. G., Merkle, H., and Ugurbil, K. (1992) Intrinsic signal changes accompanying sensory stimulation: Functional brain mapping with magnetic resonance imaging. *Proc. Natl. Acad. Sci. U S A* 89: 5951–5955.

Pauling, L. and Coryell, C. (1936) The magnetic properties of and structure of hemoglobin, oxyhemoglobin, and carbonmonoxyhemoglobin. *Proc. Natl. Acad. Sci. U S A* 22: 210–216.

Roy, C. S. and Sherrington, C. S. (1890) On the regulation of the blood supply of the brain. *J. Physiol. (Lond.)* 11: 85–105.

Thulborn, K. R., Waterton, J. C., Matthews, P. M., and Radda, G. K. (1982) Oxygenation dependence of the transverse relaxation time of water protons in whole blood at high field. *Acta Biochim. Biophys.* 714: 265–270.

Tootell, R. B., Reppas, J. B., Kwong, K. K., Malach, R., Born, R. T., Brady, T. J., Rosen, B. R., and Belliveau, J. W. (1995) Functional analysis of human MT and related visual cortical areas using magnetic resonance imaging. *J. Neurosci.* 15: 3215–3230.

Turner, R. and Jezzard, P. (1995) Magnetic resonance studies of brain functional activation using echo-planar imaging. In *Functional Neuroimaging*, edited by R. Thatcher, New York: Plenum Press.

Turner, R., LeBihan, D., Jezzard, P., Despres, D., and Taylor, J. (1992) Time course imaging of blood oxygenation in cat brain. *Proc. Ann. Meet. Soc. Mag. Reson. Med.* 11: 918.

Watson, J. D., Myers, R., Frackowiak, R. S. J., Hajnal, J. V., Woods, R. P., Mazziotta, J. C., Shipp, S., and Zeki, S. (1993) Area V5 of the human brain: Evidence from a combined study using positron emission tomography and magnetic resonance imaging. *Cereb. Cortex* 3: 79–94.

Zeki, S., Watson, J. P. G., Lueck, C. J., Friston, K., Kennard, C., and Frackowiak, R. S. J. (1991) A direct demonstration of functional specialization in human visual cortex. *J. Neurosci* 11: 641–649.

8 Cortical Lesions and Attention

Diane Swick and Robert T. Knight

ABSTRACT Neurological patients have historically provided important insights into the brain mechanisms of attentive behavior. The contribution of the lesion method to understanding attentional functions is discussed with particular reference to prefrontal cortex. This brain region is a central component of the distributed neural systems engaged during sustained and phasic attention to both external environmental events and to the internal mental state. Prefrontal cortex regulates sustained attention and working memory through both inhibitory and facilitory mechanisms. Phasic attention to novel events is dependent on a prefrontal-hippocampal network. Thus, many of the observed behavioral deficits subsequent to prefrontal damage may be due to impaired function in distant neural regions under prefrontal control. Delineation of the cellular and pharmacological substrates of those pathways could lead to treatment interventions for the attention deficits observed after prefrontal damage.

For hundreds of years scientists and clinicians have made inferences about the location of cognitive functions in the human brain from observations of the behavioral deficits exhibited by persons who have suffered brain damage (Bouillard, 1825; Auburtin, 1861, as cited in Stookey, 1954; Harlow, 1868; Dejerine, 1892). Until recently, this approach—the lesion method—was one of the few techniques available for examining the neural basis of human sensory, cognitive, and motor functions.

The venerable tradition of neuropsychology entered the era of contemporary neuroscience with the advent of techniques that provide accurate, quantifiable images of the living human brain. The merger of information-processing accounts of the mind and parallel distributed processing concepts with the refined ability to localize lesions using magnetic resonance imaging (MRI) has added to knowledge of the distributed neural networks that mediate processes such as attention.

This chapter reviews the current status of the application of the lesion method to the study of attention, with special reference to the prefrontal cortex. The prefrontal cortex represents a critical component of distributed neural systems engaged during sustained and phasic attention to external and internal events.

THE LESION METHOD

Single-Case Versus Group Studies

Researchers disagree over the best way to design a research program in cognitive neuropsychology based on the lesion method. One debate concerns the importance of single-case studies versus group studies. A related issue that has generated controversy is the relative emphasis placed on localizing cognitive operations in the brain, which has been championed by those favoring the group studies approach, versus the emphasis placed on informing theoretical conceptions of normal cognitive function based on the existence of double dissociations in patients, which is a feature of the single-case approach. The single-case study camp maintains that averaging test results over a group of patients is inappropriate because brain damage can disrupt a cognitive system in a variety of ways (Caramazza, 1986, 1992; Sokol, McCloskey, Cohen, and Aliminosa, 1991). Proponents claim that the single-case approach is more likely to produce strong evidence for making inferences about normal function.

An opposing position states that limiting studies to single cases is generally an ultracognitive approach (Shallice, 1988) that ignores the importance of biological evidence in developing theories of cognition (Kosslyn and Intriligator, 1992; Robertson, Knight, Rafal, and Shimamura, 1993). Advocates of group studies contend that "[single-case studies] are of limited value in constructing a general theory of human cognitive neuropsychology because there are serious difficulties in generalizing from the behavior of one person to the behavior of all people" (Kolb and Whishaw, 1990, p. 84).

Brain structure varies from person to person and, of course, people vary in their behavior and in their cognitive capabilities. The research presented in this chapter is based on group studies of patients with unilateral, focal brain lesions, primarily due to stroke. However, we also believe that one can learn a great deal about relationships between the brain and behavior from the single-case approach (e.g., Scoville and Milner, 1957).

Indirect and Compensatory Effects of Lesions

A second important issue that must be addressed whenever neurological patients are examined, whether in single-case or in group studies, is the indirect and compensatory effects of lesions on both brain function and behavior. Recovery of function after brain damage can change the neural circuits recruited for a specific cognitive task. Damage to a particular brain area may disrupt connections to and influence the function of remote regions. However, the observation of changes remote from the site of lesion can reveal information about connectivity and modulatory interactions. For example, frontal lobe lesions can influence visual processing in extrastriate occipitotemporal areas (Kosslyn et al., 1993; Knight, 1997; Swick and Knight,

1996). Another advantage of the lesion method is that it allows determination of whether a particular brain region is necessary for a particular cognitive function. Intracerebral recordings from epilepsy patients have suggested that "full-employment [is] the brain processing policy" (Halgren et al., 1995, p. 246). Multiple cortical and limbic sites generate large potentials during simple sensory discriminations, for example, but many of those areas may be unnecessary for task performance.

With the strengths and weaknesses of the lesion method in mind, careful neuroanatomical studies in human patients have made substantial contributions to elucidation of the neural substrates of perception, attention, memory, and language (Damasio and Damasio, 1989). A series of assumptions underlies all methods used by cognitive neuroscientists, and each method has its limitations. Ultimately, converging evidence from multiple techniques will yield the most integrated and insightful models of attention. This review focuses on neuropsychological and neurophysiological data that link the frontal lobes to attention and to the control of sensory and cognitive processing. Some of the evidence implicates additional regions that comprise distributed networks for orientation and the novelty response.

DORSOLATERAL PREFRONTAL CORTEX AND ATTENTION

Dorsolateral prefrontal cortex (Brodmann's areas 6, 8, 9, 10, 44, 45, and 46) is critical for a broad range of processes, including language, motor control, attention, working memory, and executive functions. Given the extensive bidirectional connections between prefrontal cortex and numerous cortical, limbic, and subcortical regions (Goldman-Rakic, Selemon, and Schwartz, 1984; Seltzer and Pandya, 1989; Friedman and Goldman-Rakic, 1994), dorsolateral prefrontal lesions can result in a variety of cognitive disturbances. With early damage from tumors or degenerative disorders, subtle deficits in creativity and mental flexibility can be observed. Behavioral problems are more pronounced with bilateral damage or with the progression of unilateral disease, producing impairments in attention, temporal coding, metamemory, planning, judgment, and insight. Acute infarcts of prefrontal cortex are associated with a transient syndrome of attention abnormalities and global confusion. Right hemisphere lesions involving areas 8 (which includes the frontal eye fields), 9, and 46 can result in hemispatial neglect (Heilman, Watson, and Valenstein, 1994; also, see Rafal, chapter 22, this volume).

Moreover, prefrontal cortex (particularly areas 9 and 46) is crucial for the control of sustained and phasic attention to environmental events (Stuss and Benson, 1986). Knight and colleagues studied the attention, orienting, and memory abilities of neurological patients with focal prefrontal lesions using behavioral and event-related potential (ERP) recording techniques (Knight, 1984, 1991; Knight, Hillyard, Woods, and Neville, 1981; Knight, Scabini, and Woods, 1989; Knight, Scabini, Woods, and Cloworth, 1989; Swick and Knight, 1994, 1996; Yamaguchi and Knight 1990, 1991a). The primary impairments in these patients include problems with inhibitory control of sensory inputs, deficits in sustained attention, and abnormalities in the detection of novel events. The inability to gate irrelevant inputs and sustain attention, coupled with deficits in novelty detection, impairs the coding and processing of discrete external events. Similar to the role it plays in attention to external events, prefrontal cortex is crucial for attention to the internal mental representations that presumably contribute to working memory, to the use of strategies in experimental (and everyday) settings, to planning, and to decision making (Knight and Grabowecky, 1995; Stuss, Eskes, and Foster, 1994).

Sensory Gating and Prefrontal Cortex

The attention deficits and perseveration observed in patients with frontal lesions have been linked to problems with inhibitory control of posterior sensory and perceptual mechanisms (Lhermitte, 1986; Lhermitte, Pillon, and Serdaru, 1986). This relatively early sensory gating deficit, combined with abnormalities in the detection of novel events, can lead to deficits in higher-order cognitive processes such as executive control. For instance, the inability to inhibit internal representations of previous responses that are no longer correct may cause poor performance on the Wisconsin card-sorting task and on the Stroop task (Shimamura, 1995; Vendrell et al., 1995). Physiological data indicate that the lack of inhibitory control may begin with early sensory processing in primary cortical regions. Suppression of a prefrontal-thalamic gating system in cats increased the amplitudes of evoked responses in primary auditory cortex (Skinner and Yingling, 1977; Yingling and Skinner, 1977).

Prefrontal cortex can thus exert an inhibitory, top-down influence on neural activity within primary sensory cortices. Additional support for such a mechanism has been obtained from ERP recordings in stroke patients. ERPs are brain potentials that are time-locked to the occurrence of sensory, motor, or cognitive events and that are extracted from the ongoing electroencephalogram (EEG) by signal-averaging techniques (Hillyard and Picton, 1987). Because of their excellent temporal resolution, ERPs provide a valuable index of the timing of covert sensory and cognitive processing in humans that complements both the behavioral measures of cognitive psychology and the superior spatial resolution of functional neuroimaging techniques (see Corbetta, chapter 6, this volume). Application of the ERP methodology to studies of attention is discussed by Luck and Girelli (chapter 5, this volume). Constraints upon localizing the neural generators of ERP components have been obtained from lesion studies in both animals and humans (for a review, see Swick, Kutas, and Neville, 1994).

Task-irrelevant auditory and somatosensory stimuli (i.e., monaural clicks or brief electric shocks to the median nerve) were presented to patients with comparably sized lesions in dorsolateral prefrontal cortex, in the temporal-

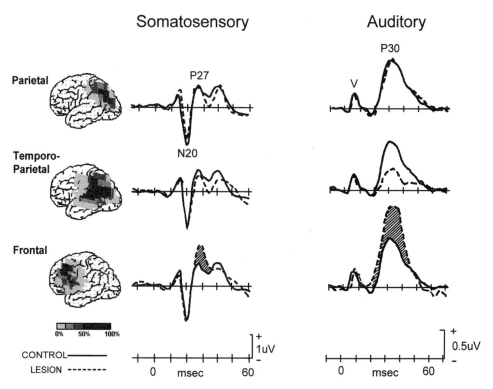

Figure 8.1 Primary cortical somatosensory and auditory evoked responses in control subjects (solid line) and patients (dashed line) with focal damage in lateral parietal cortex (top, $n = 8$), temporal-parietal junction (middle, $n = 13$), or in dorsolateral prefrontal cortex (bottom, $n = 11$). Reconstructions of the extent of damage in each patient group are shown on the left. Somatosensory potentials were elicited by square-wave pulses delivered to the median nerve at the wrist and recorded from area 3b (N20) and areas 1 and 2 (P27). Auditory evoked responses generated in the inferior colliculus (wave V) and the primary auditory cortex (P30) were elicited by clicks delivered at a rate of 13/s and a 50 dB HL intensity level. Prefrontal lesions resulted in a selective increase in the amplitudes of the P27 and P30 responses (shaded areas). See color plate 7.

parietal junction, or in lateral parietal cortex. Evoked responses from primary auditory (Kraus, Ozolamar, and Stein, 1982) and somatosensory (Leuders, Leser, Harn, Dinner, and Klem, 1983) cortices were recorded from these patients and from age-matched controls (figure 8.1 and color plate 7). Not surprisingly, damage to primary auditory or somatosensory cortex reduced the early-latency (20–40 ms) ERPs generated in those regions. Posterior association cortex lesions that spared the primary sensory regions had no effect on the amplitudes or latencies of the early potentials; thus, the patients with posterior association cortex lesions served as a brain-lesioned control group. Prefrontal damage produced disinhibition of both the primary auditory and somatosensory evoked responses (Knight, Scabini, and Woods, 1989; Yamaguchi and Knight, 1990). Spinal cord and brain stem potentials were not affected by prefrontal damage, suggesting that the amplitude enhancement was due to abnormalities in either prefrontal-thalamic or direct prefrontal-sensory cortex mechanisms.

Chronic disinhibition of sensory inputs may contribute to many of the behavioral sequelae of prefrontal damage. Distractibility has been proposed to be a major component of the delayed response deficit in animals with prefrontal lesions (Malmo, 1942; Bartus and Levere, 1977). The inability to suppress irrelevant information can lead to difficulties in target detection and match-to-sample paradigms. For example, patients with frontal resections were impaired at detecting multiple visual targets embedded among distractors (Richer et al., 1993). Likewise, patients with lesions confined to dorsolateral prefrontal cortex were impaired at matching two environmental sounds only when distractors intervened between cue and target (Chao and Knight, 1995).

Visual Attention and Prefrontal Cortex

Visual stimuli elicit a prominent, attention-sensitive N170 (N1) scalp potential that is maximal over temporal-occipital sites. Topographic and dipole modeling studies have suggested an N170 source in extrastriate cortex (Gomez Gonzalez, Clark, Fan, Luck, and Hillyard, 1994; Johannes, Munte, Heinze, and Mangun, 1995). In the auditory modality, the presence of frontal lesions reduced the N1 attention effect in a dichotic listening task (Knight et al., 1981). A recent experiment examined the influence of prefrontal cortex on the visual N1. Control subjects and patients with frontal lesions performed a visual detection task while viewing centrally presented triangles, inverted triangles, and irrelevant novel stimuli (Knight, 1997). In control subjects, N170 amplitude was largest for target stimuli. Dorsolateral prefrontal damage decreased N170 amplitude over the lesioned hemisphere for all visual stimuli, with maximal reductions seen at posterior temporal sites (figure 8.2 and color plate 8). However, the degree of target-related N1 enhancement was comparable to controls over the extrastriate cortex of both lesioned and intact hemispheres (Knight, 1997). The N2 component to targets was eliminated over the lesioned hemisphere.

The reduction of N170 in frontal lesion patients was also observed in tasks using verbal stimuli (Swick and Knight, 1996). Subjects read centrally presented words and pronounceable nonwords and performed lexical decision or recognition memory tasks. For control subjects, both stimulus types elicited a focal N170 that was maximal at posterior temporal and occipital electrodes (figure 8.3). N170 was significantly larger over the left hemisphere in both tasks, similar to previous studies with words (Neville, Kutas, Chesney, and Schmidt, 1986; Curran, Tucker, Kutas, Posner, 1993). N170 amplitude was reduced in frontal lesion patients ipsilateral to damage, but peak latency was unaffected.

Those two experiments suggest that dorsolateral prefrontal cortex provides an ipsilateral facilitory input to neural processing in extrastriate cortex that begins within 120 ms post-stimulus. Additional support for prefrontal

PFCx - Visual Modulation

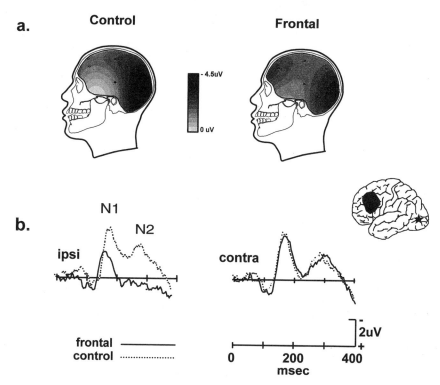

Figure 8.2 Prefrontal cortex modulates the visual N170 component. (a) Topographic maps display the scalp voltage distribution (in μV) of the N170 to targets. The extrastriate focus of the N170 in controls is reduced ipsilateral to prefrontal damage. (Inset) The gray shading on the brain shows the area of maximum lesion overlap, while the star indicates a putative N170 generator in extrastriate cortex. (b) Group averaged ERPs for target stimuli in controls and frontal patients ($n = 11$). Waveforms are from posterior temporal electrodes (T5/T6 in controls), ipsilateral (ipsi) and contralateral (contra) to the lesion. The N1 (N170) and N2 components are labeled. In this and subsequent figures, negative is up, stimulus onset occurs at 0 ms, and the scale is given in microvolts (μV). See color plate 8.

modulation of visual processing in extrastriate areas during sustained attention and spatial memory comes from blood flow data in humans (Roland, 1982), network analyses of PET results (McIntosh et al., 1994), and single-unit and lesion data in monkeys (Fuster, Bauer, and Jervey, 1985; Funahashi, Bruce, and Goldman-Rakic, 1993). Combined with the auditory ERP findings (Knight et al., 1981), these data suggest that dorsolateral prefrontal cortex is involved in multimodal control of sustained attention. However, caution is needed in comparing the current ERP results to those reported in prior visual attention studies (for a review, see Mangun, 1995). Most studies have employed lateralized stimulus arrays and divided or cued attention paradigms. Those designs allowed comparisons between attended and unattended stimuli. That design was not employed in our studies, both of which used central

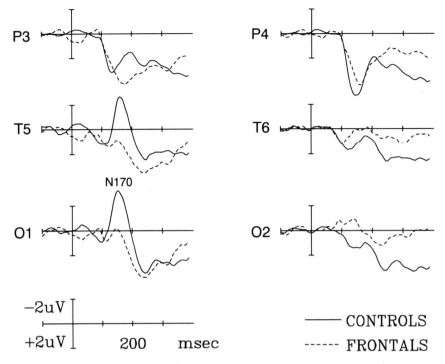

P3   P4

T5   T6

N170

O1   O2

−2uV

+2uV   200   msec

———— CONTROLS

------ FRONTALS

Figure 8.3 Grand average ERPs recorded from left and right parietal, posterior temporal, and occipital electrodes in controls and patients with prefrontal lesions (10 left, 1 right hemisphere). These ERPs were elicited by visually presented words in a recognition memory paradigm. The left lateralized N170 component was reduced by lesions of left dorsolateral prefrontal cortex.

presentation and either target detection or responses to all stimuli. Lateralized stimulation could conceivably result in signal detection deficits in the visual field contralateral to the lesioned hemisphere.

Phasic Attention and Frontal-Hippocampal Circuits

The P300 component of the human ERP is a prominent scalp-recorded response that is widely utilized to study phasic attention and memory mechanisms. The P300 potential was first reported in 1965 (Sutton, Braren, Zubin, and John, 1965; Desmedt, Debecker, and Manil, 1965) and since then has been the subject of extensive cognitive research in normal, neurological, and psychiatric populations. P300-like potentials have been described in rats (Ehlers, Wall, and Chapin, 1991), cats (Buchwald and Squires, 1982), and monkeys (Arthur and Starr, 1984; Neville and Foote, 1984; Pineda, Foote, Neville, and Holmes, 1988), supporting a broad ethological significance and leading to systematic investigations of possible neural substrates (Paller, 1994; Swick et al., 1994).

Subcomponents of the P300 have been proposed to measure engagement of early attention and working memory mechanisms. Voluntary detection of a task-relevant stimulus in the visual, auditory, or somatosensory modalities generates a large P300 response that is maximal over parietal scalp regions (P3b). P3b amplitude and latency are responsive to stimulus probability, subjective probability, stimulus meaning, and task relevance (Donchin and Coles, 1988; Johnson, 1988) and have been related to a range of cognitive processes, including context updating, information delivery, stimulus categorization, and cognitive closure. Delivery of an unexpected and novel stimulus elicits an earlier latency P300 response (P3a), which is recorded over widespread anterior and posterior scalp sites. The P3a potential has a more frontocentral scalp distribution than the P3b in all sensory modalities and has been proposed as a central marker of the orienting response (Sokolov, 1963; Courchesne, Hillyard, and Galambos, 1975; Knight, 1984; Yamaguchi and Knight, 1991b).

No clear consensus has emerged on the cognitive underpinnings of the P300 (Verleger, 1988), primarily due to the fact that P300 is not a unitary brain potential arising from a discrete brain region or cognitive process, as was initially theorized. Instead, scalp positivities generated from 300 to 700 ms post-stimulus measure activation of multiple neocortical and limbic regions dependent upon the particular stimuli and tasks used. For instance, late positive components differing in scalp topography and latency have been linked to voluntary and involuntary attention and to different aspects of memory processing. Support for these conclusions is derived from scalp data in control subjects (Courchesne et al., 1975; Squires, Squires, and Hillyard, 1975; Ruchkin, Johnson, Grafman, Canoune, and Ritter, 1992; Rugg, 1995), intracranial recording in epileptic patients (Smith, Stapleton, and Halgren, 1986; McCarthy, Wood, Williamson, and Spencer, 1989; Puce, Andrewes, Berkovic, and Bladin, 1991; Halgren et al., 1995), and lesion studies in neurological patients (Knight, 1984, 1997; Knight, Scabini, et al., 1989; Yamaguchi and Knight, 1991a; Johnson, 1995).

Lesion data recorded from patients with focal damage in dorsolateral prefrontal cortex, in temporal-parietal junction, or in lateral parietal cortex (figure 8.4) have indicated that P300 has multiple neural generators. Lesions of the temporal-parietal junction result in marked reduction of P3a and P3b at posterior scalp sites in both the auditory (Knight, Scabini, et al., 1989; Verleger, Heide, Butt, and Kompf, 1994) and somatosensory modalities (Yamaguchi and Knight 1991a), but not in the visual modality (Knight, 1997). Lateral parietal lesions had no effect on either P3a or P3b. Additionally, these studies demonstrate that modality-specific regions contribute to the scalp P3b.

Prefrontal damage produces differential effects on P3a and P3b (figure 8.4). The parietal P3b is unaffected by prefrontal damage in simple sensory discrimination tasks. However, reductions are observed in more difficult tasks, particularly when the lesions include posterior prefrontal cortex (Swick and Knight, 1994). The novelty P3a response is decreased in prefrontal patients,

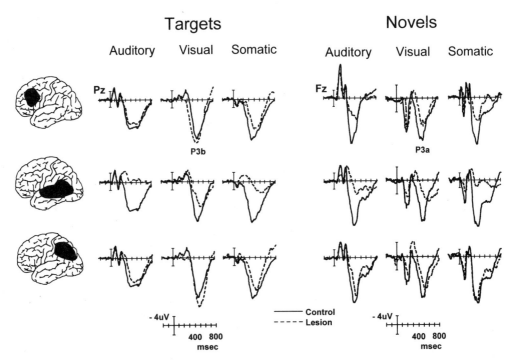

Figure 8.4 Summary of the target P3b (left) and novelty P3a components (right) in controls and three patient groups with focal cortical damage. The area of maximum lesion overlap in each group is drawn in black (far left). ERPs are shown for electrodes with the largest responses (Pz for targets, Fz for novels) to stimuli in the auditory, visual, and somatosensory modalities. Prefrontal (top) and lateral parietal damage (bottom) did not affect the latency or amplitude of P3b in simple detection tasks of any modality. Conversely, temporal-parietal lesions (middle) reduced P3b amplitude in the auditory and somatosensory modalities, with only partial reductions in the visual modality. Prefrontal and temporal-parietal lesions produced multi-modal reductions of the novelty P3a, while lateral parietal lesions had no significant effects.

with reductions observed throughout the lesioned hemisphere. Frontal lesions produce comparable P3a decrements in the auditory (Knight, 1984), visual (Knight, 1997), and somatosensory modalities (Yamaguchi and Knight, 1991a). These findings suggest that prefrontal cortex plays a critical role in the detection of novel stimuli. Furthermore, the results illustrate the importance of distributed interactions between prefrontal and posterior regions during both voluntary and involuntary attention (Mesulam, 1981).

Neural modeling (Metcalfe, 1993) and PET data (Tulving, Markowitsch, et al., 1994; Tulving, Markowitsch, Craik, Habib, and Houle, 1996) have recently implicated prefrontal and mesial temporal structures in novelty detection. Unilateral damage centered in the posterior hippocampal region has minimal effect on parietal P3b activity generated in response to auditory, visual, and somatosensory targets, but reduces front-central P3a activity to novel stimuli in all modalities (see figure 8.5 and color plate 9 for visual P3), with reductions most prominent at frontal sites (Knight, 1996). These observations

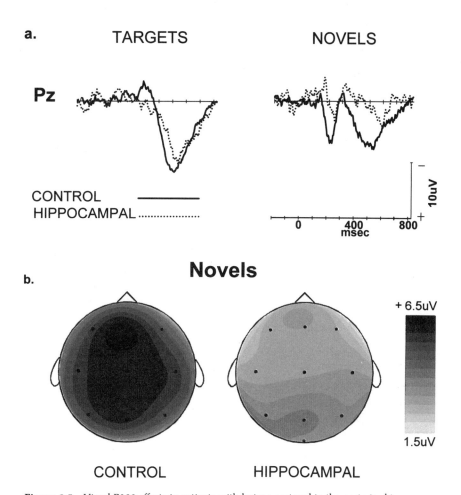

a.

TARGETS   NOVELS

Pz

CONTROL ————
HIPPOCAMPAL ·················

10uV

0   400   800
msec

b.

Novels

+ 6.5uV

1.5uV

CONTROL   HIPPOCAMPAL

Figure 8.5 Visual P300 effects in patients with lesions centered in the posterior hippocampus. (a) The target P3b (left) and novelty P3a responses (right) from control subjects and patients. Hippocampal lesions produced reductions in the P3a while sparing the P3b. (b) Scalp voltage maps illustrate the widespread decrease in the novelty P3a after hippocampal damage. See color plate 9.

support involvement of a prefrontal-hippocampal system in the detection of deviancies in the ongoing sensory stream. Reciprocal intra- and interhemispheric pathways (Amaral, Insausti, and Cowan, 1984; Goldman-Rakic et al., 1984) coursing through retrosplenial cortex or the cingulate may provide the anatomical substrates for prefrontal-hippocampal interactions during novelty detection. Prefrontal-hippocampal interactions during orientation to novel stimuli may underlie the classic von Restorff effect, wherein novel or out-of-context stimuli are better remembered (von Restorff, 1933; Karis, Fabiani, and Donchin, 1984; Metcalfe, 1993). Taken together, these ERP experiments provide further evidence that P300 subcomponents reflect distributed neural activity in corticolimbic regions engaged during voluntary and involuntary responses to discrete environmental events.

Higher-Level Functions: Executive Control and the Use of Strategies

One difficulty with precise definition of the role of the frontal lobes in higher cognitive functions is deciding whether an observed impairment is a primary effect of frontal lobe damage or is secondary to deficits in more basic processes. For example, neuropsychological studies have implicated the frontal lobes in various types of human memory, including free recall (Incisa della Rocchetta and Milner, 1993; Janowsky, Shimamura, Kritchevsky, and Squire, 1989; Jetter, Posner, Freeman, and Markowitsch, 1986), source memory (Janowsky, Shimamura, and Squire, 1989), and memory for temporal order (McAndrews and Milner, 1991; Shimamura, Janowsky, and Squire, 1990). However, deficits in attention and sensory gating could contribute to an inefficient use of encoding and retrieval strategies (Gershberg and Shimamura, 1995; Stuss, Alexander, et al., 1994). Distractibility and interference effects have been cited as major contributors to the types of memory problems exhibited by frontal lesion patients (Knight, 1991; Shimamura, Jurica, Mangels, Gershberg, and Knight, 1995).

A proliferation of functional neuroimaging experiments has reported blood flow changes in frontal regions during the performance of various memory tasks (for a review, see Buckner and Petersen, 1996). Positron emission tomography (PET) studies have observed blood flow activations in right anterior prefrontal cortex during memory retrieval in word stem cued recall (Buckner et al., 1995; Squire et al., 1992), verbal recognition (Tulving, Markowitsch, Kapur, et al., 1994; Andreasen et al., 1995), and retrieval of previously studied category exemplars (Shallice et al., 1994). Other PET investigations that scanned subjects during memory encoding yielded activations in left inferior prefrontal cortex (areas 45, 46, 47, and 10; Kapur et al., 1994). Given that set of observations, the hemispheric encoding/retrieval asymmetry model (Tulving, Kapur, Craik, et al., 1994) proposed that left prefrontal cortex is preferentially involved in the encoding of novel information into episodic memory, whereas right prefrontal cortex is more involved in episodic memory retrieval.

To test that hypothesis, cued recall performance was evaluated in a group of 16 frontal lesion patients (Swick and Knight, 1996). To control for possible strategy deficits, a simple organizing framework was provided. All subjects were told they could complete the items in any order and could fill in the items they remembered first. Patients were selected on the basis of focal prefrontal cortex lesion (11 patients had lesions on the left, and 5 had lesions on the right hemisphere) and were divided into three groups (figure 8.6 and color plate 10). Left superior frontal lesions were restricted to areas 6, 8, 9, 10, and superior 46; left inferior frontal lesions also included inferior areas 44, 45, and 46; right frontal lesions included areas 6, 8, 9, 10, or 46. Left frontal lesion patients (collapsed across superior and inferior groups) recalled fewer words than did controls in the first but not in the second experiment (figure 8.7). The right frontal lesion patients were not impaired with either

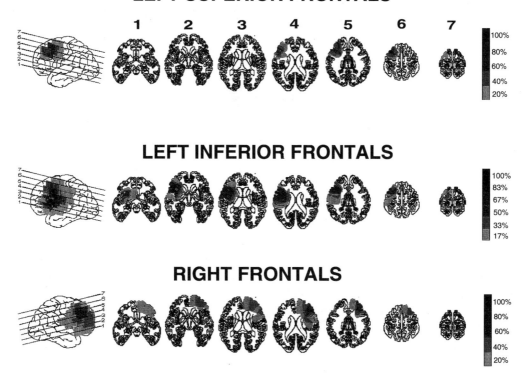

LEFT SUPERIOR FRONTALS

1   2   3   4   5   6   7

100%
80%
60%
40%
20%

LEFT INFERIOR FRONTALS

100%
83%
67%
50%
33%
17%

RIGHT FRONTALS

100%
80%
60%
40%
20%

Figure 8.6 Lesion reconstructions for frontal patients in the cued recall study, showing the degree of overlap and lesion variability. The scale refers to the percentage of patients in each group with lesions in that area. Lines through the lateral view show the level of the axial cuts from ventral (1) to dorsal (7). (Top) Patients with left frontal lesions restricted to areas 6, 8, 9, 10, and superior 46. (Middle) Patients with left frontal lesions that included inferior areas 44, 45, and 46. (Bottom) Patients with damage to right frontal areas 6, 8, 9, 10, or 46. See color plate 10.

list. Thus, the regions of prefrontal cortex activated in PET studies of young control subjects were not necessary for memory retrieval in these patients. Right prefrontal cortex could be activated by several strategic aspects of the cued recall paradigm (operating under time constraints, switching between recall of old words and generation of new words, etc.) that were minimized in our study. Hence, brain reorganization, a change in cognitive strategies, or both could be responsible for their intact performance.

CONCLUSIONS

Damage to dorsolateral prefrontal cortex produces impairments in sustained and phasic attention abilities, as well as deficits in inhibitory control of external stimuli and internal cognitive processing. Thus, the prefrontal lesion patient operates in a noisy internal environment deficient in the critical regulatory mechanisms necessary for the maintenance of working memory,

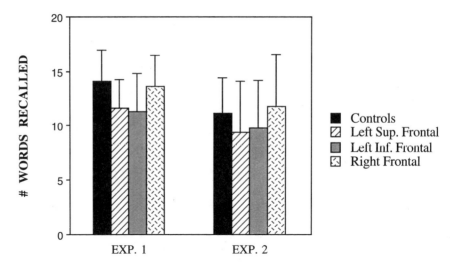

Figure 8.7 Number of words recalled (out of 20) in the word stem cued recall study. Subjects were controls and patients with left superior frontal ($n = 5$), left inferior frontal ($n = 6$), or right frontal lesions ($n = 5$). The encoding tasks were living versus nonliving (experiment 1) and concrete versus abstract discriminations (experiment 2).

executive control functions, and the use of strategies. Prefrontal cortex appears to have both inhibitory and facilitory influences on sensory and cognitive processing. Early input to primary sensory cortices is modulated by net inhibitory, prefrontal-controlled mechanisms. Conversely, later processing in association cortices is dependent on a facilitory prefrontal input. Little is known about the cellular or pharmacological substrates of these systems. This is a crucial area of research, because it has the potential to lead to treatment intervention for regulatory deficits in remote cortex secondary to prefrontal damage.

In addition to these sensory control mechanisms subserving sustained attention and working memory, a prefrontal-hippocampal network is selectively engaged during processing of novel stimuli. Based on anatomical connectivity, Nauta (1971) suggested that the prefrontal cortex is ideally suited to generate and evaluate internal models of action. It is proposed that in addition to that function and its role in sustained attention and working memory, a prefrontal-hippocampal system is crucial for detecting changes in the environment and for discriminating between internally and externally derived models of the world (Knight and Grabowecky, 1995). Deficits in those abilities may be responsible for most of the cognitive consequences of prefrontal lesions.

ACKNOWLEDGMENTS

We give special thanks to Clay C. Clayworth for technical assistance in all phases of the work. This work is supported by NINDS Javits Award

NS21135, by PO NS17778 from the NINDS, by the Veterans Administration Medical Research Service, and by the McDonnell-Pew Charitable Trust.

REFERENCES

Amaral, D. G., Insausti, R., and Cowan, W. M. (1984) The commisural connections of the monkey hippocampal formation. *J. Comp. Neurol.* 224: 307–336.

Andreasen, N. C., O'Leary, D. S., Arndt, S., Cizadlo, T., Hurtig, R., Rezai, K., Watkins, G. L., Ponto, L. L., and Hichwa, R. D. (1995) Short-term and long-term verbal memory: A positron emission tomography study. *Proc. Natl. Acad.Sci. U S A* 92: 5111–5115.

Arthur, D. L. and Starr, A. (1984) Task-relevant late positive component of the auditory event-related potential in monkeys resembles P300 in humans. *Science* 223: 186–188.

Bartus R. T. and Levere, T. E. (1977) Frontal decortication in Rhesus monkeys. A test of the interference hypothesis. *Brain Res.* 119: 233–248.

Bouillard, J. B. (1825) Recherches cliniques propres a demontrer que la perte de la parole correspond a la lesion des lobules anterieurs du cerveau. *Arch. Gen. Med.* 8: 24–45.

Buchwald, J. S. and Squires, N. K. (1982) Endogenous auditory potentials in the cat: A P300 model. In *Conditioning: Representation of Involved Neural Function*, edited by C. Woody, pp. 503–515. New York: Plenum Press.

Buckner, R. L. and Petersen, S. E. (1996) What does neuroimaging tell us about the role of prefrontal cortex in memory retrieval? *Sem. Neurosci.* 8: 47–55.

Buckner, R. L., Petersen, S. E., Ojemann, J. G., Miesin, F. M., Squire, L. R., and Raichle, M. E. (1995). Functional anatomical studies of explicit and implicit memory retrieval tasks. *J. Neurosci.* 15: 12–29.

Caramazza, A. (1986) On drawing inferences about the structure of normal cognitive processes from patterns of impaired performance: The case for single-patient studies. *Brain Cogn.* 5: 41–66.

Caramazza, A. (1992) Is cognitive neuropsychology possible? *J. Cog. Neurosci.* 4: 80–95.

Chao, L. L. and Knight, R. T. (1995) Human prefrontal lesions increase distractibility to irrelevant sensory inputs. *Neuroreport* 6: 1605–1610.

Courchesne, E., Hillyard, S. A., and Galambos, R. (1975) Stimulus novelty, task relevance, and the visual evoked potential. *Electroencephalogr. Clin. Neurophysiol.* 39: 131–143.

Curran, T., Tucker, D. M., Kutas, M., and Posner, M. I. (1993) Topography of the N400: Brain electrical activity reflecting semantic expectancy. *Electroencephalogr. Clin. Neurophysiol.* 88: 188–209.

Damasio, H. and Damasio, A. R. (1989) *Lesion Analysis in Neuropsychology*. New York: Oxford University Press.

Dejerine, J. (1892) Contribution a l'etude anatomopathologique et clinique des differentes varietes de cecite verbale. *Compt Rend Hebdomadaires Seances Mem. Soc. Biol.* 4: 61–90.

Desmedt, J. E., Debecker, J., and Manil, J. (1965) Mise en evidence d'un signe electrique cerebral associe a la detection par le sujet d'un stimulus sensoriel tactile. *Bull. Acad. R. Med. Belg.* 5: 887–936.

Donchin, E. and Coles, M. G. H. (1988) Is the P300 component a manifestation of context updating? *Behav. Brain Sci.* 11: 357–374.

Ehlers, C. L., Wall, T. L., and Chapin, R. I. (1991) Long latency event-related potentials in rats: Effects of dopaminergic and serotonergic depletions. *Pharm. Biochem. Behav.* 38: 789–793.

Friedman, H. R. and Goldman-Rakic, P. S. (1994) Coactivation of prefrontal and inferior parietal cortex in working memory tasks revealed by 2DG functional mapping in the Rhesus monkey. *J. Neurosci.* 14: 2775–2788.

Funahashi, S., Bruce, C. J., and Goldman-Rakic, P. S. (1993) Dorsolateral prefrontal lesions and oculomotor delayed-response performance: Evidence for mnemonic "scotomas." *J. Neurosci.* 13: 1479–1497.

Fuster, J. M., Bauer, R. H., and Jervey, J. P. (1985) Functional interactions between inferotemporal and prefrontal cortex in a cognitive task. *Brain Res.* 330: 299–307.

Gershberg, F. B. and Shimamura, A. P. (1995) Impaired use of organizational strategies in free recall following frontal lobe damage. *Neuropsychologia* 33: 1305–1333.

Goldman-Rakic, P. S., Selemon, L. D., and Schwartz, M. L. (1984) Dual pathways connecting the dorsolateral prefrontal cortex with the hippocampal formation and parahippocampal cortex in the Rhesus monkey. *Neuroscience* 12: 719–743.

Gomez Gonzalez, C. M., Clark, V. P., Fan, S., Luck, S. J., and Hillyard, S. A. (1994) Sources of attention-sensitive visual event-related potentials. *Brain Topogr.* 7: 41–51.

Halgren, E., Baudena, P., Clarke, J. M., Heit, G., Marinkovic, K., Devaux, B., Vignal, J. P., and Biraben, A. (1995) Intracerebral potentials to rare target and distractor stimuli. II. Medial, lateral and posterior temporal lobe. *Electroencephalogr. Clin. Neurophysiol.* 94: 229–250.

Harlow, J. M. (1868) Recovery from the passage of an iron bar through the head. *Publ. Mass. Med. Soc.* 2: 327–346.

Heilman, K. M., Watson, R. T., and Valenstein, E. (1994) Localization of lesions in neglect and related disorders. In *Localization and Neuroimaging in Neuropsychology*, edited by A. Kertesz, pp. 495–524. San Diego: Academic Press.

Hillyard, S. A. and Picton, T. W. (1987) Electrophysiology of cognition. In *Handbook of Physiology: The Nervous System* (Vol. 5), edited by F. Plum, pp. 519–584. Bethesda, MD: American Physiological Society.

Incisa della Rocchetta, A. and Milner, B. (1993) Strategic search and retrieval inhibition: The role of the frontal lobes. *Neuropsychologia* 31: 503–524.

Janowsky, J. S., Shimamura, A. P., Kritchevsky, M., and Squire, L. R. (1989) Cognitive impairment following frontal lobe damage and its relevance to human amnesia. *Behav. Neurosci.* 103: 548–560.

Janowsky, J. S., Shimamura, A. P., and Squire, L. R. (1989) Source memory impairment in patients with frontal lobe lesions. *Neuropsychologia* 27: 1043–1056.

Jetter, W., Poser, U., Freeman, R. B., and Markowitsch, H. J. (1986) A verbal long term memory deficit in frontal lobe damaged patients. *Cortex* 22: 229–242.

Johannes, S., Munte, T. F., Heinze, H. J., and Mangun, G. R. (1995) Luminance and spatial attention effects on early visual processing. *Cogn. Brain Res.* 2: 189–205.

Johnson, R., Jr. (1988) The amplitude of the P300 component of the event-related potential: Review and synthesis. In *Advances in Psychophysiology* (Vol. 3) edited by P. K. Ackles, J. R. Jennings, and M. G. H. Coles, Greenwich, CT: JAI Press.

———. (1995) On the neural generators of the P300: Evidence from temporal lobectomy patients. *Electroencephalogr. Clin. Neurophysiol. Suppl.* 44: 110–129.

Kapur, S., Craik, F. I. M., Tulving, E., Wilson, A. A., Houle, S., and Brown, G. M. (1994) Neuroanatomical correlates of encoding in episodic memory: Levels of processing effect. *Proc. Natl. Acad. Sci. U S A* 91: 2008–2011.

Karis, D., Fabiani, M., and Donchin, E. (1984) "P300" and memory: Individual differences in the von Restorff effect. *Cognit. Psychol.* 16: 177–216.

Knight, R. T. (1984) Decreased response to novel stimuli after prefrontal lesions in man. *Electroencephalogr. Clin. Neurophysiol.* 59: 9–20.

Knight, R. T. (1991) Evoked potential studies of attention capacity in human frontal lobe lesions. In *Frontal Lobe Function and Dysfunction,* edited by H. Levin, H. Eisenberg, and F. Benton, pp. 139–153. New York: Oxford University Press.

Knight, R. T. (1996) Contribution of human hippocampal region to novelty detection. *Nature.* 383: 256–259.

Knight, R. T. (1997) Distributed cortical network for visual stimulus detection. *J. Cog. Neurosci.* 9: 75–91.

Knight, R. T. and Grabowecky, M. (1995) Escape from linear time: Prefrontal cortex and conscious experience. In *The Cognitive Neurosciences,* edited by M. S. Gazzaniga, pp. 1357–1371. Cambridge, MA: MIT Press.

Knight, R. T., Hillyard, S. A., Woods, D. L., and Neville, H. J. (1981) The effects of frontal cortex lesions on event-related potentials during auditory selective attention. *Electroencephalogr. Clin. Neurophysiol.* 52: 571–582.

Knight, R. T., Scabini, D., and Woods, D. L. (1989) Prefrontal cortex gating of auditory transmission in humans. *Brain Res.* 504: 338–342.

Knight, R. T., Scabini, D., Woods, D. L., and Clayworth, C. C. (1989) Contribution of the temporal-parietal junction to the auditory P3. *Brain Res.* 502: 109–116.

Kolb, B. and Whishaw, I. Q. (1990) *Fundamentals of Human Neuropsychology* 3rd. New York: W. H. Freeman.

Kosslyn, S. M., Daly, P. F., McPeek, R. M., Alpert, N. M., Kennedy, D. N., and Caviness, V. S., Jr. (1993) Using locations to store shape: An indirect effect of a lesion. *Cereb. Cortex* 3: 567–582.

Kosslyn, S. M. and Intriligator, J. M. (1992) Is cognitive neuropsychology plausible? The perils of sitting on a one-legged stool. *J. Cog. Neurosci.* 4: 96–106.

Kraus, N., Ozdamar, O., and Stein, L. (1982) Auditory middle latency responses (MLRs) in patients with cortical lesions. *Electroencephalogr. Clin. Neurophysiol.* 54: 275–287.

Leuders, H., Leser, R. P., Harn, J., Dinner, D. S., and Klem, G. (1983) Cortical somatosensory evoked potentials in response to hand stimulation. *J. Neurosurg.* 58: 885–894.

Lhermitte, F. (1986) Human autonomy and the frontal lobes. Part II. Patient behavior in complex and social situations: The "environmental dependency syndrome." *Ann. Neurol.* 19: 335–343.

Lhermitte, F., Pillon, B., and Serdaru, M. (1986) Human autonomy and the frontal lobes. Part I. Imitation and utilization behavior: A neuropsychological study of 75 patients. *Ann. Neurol.* 19: 326–334.

Malmo, R. R. (1942) Interference factors in delayed response in monkeys after removal of frontal lobes. *J. Neurophysiol.* 5: 295–308.

Mangun, G. R. (1995) Neural mechanisms of visual selective attention. *Psychophysiology* 32: 4–18.

McAndrews, M. P. and Milner, B. (1991) The frontal cortex and memory for temporal order. *Neuropsychologia* 29: 849–859.

McCarthy, G., Wood, C. C., Williamson, P. D., and Spencer, D. D. (1989) Task-dependent field potentials in human hippocampal formation. *J. Neurosci.* 9: 4253–4268.

McIntosh, A. R., Grady, C. L., Ungerleider, L. G., Haxby, J. V., Rapoport, S. I., and Horwitz, B. (1994) Network analysis of cortical visual pathways mapped with PET. *J. Neurosci.* 14: 655–666.

Mesulam, M. M. (1981) A cortical network for directed attention and unilateral neglect. *Ann. Neurol.* 10: 309–325.

Metcalfe, J. (1993) Novelty monitoring, metacognition, and control in a composite holographic associative recall model: Implications for Korsakoff amnesia. *Psychol. Rev.* 100: 3–22.

Nauta, W. J. H. (1971) The problem of the frontal lobe: A reinterpretation. *J. Psychiat. Res.* 8: 167–187.

Neville, H. J. and Foote, S. L. (1984) Auditory event-related potentials in the squirrel monkey: Parallels to human late wave responses. *Brain Res.* 298: 107–116.

Neville, H., Kutas, M., Chesney, G., and Schmidt, A. (1986) Event-related brain potentials during initial encoding and recognition memory of congruous and incongruous words. *J. Mem. Lang.* 25: 75–92.

Paller, K. A. (1994) The neural substrates of cognitive event-related potentials: A review of animal models of P3. In *Cognitive Electrophysiology: ERPs in Basic and Clinical Research*, edited by H. J. Heinze, T. F. Munte, and G. R. Mangun, pp. 300–333. Boston: Birkhauser.

Pineda, J. A., Foote, S. L., Neville, H. J., and Holmes, T. C. (1988) Endogenous event-related potentials in monkey: The role of task relevance, stimulus probability, and behavioral response. *Electroencephalogr. Clin. Neurophysiol.* 70: 155–171.

Puce, A., Andrewes, D. G., Berkovic, S. F., and Bladin, P. F. (1991) Visual recognition memory: Neurophysiological evidence for the role of temporal white matter in man. *Brain* 114: 1647–1666.

Richer, F., Decary, A., Lapierre, M. F., Rouleau, I., Bouvier, G., and Saint-Hilaire, J. M. (1993) Target detection deficits in frontal lobectomy. *Brain Cogn.* 21: 203–211.

Robertson, L. C., Knight, R. T., Rafal, R., and Shimamura, A. P. (1993) Cognitive neuro-psychology is more than single case studies. *J. Exp. Psychol. Learn. Mem. Cogn.* 19: 710–717.

Roland, P. E. (1982) Cortical regulation of selective attention in man. A regional cerebral blood flow study. *J. Neurophysiol.* 48: 1059–1078.

Ruchkin, D. S., Johnson, R., Jr., Grafman, J., Canoune, H., and Ritter, W. (1992) Distinctions and similarities among working memory processes: An event-related potential study. *Cogn. Brain Res.* 1: 53–66.

Rugg, M. D. (1995) Event-related potential studies of human memory. In *The Cognitive Neuro-sciences*, edited by M. S. Gazzaniga, pp. 789–801. Cambridge, MA: MIT Press.

Scoville, W. B. and Milner, B. (1957) Loss of recent memory after bilateral hippocampal lesions. *J. Neurol. Neurosurg. Psychiatry* 20: 11–21.

Seltzer, B. and Pandya, D. N. (1989) Frontal lobe connections of the superior temporal sulcus in the Rhesus monkey. *J. Comp. Neurol.* 281: 97–113.

Shallice, T. (1988) *From Neuropsychology to Mental Structure*. Cambridge, England: Cambridge University Press.

Shallice, T., Fletcher, P., Frith, C. D., Grasby, P., Frackowiak, R. S., and Dolan, R. J. (1994) Brain regions associated with acquisition and retrieval of verbal episodic memory. *Nature* 368: 633–635.

Shimamura, A. P. (1995) Memory and the frontal lobe. In *The Cognitive Neurosciences*, edited by M. S Gazzaniga, pp. 803–813. Cambridge: MIT Press.

Shimamura, A. P., Janowsky, J. S., and Squire, L. R. (1990) Memory for the temporal order of events in patients with frontal lobe lesions and amnesic patients. *Neuropsychologia* 28: 803–814.

Shimamura, A. P., Jurica, P. J., Mangels, J. A., Gershberg, F. B., and Knight, R. T. (1995) Susceptibility to memory interference effects following frontal lobe damage: Findings from tests of paired-associate learning. *J. Cog. Neurosci.* 7: 144–152.

Skinner, J. E. and Yingling, C. D. (1977) Central gating mechanisms that regulate event-related potentials and behavior. In *Progress in Clinical Neurophysiology* (Vol. 1), edited by J. E. Desmedt, pp. 30–69. Basel, Switzerland: S. Karger.

Smith, M. E., Stapleton, J. M., and Halgren, E. (1986) Human medial temporal lobe potentials evoked in memory and language tasks. *Electroencephalogr. Clin. Neurophysiol.* 63: 145–159.

Sokol, S. M., McCloskey, M., Cohen, N. J., and Aliminosa, D. (1991) Cognitive representations and processes in arithmetic: Inferences from the performance of brain-damaged subjects. *J. Exp. Psychol. Learn. Mem. Cogn.* 17: 355–376.

Sokolov, E. N. (1963) Higher nervous functions: The orienting reflex. *Annu. Rev. Physiol.* 25: 545–580.

Squire, L. R., Ojemann, J. G., Miezin, F. M., Petersen, S. E., Videen, T. O., and Raichle, M. E. (1992) Activation of the hippocampus in normal humans: A functional anatomical study of memory. *Proc. Natl. Acad. Sci. U S A* 89: 1837–1841.

Squires, N. K., Squires, K. C., and Hillyard, S. A. (1975) Two varieties of long-latency positive waves evoked by unpredictable auditory stimuli in man. *Electroencephalogr. Clin. Neurophysiol.* 38: 387–401.

Stookey, B. (1954) A note on the early history of cerebral localization. *Bull. N Y Acad. Med.* 30: 559–578.

Stuss, D. T., Alexander, M. P., Palumbo, C. L., Buckle, L., Sayer, L., and Pogue, J. (1994) Organizational strategies of patients with unilateral or bilateral frontal lobe injury in word learning tasks. *Neuropsychology* 8: 355–373.

Stuss, D. T. and Benson, D. F. (1986) *The Frontal Lobes.* New York: Raven Press.

Stuss, D. T., Eskes, G. A., and Foster, J. K. (1994) Experimental neuropsychological studies of frontal lobe function. In *Handbook of Neuropsychology* (Vol. 9) edited by F. Boller, and J. Grafman, Amsterdam: Elsevier.

Sutton, S., Braren, M., Zubin, J., and John, E. R. (1965) Evoked-potential correlates of stimulus uncertainty. *Science* 150: 1187–1188.

Swick, D. and Knight, R. T. (1994) Recognition memory and cued recall in patients with frontal cortex lesions: ERP and behavioral findings. *Soc. Neurosci. Abstr.* 20: 1003.

Swick, D. and Knight, R. T. (1996) Is prefrontal cortex involved in cued recall? A neuropsychological test of PET findings. *Neuropsychologia* 34: 1019–1028.

Swick, D. and Knight, R. T. (1996) Dorsolateral prefrontal cortex modulates visual processing in extrastriate cortex. *Soc. Neurosci. Abstr.* 22: 1107.

Swick, D., Kutas, M., and Neville, H. (1994) Localizing the neural generators of event-related brain potentials. In *Localization and Neuroimaging in Neuropsychology*, edited by A. Kertesz, pp. 73–121. San Diego: Academic Press.

Tulving, E., Kapur, S., Craik, F. I. M., Moscovitch, M., and Houle, S. (1994) Hemispheric encoding/retrieval asymmetry in episodic memory: Positron emission tomography findings. *Proc. Natl. Acad. Sci. U S A* 91: 2016–2020.

Tulving, E., Kapur, S., Markowitsch, H. J., Craik, F. I. M., Habib, R., and Houle, S. (1994) Neuro-anatomical correlates of retrieval in episodic memory: Auditory sentence recognition. *Proc. Natl. Acad. Sci. U S A* 91: 2012–2015.

Tulving, E., Markowitsch, H. J., Kapur, S., Habib, R., and Houle, S. (1994) Novelty encoding networks in the human brain: Positron emission tomography data. *Neuroreport* 5: 2525–2528.

Tulving, E., Markowitsch, H. J., Craik, F. I. M., Habib, R., and Houle, S. (1996) Novelty and familiarity activations in PET studies of memory encoding and retrieval. *Cereb. Cortex* 6: 71–79.

Vendrell, P., Junque, C., Pujol, J., Jurado, M. A., Molet, J., and Grafman, J. (1995) The role of prefrontal regions in the Stroop task. *Neuropsychologia* 33: 341–352.

Verleger, R. (1988) Event-related potentials and cognition: A critique of the context updating hypothesis and an alternative interpretation of P3. *Behav. Brain Sci.* 11: 343–427.

Verleger, R., Heide, W., Butt, C., and Kompf, D. (1994) Reduction of P3b potentials in patients with temporo-parietal lesions. *Cogn. Brain Res.* 2: 103–116.

von Restorff, H. (1933) Uber die Wirkung von Bereischsbildungen im spurenfeld. *Psychol. Forsch.* 18: 299–342.

Yamaguchi, S. and Knight, R. T. (1990) Gating of somatosensory inputs by human prefrontal cortex. *Brain Res.* 521: 281–288.

Yamaguchi, S. and Knight, R. T. (1991a) Anterior and posterior association cortex contribution to the somatosensory P300. *J. Neurosci.* 11: 2039–2054.

Yamaguchi, S. and Knight, R. T. (1991b) P300 generation by novel somatosensory stimuli. *Electroencephalogr. Clin. Neurophysiol.* 78: 50–55.

Yingling, C. D. and Skinner, J. E. (1977) Gating of thalamic input to cerebral cortex by nucleus reticularis thalami. In *Progress in Clinical Neurophysiology* (Vol. I) edited by J. E. Desmedt, pp. 70–96. Basel, Switzerland: S. Karger.

9 Computational Architectures for Attention

Ernst Niebur and Christof Koch

ABSTRACT   Visual selective attention is analyzed from a computational point of view. The functional necessity for an attentional process is explained and its implementation in biology is studied. The control processes of spatial attentional are examined and several neurobiologically relevant theories and detailed models of focal attention are discussed.

THE COMPUTATIONAL NEED FOR A SELECTION PROCESS

Selective attention is nature's solution to a computational dilemma. On the one hand, a large variety of sensors in different modalities is required to monitor ongoing events in the environment. On the other hand, the amount of information provided by the multitude of sensors far exceeds the information-processing capacity fo the brain. Likewise, a complete, verbatim storage of all sensory information would also exhaust the available storage capacity within a short period of time. Therefore, appropriate filtering to eliminate all sensory input except for a carefully selected small subset is essential for the efficient functioning of biological information processors.

Computational models of the filtering process, which is commonly known as selective attention, are examined in this chapter. Different neuroscience methods, from single-neuron recordings (Motter, chapter 4, this volume) to functional magnetic resonance imaging (Haxby, chapter 7, this volume) have been used to examine selective attention. Computational models that are guided by neuroscience data can contribute to a deeper understanding of the neural mechanisms of attention. In turn, such models offer quantitative hypotheses that can be tested using these and other empirical neuroscience methods. Moreover, computational methods may contribute to the development of future artificial information-processing systems (e.g., computer vision). Functionality similar to selective processing has been shown to be necessary for such systems once a certain level of complexity is achieved.

OVERVIEW OF COMPUTATIONAL MODELS OF ATTENTION

In recent years, considerable effort has been devoted to the understanding of attentional mechanisms, frequently with computational considerations in mind. Only those computational models that have a clear relation to the underlying biological substrate are examined here. Connectionist (or neural network) studies developed in the last years (for examples, see Fukushima, Miyaki, and Ito, 1983; Grossberg, Mingolla, and Ross, 1994; Humphreys and Müller, 1993) are not discussed in detail. In the connectionist paradigm, networks are constructed from interacting units (assumed to correspond roughly to neurons or groups of neurons), which are connected in various ways. The basic functions in many connectionist networks are, however, quite different from those of biological neurons (for instance, units may exchange information about pointers, abstract addresses, etc.). This difference makes it difficult to compare predictions of connectionist architectures with physiological observations. An additional problem is that most connectionist studies are limited in the set of data they explain. There are, however, attempts to correlate the behavior of connectionist networks with that observed in patients with attentional deficits (e.g., Mozer and Behrmann, 1990).

The following computational models are discussed. First, a recently developed framework for feature-based attention based on simple assumptions regarding the behavior of single neurons is examined. Second, a number of theories of selective attention comprise two interacting processing stages, the first being a fast and parallel preattentive module that provides input to a second stage that is slow and sequential (Hoffman, 1978, 1979; Neisser, 1967). Those theories include feature integration theory (Treisman and Gelade, 1980), attentional engagement theory (Duncan and Humphreys, 1989), and guided search (Wolfe, Cave, and Franzel, 1989; Wolfe, 1994). The link between the two stages is usually implemented by a saliency map, the modeling of which is examined. Finally, models of selective attention based on the distinction between the "what" and "where" neural pathways of vision are examined.

COVERT AND OVERT ATTENTION

Only a small fraction of the information registered by the visual system at any given time reaches levels of processing that directly influence behavior. Visual attention controls access to that privileged level and ensures that the selected information is relevant to behavioral priorities and objectives. Visual attention can be covert, or not directly observable from outside the organism, or it can be overt, as in the movements of the eyes that accompany visual monitoring. Operationally, information is said to be attended if it enters short-term memory and remains there long enough to be voluntarily reported (in principle). Thus, visual attention is closely linked to visual awareness and consciousness (Crick and Koch, 1995).

Selective attention is required because the detailed processing of all sensory information from all channels simultaneously and in time is computationally too demanding, either for biological or for physical systems. Another, closely related problem faced by animals and humans is the required spatial resolution of visual input. In that case, the conflict arises because, on the one hand, a mechanism with very high spatial resolution is needed for such perceptual tasks as hyperacuity. On the other hand, a powerful surveying capability is needed for monitoring large parts of the visual field. Both tasks are apparently necessary for survival, but it is not feasible to endow the surveying mechanism with a spatial resolution necessary for some of the finer tasks.

In the case of visual attention, the solution adopted by nature is to not fulfill all requirements simultaneously and instead to spread processing over a longer period of time. The solution amounts to the sharing of computational resources; they are allocated at one time to one task and at another time to another task. The conflicting requirements of spatial resolution are met by a similar strategy that emphasizes the spatial allocation of resources over the temporal one. The adopted solution is a spatial segregation of the visual field into a high-resolution central foveal region (Westheimer, 1979) and a periphery with progressively lower resolution that decreases approximately linearly with excentricity outside the foveal region. Because only fixated stimuli benefit from the high foveal resolution, detailed scrutiny of different parts of the environment requires that the machinery for high-resolution processing be brought in register with the region to be scanned. The fovea has thus to be moved over the visual field, an activity that is typically achieved in primates with the use of rapid eye movements (or with head movements, which are not discussed here).

The spatial selection process, or overt attention, is easily observed in the form of eye movements and is functionally quite similar to covert selective attention. Covert attention is less directly observable, although many quantitative measures have been devised to characterize it (see Marrocco and Davidson, chapter 3 this volume). Note also that the visual modality is not the only one in which it is possible to distinguish between the two types of attention; for example the motor behavior associated with exploratory touch responses (Hsiao, O'Shaughness, and Johnson, 1993) can be understood as overt attention in the somatosensory modality.

Overt and covert visual attention are not two independent functions. The maximal rate of eye movements (saccades) in humans is about five per second; most estimates for the rate of the shift of covert attention are higher by at least a factor of five. That difference supports the so-called scouting hypothesis, which states that several shifts of covert attention precede and accompany each saccade and assist in choosing the location in the visual field to where the next saccade will be made. That hypothesis is supported by recordings of eye movements following the tachistoscopic presentation of letters or numerals too fast to allow the subject to benefit from eye movements during the presentation. It was observed that the part of the display most accurately reported was the one to which the eyes jumped after the presentation (Bryden, 1961; Crovitz and Daves, 1962; for more recent data, see McPeek and Nakayama, 1995). Those data are thus consistent with the assumption that the focus of attention was shifted rapidly before the eye movement and, while allowing the subject to generate an accurate report of the stimulus in that area, also guided the eye movement towards this region. Other lines of evidence in support of this hypothesis come from electro-physiological data implying that receptive fields in parietal cortex (an area closely related to attentional control; Bushnell, Goldberg, and Robinson, 1981; Mountcastle, Andersen, and Motter, 1981) shift in anticipation of eye movements (Duhamel, Colby, and Goldberg, 1992).

COMPUTATIONAL ARCHITECTURE OF THE SELECTION PROCESS

The structure of the visual system reflects the functionality of the attentional selection process. Close to the sensory periphery, neural receptive fields are characterized by a high degree of spatial specificity, allowing for massively parallel information processing in the different parts of the visual field. Receptive fields generally become larger (i.e., have coarse spatial specificity) for cells that are higher in the cortical hierarchy. In inferotemporal (IT) cortex, cells also become more selective for stimulus features. For example, an oriented edge of a certain angle is a good stimulus for a neuron in striate cortex, provided that the edge is located in a small part of the visual field. Most neurons in the IT areas are excited best by more complex stimuli, like pictures of faces or hands, that can occur almost anywhere in the visual field. Selective attention assures that we do not perceive a superposition of all stimuli present at a given time in our visual field, by suppressing the non-attended stimuli such that only one stimulus is processed at a given time in higher cortical areas. The suppression is observed in electrophysiological recordings in extrastriate and IT areas (Moran and Desimone, 1985; Motter, 1993; also, see Motter, chapter 4 this volume). If, as is usually the case, more than one relevant stimulus is present in the visual scene at a given time, they are processed sequentially. Thus, selective attention provides an effective bottleneck between the massively parallel information processing in early cortex and the sequential processing in later stages.

Parallel and Sequential Processing

Because of the large number of elements in the sensory arrays, efficient information processing requires massive parallelism close to the sensory surfaces (e.g., retina, lateral geniculate nucleus, superior colliculus, and striate cortex). An essential task of the neurons in those structures is the extraction of elementary stimulus features, such as oriented edges in vision. Parallelism is an efficient strategy because of the limited number of such elementary features, which makes it possible to provide dedicated processors for each such feature at each location. However, only a limited amount of information can be extracted directly from such elementary stimuli, which is in general not sufficient for the needs of higher organisms. Because of the astronomical number of possible combinations of stimuli, which creates a combinatorial explosion, it is practically impossible to provide specialized detectors for each behaviorally important stimulus at every possible position, orientation, contrast, and so forth.

That impossibility leads to two consequences. The first is that not every perceptual operation is possible in parallel at every location on the sensory surface. Instead, perception becomes a hybrid of parallel and sequential processes, in which the extraction of elementary features is performed in parallel for all locations of the sensory surface, whereas more advanced processing is a sequential process. The interplay between the processes is the primary subject of this chapter. (Note, however, that it is difficult to determine from behavioral data alone, e.g., reaction time, whether a process is executed sequentially or in parallel. See Egeth, 1966; Townsend, 1972, 1990.)

The second consequence is that a pure feedforward, or bottom-up, approach is severely limited (Tsotsos, 1990). The explosion of the number of all feature combinations can be avoided by constructing an internal representation of the stimulus, which makes it possible to manipulate such abstract representations of the external world rather than enumerate all possible stimulus situations (which is called analysis by synthesis; see Neisser, 1967). Despite the obvious importance of that strategy in a behavioral context, it goes beyond the selection process commonly associated with selective attention and we will therefore not discuss it in detail in this chapter.

Although we will frequently discuss the hierarchical structure of perception, we do not want to suggest a feedforward paradigm, according to which perception can be seen as a filtering operation of more and more complex stimuli. Such a feedforward paradigm is incompatible with physiological (Douglas, Martin, and Whitteridge, 1989) and anatomical (Douglas, Koch, Mahowald, Martin, and Suarez, 1995; Sherman and Koch, 1986) evidence that shows that the majority of synaptic inputs to cortical cells (up to 90% or more of all excitatory synapses) is provided by other cortical cells and not by sensory input. This highlights the importance of top-down influences in the central nervous system but it is, nevertheless, convenient to label the different areas depending on their functional distance to the sensory input as more or less peripheral. The importance of both bottom-up and top-down processes is exemplified by Ullman's (1995) model of information flow in visual cortex for object recognition. His basic elements are counterstreams, in which multiple hypotheses about the input are explored simultaneously bottom-up and top-down until a match is found.

What and Where

The attentional bottleneck that limits the total amount of information made accessible to higher cognitive functions could be implemented in a variety of ways. Computational arguments favor a divide-and-conquer strategy, in which stimuli are classified according to subsets of their features and those subsets are then treated sequentially. Although the general arguments are valid for any segregation of features in subsets, the most commonly evoked feature subset is the spatial location of a stimulus. The strategy then amounts to the sequential treatment of different spatially defined parts of the visual field (the focus, or spotlight of attention).

The key observation is that a significant reduction of complexity is achieved if the recognition of an object (what is it?) can be separated from its localization (where is it?). Such a separation is useful because those two properties of a stimulus are often independent from each other: a given stimulus can occur in many different places in a visual scene and, conversely, a given location in a visual scene can hold a variety of different stimuli. That observation allows the decoupling of the tasks of recognition and localization. Computationally, therefore, the size of the required space is only the sum of the feature space and the locality space, rather than their (outer) product, which is in general significantly larger.

There is psychophysical evidence that space does play a special role among features (Nissen, 1985; Shih and Sperling, 1993; for a different view, however, see Bundesen, 1991). Also, most quantitative paradigms are defined in terms of a focus of attention. Furthermore, a spatially based mechanism is supported by the observed anatomical and physiological structure of the primate visual system. That system uses anatomically distinct pathways for encoding spatial information of objects in the environment and the specific features of those objects. The locations of visual stimuli are represented in the dorsal (or "where") pathway, which is also the dominant cortical pathway for any visuomotor tasks, such as controlling the eyes, reaching with the hand toward a visually identified target, visually induced body adjustements, and so forth (Goodale and Milner, 1993). Detailed feature processing and object recognition are localized in the ventral (or "what") pathway (Ungerleider and Mishkin, 1982). Tight integration of the two pathways is essential; at any time, it is necessary that the information in one pathway can be unambiguously correlated with that in the other. A later section of this chapter examines how that integration is accomplished in the framework of recently developed models. The next section reviews psychophysical data detailing the control of the spotlight of attention.

The Control Of Attention

Cued Attention Within a psychophysical context it is useful to distinguish between experiments in which attention is captured by the features of the stimulus itself (i.e., that part of the visual stimulation to which the subject has to respond) and those experiments in which a cue is provided prior to the stimulus, the function of the cue being only to attract attention. Spatial cues direct attentional resources (the spotlight) to one part of the visual field. The most elementary type of cue directly indicates that the stimulus is to be expected at or near the location at which the cue is located. Another class consists of indirect cues that provide information about the location in a form that requires further processing (e.g., an arrowhead). Direct spatial cues are impossible to ignore in situations when one of several locations is known to hold the target stimulus. This is also true when it is known that the cue is irrelevant (Jonides, 1981) and even when it is known to be misleading (Remington, Johnston, and Yantis, 1992). Irrelevant indirect cues are also effective (Müller and Rabbitt, 1989).

Are organisms at the mercy of a visual environment that constantly generates cues at various locations in the visual scene, unable to attend anywhere else but to the cued locatios? Clearly not. Yantis and Jonides (1990) showed that deliberate attention can override direct (onset) cues. When an indirect cue indicated the location of the stimulus to be presented after the appearance of the cue, participants were able to focus attention to the cued area and ignore additional direct cues.

Can the seemingly opposing effects of direct cues be reconciled? The difference between the earlier observations and those reported by Yantis and Jonides (1990) is that in the latter case the location could be selected unequivocally before the appearance of the stimulus. In contrast, in the study by Jonides (1981), the cued location was only one of several, all of which could contain the stimulus. In the Remington et al. (1992) experiment, the cued location was certain not to contain the stimulus, but again the cue did not specify unambiguously which location would hold the stimulus; again, only a set of possible locations was indicated. It seems, therefore, that participants are able to focus on one contiguous part of the visual field but they cannot exclude (or negate) such a part, nor attend to more than one area (split-brain patients are an exception; see Luck, Hillyard, Mangun, and Gazzaniga, 1994). This has immediate consequences for the implementation of top-down control in a formal model discussed later.

Feature Detection   Attentional influences exist in the absence of cues; that is, they can be based on the properties of the stimulus itself. For instance, in visual search, salient visual features guide attention to the stimuli possessing those features, and those stimuli are then selected preferentially. In particular, it is known that stimuli that differ from nearby stimuli in one or more feature dimensions can be easily found in visual search. Treisman and Gelade (1980) published an elegant theoretical explanation accounting for that observation, based on the principle that the detection of elementary features is most economically carried out by massively parallel processes early in the visual hierarchy. Because the number of possible combinations of features increases very rapidly with the number of features to be combined, there are parallel, preattentive maps only for the elementary features. Conjunctions of the features can only be processed by a central attentional authority, which gives rise to the sequential attentional process. Although Treisman and Gelade's feature integration theory explained many properties of visual search, it was shown later to be invalid in its simplest form (Egeth, Virzi, and Garbart, 1984; Wolfe et al., 1989).

Furthermore, Yantis (1996) pointed out that although many single-feature stimuli (called singletons) are efficiently detected when they are targets in visual search tasks, this is not the equivalent of capturing attention. Several psychophysical experiments have shown that singletons capture attention only if the subject is expecting a singleton (Folk, Remington, and Johnston, 1992; Jonides and Yantis, 1988). If such is the case, then any singleton (in the feature dimension in which it is expected) is capable of capturing attention (e.g., if the expected singleton is in the color domain, then any color singleton will capture attention, not only a singleton of the expected color). Bacon and Egeth (1994) called this the singleton detection mode.

Temporal Dynamics Sequential scanning of the visual scene requires movement of the focus of attention analogous to the eye movements of overt attention. Several independent sets of data indicate that the time required for one shift of attention is on the order of 30–50 ms (for a direct measurement, see Saarinen and Julesz, 1994). Note, however, that other data indicate much longer dwell times for the focus of attention (Duncan, Ward, and Shapiro, 1994). The significant differences in scan times might possibly be accounted for by the use of simultaneously flashed stimuli in the former experiment and consecutively flashed stimuli in the latter.

It has been found that the time courses of the scanning motions generated by the two types of cues (direct and indirect) are different. Direct cues provide fast, strong effects that reach a maximum about 200 ms after the cue and decay within a few hundred milliseconds. In contrast, indirect cues generate moderately enhanced performance in the cued region that persists for a longer time (Cheal and Lyon, 1991; Müller and Rabbitt, 1989; Nakayama and Mackeben, 1989). A simple architecture incorporating a persistent top-down attentional influence has been suggested recently (Usher and Niebur, 1996) and is discussed later in this chapter.

Contemplation of a static scene is more the exception than the rule; attentional processes constantly need to cope with a changing environment. It was postulated by William James (1890) that abruptly changing stimuli attract attention. (That thesis was qualified recently by Hillstro, and Yantis [1994], who observed that motion per se does not capture attention in all cases. Instead, they found capture of attention in situations when relative motion segregated a new visual object from its perceptual group.) As always in situations in which more than one stimulus is present, sequential processing requires a decision to be made about the order in which the stimuli are attended to. In the context of abruptly appearing stimuli, Yantis and Johnson (1990) found that such stimuli were treated preferentially and that their priority decayed with time. That behavior is reflected in a model discussed later.

An additional temporal effect comes into play after the focus of attention has moved away from an attended location. There is strong psychophysical evidence that the visual system tries to avoid shifting back the focus of attention to a location that it has just visited. One of the most direct observations of that behavior is in terms of reaction times, which are longer when the subject is requested to return attention to a location that had just been attended (Posner and Cohen, 1984). Kwak and Egeth (1992) showed that the inhibition of return is spatially defined; that is, the return is inhibited to the location of the last attended item, not to its other properties. Gibson and Egeth (1994) provided evidence showing that both object-based and environment-based descriptions can influence location-based inhibition of return. Such behavior is in agreement with previously mentioned data (Nissen, 1985; Shih and Sperling, 1993), which showed that spatial location has a somewhat special role among object features. A later section will examine how this temporal behavior can be taken into account computationally.

Beyond Selective Attention

Selective attention is not an isolated perceptual mechanism. Attentional processes interact, on the one hand, with sensory input and, on the other hand, with cognitive mechanisms, memory, and behavioral control. In a first approximation, the latter can be considered as the stages to which the output of selective attention is delivered, whereas sensory information provides its input. This feedforward scheme of information processing is certainly oversimplified; there is obviously an influence of motor actions on the sensory input (e.g., re-orienting of the head or body, or simply closing the eyes), which is now being exploited in a technological context (Aloimonos and Weiss, 1987; Clark and Ferrier, 1992). This chapter has focused mainly on the interaction between attention and its input, but in this section the output is briefly discussed.

The role of attention as a gatekeeper for memory and awareness, allowing only selected portions of the visual scene to enter working memory, has been alluded to previously. Working memory may be thought of as a canvas that provides intermediate storage for the different perceptual elements selected at different times. Another task of working memory is to establish spatial relations between the selected feature elements, in a more abstract and computationally more efficient form than the spatial relations between the neurons that code for the feature elements.

Unfortunately, in spite of decades of intensive research, less is known about the representations of stimuli and memory in the more central brain areas than could be desired (see Ballard, Hayhoe, and Pelz, 1995; Tiitinen, May, and Reinikainen, 1994). There is little doubt, at least, that we do not store little pictures of what we see. Rather, at some point we use abstract or symbolic representations, which implies that the representation of spatial relations between objects in higher areas is not in the form of corresponding spatial relations between neurons. In other words, the representation of visual (and other) perceptual elements in higher cortices is different from literal copies of the two-dimensional retinal image. That much is clear from computational arguments and is confirmed by the observation that such a representation is not observed in IT cortex (e.g., Young and Yamane, 1992). Ullman (1984) developed strategies for how spatial relations between different objects in the visual field can be determined and coded.

Perception and cognition are not goals that behaving organisms pursue for their own sake; instead, such goals are parts of a behavioral chain of events that eventually leads to motor actions. At some point perception and cognition end and action is required. The theoretical challenge is to join at some point the "uphill" side of perception with the "downhill" side of motor control, without requiring the services of a homunculus in-between (for a technologically oriented approach towards closing the gap between perception and action, see Ballard, 1991).

COMPUTATIONAL MODELS

Feature-Based Attention

Several computational models of selective attention have been proposed in recent years. Examined first is a model for feature-based attention that can quantitatively reproduce the temporal dynamics of neurons in monkey IT cortex during delayed match-to-sample tasks (Usher and Niebur, 1996). In that model, competing, mutually inhibitory cell assemblies are used to represent visual stimuli such as letters. Competition is implemented in terms of a shared pool of inhibition, rather than in terms of an explicit sequential mechanism, as is common in two-stage models of attention. In particular, the architecture does not require a structure corresponding to the saliency map. Instead, the parallel maps interact with each other via the inhibitory pool. A mechanism that does not require a saliency map has also been suggested by Desimone and Duncan (1995).

Each cell assembly receives input from an input layer (e.g., primary visual cortex). For each object in the input layer, activation is transmitted to a population of cell assemblies, the strength of the input being proportional to the similarity between the learned object and the shape present in the display. Based on physiological evidence (Miller, Li, and Desimone, 1993), Usher and Niebur (1996) assume the existence of an intermediate preprocessing stage that makes the input to each cell assembly in the working memory module dependent in a non-monotonic way on the number of stimuli of that type.

The weights of the excitatory connections between cells in each assembly are chosen such that they are strong enough to generate (via the inhibitory pool; see figure 9.1) strong competition between the objects. A working memory module, located presumably in prefrontal cortex and with an in-

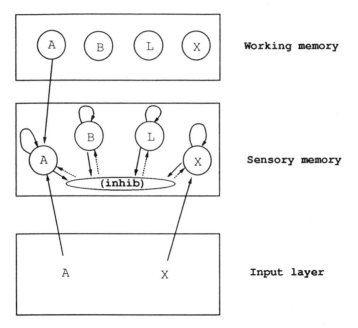

Figure 9.1 Architecture of the model for feature-oriented attention developed by Usher and Niebur (1996). Three stages (rectangles) are modeled, corresponding to sensory input, sensory memory, and working memory. Stimuli known to the system are represented by cell assemblies (circles). In the sensory memory module, those assemblies compete with each other via a pool of inhibitory neurons (ellipse). Cell assemblies in working memory provide feedback to corresponding populations in sensory memory, which biases the competition in favor of the selected stimulus. Excitatory and inhibitory synapses are shown as full and dotted arrows, respectively. In the situation shown, objects A and X are in the visual field and object A is, in addition, stored in the working memory module. Note, in particular, the absence of a control structure corresponding to the saliency map in figures 9.2 and 9.4.

ternal architecture similar to the modules in sensory memory, serves to store the response of an activated assembly for some time. Such is the case during the delay in a delayed match-to-sample task. Eventually, the activity is extinguished by a cognitive mechanism exterior to the network. The differentiation between the memory characteristics of cells in IT and prefrontal cortex is motivated by the recent finding that, unlike in IT cortical areas, the delayed activity in prefrontal cortex conveys information about targets even across intervening stimuli (Chelazzi, Miller, Lueschow, and Desimone, 1993). Usher and Niebur (1996) further assume that each working memory cell assembly sends a weak excitatory top-down projection to its associate assembly in the sensory memory area. During a search task, when a subject is searching for an expected target, the top-down feedback projection will add a weak additional input to the target assembly in the sensory memory. The architecture is displayed in figure 9.1.

The network response to a sequence of cue and target stimuli mimics the neural responses in IT visual cortex of monkeys performing a visual search task: enhanced response during the display of the stimulus, which decays but remains above a spontaneous rate after the cue disappears. When, subsequently, a display consisting of the target and several distractors is presented, the activity of all stimulus-driven cells is initially increased. After a short period of time, however, the activity of the cell assembly representing the cue stimulus is enhanced due to competition induced by the increasing activation and to a small top-down expectational input, whereas the activity of the distractors decays. The simulated response fits the measured delayed activity in IT cortex (Chelazzi, Miller, Duncan and Desimone, 1993), and Usher and Niebur (1996) suggest that such a process, which can be largely independent of the number of distractors, may be used by the visual system for selecting an expected target among distractors.

The Saliency Map

It has previously been noted that decoupling of feature dimensions is computationally advantageous. One implementation of such decoupling is sequential scanning of different parts of the visual field. This leads to the metaphor of the focus of attention and requires a spatially defined selection scheme that controls where the focus of attention is deployed at any given time. Koch and Ullman (1985) suggested that an efficient way to coordinate that control mechanism is in the form of a topographic feature map, which codes for the saliency or conspicuity of every location in the visual field. In other words, activity in the map does not indicate a green or an oriented stimulus, for example, but indicates instead a particular location in the visual scene that is salient or conspicuous with respect to its neighborhood. Psychophysical evidence indicates that the map may not be organized retinotopically but instead with a coordinate system relative to the visual environment of the observer (Posner and Cohen, 1984) or relative to the observed objects (Tipper, Driver, and Weaver, 1991). Variations of the saliency map concept have been used in multiple instances and with different terminologies (e.g., the master map of Treisman [1988] or the activation map of Wolfe [1994]).

More recently, a binary theory has been developed (see Braun, chapter 12 this volume), in which saliency is limited to stimulus (bottom-up) influences; volitional (top-down control) is exerted by a separate mechanism. Braun and Sagi (1990, 1991) suggested that the two mechanisms have different capabilities and selection criteria and they studied their interaction psychophysically. However, some researchers reject the idea of a topographic map in the brain whose *raison d'être* is the representation of salient stimuli. Thus, Desimone and Duncan (1995) proposed that selective attention is a consequence of interactions between feature maps only.

There is stronger evidence in favor of a functional saliency map than there is for a single, anatomically localized saliency map. In other words, the functionality of a saliency map may be spread over different anatomical areas. Robinson and Petersen (1992) reviewed data showing that the pulvinar nuclei of the thalamus play a significant role in the selection of visual targets. However, it seems unlikely that the pulvinar is the only location implicated in that selection process. Other candidate areas are the posterior parietal cortex (Bushnell et al., 1981; Mountcastle et al., 1981) and the superior colliculus (Goldberg and Wurtz, 1972); a possible scenario describes a saliency map distributed over several of those structures.

Within the class of models that assume the existence of a saliency map, Desimone (1992) distinguished input-gated mechanisms (e.g., Olshausen, Andersen and Van Essen, 1993) from cell gated mechanisms (Niebur, Koch, and Rosin, 1993; Niebur and Koch, 1994). In architectures of the first kind, information is channeled along precisely determined routes, providing the input to cells in higher areas. In contrast, cell-gated architectures allow information to spread with fewer restrictions; instead, those cell populations that do not code for the attended information are deactivated (suppressed).

Modeling the "Where" Pathway

Niebur and Koch (1996) developed a model of the "where" pathway that allows the autonomous selection of salient regions in a visual scene. The underlying network generates spikes at a sequence of locations in visual space, starting with the most salient location and scanning the visual input in the order of decreasing salience. Its structure is shown in figure 9.2.

Control Input   The input to the simulated network is provided in the form of digitized images from a CCD camera, which are analyzed in various feature maps. The maps are organized around the known operations in early visual cortices and are implemented at different spatial scales (Burt and Adelson, 1983) in a center-surround structure akin to visual receptive fields. Different maps code for the three principal components of primate color vision (intensity, red-green, blue-yellow), for four orientations (via convolution with Gabor filters), as well as for the locally defined temporal change. Provision is made for top-down influence, in accordance with restrictions discussed previously. In particular, such influence is always positive (i.e., increasing saliency) and is limited to a contiguous part of the visual field.

Dynamics of the Saliency Map   Once all relevant features have been computed in the various feature maps, they are combined to yield the salience. In the Niebur and Koch (1996) paper, that task is solved simply by adding the activities in the different feature maps, with constant weights. Alternatively, weight can be determined by a supervised learning algorithm (Itti, Niebur, Braun, and Koch, 1996). By definition, the activity in a given location of the saliency map represents the relative conspicuity of the corresponding location in the visual field. Because the maximum of the map is the most salient stimulus at any given time, selective attention has to be guided to that location. The maximum is selected by application of a simple

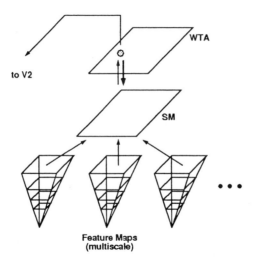

to V2

WTA

SM

Feature Maps
(multiscale)

Figure 9.2 Overview of the model "where" pathway of Niebur and Koch (1996). Features are computed as center-surround differences at four different spatial scales. The feature maps are represented as pyramids, and only three are shown. Information from all maps is added (arrows) with constant weights and provides input to the saliency map (SM). Activity in the saliency map provides input to an array of integrate-and-fire neurons with global inhibition. This array (WTA) has the functionality of a winner-take-all network. It generates a sequence of spikes in different locations (in order of decreasing saliency) that projects to the ventral pathway (V2; see figure 9.4). The WTA array also provides feedback activity (bold arrow) to the saliency map to inhibit the just-visited location. This feedback activity generates the motion of the focus of attention over the visual field and also explains the psychophysical evidence for inhibition of return.

winner-take-all (WTA) mechanism, implemented as a two-dimensional layer of integrate-and-fire neurons with strong global inhibition, in which the inhibitory population is reliably activated by any neuron in the layer.

After inspection of a given location, the next-most salient point needs to be attended. Scanning of a static or dynamic scene is implemented by introducing feedback from the WTA array. When a spike occurs in the WTA network, the integrators in the saliency map receive additional inhibitory input at the location of the winner, leading to a reduction of its associated neuronal activity. Consequently, the network automatically selects the unit in the saliency map with the next greatest activity. Such scanning of the visual scene proceeds at about 40 ms per item, compatible with some of the experimental data discussed previously. Note that the focus of attention jumps to the next location in a discontinuous motion, with a switching time independent of the distance between subsequent locations (Kwak, Dagenbach, and Egeth, 1991; Sagi and Julesz, 1985). The control mechanism is supported by recent results by Yantis and Jones (1991) showing that a certain number of onset stimuli receive priority, and that the priority decays over time.

The inhibitory feedback is central to the working of the model because it not only explains the data showing inhibition of return but is responsible for the scanning motion itself. The inhibition is consistent with the recently observed suppression of the attended location in brain area 7a of rhesus monkeys performing a match-to-sample task (Steinmetz, Connor, Constantinidis, and McLaughlin, 1994; Steinmetz and Constantinidis, 1995).

Shifter Circuits

Anderson and Van Essen (1987) proposed that the motion of the focus of attention (together with other phenomena, such as the stability of stereoscopic perception in the face of constant and relatively large disjunctive eye movements as well as the prevention of motion blur) is implemented in an explicit way by shifts of the image across cortex (connectionist models based on similar ideas were developed earlier by Hinton and Lang, 1985, and by Sandon, 1989). The shifter circuit hypothesis was refined and simulated by Olshausen et al. (1993). The authors assumed a layered network in which each cell functions as a switch that connects to two target cells in the next higher layer. The switch can either be open (in which case no information is transmitted to the higher layer) or it can connect the cell to either one of the two cells in the higher level. An elaborate control system opens and closes the switches with the effect that a scaled image of the activity in the input layer (in primary visual cortex) is transmitted over several stages (i.e., layers) to IT cortex. By opening and closing the appropriate switches, it can be demonstrated that it is possible to move the focus of attention either continuously or discontinuously and to change its size.

Olshausen et al. (1993) also showed that the numbers of cells in several of the participating structures (V1, V2, V4, and the pulvinar) are compatible with the proposed mechanism. Changes in the positions of the receptive fields in intermediate cortical areas (for a discussion of changes in area V4, see Connor, Gallant, and Van Essen, 1994) provide further support for the shifter circuit hypothesis. Olshausen et al. (1993) emphasized the fact that in the shifter circuit framework the spatial relations of stimuli within the focus of attention are conserved at all levels, all the way to IT cortex, which is not the case in many other models. For example, they pointed out that an observer would have problems recognizing the image shown in figure 9.3b even if he or she was familiar with the image in figure 9.3a.

Nevertheless, information about spatial relations can be transmitted in other ways than by coding it in the spatial relations of the neurons themselves. For example, neurons have been found that code explicitly for the relative locations of different stimuli. Nelson and Frost (1985) showed that a significant percentage (40%) of neurons in cat striate cortex fired selectively for stimuli in specific locations far outside their (classical) receptive fields (for a model of the underlying biophysical mechanism, see Stemmler, Usher, and Niebur, 1995). Spatial relations between small features are coded by neurons detecting spatially larger features (Gallant, Braun, and Van Essen, 1993). The necessity for the preservation of spatial relations in the framework of Olshausen et al. (1993) may be an artifact of the input representation used,

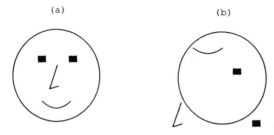

Figure 9.3 Schematic drawing of (a) a normally arranged and (b) scrambled face. Figure (a) is readily recognized as representing a face. Rearranging the features with different spatial relations, as shown in (b), makes the image meaningless and the figure is no longer recognized as a face.

which consists only of individual pixels and disregards the existing hierarchical representational structure of cortex.

Preservation of spatial relations may represent more of a problem than of a desirable feature. As was discussed previously, the spatial relations between objects in the visual environment have to be coded in an abstract representation that is presumably used in the cognitive processing of spatial relations. That representation is most certainly different from the two-dimensional patterns on the retina. The transformation between representations has to happen somewhere. In the shifter circuit paradigm, a very significant fraction of visual cortex (all areas between and including area V1 and IT cortex) is devoted to literal reproduction of a part of the retinal image, except for a change of scale and location, thereby leaving all the other work to unspecified higher areas.

Temporal Tagging

So far, attention has been considered mainly as an isolated mechanism that delivers an appropriately chosen selection of the sensory input to higher cognitive centers. The work to be discussed in this section is intended to be compatible with cognitive representations in higher areas, and eventually with mechanisms of motor control.

The underlying idea (Crick and Koch, 1990) is that the attentional selection process works by marking (or tagging) the selected stimuli, based on the temporal fine structure of neuronal spike trains. Only such tagged stimuli can access awareness and memory and only those stimuli will contribute to the decision-making process leading to motor actions. Assuming that a tagged stimulus leads to more effective neural responses, a tagged stimulus not only survives the perceptual selection process but will also lead to a motor action. In contrast, unattended (nontagged) simultaneously present stimuli do not have behavioral consequences. Suppression of unattended stimuli was observed directly by Moran and Desimone (1985) in macaque V4 cortex.

Niebur et al. (1993) showed how such tagging might be accomplished using spiking neurons: cells in early visual cortex (area V2) respond to visual stimuli with a spike train with a stochastic distribution of interspike intervals with an appropriate, stimulus-dependent mean firing rate. The spike trains of neurons whose receptive fields do not overlap with the focus of attention are distributed according to a stochastic process called the homogeneous Poisson process; Moore, Perkel, and Segundo, 1967), which is memoryless except for a refractory period after each spike. In contrast, spike trains of cells with receptive fields within the focus of attention are distributed according to a probabilistic distribution with a different time structure, which is generated by modulatory influences from the saliency map. Niebur et al. (1993) proposed that the modulated time structure of each spike train is realized as a periodic repetition with a frequency in the gamma, or 40 Hz, range. Niebur and Koch (1994) suggested that no specific time structure is imposed on spike trains from any one single cell but that the modulation is manifest in the form of correlations (or synchronization) between spike trains of cells responding to an attended stimulus. In both cases, the average firing rate in early cortex is the same inside and outside the focus of attention, but the different time structure enables neurons in higher cortical areas to distinguish between attended and unattended stimuli. In both cases, quantitative agreement with observed neurophysiological results was obtained, and both models make explicit predictions about the time structure of neural signals inside and outside the focus of attention. This makes it possible to decide experimentally which one of the models (if any) corresponds to biological reality.

How can the modulatory input from the saliency map be generated? In the case of imposed synchronicity (imposed periodicity can be implemented similarly), the modulation is most easily generated by common input to all cells that respond to attended stimuli. Such excitatory input will increase the propensity of postsynaptic cells to fire for a very short time after receiving the input, and will thereby increase the correlation between spike trains (for details, see Niebur and Koch, 1994). Suitable modulatory input is produced by the saliency map implementation discussed previously, which generates a train of spikes at the location of the currently most salient location.

It should be emphasized again that the temporal tagging paradigm transcends the task of modeling selective attention as a perceptual filter. In Niebur and Koch's (1994) model (figure 9.4), a subpopulation of neurons in higher cortical areas is assumed to function as coincidence detectors and therefore should respond preferentially to synchronous input. This allows for segregation of attended (or aynchronous) from unattended (or asynchronous) stimuli throughout the visual system and beyond, possibly into motor control structures. Because unattended stimuli are suppressed by the mechanism, only attended stimuli lead to behavioral responses. This makes any homunculus superfluous.

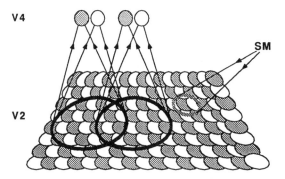

Figure 9.4 Architecture of the "what" pathway in the model of Niebur and Koch (1994). Receptive fields of V2 cells are represented by overlapping circles arranged in a two-dimensional tiling array. White and gray circles represent cells receptive to the two features considered in the text. The two unfilled black circles denote the receptive fields of V4 cells; that is, all cells in a stack in V4 receive input from all V2 cells in the corresponding circle (arrows) with the same feature selectivity. The shaded unfilled circle indicates the focus of attention; the activity of all V2 cells inside this circle is subjected to temporal modulation by the saliency map (SM). In area V4 (and in higher cortical areas), cells distinguish between modulated and unmodulated spike trains and suppress unmodulated responses. The arrows labeled SM in the present figure correspond to the arrow labeled "to V2" in figure 9.2; that is, the "where" pathway in figure 9.2 provides the input for the "what" pathway shown here.

CONCLUSIONS

The computational approach to selective attention discussed in this chapter provides a framework for understanding psychophysical and neuroscience research, and should eventually yield concrete models of visual information processing. Furthermore, it can be expected that machine vision systems will greatly benefit from insights into the computational mechanisms of biological vision systems, because the biological systems have been honed by evolution over the last 500 million years to survive in a very competitive world.

Almost any information-processing system with finite resources operating in the real world requires an attentive mechanism, because the multitude of sensors would overwhelm its computational capabilities if all sensory input were processed simultaneously. Efficient processing requires careful selection of the most relevant stimuli and suppression of all others. If, as is usually the case in a realistic scenario, multiple relevant stimuli are presented simultaneously, then they must be processed sequentially. That situation requires a dynamical control of the attended part of the visual field. The sequential treatment of different parts of the visual field has the further advantage of contributing to the decoupling of stimulus features, which significantly reduces the complexity of the recognition task.

Several detailed models of selective attention were presented. Shifter circuits solve the problem of generating a standardized representation of objects by abstracting from the size and location of the object in a feedforward filtering operation. A very significant part of all cortical areas from V1 to IT is required for that scaling operation, which limits the areas available for higher cognitive processing.

Another set of work is based on the temporal tagging of attended stimuli. The basic assumption is that the time structure of spike trains representing attended stimuli is subtly different from the time structure of spike trains representing unattended stimuli. The mechanism is compatible with the transformation of sensory stimuli towards more abstract representations, as well as with feedforward and feedback. Temporal tagging signals occur naturally from a control mechanism for the focus of attention. Autonomous control of selective attention entirely within that framework has been demonstrated. The mechanism can be extended to perceptual hierarchies throughout the visual system and beyond, possibly including behavioral (motor) responses.

Although bottom-up selection processing has been emphasized throughout this chapter, complexity arguments indicate that top-down processes are indispensable for the processing of complex stimuli. One architecture with a strong top-down component was presented. That model represents a simple theory for feature-oriented attention and is in agreement with recent recordings in IT cortex.

Although the described studies are very promising approaches to the understanding of perceptual processes, they are clearly only a beginning. For example, the described mechanisms neglect all finer forms of the attentional set. This implies, for instance, that singletons are always salient features in the models and (if strong enough) will always capture attention. In other words, the system is always in singleton detection mode. We expect that future work will overcome such limitations.

ACKNOWLEDGMENTS

The research reported in this chapter was performed while both authors were at the California Institute of Technology and supported by the Office of Naval Research, the Air Force Office of Scientific Research, the National Science Foundation, the Center for Neuromorphic Systems Engineering as a part of the National Science Foundation Engineering Research Center Program, and by the Office of Strategic Technology of the California Trade and Commerce Agency. Christof Koch thanks the Institute for Theoretical Physics at the Eidgenössische Technische Hochschule in Zurich for the kind hospitality extended to him during the preparation of this manuscript.

REFERENCES

Aloimonos, J. and Weiss, I. (1987) Active vision. *Proc. DARPA Image Understanding Workshop*, 35–54.

Anderson, C. and Van Essen, D. (1987) Shifter circuits: A computational strategy for dynamic aspects of visual processing. *Proc. Natl. Acad. Sci. USA* 84: 6297–6301.

Bacon, W. F. and Egeth, H. E. (1994) Overriding stimulus-driven attentional capture. *Percept. Psychophys.* 55: 485–496.

Ballard, D. (1991) Animate vision. *Artif. Intell.* 48: 57–86.

Ballard, D., Hayhoe, M., and Pelz, J. (1995) Memory representations in natural tasks *J. Cog. Neurosci.* 7: 66–90.

Braun, J. and Sagi, D. (1990) Vision outside the focus of attention. *Percept. Psychophys.* 48: 45–58.

Braun, J. and Sagi, D. (1991) Texture-based tasks are little affected by second tasks requiring peripheral or central attentive fixation. *Perception* 20: 483–500.

Bryden, M. (1961) The role of post-exposural eye movements in tachistoscopic perception. *Canad. J. Exp. Psychol.* 15: 220–225.

Bundesen, C. (1991) Visual selection of features and objects: Is location special? A reinterpretation of Nissen's (1985) findings. *Percept. Psychophys.* 50: 87–89.

Burt, P. J. and Adelson, E. H. (1983) The Laplacian pyramid as a compact image code. *IEEE Trans. Communi.* 31: 532–540.

Bushnell, M. C., Goldberg, M. E., and Robinson, D. L. (1981) Behavioral enhancement of visual responses in monkey cerebral cortex. I. Modulation in posterior parietal cortex related to selective visual attention. *J. Neurophysiol.* 46: 755–772.

Cheal, M. and Lyon, R. (1991) Central and peripheral precuing of forced-choice discrimination. *Q. J. Exp. Psychol.* 43A: 859–880.

Chelazzi, L., Miller, E., Duncan, J., and Desimone, R. (1993) A neural basis for visual search in inferior temporal cortex *Nature* 363: 345–347.

Chelazzi, L., Miller, E., Lueschow, A., and Desimone, R. (1993) Dual mechanisms of short-term memory: Ventral prefrontal cortex. *Soc. Neurosci. Abstr.* 19: 975.

Clark, J. and Ferrier, N. (1992) Attentive visual servoing. In *An introduction to active vision*, edited by A. Blake, and A. Yuille. Cambridge, MA: MIT Press.

Connor, C. E., Gallant, J. L., and Van Essen, D. C. (1994) Modulation of receptive field properties in area V4 by shifts in focal attention. *Invest. Ophthalmol. Vis. Sci.* 35: 2147.

Crick, F. and Koch, C. (1990) Some reflections on visual awareness. *Cold Spring Harb. Symp. Quant. Biol.* 55: 953–962.

Crick, F. and Koch, C. (1995) Are we aware of neural activity in primary visual cortex? *Nature* 375: 121–123.

Crovitz, H. and Daves, W. (1962) Tendencies to eye movement and perceptual accuracy. *J. Exp. Psychol.* 63: 495–498.

Desimone, R. (1992) Neural circuits for visual attention in the primate brain. In *Neural Networks for Vision and Image Processing*, edited by G. Carpenter and S. Grossberg. Cambridge, MA: MIT Press.

Desimone, R. and Duncan, J. (1995) Neural mechanisms of selective visual attention. *Annu. Rev. Neurosci.* 18: 193–222.

Douglas, R., Koch, C., Mahowald, M., Martin, K., and Suarez, H. (1995) Recurrent excitation in neocortical circuits. *Science* 269: 981–985.

Douglas, R. J., Martin, K. A., and Whitteridge, D. (1989) A canonical microcircuit for neocortex. *Neural Comput.* 1: 480–488.

Duhamel, J. R., Colby, C. L., and Goldberg, M. E. (1992) The updating of the representation of visual space in parietal cortex by intended eye movements. *Science* 255: 90–92.

Duncan, J. and Humphreys, G. (1989) Visual search and stimulus similarity. *Psychol. Rev.* 96: 433–458.

Duncan, J., Ward, R., and Shapiro, K. (1994) Direct measurement of attentional dwell time in human vision. *Nature* 369: 313–315.

Egeth, H. (1966) Parallel versus serial processes in multidimension stimulus discrimination. *Percept. Psychophys.* 1: 245–252.

Egeth, H., Virzi, R., and Garbart, H. (1984) Searching for conjunctively defined targets. *J. Exp. Psychol. Hum. Percept. Perform.* 10: 32–39.

Folk, C. L., Remington, R. W., and Johnston, J. C. (1992) Involuntary covert orienting is contingent on attentional control setting. *J. Exp. Psychol. Hum. Percept. Perform.* 18: 1030–1044.

Fukushima, K., Miyake, S., and Ito, T. (1983) Neocognitron: A neural network model for a mechanism of visual pattern recognition. *IEEE Trans. Syst. Man Cyber.* 13: 826–834.

Gallant, J., Braun, J., and Van Essen, D. (1993) Selectivity for polar, hyperbolic, and cartesian gratings in macaque visual cortex. *Science* 259: 100–103.

Gibson, B. and Egeth, H. (1994) Inhibition of return to object-based and environment-based locations. *Percept. Psychophys.* 55: 323–339.

Goldberg, M. E. and Wurtz, R. H. (1972) Activity of superior colliculus in behaving monkey. II. The effect of attention on neuronal responses. *J. Neurophysiol.* 35: 560–574.

Grossberg, S., Mingolla, E., and Ross, W. (1994) A neural theory of attentive visual search: Interactions at boundary, surface, spatial and object recognition. *Psychol. Rev.* 101: 470–489.

Hillstrom, A. P. and Yantis, S. (1994) Visual motion and attentional capture. *Percep. Psychophys.* 55: 399–411.

Hinton, G. and Lang, K. (1985) Shape recognition and illusory conjunctions. *Proc. Ninth Intl. Joint Conf. Artif. Intell.*, 252–259.

Hoffman, J. E. (1978) Search through a sequentially presented visual display *Percept. Psychophys.* 23: 1–11.

Hoffman, J. E. (1979) A two-stage model of visual search. *Percept. Psychophys.* 25: 319–327.

Hsiao, S. S., O'Shaughness, D. M., and Johnson, K. O. (1993) Effects of selective attention on spatial form processing in monkey primary and secondary somatosensory cortex. *J. Neurophysiol.* 70: 444–447.

Humphreys, G. and Muller, H. (1993) Search via recursive rejection (SERR): A connectionist model of visual search. *Cognit. Psychol.* 25: 43–110.

Itti, L., Niebur, E., Braun, J., and Koch, C. (1996). A trainable model of saliency-based visual attention. *Soc. Neurosci. Abst.* 22: 270.

James, W. (1890) *The Principles of Psychology*. New York: Henry Holt.

Jonides, J. (1981) Voluntary versus automatic control over the mind's eye's movement. In *Attention and Performance IX*, edited by J. Long, and A. Baddeley, pp. 187–203. Hillsdale, NJ: Lawrence Erlbaum.

Jonides, J. and Yantis, S. (1988) Uniqueness of abrupt visual onset in capturing attention. *Percept. Psychophys.* 43: 346–354.

Koch, C. and Ullman, S. (1985) Shifts in selective visual attention: Towards the underlying neural circuitry. *Hum. Neurobiol.* 4: 219–227.

Kwak, H., Dagenbach, D., and Egeth, H. (1991) Further evidence for a time-independent shift of the focus of attention. *Percept. Psychophys.* 49: 473–480.

Kwak, H. and Egeth, H. (1992) Consequences of allocating attention to locations and to other attributes. *Percept. Psychophys.* 51: 455–464.

Milner, A. D., and Goodale, M. A. (1995) *The visual Brain in Action.* New York: Oxford University Press.

Luck, S., Hillyard, S., Mangun, G., and Gazzaniga, M. (1994) Independent attentional scanning in the separated hemispheres of split-brain patients. *J. Cog. Neurosci.* 6: 84–91.

McPeek, R. M. and Nakayama, K. (1995) Linkage of attention and saccades in a visual search task. *Invest. Opthalmol. Vis. Sci.* 36: S354.

Miller, E., Li, L., and Desimone, R. (1993) Activity of neurons in anterior inferior temporal cortex during a short-term memory task. *J. Neurosci.* 13: 1460–1478.

Moore, G., Perkel, D., and Segundo, J. (1967) Statistical analysis and functional interpretation of neuron spike data. *Annu. Rev. Physiol.* 28: 493–522.

Moran, J. and Desimone, R. (1985) Selective attention gates visual processing in the extrastriate cortex. *Science* 229: 782–784.

Motter, B. (1993) Focal attention produces spatially selective processing in visual cortical areas V1, V2, and V4 in the presence of competing stimuli. *J. Neurophysiol.* 70: 909–919.

Mountcastle, V., Andersen, R., and Motter, B. (1981) The influence of attentive fixation upon the excitability of the light-sensitive neurons of the posterior parietal cortex. *J. Neurosci.* 1: 1218–1232.

Mozer, M. and Behrmann, M. (1990) On the interaction of selective attention and lexical knowledge: A connectionist account of neglect dyslexia. *J. Cog. Neurosci.* 2: 96–123.

Muller, H. and Rabbitt, P. (1989) Reflexive and voluntary orienting of visual attention: Time course of activation and resistance to interruption. *J. Exp. Psychol. Hum. Percept. Perform.* 15: 315–330.

Neisser, U. (1967) *Cognitive Psychology.* New York: Appleton-Century-Crofts.

Nelson, J. and Frost, B. (1985) Intracortical facilitation among co-oriented, co-axially aligned simple cells in cat striate cortex. *Exp. Brain Res.* 61: 54–61.

Niebur, E. and Koch, C. (1994) A model for the neuronal implementation of selective visual attention based on temporal correlation among neurons. *J. Comput. Neurosci.* 1: 141–158.

Niebur, E. and Koch, C. (1996) Control of selective visual attention: Modeling the "where" pathway. In *Advances in Neural Information Processing Systems* (Vol. 8) edited by D. S. Touretzky, M. C. Mozer, and M. E. Hasselmo, pp. 802–808. Cambridge, MA: MIT Press.

Niebur, E., Koch, C., and Rosin, C. (1993) An oscillation-based model for the neural basis of attention. *Vis. Res.* 33: 2789–2802.

Nissen, M. (1985) Accessing features and objects: is location special? In *Attention and Performance XI,* edited by M. Posner and O. Marin, pp. 205–219. Hillsdale, NJ: Lawrence Erlbaum.

Olshausen, B., Andersen, C., and Van Essen, D. (1993) A neural model of visual attention and invariant pattern recognition *J. Neurosci.* 13: 4700–4719.

Posner, M. I. Cohen, Y. (1984) Components of visual orienting. In *Attention and Performance X,* edited by H. Bouma, D. G. Bouwhuis, pp. 531–556. Hillsdale, NJ: Lawrence Erlbaum.

Remington, R., Johnston, J., and Yantis, S. (1992) Involuntary attention capture by abrupt onsets *Percept. Psychophys.* 51: 279–290.

Robinson, D. L. and Petersen, S. E. (1992) The pulvinar and visual salience. *Trends Neuroci.* 15: 127–132.

Saarinen, J. and Julesz, B. (1991) The speed of attentional shifts in the visual field *Proc. Natl. Acad. Sci. USA* 88: 1812–1814.

Sagi, D. and Julesz, B. (1985) Fast noninertial shifts of attention. *Spat. Vis.* 2, 141–149.

Sandou, P. A. (1989) Simulating visual attention. *J. Cog. Nousosci.* 2: 213–231.

Sherman, S. M. and Koch, C. (1986) The control of retinogeniculate transmission in the mammalian lateral geniculate nucleus. *Exp. Brain Res.* 63: 1–20.

Shih, S. and Sperling, G. (1993) Visual search, visual attention and feature-based stimulus selection. *Invest. Ophthalmol. Vis. Sci.* 34: 1288.

Steinmetz, M., Connor, C. E., Constantinidis, C., and McLaughlin, J. (1994) Covert attention suppresses neuronal responses in area 7A of the posterior parietal cortex *J. Neurophysiol.* 72: 1020–1023.

Steinmetz, M. and Constantinidis, C. (1995) Neurophysiological evidence for a role of posterior parietal cortex in redirecting visual attention *Cereb. Cortex* 5: 448–456.

Stemmler, M., Usher, M., Niebur, E. (1995) Lateral Interactions in Primary Visual Cortex: A Model Bridging Physiology and Psychophysics. *Science* 269: 1877–1880.

Tiitinen, H., May, P., Reinikainen, K. (1994) Attention novelty detection in humans is governed by pre-attentive sensory memory. *Nature* 372: 90–92.

Tipper, S. P., Driver, J., Weaver, B. (1991) Short report: object-centered inhibition or return of visual attention *Q. J. Exp. Psychol.* 43A: 289–298.

Townsend, J. (1972) Some results concerning the identifiability of parallel and serial search *Br. J. Math. Stat. Psychol.* 25: 168–199.

Townsend, J. (1990) Serial vs. parallel processing: Sometimes they look like tweedledum and tweedledee but they can (and should) be distinguished. *Psychol. Sci.* 1: 46–54.

Treisman, A. (1988) Features and objects: The fourteenth Bartlett memorial lecture. *Q. J. Exp. Psychol.* 40A: 201–237.

Treisman, A. and Gelade, G. (1980) A feature-integration theory of attention. *Cognit. Psychol.* 12: 97–136.

Tsotsos, J. (1990) Analyzing vision at the complexity level. *Behav. Brain Sci.* 13: 423–469.

Ullman, S. (1984) Visual routines. *Cognition* 18: 97–159.

Ullman, S. (1995) Sequence seeking and counter streams: A computation model for bidirectional flow in the visual cortex. *Cereb. Cortex* 5: 1–11.

Ungerleider, L. G. and Mishkin, M. (1982) Two cortical visual systems. In *Analysis of Visual Behavior*, edited by D. J. Ingle, M. A. Goodale, and R. J. W. Mansfield, pp. 549–586. Cambridge, MA: MIT Press.

Usher, M. and Niebur, E. (1996) A neural model for parallel, expectation-driven attention for objects. *J. Cog. Neurosci.* 8: 305–321.

Westheimer, G. (1979) Scaling of visual acuity measurements. *Arch. Ophthalmol.* 97: 327–330.

Wolfe, J. (1994) Guided Search 2.0: A revised model of visual search. *Psychon. Bull. Rev.* 1: 202–238.

Wolfe, J., Cave, K., and Franzel, S. (1989) Guided search: An alternative to the feature integration model for visual search. *J. Exp. Psychol Hum. Percept. Perform.* 15: 419–433.

Yantis, S. (1996) Attentional capture in vision. In *Converging Operations in the Study of Visual Selective Attention*, edited by A. Kramer, G. Logan, and M. Coles, Washington, DC: American Psychological Association.

Yantis, S. and Johnson, D. (1990) Mechanisms of attentional priority. *J. Exp. Psychol. Hum. Percept. Perform.* 16: 812–825.

Yantis, S. and Jonides, J. (1990) Abrupt visual onsets and selective attention: Voluntary versus automatic allocation. *J. Exp. Psychol. Hum. Percept. Perform.* 16: 121–134.

Young, M. and Yamane, S. (1992) Sparse population coding of faces in the inferotemporal cortex. *Science* 256: 1327–1331.

III Varieties of Attention

10 Arousal and Attention: Psychopharmacological and Neuropsychological Studies in Experimental Animals

Trevor W. Robbins

ABSTRACT Psychopharmacological and neuropsychological analyses of arousal and attentional mechanisms in experimental animals are reviewed, especially from the perspective of their comparability with paradigms used with human subjects. Several varieties of attentional processing are considered, including sustained attention and vigilance, divided attention, and selective attention. The five-choice serial reaction time task for the rat is considered as an analog of the human continuous performance test, and manipulations of central noradrenergic, dopaminergic, serotoninergic, and cholinergic function are compared in the context of effects produced by discrete lesions to cortical structures. Those results are integrated with data from other tasks employing analogs of human vigilance, divided attention, and covert orienting paradigms. Clinical applications considered include modeling of human neglect syndromes and schizophrenic attentional dysfunction. The utility of using experimental animals in the analysis of arousal and attention is discussed, as well as the continuing need to set the studies into the theoretical context of cognitive neuroscience.

The study of attention in experimental animals has only recently gained a measure of respectability. Some investigators still prefer to describe behavioral phenomena apparently relevant to attentional mechanisms with terms such as "stimulus control" from the more theoretically neutral language of operant psychology (e.g., Heise and Milar, 1984). The various processes of attention to be classified in this chapter largely derive from research in human experimental psychology, often in applied or psychopathological contexts. However, the rise of cognitive neuroscience and the concomitant interest in the functions of the healthy or damaged cerebral cortex have necessitated the development of animal models of attentional processes in order to explore their neural correlates. There has also been an impetus to understand the functions of chemical neurotransmitter arousal systems that innervate the cortex and other forebrain structures because of conjectures that those systems play important roles in attention and arousal in all mammalian species.

These different lines of research essentially represent the convergence of neuropsychological and psychopharmacological approaches to the study of arousal and attention, a convergence that forms the basis of this chapter. Both approaches are enriched by advances in animal learning theory, which have addressed the important issue of how attentional processes interact with associative or learning mechanisms. It is also worth noting that much therorizing about attentional functioning in animals comes from a study of behavioral performance in test situations that are not designed expressly to measure specific aspects of attention. From a theoretical point of view it is of course desirable to integrate such findings into an explanatory framework that may have a more explicit basis in known attentional paradigms.

Mechanisms of attention enable animals to allocate processing resources efficiently when responding to important environmental events. Attention cannot be considered a unitary construct in humans: so too in other animals. For example, one form of attention is *sustained attention* or *vigilance*, a continuous allocation of processing resources for the detection of rare events. Another is *divided attention*, where an animal has to simultaneously monitor several different sensory channels, perhaps in order to perform different types of tasks, which requires optimal allocation of limited information-processing resources. A third form of attention is *selective (focused) attention*, where an animal has to focus resources on a restricted number of sensory channels while ignoring the rest. In practice, many situations require a mixture of those different processes. This chapter focuses on experimental tests with animals that attempt to make clear links with human paradigms.

AROUSAL, ACTIVATION, AND ATTENTION

Mechanisms of attention are related to energetic constructs such as arousal and activation, which generally connote some level of nonspecific neuronal excitability deriving from the structures formerly known as the reticular formation but now generally referred to as specific chemically defined or thalamic systems that innervate the forebrain (Robbins and Everitt, 1995a). Activity in some of those systems, especially the monoaminergic or cholinergic systems, is often correlated with higher levels of arousal such as active wakefulness or response to stress. As a consequence of such activity, those systems can modulate the functioning of neuronal networks in their terminal domains by adjusting the signal-to-noise ratios of evoked potentials triggered by forebrain processing. The relative capacities and forms of processing affected by the functioning of the monoaminergic and cholinergic systems have been considered previously (e.g., Robbins and Everitt, 1995a); their relevance to the present chapter is that many of these effects can be interpreted as the operation of crude attentional processes.

Some of the initial rationale for studying attentional function in animals came from the problem of characterizing effects of psychoactive drugs of various classes, including stimulants and sedative and tranquilizing agents, administered via the systemic route (Uhr and Miller, 1960). This is still an important goal, but the greater understanding of how such drugs affect central neurotransmitters has enabled more precise questions to be asked about the functions of those systems. It is probably unwise to assume that the functions of those systems map onto the conceptualizations of different attentional processes in a simple way, because research in that area is still at a relatively early stage and has rarely employed tasks that completely isolate elementary attentional mechanisms. Thus, the material is considered in terms of paradigm rather than in terms of discrete systems or discrete attentional mechanisms. However, working hypotheses are used to summarize any emergent consensus, wherever appropriate.

ATTENTIONAL PARADIGMS IN EXPERIMENTAL ANIMALS

Sustained Attention: Continuous Performance Tasks

Continuous attention tasks appear to have several origins and are generally termed tests of "sustained attention," although the test requirements often fall short of what is normally regarded as vigilance (see Parasuraman, Warm, and See, chapter 11, this volume), and other nonattentional, as well as attentional, components can clearly influence performance. Rosvold, Mirsky, Sarason, Bransome, and Beck, (1956) designed a test in which human subjects had to continually make decisions about the occurrence of target events versus nontarget items. In one version of the task the occurrence of target stimulus X had to be reported by a key press; in a related version, responding to X was only correct if X was preceded by another stimulus, A. That test became useful for investigating apparent attentional dysfunction in schizophrenia (see Nestor and O'Donnell, chapter 23, this volume). More modern variants have included the so-called rapid visual information-processing (RVIP) task, in which a subject is required to report the occurrence of specified sequences of digits presented at 100/s on a computer screen (Wesnes and Warburton, 1983). The task was also the basis of animal models in which the effects of reticular stimulation were counteracted by treatment with the major tranquilizer chlorpromazine (Kornetsky and Eliasson, 1969). A possible problem of interpretation was that the test was of the "go-no-go" type; that is, the percentage-correct measure included responses prior to the occurrence of the stimulus.

In the United Kingdom, Wilkinson (e.g., 1963) devised the five-choice serial reaction time task, in which subjects again had to continually monitor the location of a visual target stimulus in one of five locations over repeated trials. Immediately upon reporting its occurrence, another of the five locations was randomly chosen as the next target. The task, thus, has elements of a continuous performance test, but also has an obvious spatial component. The main application of the test was in measuring the effects of stressors and other agents, including drugs, that affected arousal; results formed some of the empirical basis for Broadbent's influential work *Decision and Stress* (1971).

Some of our own early attempts to examine attentional processes in animals (Carli, Robbins, Evenden, and Everitt, 1983) were based on that task, which we configured in a specially designed apparatus in which the rat had to monitor the occurrence of a brief (0.5 s) target stimulus (light) projected at the rear of one of five holes set in an arc of nine holes at the front of the chamber. Nose-poke responses in the holes were monitored by infrared photocell beams placed at their entrances. Correct responses were rewarded by the presentation of food pellets in a magazine at the rear of the chamber, which was monitored by a movable flap with a microswitch attached. Errors of commission (responding in a hole in which the stimulus had not been presented), errors of omission (failing to respond to the occurrence of a stimulus within a prescribed time limit), and premature responses (prior to the onset of the target stimulus or in the 5 s intertrial interval) were all punished by a brief period of darkness (time-out), after which the trial had to be initiated by a response in the food magazine.

The basic task essentially tests the ability of the rat to sustain spatial attention divided among a number of locations over a large number of trials (100). The difficulty of the task can be varied by reducing or increasing the duration of the target visual stimuli. However, the task parameters can also be manipulated in order to probe other aspects of attention or more general performance factors. For example, the stimuli can be made temporally as well spatially unpredictable, a manipulation that is equivalent to the unpaced version of the continuous performance task (versus the standard, or paced, version, in which stimuli come at predictable intervals). The less predictable schedule, or event/stimulus onset asynchrony (SOA), means that the rat or human cannot rely on automatic processing to control orientation to the location of the stimuli at a particular time and thus has to monitor readiness to respond on a continuous basis. Alternatively, distracting stimuli, such as bursts of white noise, can be interpolated into the intertrial interval in order to distract the rat from the target visual stimuli (this could also be done in the visual modality by presenting irrelevant visual stimuli in the four locations not used for presenting targets, or by dimming the house light). Such manipulations clearly test the ability of the animal to screen out irrelevant stimuli and thus constitutes a test of selective attention. Finally, the luminance of the stimuli can also be varied to test for basic changes in sensory threshold, and various other measures such as the latency to collect food pellets provide important internal controls for factors such as motor incapacity and motivation. One common problem with this type of paradigm is that it is difficult to separate out possible effects of vigilance decrement (Parasuraman, Warm, and Dember, 1987) from simple satiety, due to the ability of the rat to earn large numbers of food pellets by working for long periods over large numbers of trials.

Five-Choice Task: Intracerebral Psychopharmacology This paradigm has been used to test the effects of a large number of neuropharmacological manipulations (see table 10.1). The major findings are the dissociable effects observed following selective lesions to each of the monoaminergic neurotransmitter systems (noradrenergic, dopaminergic, and serotoninergic) as well as to the cholinergic (acetylcholine, ACh) system. Thus, excitotoxic

Table 10.1 Summary of main neuropharmacological effects on performance of the five-choice task and of interactions with behavioral manipulations on measures of choice accuracy and impulsivity

	Baseline Task	Variations of Brightness	Variability of Intertrial Interval	Reduced Duration of Visual Target	Bursts of White Noise	Systemic D-Amphetamine
			percent correct			
DNAB	0	0	↓	NT	↓[a]	↓[b]
NBM-ACh	↓	0	0	↓	↓[c]	0
VS-DA	0	0[d]	0[e]	NT	0	0
5-HT	↑[f]	0	0[g]	0	↓[c]	0
			premature responses			
DNAB	0	0	↓[h]	NT	0[i]	0[i]
NBM-ACh	↑[j]	0	0	0	0	0
VS-DA	↓	0	0	NT	↓	↓
5-HT	↑	↑	↑	↑	↑[k]	↓[l]

Key to effects (relative to sham control): ↑ = increase; ↓ = decrease; 0 = no difference; NT = not tested.
Key to treatments: DNAB = dorsal noradrenergic bundle lesion (Carli et al., 1983; Cole and Robbins, 1992); NBM-ACh = excitotoxic lesions of cholinergic projections of NBM (Robbins et al. 1989; Muir et al., 1994, 1995); VS-DA = ventral striatal dopamine depletion (Cole and Robbins, 1989); 5-HT = global and profound depletion of forebrain 5-HT (Harrison et al., 1997; Harrison et al., 1997 in press, a, b).
[a] Only when the white noise occurred just prior to target presentation.
[b] At higher doses.
[c] When presented just prior to the visual target; effect not replicated with selective dorsal or median raphé lesions.
[d] Small improvement at lowest level.
[e] Small improvement at shortest ITI.
[f] Transient improvement following dorsal raphe lesions only.
[g] Performance improved at short ITIs following median raphe lesions.
[h] At certain ITIs.
[i] White noise or D-amphetamine increased premature responses equally in lesioned and in sham rats.
[j] Transient effect; not always replicated.
[k] Less increase in 5-HT lesioned rats just prior to presentation of visual target.
[l] Less increase in 5-HT lesioned rats with increasing doses.

lesions of the nucleus basalis magnocellularis (NBM) in rats (using initially quisqualic acid, and later AMPA) produce impairments of basic discrimination performance (Robbins et al., 1989; Muir, Robbins, and Everitt, 1994), especially if the duration of the stimuli is reduced, although the impairments cannot be attributed to sensory loss per se. The deficit is reduced when the duration of the stimuli is lengthened (Muir et al., 1994). There are ancillary deficits in the accuracy of responding when bursts of white noise are presented simultaneously with the discriminanda, but not during other variations of the task (Robbins et al., 1989; Muir et al., 1994). The effects of basal forebrain lesions are remediated by systemic treatment with physostigmine or nicotine, supporting a cholinergic basis for the effects (Muir, Robbins, and Everitt, 1995).

By contrast, virtually complete depletion of cortical noradrenaline (NA), achieved by infusions of the catecholamine selective neurotoxin 6-hydroxydopamine into the trajectory of the dorsal noradrenergic ascending bundle (DNAB), only produced accuracy deficits under certain conditions (table 10.1). These conditions occurred when the stimuli were presented unpredictably in time, when distracting bursts of noise occurred just prior to the target stimuli, and when the behaviorally activating drug D-amphetamine was infused into the region of the nucleus accumbens. A working hypothesis was developed to accomodate those findings, namely that cortical NA was engaged in conditions of high arousal to preserve attentional selectivity (for a reappraisal of this hypothesis in the light of subsequent evidence, see Robbins and Everitt, 1995b). A later study replicated and extended most of the original findings of the effects of DNAB lesions on performance of the five-choice task. Of particular interest was the finding that the disruptive effects of white noise on choice accuracy were of similar magnitude over several values of illuminance for the visual signals, suggesting an effect of NA depletion relatively late in the course of processing, perhaps at the level of response preparation (Cole and Robbins, 1992).

The consequences of manipulating central dopaminergic transmission on performance of the task have been restricted mainly to the ventral striatum, including the nucleus accumbens. Depletion of dopamine in that region mainly affected indices of response vigor: the number of errors of omission were increased and response latencies were lengthened, whereas response accuracy was largely unaffected, as shown in table 10.1 (Cole and Robbins, 1989). Intra-accumbens infusions of the drug D-amphetamine had almost the opposite effects (Cole and Robbins, 1987). Dose-dependent increases in impulsive (premature) responses were the main effect, with no obvious change in response accuracy until relatively high doses of the drug were used. Depletion of nucleus accumbens dopamine reduced the impulsive responses produced both by systemic d-amphetamine and bursts of white noise (Cole and Robbins, 1989). Both of the latter agents mainly enhanced the response vigor, but unlike cholinergic and noradrenergic treatments did not significantly affect discrimination or choice accuracy.

The effects of forebrain 5-hydroxytryptamine (5-HT) depletion following intraventricular administration of the neurotoxin 5,7 dihydroxytryptamine (DHT) provide a complex pattern that contrasts with the pattern resulting from manipulations of the other neurochemical systems. The most striking and seemingly permanent effects are increased impulsive responses, similar to effects seen with intra-accumbens amphetamine. Additional effects include a speeding of the latency to collect food pellets; that result, however, does not appear to result merely from enhanced primary motivation. More selective patterns of depletion, produced by infusions of 5,7 DHT from the medial and dorsal raphe nuclei, lead to dissociable profiles of effects. The enhancement of impulsivity is especially apparent following infusions in the dorsal raphe, which mainly innervates the neocortex and striatum, but this depletion also uncovers a transient but significant enhancement of choice accuracy. Median raphe lesions, by contrast, which produce widespread 5-HT depletions in the forebrain, especially in the hippocampal region, are probably responsible for the speeded latencies to collect earned food pellets (Harrison, Everitt, and Robbins, 1997a, b). These varied effects of 5-HT depletion clearly indicate that this neurotransmitter has multiple functions in different aspects of the task, depending upon the anatomical locus of depletion. The results further suggest the likelihood of interactions with each of the other neurochemical systems considered. The results have to be assessed in the context of other studies that sometimes employ systemic drug treatments with this paradigm, or with others that attempt to isolate different aspects of attentional processing, as well as in comparison with the relevant human literature.

Five-Choice Task: Systemic Psychopharmacology How well do the above findings agree with those of other investigations that used related five-choice paradigms in which the neurochemical systems were manipulated peripherally? Considering the cholinergic effects on reduced choice accuracy, it is salient that Jones, Barnes, Kirkby, and Higgins (1995) have recently reported very similar effects in aged rats that were exacerbated by systemic treatment with scopolamine, the antimuscarinic agent, or with mecamylamine, the nicotine receptor antagonist. However, similar treatment with scopolamine did not greatly impair choice accuracy in young rats except in the added white noise condition (Jones and Higgins, 1995). The increase in distractibility may explain the deleterious effects of a single dose of scopolamine on the accuracy of detecting one of three spatially separated visual stimuli observed by the rat after it inserts its head into an observation tunnel (Skjoldager and Fowler, 1991).

It is of considerable interest that the anticholinesterase tacrine improved attentional performance of patients with probable dementia of the Alzheimer's type (DAT) in a direct analog of the five-choice task (Sahakian et al., 1993), and that subcutaneous nicotine similarly improved performance in terms of both accuracy and latency in the RVIP task described above both for elderly patients and also for those diagnosed with DAT (Sahakian, Jones, Levy, Warburton, and Grey, 1989; Jones, Sahakian, Warburton, and Gray, 1992).

For noradrenaline, only effects of systemic adrenergic alpha-1 and alpha-2 agonists and antagonists have been reported. Systemic doses of dexmedetomidine, an alpha-2 agonist that probably reduces central NA-ergic function, mainly increased omissions and reduced premature responses. There is thus a mismatch between those findings and those that are seen following DNAB lesions (Sirvio et al., 1994). In comparison, the alpha-2 antagonist atipamezole, when administered at doses that might be expected to enhance central noradrenergic function, improved detection of visual signals when their brightness was reduced. There were, however, no significant effects when the signals were made unpredictable by varying the intertrial interval (ITI) except at the highest doses, which impaired performance (Sirvio et al., 1993). Those effects are not easily integrated with those reported for another alpha-2 antagonist, idazoxan, which produced a complicated pattern of results in a related paradigm in which the drug modulated the propensity to make a premature response under certain distracting conditions, an effect that appeared to depend upon individual baselines of performance (Bunsey and Strupp, 1995). These findings in rats are of interest in comparison to the apparently ameliorative effects of systemically administered alpha-2 agonists such as clonidine and guanfacine in reducing disruptive effects of interpolated white noise during the delay period of a delayed response task in monkeys (Arnsten and Contant, 1992).

Neither set of results is what might have been expected, based on the effects of DNAB lesions (Carli et al., 1983; Cole and Robbins, 1992). However, it is clear that manipulation of a single receptor cannot be expected to have directly comparable effects, especially when the manipulation is done via peripheral administration, because of the multiplicity of systems affected, both centrally and peripherally. A recent study (Puumala, Riekkinen, and Sirvio, 1997) showed that St-587, a putative alpha-1 agonist, produced a small but significant improvement in choice accuracy when the presentation duration of the visual stimuli was shortened, which suggests that the drug enhanced attentional performance (cf. Muir et al., 1994). No data exist for the effects of DNAB lesions under those conditions. Prazosin, the alpha-1 receptor antagonist, produced a mild disruptive effect on accuracy at certain doses. In order to reconcile the effects of the systemically administered adrenergic agents and central NA depletion, it will be necessary in future studies to infuse the agents at specific CNS locations and to employ testing conditions that reveal effects of DNAB lesions (e.g., choice accuracy under unpredictable and distracting conditions).

The systemic effects of the indirectly acting catecholamine agonist D-amphetamine were generally similar to those of the drug when it was infused intra-accumbens, except that the latency to respond correctly was speeded by systemic amphetamine and was slowed by intra-accumbens amphetamine (Cole and Robbins, 1987). That intriguing difference presumably reflects an alternative site to the ventral striatum for some of the behavioral effects of amphetamine in that situation. Another discrepancy to emphasize, however, is that it has not proven possible to detect the improvements in choice accuracy with D-amphetamine in human subjects, which have been the empirical basis of tests of connectionist models of the functions of the central catecholamines (Servan-Schrieber, Printz, and Cohen, 1990). This is probably because the apparent improvements seen following D-amphetamine infusion in humans have been generally observed in vigilance situations, it having long been known that D-amphetamine counteracts the effects of fatigue and the so-called vigilance decrement (Mackworth, 1965). As noted above, it has proved quite difficult to devise comparable paradigms for the rat, but the issue will be considered further below. In results that are complementary to the effects of d-amphetamine, systemic haloperidol was reported to lengthen response latency and increase errors of omission (Carli and Samanin, 1992). The latter findings are consistent with the effects of haloperidol, a dopamine and noradrenaline receptor antagonist, in a related task in which motor requirements were minimized (see above) (Skjoldager and Fowler, 1991).

Finally, the diverse behavioral effects of agents affecting 5-HT transmission on the five-choice task are broadly consistent with what has been seen following central 5-HT depletion: for example, deficits in accuracy following lysergic acid diethylamide (LSD) and quipazine that are remediated by the 5-HT2 receptor antagonist ritanserin; and effects on magazine latency and impulsive responding following the 5-HT–releasing agent fenfluramine and the 5-HT1B receptor agonist m-CPP (Carli and Samanin, 1992). Overall, consideration of these findings shows that caution must still be exercised in attempts to reach conclusions about the functions of these neurotransmitter systems. However, it seems likely that systemic drug treatments are quite likely to produce a mixture of the distinct effects that are observed following the discrete and localized manipulation of anatomically distinct components of central systems (also, see Marrocco and Davidson, chapter 3, this volume).

Five-Choice Task: Effects of Cortical Lesions   The pattern of effects on the variants of the five-choice task obtained from the manipulations of specific neurotransmitter systems presumably results from the disruption of modulation of particular neural systems in their terminal domains. Muir, Everitt, and Robbins (1996) tested that hypothesis by observing the effects on attentional performance of more direct interference with the functioning of those systems by lesioning discrete neocortical regions with the cell body excitotoxin quinolinic acid, which largely spares fibers of passage. The main results are summarized in figure 10.1. There were transient deficits in choice accuracy following lesions of the medial prefrontal cortex (PFC), cingulate cortex, and parietal cortex. The deficits were significant and substantial in the case of the medial PFC lesion; because the medial PFC is one of the cortical targets of the cholinergic NBM, it would appear to be the likely substrate of the similar behavioral effects of lesions of the NBM, which lead to profound cholinergic loss in that cortical region. After performance recovered to control levels, rats with medial PFC lesions showed a strong tendency towards impairment following shortening of the stimulus and presentation of the noise just prior to the visual target—two other manipulations that can expose further impairments in the NBM-lesioned rats. However, the most striking effect of those challenges was seen in the latencies of the lesioned animals, which lengthened specifically and significantly in each case, suggesting that the lesion created deficits that caused the animals to trade speed for accuracy. Although the anterodorsal PFC–lesioned rats had no deficits on the baseline, they too responded to the attentional challenges with significantly lengthened latencies in two cases: unpredictable or abbreviated stimuli, and interpolated bursts of white noise in the ITI. None of the lesioned

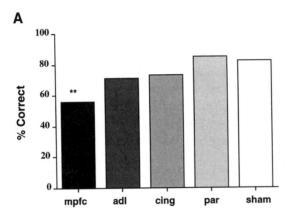

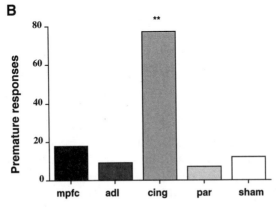

Figure 10.1 Summary of initial effects (first 10 sessions postoperative) of various cortical lesions in the rat in measures of performance (accuracy and impulsivity) on the five-choice serial reaction time task. Key: mpfc, medial prefrontal cortex; adl, antero-dorsolateral frontal cortex; cing, anterior cingulate; par, parietal cortex; sham, sham-operated controls. ** = P < 0.001 versus the other groups. (See also Muir et al., 1996.)

groups exhibited disproportionate impairments when the brightness of the discriminanda was varied.

Of the other cortical areas studied, the most clear-cut results were found following lesions to the cingulate cortex, which produced long-lasting and significant increases in impulsive responding, even though no other aspect of attentional performance was affected (figure 10.1). From the above analysis of effects of manipulating the different neurotransmitter systems, it will be plain that similar effects are produced by depletion of forebrain 5-HT and by intra-accumbens d-amphetamine via actions on the mesolimbic DA system. Either of these effects can plausibly be linked to dysfunction of neural circuitries under the control of the cingulate cortex.

The most surprising results from the study by Muir et al. (1996) are the apparent lack of effects of parietal cortex lesions, given that this region is known to be a major presumed locus of Posner and Petersen's "posterior attentional system" (1990)—and given that much evidence links it to attentional disturbances such as neglect. However, it is possible that neither the exact locus of damage in this study (designed to mimic the region of ACh depletion after NBM lesions) nor the attentional requirements of the five-choice task were appropriate for exposing attentional dysfunction dependent on the parietal cortex.

Vigilance

Early Attempts at Measurement The distinction between sustained attention and vigilance is a subtle one, the latter normally being described as a state of readiness to detect and respond to unpredictable and rare events (e.g., Broadbent, 1971; Mackworth, 1957). The need for sensitive measures of vigilance in experimental animals has been highlighted by recent theories, based largely on electrophysiological data, that postulate important roles for the noradrenergic locus coeruleus in behavioral vigilance, as measured in a "go-no-go" oddball paradigm (Aston-Jones, Chiang, and Alexinsky, 1991).

Previous attempts to measure vigilance in animals generally used discrete trial procedures in which a signal (generally a tone or light) from a single source had to be detected against a background condition by a single appropriate response (e.g., Stephens and Sarter, 1988; Sahgal, 1988; Dudchenko, Paul, and Sarter, 1992; Callahan, Kinsora, Harbaugh, Reeder, and Davis, 1993). As Posner and Boies (1971) pointed out, the foreperiod of a reaction time task may be considered as a miniature vigilance situation, albeit one that confounds measures of response preparation, and early studies such as those by Warburton and colleagues (for a review, see Warburton, 1977) used weak sensory signals in such tasks to measure attentional function in the rat. This permitted the application of signal detection theory (SDT) for separating effects on discriminative sensitivity—measured by such indices as d' or the nonparametric indices A' (Grier, 1971) or by the sensitivity index (SI) (Frey and Colliver, 1973)—from effects on response bias (β, B'', or responsivity index, RI). SDT is particularly useful for correcting percentage-correct measures for effects of changes in response bias, although there remain problems of interpretation. Does a change in the sensitivity index, for example, reflect altered sensory, perceptual, attentional, or even mnemonic processing? The most parsimonious interpretation of such effects is that they reflect altered information transmission within the CNS. It is even more difficult to interpret the meaning of changes in response bias, especially as those changes typically fluctuate more than the sensitivity index. A change in β could, for example, reflect motivational or perceptual biasing effects or even levels of response inhibition or disinhibition (as was pointed out by Frey and Colliver, 1973). A further problem is that the changes in both indices—a common sequelae of high doses of systemically administered drugs—are difficult to interpret. However, Warburton (1977) circumvented the latter problem by demonstrating that low doses of systemically administered cholinergic agents such as physostigmine and scopolamine preferentially affected the sensitivity measure in discriminations involving either exteroceptive or interoceptive events. A complementary study by Robbins and Iversen (1973), employing similar analytical techniques, found that low doses of systemic amphetamine (which presumably affected catecholaminergic systems) affected response bias more than it affected sensitivity.

Aside from problems of interpretation, the difficulties of applying and interpreting SDT analyses are compounded by overall changes in response rate (for example, even within the intertrial interval) that may confound the calculation of the p(hit) and p(false alarm) parameters that are necessary to compute SDT indices. One way around the problem is to employ two-lever discrimination tasks, in which one response is appropriate to report the occurrence of the target stimulus or signal stimulus, and another is appropriate to report noise. Appel and Dykstra (1977) reviewed some studies that employed this method for quantifying effects of systemically administered drugs on temporal discrimination; those studies are, however, largely beyond the scope of this review.

Recent Advances   Bushnell, Kelley, and Crofton (1994) employed a two-lever operant procedure that tackled some of the methodological problems of measuring vigilance in experimental animals such as the rat. In their task, there was a successive presentation over discrete trials of changes (i.e., signals) or no changes (i.e., noise) in the intensity of continuously delivered white noise. Hits were recorded by responses on one lever, and correct rejections by responses on the other. McGaughy and Sarter (1995) describe several modifications of this procedure, including the use of visual stimuli in a study of face validity in which signal intensity, background illumination, event rate, and signal asynchrony were all varied in order to determine the validity of various measures of performance in terms of human vigilance paradigms (e.g., Parasuraman et al., 1987). Predictable reductions in an SDT measure of vigilance performance based on SI were shown as a consequence of reducing the signal length from 500 to 25 ms and of adding background illumination. In one experiment, a vigilance decrement was found over three blocks of trials after an increase in signal event rate, as has been reported in human studies. There were, however, no major effects of varying the intertrial interval. Aged rats were shown to be impaired in their ability to discriminate short signals (results similar to those of Jones et al., 1995, which were reviewed previously).

In the experiments of McGaughy and Sarter (1995), systemic administration of the benzodiazepine receptor (BZP-R) agonist chlordiazepoxide also impaired performance in a similar manner. The inverse BZP-R agonists ZK 93426 and β-carboline did not affect performance. However, the partial inverse BZP-R agonist RU 33965 and amphetamine impaired vigilance performance in a dose-dependent manner, though via different relative effects on hits and misses. The effects of the BZP-R agents may be relevant to the functioning of the cholinergic basal forebrain because of interactions of GABAergic mechanisms with this system (e.g., Muir, Robbins, and Everitt, 1992; Sarter, 1994). Indeed, Holley, Turchi, Apple, and Sarter (1995) showed that infusions of chlordiazepoxide into the basal forebrain initially increased misses for short signals, and, later in the session, for long signals also. Although there were a few differences from the effects of systemic treatment, some of the effects of peripherally administered chlordiazepoxide are presumably mediated via that neural pathway.

The vigilance paradigm has also been used to assess the effects of cholinergic agents more directly. Turchi, Holley, and Sarter (1995) showed that the nicotine receptor antagonist mecamylamine potently impaired performance, while also increasing errors of omission. However, perhaps surprisingly in view of the human data (e.g., Wesnes and Warburton, 1983; Jones et al., 1992), there were no main effects of nicotine, although this is broadly consistent with the findings of Muir et al. (1995) in intact rats.

A more recent study (McGaughy et al., 1996) has shown that impairments in discriminative performance on the vigilance task result from immunotoxic lesioning of the cholinergic neurons leading to substantial loss of indices of cholinergic fiber density throughout the neocortex. Those effects contrast with the lack of effects of profound cortical depletion of noradrenaline resulting from 6-OHDA induced lesions of the dorsal noradrenergic ascending bundle (Ruland, Ronis, Bruno, and Sarter, 1995), confirming the conclusion that deficits are seen only under special circumstances (table 10.1).

Unfortunately, however, in all of these studies firm conclusions about specific effects on vigilance as opposed to signal detection were made difficult by the lack of any consistent interaction between the various treatments and trial block, and indeed sometimes by the lack of a significant decrement in untreated animals (see also Parasuraman et al., chapter 11, this volume). The two-lever paradigm is perhaps one of the most sophisticated to date for analyzing vigilance decrements, and so it is hoped that its distinguishing criterion will be specifically employed in future studies that examine the specific effects of these manipulations on vigilance. Moreover, as the authors of these studies recognize, even with a two-lever procedure there are potential problems that can compromise purely attentional interpretations of the results; for example, drugs such as amphetamine tend to produce higher-order forms of response bias, resulting, for example, in the capacity of the drug to cause changes in response output such as perseveration or switching (Koek and Slangen, 1983; Evenden and Robbins, 1983; Sahgal, 1988).

An alternative paradigm for measuring sustained attention has been employed by Pang, Merkel, Egeth, and Olton, (1992), However, their paradigm placed more emphasis on expectancy components of sustained attention than it placed on the vigilance decrement. They compared the effects of varying the stimulus frequency in rats and humans in a two-alternative forced-choice paradigm that allowed the computation of (STD) indices. Rats were trained to release one of two levers in response to either a visual or an auditory stimulus. As stimulus probability or repetition increased, response times and errors were reduced, in parallel with predictable shifts in response bias and with no significant effects on discriminability. In an experiment using this task to examine the effects of the inactivation of the cholinergic NBM via intra-NBM infusions of the GABA-A agonist muscimol, impairments in stimulus detection were observed (Pang, Williams, Egeth, and Olton, 1994), comparable to those observed in the five-choice task (Muir et al., 1992).

Divided Attention

The divided attention construct assumes that the brain is limited in its ability to monitor in parallel more than a finite number of inputs, and thus requires a switching mechanism to enable effective time-sharing of activities. Of course, the notion may also be applied at the level of response selection, as in dual task performance. There have been several attempts to measure divided attention in experimental animals. Robbins et al. (1986) required rats with ventral striatal dopamine depletion to detect which of two visual stimuli, presented separately to the two eyes, terminated first. Manipulating the offset of one of the stimuli relative to the other made it possible to infer the hypothetical minimum switching time between the two inputs; their method was analogous to that employed by Kristofferson (1967) with human subjects. In fact, it was difficult to reveal deficits produced by ventral striatal dopamine loss using this method, although the general disruptive effects of systemic amphetamine on responses in the task were completely blocked by the lesion.

A rather different approach to the problem of measuring divided attention is one in which rats have to continuously track a stimulus that is presented at two different locations in an operant paradigm (Evenden and Robbins, 1985). Each of several systemic stimulants (D-amphetamine, caffeine, nicotine, cocaine, and apomorphine) produced some improvement in tracking efficiency at certain doses; the rank order of the consistency and magnitude of the effects corresponded to the descending order of the listed drugs. These effects could not be ascribed simply to the general tendency of the drugs to enhance response switching behavior (Evenden, Turpin, Oliver, and Jennings, 1993).

Another attempt to measure divided attention in rats employed a paradigm derived from scalar timing theory in which rats were exposed to temporal discriminations that sometimes required them to divide attention between two simultaneous stimuli (Olton, Wenk, Church, and Meck, 1988). Rats with aspirative lesions of the entire prefrontal cortex or with nonspecific excitotoxic lesions of the NBM were specifically impaired in the ability to time two stimuli simultaneously; these results suggest deficits in divided attention that are possibly similar to those observed in the five-choice task (see above; Muir et al., 1996). A further method has been introduced recently in which rats are trained consecutively in operant auditory and visual conditional discrimination tasks before being placed onto a schedule with blocks initially of 20 unimodal trials followed by 60 bimodal trials with both conditional discriminations in operation (McGaughy, Turchi, and Sarter, 1994). In rats trained under this test procedure, scopolamine produced proportionately greater response latency increases in the bimodal as opposed to the unimodal conditions than did the benzodiazepine chlordiazepoxide; neither drug significantly affected response accuracy. The authors interpreted the results as reflecting enhanced costs of switching between modalities in the crossmodal trials caused by the muscarinic receptor blocker; these costs were generally higher for visual than for auditory stimuli. However, as the authors themselves conceded, it is possible that the selective deficit produced by scopolamine may have arisen from an interaction of the drug with more general factors present in the mixed condition that were unrelated to the crossmodal shift per se.

To my knowledge, there have been few, if any, attempts to measure effects of manipulations on genuine dual task performance in experimental animals; this might represent a challenge for the future.

Selective Attention: Overt and Covert Orienting and Shifting of Attention

Posner and Petersen (1990) identified several related mechanisms of spatial attention by using a deceptively simple paradigm that is described elegantly and in detail by Marrocco and Davidson (chapter 3, this volume). The main procedure requires the subject to fixate a central location and then respond to briefly presented cues in the periphery with variable stimulus onset asynchrony. Attention can be summoned covertly (i.e., in the absence of eye movements) by spatial cues presented in the periphery or by central symbolic cues, as shown by the speeding of reaction time to the visual target. Peripheral cues are assumed to summon attention to the target location automatically, whereas central cues presumably require cognitive processing. Similarly, the shifting of spatial attention can be studied by the use of invalid cues that incorrectly predict the location of targets on a proportion of trials. The time it takes to shift away from the invalid cue to respond correctly is taken as an index of attentional disengagement. The difference in performance between the valid and invalid trials is termed the validity effect. As Marrocco and Davidson describe, it is also possible to obtain estimates of the general alerting properties of the cue by including conditions with neutral cues that precede the target but provide no information about its location. This alerting effect is generally evident as a reduction in response time as the interval between cue and target increases. This paradigm has been applied with considerable success to the investigation of human patients with brain damage (see Rafal and Robertson, 1995) and also to the investigation of effects of psychoactive drugs such as clonidine and neuroleptics on normal human attentional functions (Clark, Geffen, and Geffen, 1986).

Some progress has been made in applying this paradigm, partly in order to examine in further detail the underlying neural and neuronal mechanisms of selective spatial attention, to experimental animals such as pigeons (Shimp and Friedrich, 1993), rats (Bushnell, in press), and monkeys (Bowman, Brown, Kertzman, Schwarz, and Robinson, 1993; Witte, Gordon-Lickey, and Marrocco, 1992). The former of the two studies with rhesus monkeys reported only very small validity effects that declined more rapidly than those that are seen in humans, and comparisons with the rat and pigeon are complicated by the lack of control over visual fixation (the rat, of course, being afoveate) as well as over motor orienting responses. However, the study by Bushnell with rats obtained qualitatively similar effects using auditory cues. He also made a substantial attempt to validate his procedure by varying SOA, by providing a neutral cue condition to control for alerting effects (see Marrocco and Davidson, chapter 3, this volume), and by varying the salience of the target and probability of the invalid cue. He concluded that the validity effects could not be explained by stimulus additivity or by response preparation mechanisms, whereas a cue-independent alerting effect may have affected response preparation.

Initial progress in understanding the psychopharmacology of covert orienting in the monkey is covered by Marrocco and Davidson (chapter 3, this volume). Two recent studies of obvious relevance to the understanding of the functions of the cholinergic NBM are by Voytko et al. (1994) with monkeys and by Chiba, Bushnell, Oshiro, and Gallagher, (1995) using Bushnell's (1996) paradigm for rats. In the former experiment, three rhesus monkeys with ibotenic acid–induced lesions of the NBM and two sham-operated controls performed in an orienting paradigm in which the valid (80% of trials) or invalid (20% of trials) cue was presented 200 ms before the visual target and 1–3 s after depression of an illuminated center screen. "Catch trials," in which no target was presented, required the monkey to continue to depress the central screen. The main responses monitored were premature release of the central screen, choice accuracy, reaction time (to release the central screen when the target appeared), and time taken to respond from that point in time to the appropriate stimulus ("hit time"). The lesioned monkeys had slower reaction times, especially in invalid trials, but the validity X group interaction failed to reach significance. If anything, the lesioned monkeys had quicker hit times, but not significantly so. The lesioned monkeys also made fewer premature responses, but choice accuracy was equivalent between the two groups. These effects were obtained in the context of the presence of no deficits in many other learning and memory tasks.

In the study with rats, Chiba et al. (1997) showed that in trials in which a target was preceded either by a valid cue or by no cue, performance of the lesioned rats was no different from performance in controls. However, in invalid trials, the NBM-lesioned rats exhibited impaired choice accuracy and longer response latencies, suggesting difficulties in attentional shifting. It may be premature to attempt to integrate these data with the effects of systemic cholinergic agents in the covert orienting paradigm for rhesus monkeys, which are described by Marrocco and Davidson (chapter 3, this volume; also, see Witte and Marrocco, 1993). However, it is noted that low doses of muscarinic receptor antagonists appear to have no serious deleterious effects on the task, whereas nicotine appears to promote attentional shifting by reducing the cost of the invalidity effect; this might be consistent with the effects of cortical cholinergic depletion in rats described above. It is of interest that systemic adrenergic and dopaminergic agents in the same paradigm appear to affect different aspects of alerting functions rather than affecting orienting per se (see Marrocco and Davidson, chapter 3, this volume).

The psychopharmacological results will ultimately have to be interpreted in the context of the literature supporting the existence of several attentional networks in the primate brain (Posner and Peterson, 1990). Three regions of the primate brain appear to play unique roles in attentional shifts: the midbrain, including the superior colliculus (in the control of visual saccades and the movement of attention); the lateral pulvinar of the thalamus, which mediates the engagement of attention at a novel attentional focus; and the posterior parietal cortex, which probably mediates the disengagement of attention from a given location and which may accouint for some of the deficits observed in the neglect syndromes.

MODELING ATTENTIONAL DYSFUNCTIONS IN CLINICAL SYNDROMES

Attentional Neglect

Another important source of data concerning possible attentional mechanisms within the CNS has arisen from animal studies of the neglect syndrome, in which stimuli on one side of the sensory world are ignored; the syndrome is generally produced by lesions to the contralateral brain either at the cortical or subcortical level. The exact explanation of neglect in human subjects is still a controversial matter, as there are accounts based on impairments of spatial representation and accounts based on specific attentional deficits such as "attentional disengagement" (for a review, see Shallice, 1988). Neglect-like phenomena following unilateral brain damage in regions including the parietal and frontal cortex, basal ganglia, and superior colliculus have been reported in experimental animals, as reviewed by Milner (1987). The main interpretation problem is the separation of motor or output forms of neglect, in which the animal is capable of attending to a particular stimulus channel but is unable to initiate responses toward the stimulus because of hemi-akinetic or hemispatial problems. Indeed, Rizzolatti and

Camarda (1987) opt for a premotor theory of selective attention in order to accommodate the congruence of motor and attentional deficits that is often observed.

Attentional Neglect Arising from Subcortical Lesions in Animals The difficulty of distinguishing sensory attentional deficits from output-related deficits is especially problematic in the case of unilateral lesions to the basal ganglia, either of the ascending dopaminergic projections from the substantia nigra (produced, for example, either with 6-OHDA or with electrolytic lesions of the medial forebrain bundle at the level of the lateral hypothalamus) or of the dorsal striatum (caudate-putamen) itself. Early studies using a neurological sensorimotor test battery seemed to conclude that such lesions produced sensory inattention (e.g., Marshall and Teitelbaum, 1974). However, when attempts were made to separate out possible effects of sensory neglect versus response-related deficits in orienting, following either unilateral striatal dopamine depletion (Carli, Evenden, and Robbins, 1985; Carli, Jones, and Robbins, 1989), unilateral lateral hypothalamic lesions (Hoyman, Weese, and Frommer, 1979), or unilateral lesions of the striatum itself (Mittleman, Brown, and Robbins, 1988; Brown and Robbins, 1989a), no convincing evidence for sensory loss per se was observed, although it remains difficult to distinguish explanations based on hemispatial as opposed to hemi-akinetic deficits (Brown and Robbins, 1989b). A typical set of findings was that rats with unilateral dopamine depletion from the dorsal but not the ventral striatum were slower to initiate responses in space contralateral to the lesioned side, regardless of whether the animals were responding to visual stimuli on the ipsilateral or contralateral sides (Carli et al., 1989). However, when rats were required to detect stimuli with unlateralized responses, no deficits were observed (Carli et al., 1985). Other evidence is apparently consistent with this view: for example, observational evidence has suggested that the recovery of contralateral responsiveness may reflect a form of compensatory learning (Schallert and Hall, 1988). A further study has clarified some of the nature of the deficit arising from dopaminergic lesions: rats with unilateral striatal dopamine depletion were shown not to hasten their response times as the foreperiod preceding the imperative signal was lengthened. However, they continued to show a normal benefit of advance information for response choice (Brown and Robbins, 1991). That pattern of results suggests an impairment in response preparation rather than in response programming. Specifically, it is proposed that rats with unilateral striatal dopamine depletion have deficits in the readiness to respond appropriately. Furthermore, this concept can be applied to responses controlled by spatial as well as by temporal factors (Robbins and Brown, 1990; see also Ward and Brown, 1996).

Overall, although it cannot be excluded that unilateral striatal lesions produce some attentional impairments analogous to those observed in human neglect syndromes, it is evident that a major component of the impairments is most comparable to what has been termed output or intentional neglect in the clinical literature (Valenstein and Heilman, 1981).

Attentional Neglect Arising from Cortical Lesions in Animals Milner (1987) has reviewed evidence of the effects of neglect following unilateral cortical lesions in animals. Despite the efforts of many investigators (e.g., Crowne, Yeo, and Steele-Russell, 1981; Crown and Pathria, 1982), it remains difficult to decide if the transient neglect syndromes observed are equivalent to the syndromes observed clinically. Indeed, there is only inferential evidence that a genuine sensory attentional form of neglect exists that is clearly distinct from problems of initiating contralateral responses. One potentially important dissociation was obtained following unilateral parietal cortical lesions in the rat; such lesions produced contralateral neglect but also rotation towards the contralateral (rather than toward the ipsilateral) lesioned side (Crowne, Richardson, and Dawson, 1986).

A second study focused on the extinction phenomenon characteristic of neglect. Bilateral, simultaneous somatosensory stimulation in recovered hemidecorticate rats led to a slower response to stimuli presented contralaterally to the lesioned side (Schallert and Whishaw, 1984). However, even in that case it is possible that the asymmetry arose from response-related factors; for example, it is generally quicker to use the ipsilateral limb to respond to an ipsilateral stimulus.

There are only a few direct comparisons of the effects of unilateral subcortical and cortical lesions. Dopamine-depleted rats and monkeys showed tactile extinction (Schallert et al., 1982; Annett, Rogers, Hernandez, and Dunnett, 1992). However, Schallert and Hall (1988) failed to observe significant tactile extinction deficits in rats recovered from initial effects of unilateral dopamine depletion, although the lesioned rats did display disengagement deficits in responding to contralateral cues when already performing other types of behavior. Brown, Bowman, and Robbins (1991) used the same paradigm for disconfounding sensory and motor requirements in a response time task as employed by Carli et al. (1989) and by Brown and Robbins (1989a) for assessing neglect in rats with unilateral lesions of the agranular frontal cortex (Zilles' Fr2 region; 1985). They again found evidence for lasting deficits in initiation of reponse into contralateral space rather than for in detection of the sensory signals. It is of interest that these rats also exhibited the tactile extinction phenomenon reported by Schallert and Whishaw (1984) for hemidecorticate rats.

Prepulse Inhibition and Sensory Gating

An experimental index of central inhibitory, automatic mechanisms of attention is the prepulse inhibition (PPI) of the acoustic startle response. This reflex is a widespread contraction of the muscles in response to a sudden loud sound; its magnitude may be significantly diminished if preceded by 30–500 ms by a much weaker stimulus from any modality (though typically the weaker stimulus also comes from the auditory modality) (Ison, Hammond, and Krauter, 1973). The phenomenon occurs in humans as well as in other animals, and can be used as a direct comparative index of the ability to "gate" sensory stimuli in patients with psychopathology such as schizophrenia. The convenience of the measure and the ease of generating detailed parametric data—for example, as a function of the interval between the prepulse and startle stimuli—have enabled it to be used as a useful animal model of human attentional deficits, to establish the neural systems underlying gating phenomena (Braff and Geyer, 1992).

Although the primary acoustic startle reflex is known to be controlled by brainstem nuclei, and although it is likely that PPI is mediated at the same level via inputs to the ventral cochlear nucleus and to the nucleus reticularis pontis caudalis, PPI is affected by manipulations of forebrain structures such as the hippocampus and ventral striatopallidal circuitry that target the pedunculopontine tegmental nuclei (see Swerdlow, Caine, Braff, and Geyer, 1992; Swerdlow, 1996); an analogous form of PPI persists, however, even after transcollicular decerebration (Davis and Gendelman, 1977). The ventral striatum has been particularly implicated in PPI by the observation that the direct infusion of dopamine agonists or of dopamine itself into that structure attenuates PPI, and excitotoxic lesions of the ventral striatum similarly decrease it (Swerdlow et al., 1992; Kodsi and Swerdlow, 1994). However, other regions of the striatum and pallidum also participate in this downstream modulation of PPI, lesions of the caudal portions of the striatum and pharmacological manipulation of the dorsal pallidum also being effective (Kodsi and Swerdlow, 1995).

It is clearly difficult to relate these interesting findings to conventional notions of attention, although links to aspects of selective attention are perhaps the most obvious. The phenomenon of PPI itself appears to represent an automatic mechanism for regulation of reflexive responsiveness. Its modulation by forebrain structures may represent another example of "set" or of readiness, which presumably operates at several levels to control both voluntary responses, as occur in response time tasks, as well as reflexive activity. One way of testing that hypothesis is to make systematic comparisons with effects of those neural manipulations that affect distinct aspects of attention. Thus, for example, ventral striatal dopamine depletion markedly affects the overall propensity to respond; the effect includes the blockade of premature responses produced in the five-choice task following the introduction of bursts of white noise or following systemic D-amphetamine (Cole and Robbins, 1989; also, see above).

Attention in Relation to Associative Learning

In the last two decades, some animal learning theorists have begun to reexamine attentional constructs in attempting to account for behavioral phenomena (e.g., Mackintosh, 1975; Shimp and Friedrich, 1993), although some apparently attentional effects can profitably be viewed as products of memory and associative learning. Much research activity has focused on Pavlovian procedures such as latent inhibition, blocking, and overshadowing to make inferences about selective attentional processes (Mackintosh, 1983), because those procedures have the advantage of a substantial theoretical framework. Chiba, Bucci, Holland, and Gallagher (1995) provide a recent, particularly elegant example of this approach; however, for reasons of space it will be illustrated here by a simplified treatment of two standard paradigms.

Latent inhibition (LI) occurs when the repeated nonreinforced presentation of a stimulus retards the subsequent conditioning to that stimulus (Lubow, 1989; Mackintosh, 1983). Therefore, an LI experiment typically has two main stages. The first stage pre-exposes the to-be-conditioned CS and the second examines the effects of the pre-exposure on conditioning to the CS. The typical LI effect is that the pre-exposed group shows retarded conditioning to the CS compared with a control group that did not receive pre-exposures. This means that impairments in LI are expressed by superior conditioning in the non-pre-exposed control group. Impaired LI is shown when the pre-exposed group does not show retarded conditioning, that is, when their performance is significantly better than usual (for idealized data, see Robbins, Muir, Killcross, and Pretsell, 1993). This is a convenient outcome when studying the effects of neural manipulations such as drugs or lesions because it rules out nonspecific deficits produced by neural manipulations, such as sensory loss or lack of motivation, in explaining the results.

A simple interpretation of the LI phenomenon is that it results from an inability to screen out irrelevant stimuli (in this case, the pre-exposed CS). A prominent theory of LI refers to learned inattention as a mediating intervening variable (Lubow, 1989). Several groups have capitalized on this hypothesis to advance LI as a model for attentional dysfunction in schizophrenia (see Gray et al., 1995). Central to their theorizing is the finding that systemic treatment of rats with amphetamine reduces LI, whereas similar treatment with dopamine receptor blocking drugs such as haloperidol enhances it. These effects are related to other results that implicate hippocampal–ventral striatum circuitry in the mediation of LI (for a review, see Gray et al., 1995). However, there is some contradictory evidence—notably, manipulations that enhance ventral striatal dopamine function, such as intra-accumbens amphetamine or rearing in social isolation, without affecting LI (Killcross and Robbins, 1993; Wilkinson et al., 1994). It is of interest that both of those manipulations have been shown to affect prepulse inhibition (Wilkinson et al., 1994; also, see preceding section). It is beyond the scope of this chapter to consider this controversy in more detail—and certain considerations suggest that it is inappropriate to devote much more space to LI here. In particular, there is currently theoretical debate about the exact interpretation of LI, and explanations other than those that consider solely attentional, as distinct from associative, factors need further investigation (see Hall, 1992). One set of findings that may complicate the psychological interpretation of LI is that motivational manipulations, such as changes in the concentration or level of the appetitive or aversive reinforcers employed, appear to alter the effects of drugs such as systemic amphetamine or neuroleptics (Killcross et al., 1994a,b)—suggesting that disruptions of LI, whatever their precise relevance to schizophrenia, may not be attributable to changes in selective attention.

Extra-Dimensional Shift

A final example of a paradigm derived from animal learning theory that may have relevance for the study of attentional control is the extradimensional shift (EDS), in which a subject is trained to respond to one stimulus dimension (e.g., color or form) of a compound stimulus composed of several dimensions and is then required to respond instead to the alternative stimulus dimension. Slamecka (1968) carefully described the criteria for establishing whether performance in an EDS paradigm in fact corresponds to a shift in selective response to a given stimulus dimension rather than to a more general response to altered contingencies. The critical comparisons are with another form of shift termed intradimensional shift (IDS), in which subjects are required to transfer responses toward different exemplars of stimuli within the same stimulus dimension; essentially, in this paradigm, subjects are learning set. If transfer is quicker for IDS compared with EDS, then it can be concluded that the subject attended selectively to a particular dimension before transferring to the alternative one (for further explanation, see Slamecka, 1968; Roberts, Everitt, and Robbins, 1988).

The salient features of the EDS for present discussion are that (1) it constitutes the main requirement in the Wisconsin Card Sorting Test commonly used in the neuropsychological assessment of patients with frontal lobe dysfunction and schizophrenia, and that (2) a parallel version has been devised for testing monkeys as well as humans (Roberts et al., 1988). Using the parallel version it has been shown that lesions to the prefrontal cortex (Brodmann's area 9) in marmosets selectively impair EDS performance without affecting IDS performance (Dias, Robbins, and Roberts, 1996). The EDS task may also be differentially sensitive to lesions of the cholinergic or dopaminergic projections to the prefrontal cortex in marmosets (Roberts, Robbins, Everitt, and Muir, 1992; Roberts et al., 1994), but firm conclusions await converging evidence from other manipulations of these systems. The relevance to human attentional deficits produced by neurological and neuropsychiatric factors is shown from the fact that neurosurgical lesions of the prefrontal cortex, but not of the temporal cortex, produce disproportionate deficits on the EDS compared with the IDS condition (Owen, Roberts, Polkey, Sahakian, and Robbins, 1991). Moreover, a similar selective effect on the EDS task has been shown in chronic schizophrenics (Elliott, McKenna, Robbins, and Sahakian, 1995).

The EDS task reflects some form of selective attention, probably one that is expressed at the level of executive control over response output—possibly related to the types of function performed by the anterior attentional system of Posner and Petersen (1990). Such a relationship could explain the susceptibility of EDS task performance to damage to the frontal cortex.

CONCLUSIONS

There is considerable interest in the attentional capacities of experimental animals because of the useful perspective that they provide on the neural substrates of attention. Data from animal tests supplement, for example, studies of brain-damaged patients and functional neuroimaging studies of normal volunteers. It is difficult to see, for example, how such specific information on attentional processing as a function of chemical neurotransmitter systems and neuroanatomical location could be obtained using human subjects alone. A major concern, however, is how well findings on the neural substrates of attention in experimental animals can be extrapolated to humans. Although a wealth of detailed theory exists concerning attentional function in human subjects, derived from cognitive psychology paradigms, animal researchers are only just beginning to capitalize upon those theories. This chapter has attempted to summarize what has been achieved in the field, especially by investigators who have adapted human paradigms suitable for investigating different aspects of attention such as vigilance, divided attention, sustained attention, and selective attention. In some cases (e.g., prepulse inhibition and latent inhibition), the process has actually worked in reverse. In many areas, the status of the field is empirical, especially as investigators are intent on validating the test procedures and do not have very precise hypotheses about the exact nature of the suspected attentional functions of particular brain regions or neurochemical systems. It is in the latter sphere that neurochemical and psychopharmacological studies in animals are of especial value. Although consensus certainly cannot be said to have been achieved in many areas, there is a substantial amount of data in certain instances to offer considerable encouragement for hypothesis-testing studies in the future, and also to point out suitable directions for studies with human subjects that otherwise may not be undertaken.

In the case of the cholinergic systems, recent studies of lesions of the cholinergic basal forebrain or of the effects of systemic muscarinic receptor antagonists in both rats and monkeys have suggested deficits in several different paradigms for measuring attention, including sustained and divided attention (Olton et al., 1988; Robbins et al., 1989; Muir et al., 1994; Jones et al., 1995; McGaughy, Kaiser, and Sarter, 1996) and selective spatial attention (Voytko et al., 1994; Chiba et al., 1997). Thus, there is general agreement that the projection from the cholinergic basal forebrain to the neocortex (primarily the anterior regions) plays a role in attention, but it is not very clearly linked to particular attentional processes. The discovery that micro-iontophoretic application of acetylcholine leads to enhanced signal-to-noise ratios for evoked potentials recorded from the several different regions of neocortex (e.g., Sillito, 1987) suggests a possible involvement in different forms of attentional process controlled, for example, by posterior and anterior cortical regions. Alternatively, the range of effects described may indicate that the cortical cholinergic system is implicated in a more basic attentional mechanism.

The striatal dopaminergic systems appear be involved in attentional processes such as readiness that may operate at the output stage on mechanisms related to response preparation (e.g., Brown and Robbins, 1991). This appears to be consistent with the effects of dopamine receptor blocking drugs, which tend to selectively impair reaction times in the absence of alerting stimuli (see Marrocco and Davidson, chapter 3, this volume). However, it is of interest that several investigators have also shown effects of manipulating central dopaminergic systems on rather different attentional functions, including that of sensory gating (in the case of prepulse inhibition) and other forms of selective attention that are hypothetically engaged during LI. Much less is known in the case of the central 5-HT systems, although many of the effects of depletion of central 5-HT seem to be in functional opposition to those produced by manipulation of the central monoaminergic and cholinergic systems.

Understanding the functions of the coeruleo-cortical noradrenergic projections presents the greatest challenge in view of the lack of consistent findings across different laboratories. There are apparently strong grounds, based on electrophysiological data, for hypothesizing a specific role for this projection in vigilance (Aston-Jones et al., 1991), but other data—for example, from the five-choice task (Cole and Robbins, 1992)—suggest an involvement in a wider range of attentional processes. As reviewed in this chapter, studies with systemically administered adrenergic agents in experimental animals (and human volunteers) do not always agree with the effects of local manipulations of the noradrenergic system. Resolving these controversies may depend on systematic comparisons of the effects of the different pharmacological methods of influencing central noradrenergic activity in the same test setting, perhaps in combination with electrophysiological recording from locus coeruleus neurons, especially as it is sometimes difficult to be confident of the precise net impact of these treatments on central noradrenergic function. Resolution may also depend on the formulation of novel principles underlying certain forms of attention. It will also be important to distinguish precise functions of the noradrenergic neurons in attentional processes that are distinct from, for example, the cholinergic or dopaminergic innervations of the cerebral cortex. Finally, it will be essential to compare the roles of these somewhat diffuse systems with what has been discovered about the functioning of the neural networks in control of attention at a thalamocortical level (e.g., Corbetta, Shulman, Miezin, and Petersen, 1995; Desimone,

Miller, Chelazzi, and Leuschow, 1995; Maunsell, 1995), using rather complementary approaches to those discussed here.

ACKNOWLEDGMENTS

I thank my colleagues for their contributions to the studies discussed and R. D. Rogers for helpful comments on the manuscript. The work described was supported mainly by grants from the Medical Research Council (U.K.) and from the Wellcome Trust.

REFERENCES

Annett, L. E., Rogers, D. C., Hernandez, T. D., and Dunnett, S. B. (1992) Behavioral analysis of unilateral monoamine depletion in the marmoset. *Brain* 115: 825–856.

Appel, J. B. and Dykstra, L. A. (1977) Drugs, discrimination, and signal detection theory. In *Advances in Behavioral Pharmacology* (Vol. 1), edited by T. Thompson and P. B. Dews, pp. 139–166. New York: Academic Press.

Arnsten, A. F. T. and Contant, T. A. (1992) Alpha-2 adrenergic agonists decrease distractibility in aged monkeys performing the delayed response task. *Psychopharmacology* 108: 159–169.

Aston-Jones, G., Chiang, C., and Alexinsky, T. (1991) Discharge of noradrenergic locus coeruleus neurons in behaving rats and monkeys suggests a role in vigilance. *Prog. Brain Res.* 88: 501–520.

Bowman, E. M., Brown, V. J., Kertzman, C., Schwarz, U., and Robinson D. L. (1993) Covert orienting of attention in macaques. I. Effects of behavioral context. *J. Neurophysiol.* 70: 431–443.

Braff, D. L. and Geyer, M. A. (1992) Sensorimotor gating and schizophrenia: Human and animal model studies. *Arch. Gen. Psychiatry* 47: 181–188.

Broadbent, D. E. (1971) *Decision and Stress.* London: Academic Press.

Brown, V. J., Bowman, E. M., and Robbins, T. W. (1991) Unilateral and bilateral effects of unilateral lesions of medial agranular cortex of the rat. *Behav. Neurosci.* 105: 567–578.

Brown, V. J. and Robbins, T. W. (1989a) Elementary processes of response selection mediated by distinct regions of the striatum. *J. Neurosci.* 9: 3760–3765.

Brown, V. J. and Robbins, T. W. (1989b) Disruption of response space following unilateral striatal dopamine depletion. *J. Neurosci.* 9: 983–989.

Brown, V. J. and Robbins, T. W. (1991) Simple and choice reaction time performance following unilateral striatal dopamine depletion in the rat: Impaired motor readiness but preserved response preparation. *Brain* 114: 513–525.

Bunsey, M. D. and Strupp, B. J. (1995) Specific effects of idazoxan in a distraction task: Evidence that endogenous norepinephrine plays a role in selective attention in rats. *Behav. Neurosci.* 109: 903–911.

Bushnell, P. J. (1995) Overt orienting in the rat: Parametric studies of cued detection of visual targets. *Behav. Neurosci.* 109: 1095–1105.

Bushnell, P. J., Kelley, K. L., and Crofton, K. M. (1994) Effects of toluene inhalation on detection of auditory signals in rats. *Neurotoxicol. Teratol.* 16: 149–160.

Callahan, M. J., Kinsora, J. J., Harbaugh, R. E., Reeder, T. M., and Davis, R. E. (1993) Continuous ICV infusion of scopolamine impairs sustained attention of rhesus monkeys. *Neurobiol. Aging* 14: 147–151.

Carli, M., Evenden, J. L., and Robbins, T. W. (1985) Depletion of unilateral striatal dopamine impairs initiation of contralateral actions and not sensory attention. *Nature* 313: 679–682.

Carli, M., Jones, G. H., and Robbins, T. W. (1989) Effects of 6-OHDA lesions of the dorsal and ventral striatum on visual neglect in the rat. *Neuroscience* 29: 309–327.

Carli, M., Robbins, T. W., Evenden, J. L., and Everitt, B. J. (1983) Effects of lesions to ascending noradenergic neurones on performance of a 5-choice serial reaction task in rats: Implications for theories of dorsal noradenergic bundle function based on selective attention and arousal. *Behav. Brain Res.* 9: 361–380.

Carli, M. and Samanin, R. (1992) Serotonin2 receptor agonists and serotonergic anorectic drugs affect rats' performance differently in a five-choice serial reaction time task. *Psychopharmacology* 106: 228–234.

Chiba, A. A., Bucci, D. J., Holland, P. C., and Gallagher, M. (1995) Basal forebrain lesions disrupt increments but no decrements in conditioned stimulus processing. *J. Neurosci.* 15: 7315–7322.

Chiba, A. A., Bushnell, P. J., Oshiro, W. M., and Gallagher, M. (1997) Selective removal of cholinergic neurons in the basal forebrain alters cued target detection in rat. *Neuroreport*, in press.

Clark, C. R., Geffen, G. M., and Geffen, L. B. (1986) Catecholamines and the covert orienting of attention. *Neuropsychologia* 27: 131–140.

Cole, B. J. and Robbins, T. W. (1987) Amphetamine impairs the discrimination performance of rats with dorsal bundle lesions on a 5-choice serial reaction time task: New evidence for central dopaminergic-noradrenergic interactions. *Psychopharmacology* 91: 458–466.

Cole, B. J. and Robbins, T. W. (1989) Effects of 6-hydroxydopamine lesions of the nucleus accumbens septi on performance of a 5-choice serial reaction time task in rats: Implications for theories of selective attention and arousal. *Behav. Brain Res.* 33: 165–179.

Cole, B. J. and Robbins, T. W. (1992) Forebrain norepinephrine: Role in effortful but not automatic processing in the rat. *Neuropsychopharmacology* 7: 129–142.

Corbetta, M., Shulman, G. L., Miezin, F. M., and Petersen, S. E. (1995) Superior parietal cortex activation during spatial attention shifts and visual feature conjunction. *Science* 270: 802–805.

Crowne, D. P. and Pathria, M. N. (1982) Some attentional effects of unilateral frontal lesions in the rat. *Behav. Brain Res.* 6: 25–39.

Crowne, D. P., Richardson, C. M., and Dawson, K. A. (1986) Parietal and frontal eye field neglect in the rat. *Behav. Brain Res.* 22: 227–231.

Crowne, D. P., Yeo, C. H., and Steele-Russell, I. S. (1981) The effects of unilateral frontal eye field lesions in the monkey: Visuomotor guidance and avoidance behavior. *Behav. Brain Res.* 7: 165–185.

Davis, M. and Gendelman P. M. (1977) Plasticity of the acoustic startle reflex in acutely decerebrate rats. *J. Comp. Physiol. Psychol.* 4 : 241–263.

Desimone, R., Miller, E. K., Chelazzi, L., and Leuschow A. (1995) Multiple memory systems in the visual cortex. In *The Cognitive Neurosciences*, edited by M. S. Gazzaniga, pp. 475–486. Cambridge, MA: MIT Press.

Dias, R., Robbins, T. W., and Roberts, A. (1996) Dissociation of affective and attentional shifting by selective lesions of prefrontal cortex. *Nature.* 380: 69–72.

Dudchenko, P., Paul, B., and Sarter, M. (1992) Dissociation between the effects of benzodiazepine receptor agonists on behavioral vigilance and responsivity. *Psychopharmacology* 109: 203–211.

Elliott, R., McKenna, P. J., Robbins, T. W., and Sahakian, B. J. (1995) Neuropsychological evidence for fronto-striatal dysfunction in schizophrenia. *Psychol. Med.* 25: 619–630.

Evenden, J. L. and Robbins, T. W. (1983) Increased response switching, perseveration and perseverative switching following d-ampetamine in the rat. *Psychopharmacology* 80: 67–73.

Evenden, J. L. and Robbins, T. W. (1985) The effects of d-amphetamine, chlordiazepoxide and alpha-flupenthioxol on food-reinforced tracking of a visual stimulus by rats. *Psychopharmacology* 85: 361–366.

Evenden, J. L., Turpin, M., Oliver, L., and Jennings C. (1993) Caffeine and nicotine improve visual tracking by rats: A comparison with amphetamine, cocaine and apomorphine. *Psychopharmacology* 110: 169–176.

Frey, P. W. and Colliver, J. A. (1973) Sensitivity and responsivity measures for discrimination learning. *Learn. Motiv.* 4: 327–342.

Gray, J. A., Joseph, M. H., Hemsley, D. R., Young, A. M. J., Warburton, E. C., Boulengeuz, P., Grigoryan, G. A., Peters, S. L., Rawlins, J. N. P., Taib, C. T. Yee, B. K., Cassaday, H. H., Weiner, I., Gal, G., Gusak, O., Joel, D., Shadach, E., Shalev, U., Tarrasch, R., and Feldon, J. (1995) The role of mesolimbic dopaminergic and retrohippocampal afferents to the nucleus accumbens in latent inhibition: Implications for schizophrenia. *Behav. Brain Res.* 71: 19–31.

Grier, J. B. (1971) Nonparametric indices for sensitivity and bias: Computing formulas. *Psychol. Bull.* 75: 424–429.

Hall, G. (1992) *Perceptual and Associative Learning.* Oxford: Clarendon Press.

Harrison, A. A., Everitt, B. J., and Robbins, T. W. (1997a) Central 5-HT depletion enhances impulsive responding without affecting the accuracy of attentional performance: Interactions with dopaminergic mechanisms. *Psychopharmacology,* 133: 329–342.

Harrison, A. A., Everitt B. J., and Robbins, T. W. (1997b) Doubly dissociable effects of selective median raphé and dorsal raphé lesions on performance of the five-choice serial reaction time test of attention in rats. *Behav. Brain. Res.,* in press.

Heise, G. A. and Milar, K. S. (1984) Drugs and stimulus control. In *Handbook of Psychopharmacology: Drugs, Neurotransmitters, and Behaviour* (Vol. 18) edited by L. L. Iversen, S. D. Iversen, and S. H. Snyder, pp. 129–190. New York: Plenum Press.

Holley, L. A., Turchi, J., Apple, C., and Sarter M. (1995) Dissociation between the attentional effects of infusions of a benzodiazepine receptor agonist and an inverse agonist into the basal forebrain. *Psychopharmacology* 120: 99–108.

Hoyman, L., Weese, G. D., and Frommer, D. P. (1979) Tactile discrimination performance deficits following neglect-producing unilateral lateral hypothalamic lesions in the rat. *Physiol. Behav.* 22: 139–147.

Ison, J. R., Hammond, G. R., and Krauter, E. E. (1973) Effects of experience on stimulus-produced reflex inhibition in the rat. *J. Comp. Physiol. Psychol.* 83: 324–336.

Jones, D. N. C., Barnes, J. C., Kirkby, D. L., and Higgins, G. A. (1995) Age-associated impairments in a test of attention: Evidence for involvement of cholinergic systems. *J. Neurosci.* 15: 7282–7292.

Jones, D. N. C. and Higgins G. A. (1995) Effects of scopolamine on visual attention in rats. *Psychopharmacology* 120: 142–149.

Jones, G. M. M., Sahakian, B. J., Warburton, D. M., and Gray, J. A. (1992) Effects of acute subcutaneous nicotine on attention, information processing and short-term memory in Alzheimer's disease. *Psychopharmacology* 108: 485–494.

Killcross, A. S., Dickinson, A., and Robbins, T. W. (1994a) Amphetamine-induced abolition of latent inhibition are reinforcer-mediated: Implications for animal models of schizophrenic attentional dysfunction. *Psychopharmacology* 115: 185–195.

Killcross, A. S., Dickinson, A. and Robbins, T. W. (1994b) Effects of the neuroleptic α-flupenthixol on latent inhibition in aversively and appetitively motivated paradigms: Evidence for dopamine-reinforcer interactions. *Psychopharmacology* 115: 196–205.

Killcross, A. S. and Robbins, T. W. (1993) Differential effects of intra-accumbens and systemic amphetamine on latent inhibition using an on-baseline, within subject conditioned suppression paradigm. *Psychopharmacology* 110: 479–489.

Kodsi, M. H. and Swerdlow, N. R. (1994) Quinolinic acid lesions of the ventral striatum reduce sensorimotor gating of acoustic startle in rats. *Brain Res.* 643: 59–65.

Kodsi, M. H. and Swerdlow, N. R. (1995) Prepulse inhibition in the rat is regulated by ventral and caudodorsal striato-pallidal circuitry. *Behav. Neurosci.* 109: 1–17.

Koek, W. and Slangen, J. L. (1983) Effects of d-amphetamine and morphine on discrimination: Signal detection analysis and assessment of response repetition in the performance deficits. *Psychopharmacology* 80: 125–128.

Kornetsky, C. and Eliasson, M. (1969) Reticular stimulation and chlorpromazine: An animal model for schizophrenic overarousal. *Science* 165: 1273–1274.

Kristofferson, A. B. (1967) Attention and psychophysical time. *Acta Psychol.* 27: 93–100.

Lubow, R. E. (1989) *Latent Inhibition and Conditioned Attention Theory.* Cambridge, England: Cambridge University Press.

Mackintosh, N. J. (1975) A theory of attention: Variations in the associability of stimuli with reinforcement. *Psychol. Rev.* 4: 276–298.

Mackintosh, N. J. (1983) *Conditioning and Associative Learning.* Oxford: Clarendon Press.

Mackworth, J. F. (1965) The effect of amphetamine on the detectability of signals in a vigilance task. *Can. J. Psychol.* 19: 104–109.

Mackworth, N. H. (1957) Some factors affecting vigilance. *Adv. Sci.* 53: 389–393.

Marshall, J. F. and Teitelbaum, P. (1974) Further analysis of sensory inattention following lateral hypothalamic damage in rats. *J. Comp. Physiol. Psychol.* 86: 375–395.

Maunsell, J. (1995) The brain's visual world: Representation of visual targets in cerebral cortex. *Science* 270: 764–769.

McGaughy, J., Kaiser, T., and Sarter, M. (1996) Behavioral vigilance following infusions of 192 IgG-saporin into the basal forebrain: Selectivity of the behavoral impairment and relation to cortical AChE-positive fiber density. *Behav. Neurosci.* 110: 247–265.

McGaughy, J. and Sarter, M. (1995) Behavioral vigilance in rats: Task validation and effects of age, amphetamine, and benzodiazepine receptor ligands. *Psychopharmacology* 11: 340–357.

McGaughy, J., Turchi, J., and Sarter, M. (1994) Crossmodal divided attention in rats: Effects of chlordiazepoxide and scopolamine. *Psychopharmacology* 115: 213–220.

Milner, A. D. (1987) Animal models for the syndrome of spatial neglect. In *Neurophysiological and Neuropsychological Aspects of Spatial Neglect,* edited by M. Jeannerod, pp. 259–392. Amsterdam: Elsevier Science Publishers.

Mirsky, A. F. and Rosvold, H. E. (1960) The use of psychoactive drugs as a neuropsychological tool in studies of attention in man. In *Drugs and Behavior,* edited by L. Uhr and J. G. Miller, pp. 375–392. New York: Wiley.

Mittleman, G., Brown, V. J., and Robbins, T. W. (1988) Intentional neglect following unilateral ibotenic acid lesions of the striatum. *Neurosci. Res. Commum.* 2: 1–8.

Muir, J. L., Robbins, T. W., and Everitt, B. J. (1992) Disruptive effects of muscimol infused into the basal forebrain: Differential interaction with cholinergic mechanisms. *Psychopharmacology* 107: 541–550.

Muir, J. L., Robbins, T. W. and Everitt, B. J. (1994) AMPA-induced lesions of the basal forebrain: A significant role for the cortical cholinergic system in attentional function. *J. Neurosci.* 14: 2313–2326.

Muir, J. L., Robbins, T. W. and Everitt, B. J. (1995) Reversal of visual attentional dysfunction following lesions of the cholinergic basal forebrain by physostigmine and nicotine but not the 5HT-3 antagonist, ondansetron. *Psychopharmacology* 118: 82–92.

Muir, J. L., Everitt, B. J. and Robbins, T. W. (1996) The cerebral cortex of the rat and visual attentional function: Dissociable effects of mediofrontal, cingulate, anterior dorsolateral and parietal cortex lesions on a 5-choice serial reaction time task. *Cereb. Cortex.* 6: 470–481.

Olton, D. S., Wenk, G. L., Church, R. M., and Meck, W. H. (1988) Attention and the frontal cortex as examined by simultaneous temporal processing. *Neuropsychologia* 26: 307–318.

Owen, A. M., Roberts, A. C., Polkey, C. E., Sahakian, B. J., and Robbins, T. W. (1991) Extra-dimensional versus intradimensional set shifting performance following frontal lobe excisions, temporal lobe excisions or amygdalo-hippocampectomy in man. *Neuropsychologia* 29: 993–1006.

Pang, K., Merkel, F., Egeth, H., and Olton, D. S. (1992) Expectancy and stimulus frequency: A comparative analysis in rats and humans. *Percept. Psychophys.* 51: 607–615.

Pang, K., Williams, M. J., Egeth, H., and Olton, D. S. (1994) Nucleus basalis magnocellularis and attention: Effects of muscimol infusions. *Behav. Neurosci.* 107: 1031–1038.

Parasuraman, R., Warm, J. S., and Dember, W. N. (1987) Vigilance: Taxonomy and utility. In *Ergonomics and Human Factors*, edited by L. S. Mark, J. S. Warm., and R. L. Huston, pp. 11–32. New York: Springer.

Posner, M. I. and Boies, S. J. (1971) Components of attention. *Psychol. Rev.* 78: 391–408.

Posner, M. I. and Petersen, S. E. (1990) The attention system of the human brain. *Ann. Rev. Neurosci.* 13: 25–42.

Posner, M. I., Walker, J. A., Friedrich, F. J., and Rafal, R. D. (1984) Effects of parietal injury on covert orienting of attention. *J. Neurosci.* 4: 1863–1874.

Puumala, T., Riekkinen, P., and Sirvio, J. (1997) Modulation of vigilance and behavioral activation by alpha-1 adrenoceptors in the rat. *Pharmacol. Biochem. Behav.,* 56: 705–712.

Rafal, R. and Robertson, L. (1995) The neurology of visual attention. In *The Cognitive Neurosciences*, edited by M. S. Gazzaniga, pp. 625–648. Cambridge, MA: MIT Press.

Rizzolatti, G. and Camarda, R. (1987) Neural circuits for spatial attention and unilateral neglect. *In Neurophysiological and Neuropsychological Aspects of Spatial Neglect*, edited by M. Jeannerod, pp. 289–313. Amsterdam: Elsevier.

Robbins, T. W. (1984) Cortical noradrenaline, attention and arousal. *Psychol. Med.* 14: 13–21.

Robbins, T. W. and Brown, V. J. (1990) The role of the striatum in the mental chronometry of action: A theoretical review. *Rev. Neurosci.* 2: 181–213.

Robbins, T. W., Evenden, J. L., Ksir, C., Reading, P., Wood, S., and Carli, M. (1986) The effects of d-amphetamine, alpha flupenthixol and mesolimbic dopamine depletion on a test of attentional switching in the rat. *Psychopharmacology* 90: 72–78.

Robbins, T. W. and Everitt, B. J. (1995a) Arousal systems and attention. In *The Cognitive Neurosciences*, edited by M. S. Gazzaniga, pp. 703–725. Cambridge, MA: MIT Press.

Robbins, T. W. and Everitt, B. J. (1995b) Central norpinephrine neurons and behaviour. In *Psychopharmacology: Fourth Generation of Progress*, edited by F. E. Bloom and D. Kupfer, pp. 363–372. New York: Raven Press.

Robbins, T. W., Everitt, B. J., Marston, H. M., Wilkinson, J., Jones, G. H., and Page, K. J. (1989) Comparative effects of ibotenic acid– and quisqualic acid–induced lesions of the substantia innominata on attentional function in the rat: Further implications for the role of the cholinergic neurons of the nucleus basalis in cognitive processes. *Behav. Brain Res.* 35: 221–240.

Robbins, T. W. and Iversen, S. D. (1973) Amphetamine-induced disruption of temporal discrimination by response disinhibition. *Nature: New Biology* 245: 191–192.

Robbins, T. W., Muir, J. L., Killcross, A. S., and Pretsell, D. O. (1993) Methods for assessing attention and stimulus control in the rat. In *Behavioral Neuroscience: A Practical Approach*, edited by A. Sahgal, pp. 13–47. New York: Oxford University Press.

Roberts, A. C., De Salvia, M., Wilkinson, L. S., Collins, P., Muir, J. L., Everitt, B. J., and Robbins, T. W. (1994) 6-hydroxydopamine lesions of the prefrontal cortex in monkeys enhance performance on an analogue of the Wisconsin card sorting test: Possible interactions with subcortical dopamine. *J. Neurosci.* 14: 2531–2544.

Roberts, A., Everitt, B. J., and Robbins, T. W. (1988) Extra- and intradimensional shifts in man and marmoset. *Q. J. Exp. Psychol.* 40B: 321–342.

Roberts, A. C., Robbins, T. W., Everitt, B. J., and Muir, J. L. (1992) A specific form of cognitive rigidity following excitotoxic lesions of the basal forebrain in monkeys. *Neuroscience* 47: 251–264.

Rosvold, H. E., Mirsky, A. F., Sarason, I., Bransome, E. D., and Beck, L. H. (1956) A continuous performance test of brain damage. *J. Consult. Psychol.* 20: 343–350.

Ruland, S., Ronis, V., Bruno, J. P., and Sarter, M. (1995) Effects of lesions of the dorsal noradenergic bundle on behavioral vigilance. *Soc. Neurosci. Abst.* 21: 763.3.

Sahakian, B. J., Jones, G., Levy, R., Warburton, D., and Gray, J. (1989) The effects of nicotine on attention, information processing, and short term memory in patients with dementia of the Alzheimer type. *Br. J. Psychiatry* 154: 797–800.

Sahakian, B. J., Owen, A. M., Morant, N. J., Eagger, S. A., Boddington, S., Crayton, L., Crockford, H. A., Hill, K., and Levy, R. (1993) Further analysis of the cognitive effects of tetrahydroaminoacridine (THA) in Alzheimer's disease: Assessment of attentional and menomonic function using CANTAB. *Psychopharmacology* 110: 395–401.

Sahgal, A. (1988) Vasopressin and amphetamine, but not desglycinamide vasopressin, impair positively reinforced visual attention performance in rats. *Behav. Brain Res.* 29: 35–42.

Sarter, M. (1994) Neuronal mechanisms of the attentional dysfunctions in senile dementia and schizophrenia: Two sides of the same coin? *Psychopharmacology* 114: 539–550.

Schallert, T. and Hall, S. (1988) "Disengage" sensorimotor deficit following apparent recovery from unilateral dopamine depletion. *Behav. Brain Res.* 30: 15–24.

Schallert, T., Upchurch, M., Lobaugh, N., Farrar, S. B., Spirduso, W. W., Gillam, P., Vaughan, D., and Wilcox, R. E. (1982) Tactile extinction: Distinguishing between sensorimotor and motor asymmetries in rats with unilateral nigrostriatal damage. *Pharmacol. Biochem. Behav.* 16: 455–462.

Schallert, T. and Whishaw, I. Q. (1984) Bilateral cutaneous stimulation of the somatosensory system in hemidecorticate rats. *Behav. Neurosci.* 98: 518–540.

Servan-Schrieber, D., Printz, H., and Cohen, J. D. (1990) A network model of catecholamine effects: Gain, signal-to-noise ratio, and behavior. *Science* 249: 892–895.

Shallice, T. (1988) *From Neuropsychology to Mental Structure*. New York: Cambridge University Press.

Shimp, C. P. and Friedrich, F. J. (1993) Behavioral and computational models of spatial attention. *J. Exp. Psychol. Anim. Behav. Proc.* 19: 26–37.

Sillito, A. M. (1987) Synaptic processes and neurotransmitters operating on the central visual system: A systems approach. In *Synaptic Function*, edited by G. M. Edelman, W. E. Einar, and W. M. Cowan, pp. 329–371. New York: Wiley.

Sirvio, J., Jakala, P., Mazurkiewicz, M., Haapalinna, A., Riekkinen, P. and Riekkinen, P. J. (1993) Dose- and parameter-dependent effects of atipamezole, an α_2-antagonist, on the performance of rats in a five-choice serial reaction time task. *Pharmacol. Biochem. Behav.* 45: 123–129.

Sirvio, J., Mazurkiewicz, M., Haapalinna, A., Riekkinen, P., Lahtinen, H., and Riekkinen P. J. (1994) The effects of selective alpha-2 adrenergic agents on the performance of rats in a 5-choice serial reaction time task. *Brain Res. Bull.* 5: 451–455.

Skjoldager, P. and Fowler, S. C. (1991) Scopolamine attenuates the motor disruptions but not the attentional disturbances induced by haloperidol in a sustained attention task in the rat. *Psychopharmacology* 105: 93–100.

Slamecka, N. J. (1968) A methodological analysis of shift paradigms in human discrimination learning. *Psychol. Bull.* 69: 423–438.

Stephens, D. N. and Sarter, M. (1988) Bidirectional nature of benzodiazepine receptor ligands extends to effects on vigilance. In *Benzodiazepine Receptor Ligands, Memory and Information Processing*, edited by I. Hindmarch, and H. Ott, pp. 205–217. Berlin: Springer.

Swerdlow, N. R. (in press) Cortico-striatal substrates of cognitive, motor and sensory gating: Speculations and implications for psychological function and dysfunction. In *Advances in Biological Psychiatry* (Vol. 2) edited by J. Panksepp. New York: JAI Press.

Swerdlow N. R., Caine, S. B., Braff, D. L., and Geyer, M. (1992) Neural substrates of sensorimotor gating of the startle reflex: Preclinical findings and their implications. *J. Psychopharm.* 6: 176–190.

Turchi, J., Holley, L. A., and Sarter, M. (1995) Effects of nicotinic acetylcholine receptor ligands on behavioral vigilance in rats. *Psychopharmacology* 118: 195–205.

Uhr, L. and Miller, J. G. (1960) *Drugs and Behavior*. New York: Wiley.

Valenstein, E. and Heilman, K. M. (1981) Unilateral hypokinesia and motor extinction. *Neurology* 31: 445–448.

Voytko, M. L., Olton, D. S., Richardson, R. T., Gorman, L. K., Tobin, J. R., and Price, D. L. (1994) Basal forebrain lesions in monkeys disrupt attention but not learning and memory. *J. Neurosci.* 14: 167–186.

Warburton D. M. (1977) Stimulus selection and behavioral inhibition. In *Handbook of Psychopharmacology* (Vol. 8), edited by L. L. Iversen, S. D. Iversen, and S. H. Snyder, pp. 385–431. New York: Plenum Press.

Ward, N. M., and Brown, V. J. (1996) Covert orienting of attention in the rat and the role of striatal dopamine. *J. Neurosci.* 16: 3082–3088.

Wesnes, K. and Warburton, D. M. (1983) Effects of smoking on rapid information processing performance. *Neuropsychobiology* 9: 223–229.

Wilkinson, L. S., Killcross, A. S., Humby, T., Hall, F. S., Geyer, M. A., and Robbins, T. W. (1994) Social isolation produces developmentally specific deficits in prepulse inhibition of the acoustic startle response but does not disrupt latent inhibition. *Neuropsychopharmacology* 10: 61–72.

Wilkinson, R. T. (1963) Interaction of noise with knowledge of results and sleep deprivation. *J. Exp. Psychol.* 66: 332–337.

Witte, E. A., Gordon-Lickey, M. E., and Marrocco, R. T. (1992) Pharmacological depletion of catecholamines modifies covert orienting in rhesus monkeys. *Soc. Neurosci. Abstr.* 18: 226–11.

Witte, E. A. and Marrocco, R. T. (1993) Pharmacological manipulation of brain cholinergic activity modifies covert orienting in rhesus monkeys. *Soc. Neurosci. Abstr.* 19: 562.

Zilles, K. (1985) *The Cortex of the Rat.* Berlin: Springer Verlag.

11 Brain Systems of Vigilance

Raja Parasuraman, Joel S. Warm, and Judi E. See

ABSTRACT Neurophysiological, lesion, and functional brain-imaging studies are discussed with respect to two major issues: the relationship between vigilance and brain systems that regulate cortical arousal; and the brain structures and networks associated with vigilance decrement. The evidence indicates that vigilance is related to but also distinct from cortical arousal, and unified arousal theory is viable only for the overall level of vigilance, and not for the vigilance decrement. The noradrenergic reticular formation, intralaminar thalamic nuclei, basal forebrain cholinergic system, and the right prefrontal cortex are involved in the overall level of vigilance. However, evidence of the functional role of those brain regions in vigilance decrement is weak. Future research should examine the effects of psychophysical and task factors on putative brain mechanisms of vigilance decrement. Such studies are needed to develop a neurobiology of vigilance that is not context limited and therefore potentially superficial.

A vigilant animal can alertly and freely explore its environment; such exploration allows it to learn, adapt, and survive. In that sense, vigilance can be considered to be a basic, primitive form of attention, without which many other perceptual and cognitive functions would be compromised. It is therefore quite natural to ask what neural systems support this vital activity and how those systems evolve (Dimond and Lazarus, 1974; Jerison, 1977). The question is not new, having been first posed by Head (1923) in his examination of patients suffering from aphasia. Clinical interest in vigilance persists because deficits in vigilance occur in many disorders, including epilepsy, closed head injury, hyperactivity, neglect, and schizophrenia (Berch and Kanter, 1984; Mirsky, 1987; Nestor, Faux, McCarley, Shenton, and Sands, 1990; Parasuraman, Mutter, and Molloy, 1991; Robertson, Tegner, Tham, Lo, and Nimmo-Smith, 1995).

Some time following Head's investigations, Moruzzi and Magoun (1949) carried out their classic studies of the brainstem reticular formation, which they characterized as a cortical activation or arousal system. Vigilance was seen as the manifestation of an energetic aspect of the central nervous system, a view later extended and refined by the neurologist Norman Mackworth, who defined vigilance as a "state of readiness to detect and respond to certain small changes occurring at random time intervals in the environment" (Mackworth, 1957, pp. 389–390).

THE MEASUREMENT OF VIGILANCE

Experience indicates that it is easy to be briefly attentive to a conspicuous and predictable event, such as a traffic light changing from red to green or the factory whistle heralding the end of another workday. It is another matter, however, to maintain attention to some source of information to detect the occurrence of infrequent, unpredictable events over long periods of time. Tasks requiring detection of transient signals in that way are known as vigilance or sustained attention tasks (Davies and Parasuraman, 1982; Warm, 1984). In situations such as these, the quality of attention is fragile—it declines over time—an outcome known as the vigilance decrement.

Vigilance Decrement

Mackworth's experiments with the clock test (1950) initiated the formal study of human vigilance. That test consisted of a 2-hour discrimination task in which observers had to distinguish infrequent, unpredictable double jumps of a clock pointer (signals) from more frequent single jumps (nonsignals). In those studies, as in most that have followed, observers were tested individually in a prolonged and continuous task, signals were clearly perceivable when observers were alerted to them but were not otherwise compelling changes in the environment, and the signals appeared with low probability (approximately 3% to 5% of the time) in an unpredictable manner. Mackworth found that signal detection declined markedly from the first to the second half-hour of watch and more gradually thereafter. In general, the major portion of the decrement appears within the first 15 minutes of watch (Teichner, 1974). However, Nuechterlein, Parasuraman, and Jiang (1983) showed that under especially demanding circumstances, for instance when stimuli were perceptually degraded, the decrement could be seen within the first 5 minutes of monitoring. The temporal fragility of vigilance has not only been observed with human observers but also with animals such as monkeys and rats (Jerison, 1965; McGaughy and Sarter, 1995).

The vigilance decrement can be indexed either by a decline over time in detection rate or by an increment in response time for detection (Parasuraman and Davies, 1976; figure 11.1). In addition, in vigilance tasks, as in other psychophysical tasks, an observer's affirmation of the presence or the absence of a signal is dependent not only upon perceptual factors but also upon decision factors involved in the observer's detection goals, expectations about the nature of the stimuli, and the anticipated consequences of correct and incorrect responses. From the standpoint of signal detection theory (Macmillan and Creelman, 1991; Green and Swets, 1974), those factors comprise the observer's response criterion or willingness to emit a detection response. A fundamental issue is to ascertain whether the vigilance decrement is due to a loss in sensitivity to signals (d') or to changes in the decision criterion (β) (figure 11.2).

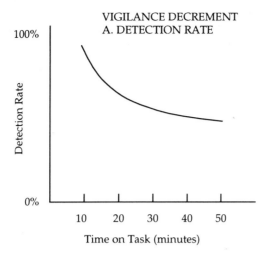

VIGILANCE DECREMENT
A. DETECTION RATE

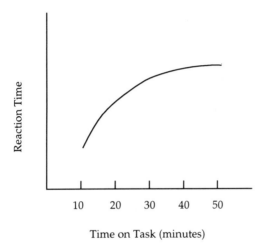

VIGILANCE DECREMENT
B. REACTION TIME

Figure 11.1 Measurement of vigilance decrement. The decrement is indexed by (A) a decline in detection rate of critical targets (hits) over time on task, or alternatively by (B) an increase over time in the mean reaction time to detect signals.

A similar question has been asked in the analysis of other varieties of attention. For example, a basic issue in the study of spatial selective attention is whether the focusing of attention to a given location enhances perceptual sensitivity to signals presented there (compared to other locations) or whether such spatial focusing only reduces the decision criterion for responding to signals at that location (Posner, 1980; Shaw, 1984). Converging evidence from psychophysical, electrophysiological, and functional brain-imaging studies indicates that allocating attention over space seems to have a primary effect on sensitivity (Hawkins et al., 1990; Heinze et al., 1994).

Parasuraman, Warm, & See: Brain Systems of Vigilance

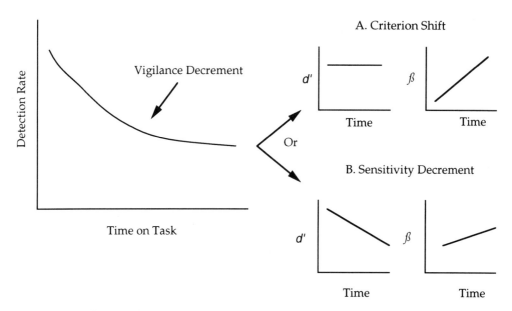

Figure 11.2 Schematic representation of the application of signal detection theory to vigilance. The vigilance decrement in detection (hit) rate may (A) reflect an increase over time in the response criterion (β) with sensitivity (d') remaining stable. Alternatively, the decrement may (B) be associated with a true decrement in sensitivity (criterion may increase or decrease). Thus, the vigilance decrement may reflect either criterion or sensitivity shifts (or both) over time.

Similarly, one can ask whether changes in the allocation of attention over time are associated primarily with changes in sensitivity or in decision criteria.

Unlike spatial selective attention, where effects have been obtained primarily with regard to sensitivity, both sensitivity and criterion changes have been observed during sustained attention. In many cases, the vigilance decrement in detection rate does not involve a decline in perceptual efficiency during a vigil (a drop in d'). Rather, it reflects a shift to a more conservative response criterion (elevation in β), either because experience with the task leads observers to develop more rational expectations of the actual (generally very low) signal probability in force during the vigil (Davies and Parasuraman, 1982; Warm and Jerison, 1984), or because they adopt a probability matching strategy (Craig, 1978). In other task conditions, however, a true drop in sensitivity occurs. Those alternative possibilities are illustrated in figure 11.2. When a sensitivity decrement occurs, it is generally restricted to demanding tasks that combine a fast event rate (the rate of presentation of stimulus events that need to be inspected for the possibility that they are critical signals) with a memory load and low signal salience (Parasuraman, 1979; Parasuraman, Warm, and Dember, 1987; See, Howe, Warm, and Dember, 1995). Thus, the vigilance decrement in detection rate may be due either to a sensitivity decrement or to a criterion shift over time. Those findings indicate that the vigilance decrement reflects multiple underlying processes.

Vigilance: Short or Long Duration?

How long should a vigilance task be? This seemingly simple question turns out to involve some complexities that have yet to be fully resolved. The issue needs serious examination because of some confusion that may exist with respect to the appropriate experimental paradigms that define vigilance.

In Mackworth's (1950) seminal investigations, as in the many studies that have followed (Davies and Parasuraman, 1982), vigilance was assessed over relatively long periods of time that extended from 30 minutes to several hours. Therefore, vigilance has traditionally been associated with relatively long-term performance. In so far as the laboratory study of vigilance hopes to have implications for the understanding of human and animal vigilance in natural settings, such time periods seem appropriate.

There is another, more recent, tradition of research that is also sometimes (but not exclusively) referred to as vigilance, in which tasks of much shorter duration (1–10 s) have been used. The task commonly used in this paradigm is one of simple or choice reaction time (RT) to a stimulus preceded by a warning signal with a variable warning interval or foreperiod (Welford, 1962). RT generally is high for very short and for long warning intervals and is low at intermediate foreperiods of about 0.5 to 1 s (Posner, 1978). That result has been interpreted as reflecting the buildup of phasic alertness following a warning signal. The increase in RT with very long foreperiods has been attributed to a difficulty in maintaining the alert state, or vigilance, beyond the optimal foreperiod. Posner (1978) proposed that the mechanisms underlying alerting in short-duration RT tasks were not fundamentally different from those operating in long-term vigilance tasks. Subsequently, many researchers have conducted neurobiological studies of vigilance using such short-duration warned RT tasks. In those studies, the vigilance effect is typically assessed as the difference in RT to a stimulus when it is preceded by a warning signal compared to when no warning is provided. Thus, for example, vigilance as measured in this paradigm has been analyzed with respect to the influence of drugs that target specific neurotransmitter systems (Marrocco and Davidson, chapter 3, this volume), subcortical regions involved in the control of vigilance (Kinomura, Larsson, Gulyas, and Roland, 1996), and hemispheric differences (Whitehead, 1991).

Is vigilance as measured by changes in RT to a signal following a warning stimulus over the course of a few seconds the same as vigilance as reflected in the decline in detection rate of signals over periods of tens of minutes or hours? Posner (1978) argued for communality between the two paradigms. Yet there is little empirical evidence to either support or reject that view (for an exception, see the subsequent discussion of the study by Rueckert and Levy [1996], who found evidence of association). In favor of the hypothesis is the fact that setting any definitive time period for measuring changes in vigilance is arbitrary. After all, even in traditional vigilance tasks, vigilance decrement has been assessed over periods of time as low as 5 minutes

(Nuechterlein et al., 1983) to as long as 24 hours (Krueger, 1989). In principle, therefore, there is no reason why vigilance decrement could not be assessed over periods of time as short as 10 seconds. However, in such short-duration tasks, vigilance failures, that is, missed signals, are virtually never observed in healthy individuals, in contrast to observations in the long-term vigilance task. In warned-RT tasks with adults, speed of response varies with the alerting properties of the warning cue and with the ability of the participant to maintain alertness over the duration of the foreperiod, but detection failures are typically never observed.

Many researchers have followed the lead of Posner (1978; Posner and Petersen, 1990) in using warned-RT tasks to measure vigilance. The terminological overlap in the concepts of vigilance and arousal, as discussed further in a later section of this chapter, has also contributed to that association. However, those tasks are probably more appropriately viewed as assessing changes in phasic alertness. Thus, neurophysiological or brain-imaging studies that have used such tasks (e.g., Kinomura et al., 1996) should be viewed as studies of phasic alertness or cortical arousal rather than of vigilance. As such, any finding that associates performance on such tasks with the activation of particular brain regions indicates that those regions are involved in phasic alertness, or in the buildup and short-term maintenance of cortical arousal. A later section of this chapter examines whether those findings also bear on the issue of the brain regions involved when vigilance fails, that is, in long-term vigilance tasks.

TWO QUESTIONS FOR A NEUROBIOLOGY OF VIGILANCE

The major issues for a neurobiology of vigilance are to describe the neural mechanisms associated with the vigilance decrement and the overall level of vigilance. Those issues can be addressed within the framework of two questions. What is the relationship between vigilance and the brain systems that regulate cortical arousal? What are the brain regions mediating vigilance and how are they functionally related?

To address those questions, studies falling into three broad categories are reviewed: electrophysiological experiments, lesion and laterality studies, and studies using functional brain-imaging techniques. Except in passing, pharmacological or neurochemical studies of vigilance and attention are not discussed; for reviews, see Koelega (1993), Robbins (chapter 10, this volume), and Sarter (1994).

VIGILANCE AND CORTICAL AROUSAL

One explanation for the vigilance decrement is that detection failures result from an inability of participants to maintain the level of cortical arousal necessary for efficient performance (Mackworth, 1969). Many studies have therefore attempted to relate vigilance to the concept of arousal or alertness. Arousal refers to a variety of physiological and behavioral changes characterized by a degree of excitation or energy mobilization (Duffy, 1962). Initially, arousal was viewed as a unidimensional construct that was mediated by the ascending reticular activating system (Moruzzi and Magoun, 1949). The unity of the arousal concept was subsequently questioned (Lacey, 1967), and recent studies have shown unequivocally that brain arousal systems are fractionated into many subsystems that differ widely in their innervation patterns and neurochemical characteristics (Marrocco and Davidson, chapter 3, this volume).

What is the relation between vigilance and cortical arousal? This is the first of the two questions that a neurobiology of vigilance must answer. The question is addressed first by briefly examining the evidence for multiple subcortical arousal systems, and then by discussing electrophysiological and functional brain-imaging studies of vigilance in humans. Those studies provide a basis for addressing the issue of the viability of an arousal account of the vigilance decrement.

Subcortical Regulation of Cortical Arousal: Multiple Arousal Systems

The classic studies of the reticular formation by Moruzzi and Magoun (1949) established the importance of the reticular formation in the regulation of cortical arousal. Lesions of this area produce coma and the absence of electroencephalographic (EEG) desynchronization to stimuli (Lindsley, 1960). On the other hand, when the reticular formation and the intralaminar thalamic nuclei to which it projects are electrically stimulated, EEG desynchronization and behavioral arousal are evoked in the animal (Steriade, 1996; Steriade and Llinas, 1988). Those findings led to the concept of a reticular activating system for the regulation of cortical arousal. More recent work has shown the notion of a unitary reticular activating system to be incorrect, there being multiple ascending pathways from subcortical nuclei, each associated with different neurotransmitters and neuromodulators that have different properties and different cortical innervation patterns (Robbins and Everett, 1995).

A detailed review of the anatomical, neurochemical, and functional characteristics of the various subcortical arousal systems is beyond the scope of this chapter (for reviews, see Marrocco and Davidson, chapter 3, this volume; Robbins and Everett, 1995), but some major points can be noted here. Four main projection systems have been identified as playing functional roles in arousal and attention: the cholinergic basal forebrain, the noradrenergic nucleus locus coerulus (LC), the dopaminergic median forebrain bundle, and the serotonergic dorsal raphe nucleus. Apart from those brainstem and midbrain structures, and in addition to the intralaminar nuclei, two other thalamic nuclei, the reticular nucleus (Skinner and Yingling, 1977) and the pulvinar (LaBerge and Buchsbaum, 1990), have been implicated in attention and arousal. The functions of those subcortical arousal systems, their interactions, and the specific role each plays in attention and in other cognitive processes are still active areas of investigation. Because of evidence that the basal forebrain cholinergic and the LC noradrenergic systems may be especially important for vigilance and phasic alertness to stimuli, those subcortical systems are briefly considered at this point.

The Basal Forebrain Cholinergic System Several pharmacological studies in animals and in humans have contributed to the view that the cholinergic system plays an important role in attention and arousal processes (Robbins and Everett, 1995; Sarter, 1994; Warburton, 1977). Sarter and colleagues specifically examined the role of that system in vigilance by using a sensitive long-duration vigilance task with rats (McGaughy and Sarter, 1995; Moore, Dudchenko, Bruno, and Sarter, 1992). Administration of the benzodiazepine receptor (BZR) agonist chlordiazepoxide (CDP) potently impaired performance on that task. Other studies have shown that, when infused directly into the basal forebrain, CDP blocks the stimulated cortical release of acetylcholine (Moore, Sarter, and Bruno, 1993). McGaughy and Sarter (1995) therefore concluded that the impairment of vigilance performance is linked to GABAergic modulation of cortical acetylcholine release.

The LC Noradrenergic System Neurophysiological studies in animals have pointed to the role of the noradrenergic system in cortical arousal (Aston-Jones, Rajkowski, Kubiak, and Alexinsky, 1994). Activation of LC cells in awake monkeys and rats results in a widespread release of norepinephrine to cortical targets; and LC cellular activity is greater during periods of behavioral alertness (Aston-Jones, Chiang, and Alexinsky, 1991). Further, LC discharge is associated with EEG desynchronization and reduction in EEG amplitude, both of which are generally correlated with increased behavioral arousal (Lindsley, 1960). Thus, the alert waking state associated with high-frequency, low-amplitude, asynchronous cortical EEG appears to reflect an increase in subcortical noradrenergic activity during which subcortical afferent inputs are relayed to the cortex in an efficient manner. On the other hand, low-frequency, high-amplitude, synchronous EEG, which accompanies states of drowsiness and sleep, is associated with decreased noradrenergic activity and with a blockade of sensory-afferent thalamic input to the cortex (Steriade, 1996).

A recent drug study also supports the role of central noradrenaline in sustained attention in humans. Administration of clonidine, an alpha-2 adrenoceptor agonist that acts presynaptically to reduce noradrenaline release, increased the number of very long RTs ("attentional lapses") in a two-choice RT task; this effect was reversed by idazoxan, a selective alpha-2 adrenoceptor antagonist (Smith and Nutt, 1996).

Electrophysiology of Arousal and Vigilance

The neurophysiological studies discussed in the previous section suggest that an assessment of brain electrical activity by means of the EEG might provide an indirect index of subcortical regulation of cortical arousal and its role in vigilance. To that end, a number of studies have examined EEG and event-related potential (ERP) activity during vigilance performance. In humans, a state of alert attentiveness is associated with fast EEG beta (14–30 Hz) activity, whereas relaxed wakefulness in which attentiveness per se is not necessary is characterized by slower alpha (8–13 Hz) activity. A state of drowsiness leads to even slower theta (4–7 Hz) and delta (1–3 Hz) activity. The EEG generally shifts from higher to lower frequencies over the course of vigilance tasks (Davies and Krkovic, 1965; Gale, 1977; Makeig and Inlow, 1993; O'Hanlon and Beatty, 1977). The presence of slower EEG activity has been correlated with poor performance. For example, using an auditory vigilance task, Davies and Krkovic (1965) found that EEG alpha activity predominated during the pretest but declined to 87% of its initial value by the end of the task, as did the detection rate.

Several studies have attempted to examine more closely the relationship between vigilance performance and EEG activity by analyzing the correspondence between the EEG and correct and incorrect responses (Belyavin and Wright, 1987; Daniel, 1967; Horvath, Frantik, Kopriva, and Meissner, 1975; Makeig and Inlow, 1993; Pennekamp, Bosel, Mecklinger, and Ott, 1994; Strauss et al., 1984; Valentino, Arruda, and Gold, 1993). For example, in one early investigation, observers were found to be more likely to miss critical signals when theta activity was predominant in the EEG record (Daniel, 1967). Makeig and Inlow (1993) recently carried out a more sophisticated study in which they computed coherences between error rate and different EEG frequencies for a 28-minute auditory detection task that participants performed with their eyes closed. Critical signals for detection were slightly more intense bursts of noise embedded in a background of white noise. Targets were presented at a very high rate of 10 per minute so that a fine-grained inspection of the relation between the EEG and performance could be completed. The performance measure used was the local error rate: the fraction of undetected targets within a moving 32.8-second window that was advanced through the data in steps of 1.64 seconds. Local error rate fluctuated considerably but showed a general increase over time. That vigilance decrement was accompanied by a reduction in alpha activity and an increase in theta and delta activity. Those trends are shown in figure 11.3, which also indicates the slowing in EEG frequency from early (A) to late (B) in the task. Coherence analysis suggested that there was a linear relationship between error rate and spectral density at specific EEG frequencies. Similar findings were reported in a subsequent study in which subjects performed both visual and auditory detection with their eyes open (Makeig and Jung, 1995).

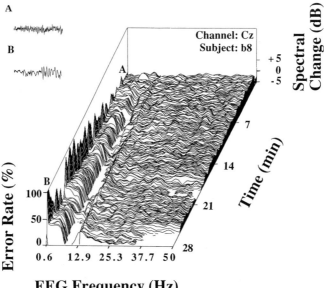

A

B

Channel: Cz
Subject: b8

Spectral Change (dB)

+5
0
-5

7

Time (min)

14

21

28

Error Rate (%)

A

B

100

50

0

0.6 12.9 25.3 37.7 50

EEG Frequency (Hz)

Figure 11.3 Changes in local error rate (averaged over a moving window of 33 s) and EEG spectral power over the course of 28-minute auditory vigilance task. Increases in error rate are accompanied by increased power in lower EEG frequencies, as also illustrated by 4 s examples of EEG activity taken early (A) and late (B) in the vigil. From Makeig and Inlow (1993). Reprinted with permission.

ERPs have also been used to examine the relation of cortical arousal to vigilance. The measurement of ERPs in the EEG constitutes a method for separating evoked responses to external stimulation or internal cognitive events from the background of continuous spontaneous electrical activity of the brain in the EEG record (see Luck and Girelli, chapter 5, this volume). ERPs provide an opportunity to examine whether the vigilance decrement is associated with a general reduction in the amplitude of evoked brain activity or whether only certain ERP components change in association with changes in vigilance. The former result would be consistent with a generalized arousal account of the decrement.

In one of the first ERP studies of vigilance, Haider, Spong, and Lindsley (1964) reported that "the principal negative component of the ERP to visual stimuli" (likely to be a negative ERP component with a latency of 160 ms) decreased in amplitude with time on task. That N160 component was also larger for detected than for missed signals. The results were interpreted as reflecting a reduction in cortical arousal over time. Other early ERP studies reached a similar conclusion with auditory stimuli (Wilkinson, Morlock, and Williams, 1966). In those early studies, ERP component analyses were incomplete, and ERPs were not separately analyzed for all response outcomes (hits, misses, false alarms, and correct rejections). Later studies showed that not all ERP components show a parallel decline in amplitude with vigilance decrement. Davies and Parasuraman (1977) examined ERPs to signals and nonsignals (N100, P200, N200, and P300 components) not only for hits and misses but also for correct rejections and false alarms in a 45-minute visual vigilance task wherein participants were required to respond "yes" (signal) or "no" (no signal) to each stimulus presentation. Signals consisted of flashes of light that were slightly less intense than nonsignal light flashes. All four ERP components declined in amplitude with time on task. However, only the "late" components, N200 and P300, were related to detection performance. The amplitudes of both ERP components were greater for detected than for missed signals. Davies and Parasuraman (1977) concluded that the results were not consistent with a generalized arousal account of vigilance performance. Instead, they proposed a signal detection theory account of changes in vigilance and suggested that only the late ERP components reflected changes in decision processes in vigilance. In a later study using the degraded digit-discrimination task developed by Nuechterlein et al. (1983), Rohrbaugh et al. (1987) also found that only late ERP components showed amplitude and latency changes over time on task that paralleled the vigilance decrement (figure 11.4). Finally, Koelega et al. (1992) also found that the relation between time-based trends in ERP amplitudes and vigilance performance appeared primarily for components occurring 250–650 ms after stimulus presentation.

Overall, studies of brain electrical activity and vigilance suggest two trends: (1) EEG activity shifts to slower-frequency bands and ERP component amplitudes decrease over the course of a vigilance task; (2) the shift to slower activity and the reduced amplitude of ERP components are correlated with decreased detection performance. The coherence analysis carried out by Makeig and Inlow (1993) strongly suggests that vigilance performance and EEG frequency changes are functionally related. Nevertheless, there is unfortunately little evidence to support the view that such changes in brain electrical activity are *necessary* for the vigilance decrement. Moreover, EEG and ERP findings provide only weak support for an arousal theory of vigilance decrement. Brain electrical changes during vigilance tasks are certainly indicative of reductions in arousal, but as discussed further in the next section, there is no evidence that such changes in arousal are causal to the decline in detection performance.

Cortical Arousal and Vigilance Decrement

In neurobiological research, vigilance is often seen as indistinguishable from arousal. The English word *arousal* is generally translated as *vigilance* in French and *vigilanz* in German. Scientists who write in English, particularly those in medicine and neurobiology, also often use *vigilance* to refer to a general state of wakefulness that we would characterize as arousal or alertness. As discussed earlier, a link between long-term vigilance and short-term phasic alertness as assessed using warned RT tasks has also been postulated (Posner,

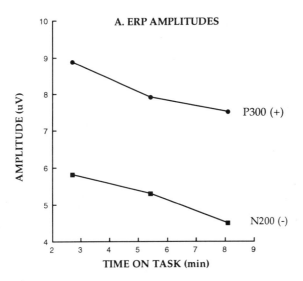

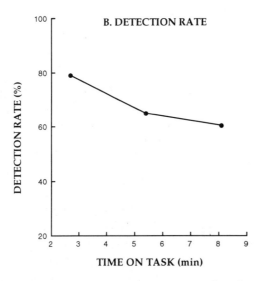

Figure 11.4 (A) Changes over time on task in the amplitudes of the N200 and P300 ERP components for a visual, degraded digit-discrimination task. (B) These changes parallel the decrease in detection rate over time in this task. (Based on data from Rohrbaugh et al., 1987.)

1978). The overlap between the concepts of arousal and vigilance is perhaps not surprising given that both Head (1923), who first used vigilance as an explanatory concept, and later Mackworth (1950) emphasized an energetic state of the central nervous system as a key feature of vigilance. Moruzzi and Magoun's (1949) research also focused on the alerting function of the reticular formation and its role in the maintenance of the animal's vigilance. Many studies conducted since that time, including the electrophysiological studies reviewed in the previous section, have also established that arousal and vigilance are related. However, while the two concepts are related, they are not identical, and they can be differentiated in particular cases.

Parasuraman (1984) reviewed studies that bear on the relation between cortical arousal and vigilance and found evidence for both association and dissociation. In general, any factor that increases or reduces the observer's arousal level correspondingly increases or decreases the overall level of vigilance. For example, sleep-deprived participants have poorer overall detection rates on vigilance tasks than do those who have had sufficient sleep (Stickgold, Baker, Kosslyn, and Hobson, 1995); that association is sufficiently robust for vigilance tasks to be used as a behavioral test for sleep deprivation (Wilkinson, 1969). On the other hand, mild stressors that increase arousal, such as limited exposure to mild heat, can improve the level of vigilance (Hancock, 1984).

In contrast to the evidence for a direct association between arousal and the overall level of vigilance, the evidence for a link between arousal and the vigilance decrement is much weaker. Parasuraman (1984) found little evidence to support a direct relationship between changes in arousal over time and the vigilance decrement. Several studies, reviewed in the previous section, found that EEG and ERP measures of cortical activity recorded during a vigilance task typically show changes over time indicative of a reduction in arousal. Such changes in arousal can be associated with vigilance decrement, and some studies also reported correlations between such electrophysiological measures and changes in vigilance performance over time. However, a reduction in cortical arousal over time can also occur under task conditions in which no decrement occurs, when participants perform other prolonged tasks, or indeed when no task is performed for a comparable period of time (Parasuraman, 1984). Such findings suggest that the vigilance decrement cannot be wholly dependent upon a reduction in cortical arousal and must also reflect other factors. In a review of theories of vigilance, Loeb and Alluisi (1984) reached a similar conclusion: "it appears unlikely either that vigilance is an entirely unitary concept or that all of the changes observed in vigilance situations can be accounted for in terms of arousal in any of its forms" (p. 187).

Those findings suggest that arousal influences the overall level of vigilance but is not a causal factor in the vigilance decrement over time. It is worth emphasizing, however, that the results reject only the unidimensional arousal theory of vigilance. Newer conceptualizations of arousal have been proposed at both the cognitive and physiological levels. For example, Humphreys and Revelle (1984) have linked arousal to attentional resource theory and have suggested that arousal can influence resource availability in resource-limited but not data-limited tasks. Norman and Bobrow (1975) and Matthews, Davies, and Lees (1990) have provided support for that view in the context of vigilance tasks. It is possible that an arousal theory of vigilance decrement based on allocation of attentional resources may fare better than traditional arousal theory.

At the physiological level, the fractionation of the unitary reticular activating system into different subcortical arousal systems may also provide testable hypotheses concerning the role of specific neurochemical systems in vigilance decrement. A recent study by Aston-Jones et al. (1994) examined changes in the firing patterns of LC neurons in monkeys performing prolonged vigilance tasks. The monkeys were trained to discriminate between horizontal and vertical lines. A line with one orientation served as the infrequent, critical target (with a probability of 10–20%), and the other orientation defined a nontarget. There was evidence of a vigilance decrement, although it was not substantial in magnitude. RT to detected targets increased from 294 ms to 318 ms from the first 30 minutes to the last 30 minutes of a 2-hour vigil, and false alarms increased from 1.2% to 2.2%. Hit rate in the task was close to 100% for all monkeys. LC neurons were selectively activated by targets but not by nontargets. Furthermore, the mean response magnitude of LC neurons decreased significantly from the first to the last 30 minutes of the task. Thus, the phasic activation of LC neurons in response to critical targets decreased concomitantly with the behavioral vigilance decrement. Additional studies of this kind, in which key psychophysical and task factors are manipulated, would help considerably in determining the precise functional significance of the decline in LC activation.

The study by Aston-Jones et al. (1994) provides evidence to implicate decreases in the activation of a specific subcortical arousal system in the vigilance decrement. Nevertheless, in one sense the data from that study are similar to the weaker evidence provided by less-specific measures of arousal—for example, the EEG studies reviewed earlier. Both LC activation to targets and the spontaneous EEG show changes over time on task that parallel the vigilance decrement, but neither physiological measure has been shown to be necessary for vigilance decrement. As Aston-Jones et al. (1994) themselves cogently concluded, "The evidence for LC activation in either selective attention or vigilance is correlative, and cannot establish whether, and to what extent, changes in the LC cause changes in performance. Direct manipulations of LC activity and measurement of behavioral effects in this task will be needed to test this possibility and to clarify the causal role of the LC system in attention and vigilance" (p. 4478). It is difficult not to agree with those sentiments.

Neural Habituation and the Vigilance Decrement

Given that a unitary arousal explanation of the vigilance decrement is not viable, can the related concept of habituation offer an alternative? One possible interpretation of the parallel decline in electrophysiological activity over time and vigilance decrement is that they are both due to neural habituation (Mackworth, 1969). Many ERP components habituate with repetitive presentation over long time intervals, including the N100 (Näätänen, 1992) and the 40 Hz response (May, Tiitinen, Sinkkonen, and Näätänen, 1994), which have been linked to general arousal. Such habituation is generally observed under passive conditions when participants perform no task or perform some irrelevant task, like reading a book. To link the habituation to the vigilance decrement, evidence under task conditions is required. If the habituation theory is correct, then any factor that accelerates the decrement should increase the rate of habituation and therefore increase the rate of decline in cortical responsivity. To test that hypothesis, Parasuraman (1985) recorded ERPs during an auditory vigilance task in which the rate at which listeners had to inspect stimulus events to determine if they were critical signals for detection was either high or low. Although the vigilance decrement, as reflected in a decline in the frequency of signal detections over time, was substantially greater in the high than in the low event rate condition, the rate of decline in N100 amplitude over time did not differ as a function of event rate. Similar divergence of trends over time in ERP amplitudes and performance were also noted by Rohrbaugh et al. (1987), who also concluded that the vigilance decrement was not simply due to a decrease in neural responsivity due to repetitive stimulation (see also Gale, 1977).

BRAIN REGIONS SUBSERVING VIGILANCE

The electrophysiological studies reviewed earlier support the conclusion that cortical arousal is functionally related to the overall level of vigilance but not to the vigilance decrement. That pattern of association and dissociation suggests that a similar pattern might hold with respect to brain regions subserving arousal and vigilance. The question is addressed in this section by examining lesion and functional brain-imaging studies of arousal and vigilance.

A general principle that has emerged from functional brain-imaging research is that most perceptual and cognitive processes are neurally mediated by multiple brain regions, rather than by a single area (Posner and Raichle, 1993). The evidence suggests that the multiple areas are anatomically interconnected and are linked together functionally. For example, Morecraft, Geula, and Mesulam (1993) showed that the posterior parietal, prefrontal, and cingulate cortices are interconnected by axonal projections to adjacent rather than to overlapping target sites in each area, without collateral inputs, thus defining a parallel, reciprocally connected network subserving spatial attention. The same may be true of vigilance. This section first describes the anatomical networks that have been proposed to mediate attentional functions, including vigilance. Lesion and brain-imaging evidence pertaining to those network models is then discussed.

Several authors have offered general anatomical models of attention in which attentional functions are considered to be controlled by networks of interconnected brain regions. Mesulam (1981) proposed a general architecture for attentional functions that distinguished between networks interconnecting posterior parietal, frontal, and cingulate cortices and the reticular

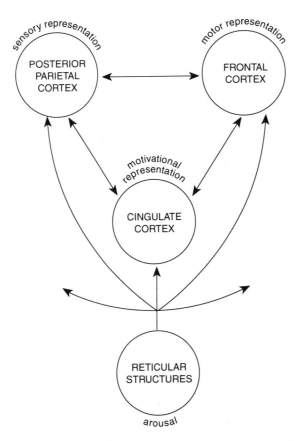

Figure 11.5 Components of a neural network involved in directed attention, including vigilance. (From Mesulam, 1981. Reprinted with permission.)

formation. In that model, parietal regions were postulated to be associated with sensory representations of the world and spatial attention, the frontal cortex with motor representations and planning, and the reticular formation with arousal and vigilance (figure 11.5). In one of the first proposals for a separate "attention system" in the brain, Mirsky (1987) argued that different attentional functions were controlled by networks comprising the inferior parietal, prefrontal, and superior temporal cortices, the reticular formation, the hippocampus, and the corpus striatum. Finally and most recently, Posner and Petersen (1990) proposed three interacting networks mediating different aspects of attention: a posterior attention system comprising parietal cortex, superior colliculus, and the pulvinar that is concerned with spatial attention; an anterior system centered on the anterior cingulate in the medial frontal lobe that mediates target detection and executive control; and a vigilance system consisting of the right frontal lobe and brainstem nuclei, principally the noradrenergic LC. Posner and Petersen (1990) also suggested that the vigilance system was right lateralized due to greater innervation of the right hemisphere by ascending noradrenergic pathways.

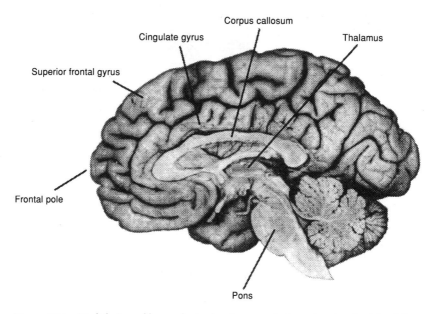

Superior frontal gyrus

Cingulate gyrus

Corpus callosum

Thalamus

Frontal pole

Pons

Figure 11.6 Medial view of human brain showing some brain regions involved in vigilance. Both subcortical (brain stem, pons) and cortical structures (frontal cortex) are shown in this view. (Adapted from DeArmond et al., 1989. Reprinted with permission.)

Each of those models identifies the brainstem reticular formation (or specific subsystems of the reticular formation) as playing an important role in vigilance, and the role of frontal cortex was also emphasized by Parasuraman (1984) and by Posner and Petersen (1990). The following sections examine the lesion and functional brain-imaging evidence pertaining to the involvement of each of those and other brain regions in vigilance, beginning with the brain stem. Figures 11.6 (medial surface of brain) and 11.7 (ventral surface of brain stem) show the location of the brain regions that have been implicated in the control of vigilance.

Brain Stem

Difficulties in concentration and maintenance of attention are often reported following diffuse injury to the brain. In an early study, Rosvold, Mirsky, Sarason, Bransome, and Beck, (1956) developed a 15-minute letter discrimination task known as the Continuous Performance Task (CPT) for use in assessing generalized brain damage. The CPT has since found wide usage as a standard neuropsychological test of sustained attention, although it is often administered or analyzed in such a way that the vigilance decrement cannot be assessed (Davies and Parasuraman, 1982). Healthy young adults typically show ceiling performance on this task. On the other hand, patients with diffuse brain damage or focal epilepsy affecting brain stem and midbrain structures typically perform poorly on the CPT (Mirsky and Orren, 1977).

Parasuraman, Warm, & See: Brain Systems of Vigilance

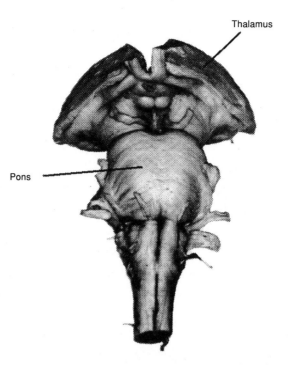

Thalamus

Pons

Figure 11.7 Ventral surface of human brain stem. The brain stem contains the reticular formation and nuclei (e.g., locus coerulus) that, in conjunction with thalamic nuclei, are involved in the subcortical control of cortical arousal. (Adapted from DeArmond et al., 1989. Reprinted with permission.)

Studies have also been carried out with persons who have suffered closed head injury, and those studies also implicate a role for brainstem structures in arousal and vigilance. In one of the earliest studies, Dencker and Lofving (1958) reported that head-injured patients were less accurate and slower to respond to stimuli in a 15-minute choice RT task compared to controls. However, the task design did not allow for the observation of the vigilance decrement (signal probability was very high), and none was found. More recent studies, in which task features designed to elicit the decrement were instituted, found that head-injured patients had lower detection rates and higher false alarm rates than did uninjured controls, but the head-injured patients did not show a greater decrement over time (Brouwer and Van Wolffelaar, 1985; Parasuraman et al., 1991). However, Whyte, Polansky, Fleming, Coslett, and Cavallucci (1995) tested more severely brain-injured patients and found evidence of a more pronounced increase in RT over time for the patients in comparison to uninjured controls for a visual vigilance task.

Because head injury produces diffuse insult to the brain, relating vigilance deficits to damage to specific brain regions is difficult. Given the role of brainstem nuclei such as the LC in arousal and vigilance, one might suppose that damage to those areas by head injury would be prominent. Direct evidence for damage to mesencephalic and diencephalic structures has proven difficult to obtain (Ommaya and Gennarelli, 1974). However, axonal shearing resulting from head injury may cause white matter damage that affects the ability of the brain stem to activate higher cortical centers. Animal models of human acceleration or deceleration head injury have indicated that brainstem structures show evidence of transient alterations in neuronal membrane permeability, axonal degeneration, and damage to the endothelium and blood-brain barrier (Jane, Steward, and Gennarelli, 1985; Povlishock, Becker, Sullivan, and Miller, 1978).

There is a long history of evidence implicating the brain stem reticular formation in arousal (beginning with Morruzzi and Magoun, 1949). Given that much of the evidence has been based on work in animals or in brain-damaged individuals, one might think that many functional imaging studies of the intact human brain would have examined the role of that region in arousal and vigilance. In fact, it is only recently that such evidence has been provided, in a single study (Kinomura et al., 1996). In part, this is because older-generation PET scanners with limited resolution had difficulty imaging small, deep structures in the brain (see figure 11.7). The development of improved PET scanners, coupled with the advent of high-resolution magnetic resonance imaging (MRI), has made imaging of those structures possible.

Kinomura et al. (1996) reported a PET study in which participants performed short-duration visual or somatosensory RT tasks. Compared to an eyes-closed condition, performance of either task was associated with activation of the midbrain tegmentum and the right intralaminar region of the thalamus. Activation of the same brain regions was found when a different control condition was used in which participants viewed the visual stimuli passively and pressed the response key in a self-paced manner. Kinomura et al. (1996) concluded that those regions were involved in the control of arousal and vigilance in the normal human brain. That conclusion is certainly valid as far as cortical arousal is concerned, and it is consistent with cellular and EEG studies that implicate the reticular formation and intralaminar thalamic nuclei in cortical arousal (Steriade, 1996). However, the significance of the results for vigilance is less clear. The vigilance decrement was not assessed in the study. Therefore, the results apply only to the initiation of the vigilant state, and do not bear on the question of whether those brainstem and thalamic areas are also involved when vigilance fails with increased time on task.

Frontal Cortex

Damage to the frontal lobes, especially right hemispheric lesions, impairs cortical arousal and the development of phasic alertness to a warning stimulus (Heilman and Van den Abell, 1979; Mesulam, 1981; Posner and

Petersen, 1990). For example, Yokoyama, Jennings, Ackles, Hood, and Boller (1987) showed that the normal deceleration of the heart rate response that occurs during the preparatory interval of a warned RT task was absent in patients with right frontal and perirolandic and frontal lesions, but was not absent in patients with left hemisphere lesions. Using an auditory task requiring participants to count sequences of tones, Wilkins, Shallice, and McCarthy (1987) reported impaired performance in right but not in left frontal-lobe lesion patients.

The impact of frontal lesions on long-duration vigilance tasks was examined by Mirsky and Rosvold (1960). They reported that patients who had undergone neurosurgery for unilateral removal of the frontal or temporal lobes did not show impairment on performance of the CPT. That is a surprising finding in view of other lesion and brain-imaging studies (reviewed later in this chapter) showing that the frontal lobe is involved in vigilance. That finding suggests either that the CPT as administered in Mirsky and Rosvold's study was insensitive or that the contralesional hemisphere was sufficient to maintain performance on the CPT in those patients. Godefroy, Cabaret, and Rousseaux (1994) also reported that patients with orbitofrontal and prefrontal lesions did not show impaired vigilance performance on a 25-minute task requiring discrimination between visual shapes (squares, crosses, and triangles). Task sensitivity may also have been a factor in that study, particularly in view of the fact that neither the brain-damaged nor the control group showed a vigilance decrement over time in either RT or detection rate.

Several functional brain-imaging studies have examined frontal lobe activation associated with arousal and vigilance (Berman and Weinberger, 1990; Buchsbaum et al., 1990; Cohen, Semple, Gross, and Holcomb, 1988; Cohen, Semple, Gross, King, and Nordahl, 1992; Deutsch, Papanicolaou, Bourbon, and Eisenberg, 1987; Pardo, Fox, and Raichle, 1991; Reivich and Gur, 1985). Such studies also provide an opportunity to identify specific regions within the very large structure that is the frontal lobe (e.g., dorsolateral prefrontal cortex). In general, those studies have found that blood flow and glucose metabolism are greater in the right versus the left frontal lobe during vigilance task performance in normal adults. For example, Berman and Weinberger (1990) compared activation patterns during performance of the CPT with those associated with several other tasks, including prototypical "frontal" tasks such as the Wisconsin Card Sorting Test. They found greater right hemisphere activation only for the CPT. In the remaining tasks, the left hemisphere exhibited greater activation than the right. Cohen and colleagues have reported two studies of auditory vigilance that also implicated right prefrontal cortex in vigilance. Cohen et al. (1988) used 18-FDG PET during a 35-minute intensity-discrimination task. They reported that glucose metabolic rate in the right middle prefrontal cortex during the performance of the auditory vigilance task was 5% to 7% higher than it was in a resting condition or in a passive somatosensory stimulation task. A subsequent study confirmed the right prefrontal activation and localized the activity to the middle prefrontal gyrus (Cohen et al., 1992).

Those imaging studies used 18-FDG and other techniques that do not permit fine-grained analysis of changes in blood flow or metabolism during the course of vigilance tasks. The half-life of 18-FDG, for example, is significantly longer than 15 minutes, within which time frame most of the vigilance decrement in detection rate occurs (Teichner, 1974). More recent studies, including the study by Kinomura et al. (1996) discussed earlier, have used PET imaging of O^{15}, which allows for assessment of blood flow within a time period of 2 minutes. Pardo et al. (1991) used O^{15} PET to study changes in regional cerebral blood flow during very brief duration somatosensory and visual vigilance tasks. In the somatosensory task, 23 observers were asked to monitor either their left or their right great toe in order to detect and keep a running count of brief pauses in a series of suprathreshold touches to the toe. In the visual task, the same group of observers was required to detect and count decreases in the intensity of a dim central fixation mark. In fact, no signals were presented at all in either task, and any responses participants made were false alarms. In both modalities, right prefrontal and superior parietal activation was observed during task performance, regardless of the laterality of sensory input.

That study was recently repeated, using gradient-echo fMRI, by Lewin et al. (1996), who used the same visual task as did Pardo et al. (1991). Task performance was associated with right frontal activation. No behavioral data were reported. The results of the two studies clearly indicate that right prefrontal activation is a correlate of the vigilant state. However, because performance was only minimally assessed in both studies (only the number of false alarms was reported by Pardo et al.), and because the design of the task did not allow for the vigilance decrement, the more interesting question of the brain systems involved when vigilance fails increasingly with time on task was not addressed by either study.

The studies discussed so far have all provided evidence that prefrontal cortex is involved in arousal and in the overall level of vigilance, but none have demonstrated that that brain area is also involved in vigilance decrement over time. However, a recent lesion study by Rueckert and Grafman (1996) has provided some evidence. They found that patients with right prefrontal and orbitofrontal lesions showed a greater increase in error rate over time on the CPT than did either left-lesioned patients or age-matched normal controls.

Cingulate Gyrus

The cingulate gyrus has also been implicated in vigilance task performance. However, unlike the brain stem and prefrontal cortex, vigilance performance has been associated with reduced activation in the anterior part of that brain region (Posner and Petersen, 1990). Lower metabolic rates in the anterior cingulate cortex were also observed during auditory CPT performance versus during rest in the previously described studies conducted by Cohen et al. (1988; 1992). In Posner and Petersen's network model of attention (1990), the anterior cingulate is postulated to be involved in active target detection and in executive control functions. Posner and Petersen (1990) speculated that reduced activation of the anterior cingulate might be necessary to optimize performance in vigilance and other tasks in which targets occur very infrequently. However, there is currently no evidence specifically linking anterior cingulate activation to vigilance decrement.

Corpus Callosum

The cingulate gyrus is a cortical area lying just above the corpus callosum, which is the nerve fiber tract that is surgically severed in split-brain patients. Studies of the vigilance performance of those individuals have indicated that intact functioning of the right hemisphere may be important for the ability to maintain attention successfully for a prolonged period of time (Dimond, 1976). Dimond (1977) studied six total commissurotomy patients who had had a complete section of the corpus callosum and hippocampal and anterior commissures. Participants performed a 30-minute visual vigilance task in which nontargets and targets were displayed in either the left or the right visual field. The total commissurotomy patients had very high false alarm rates and showed substantial decrements in detection rates over time, from 100% to 30% by the end of the session. When the same subjects completed vibrotactile and auditory vigilance tasks, their detection efficiency was observed to be higher for the right hemisphere (Dimond, 1979b). The superior detection efficiency of the right hemisphere in those investigations is consistent with the previously discussed lesion and brain-imaging evidence implicating the right frontal cortex in vigilance.

The results of laterality studies of vigilance in normal participants have not consistently favored the right hemisphere. Dimond and Beaumont (1971) found that, for the same visual vigilance tasks used in their split-brain studies, more false alarms were associated with the left hemisphere but there were no hemispheric differences in the detection rate or in the vigilance decrement. In a study in which participants listened for infrequent targets in noise bursts presented to the left or right ear, Warm, Schumsky, and Hawley (1976) also found no ear (i.e., hemisphere) differences in the vigilance decrement. However, in a subsequent study using a more fine-grained analysis of performance changes over time, Warm, Richter, Sprague, Porter, and Schumsky (1980) reported that RT to left ear signals increased with time on task, whereas RT to right ear signals remained stable, suggesting that only the right hemisphere showed a vigilance decrement. Warm et al. (1980) interpreted their findings in terms of a hemispheric cooperation model (Allen, 1983), in which the right hemisphere is postulated to show a greater initial level of performance and to show greater decrement over time, whereas the left hemisphere is proposed to show lower initial performance but less decrement over time.

Those studies suggest that, although the right frontal lobe may play a dominant role in vigilance, performance of vigilance tasks is the result of the integrated action of both cerebral hemispheres (as well as of subcortical nuclei). The hemispheric cooperation model of Warm et al. (1980) postulates that both hemispheres are involved in vigilance but that the right predominates and is the source of the vigilance decrement over time. Allen (1983) has discussed other models for hemispheric differences in attention.

All such models implicate the corpus callosum as playing a crucial role in facilitating interhemispheric coordination (Hoptman and Davidson, 1994). That would also account for the severe impairment of vigilance that occurs following total lesioning of the callosum (Dimond, 1977). Recent studies have shown that callosal efficiency may also play a role in vigilance in normal individuals. Rueckert, Sorenson, and Levy (1994) divided 6 to 10-year-old children into groups with low and high callosal efficiency as assessed by a tachistoscopic task involving stimuli presented to both visual fields. The two groups were then tested on a serial RT task in which stimuli followed each other at either short (2 s) or long (10 s) interstimulus intervals (ISIs). Rueckert et al. (1994) found that children with lower callosal efficiency had elevated RTs in the long ISI condition. That was interpreted as reflecting a deficit in the maintenance of attention following a warning stimulus, or what we have previously referred to as phasic alertness. As discussed previously, although Posner (1978) has suggested that short-term phasic alertness represents long-term vigilance in miniature, it is an open question whether the two phenomena are the same. Ideally, vigilance should be assessed over a sufficient period of time such that detection failures can be observed. That was done in a subsequent study by Rueckert and Levy (1996), who again compared the performance of children with low and high callosal efficiency (using a bimanual movement task) on a serial RT task, and also assessed performance changes over time with the 10-minute task. The previous results of Rueckert et al. (1994) were replicated. In addition, they found that, compared to high callosal efficiency children, the low callosal efficiency group had longer RTs and more missed signals in the second half of the task; both results are indicative of increased vigilance decrement. Thus, the short-term measure of phasic alertness and the long-term measure of vigilance decrement showed the same relation to callosal efficiency, thereby providing one of the few empirical verifications of Posner's suggestion (1978) that the two phenomena are the same. Rueckert and Levy (1996) concluded that the difference in the vigilance decrement between the two groups may reflect the differential contribution of the frontal lobes, a conclusion that is consistent with the lesion literature reviewed previously. Furthermore, if those results can be replicated in adults, in whom callosal maturation is complete, they would further implicate the importance of the callosum and the anterior commissure in supporting the task of the frontal lobes in the maintenance of vigilance.

Summary

The results of these lesion and brain-imaging studies substantiate existing evidence derived from studies of normal adults and behaving animals that the noradrenergic brainstem reticular formation, the intralaminar thalamic nuclei, and the right prefrontal cortex are all involved in vigilance. One limitation of the PET studies is that most—with the exception of Kinomura et al. (1996) and Pardo et al. (1991)—used the older 18-FDG technique, which does not have sufficient temporal resolution to index changes in activation over short periods of time. Furthermore, neither Pardo et al. (1991) nor Kinomura et al. (1996), who used O^{15} PET, which has a 2-minute temporal resolution, assessed changes in activation or performance over time. Thus, although the studies consistently show that regions of the right frontal lobe are involved in the initiation and maintenance of attention over periods of time, they do not directly address the question of the functional role of those areas in vigilance decrement. What is needed is a study in which the O^{15} technique or MRI is used to image functional brain activity early and late during a vigilance task in which a performance decrement occurs, in comparison to a control task in which no decrement occurs. Such a study appears not to have been conducted at this time.

PSYCHOPHYSICAL DETERMINANTS OF VIGILANCE

The neurobiological studies reviewed so far have clarified the relation between vigilance performance and cortical arousal, and have also indicated that a network of brain regions—including the LC noradrenergic system, the basal forebrain cholinergic system, the intralaminar thalamic nuclei, and the right prefrontal cortex—are involved in the initiation of the vigilant state and in cortical arousal. However, as mentioned previously, these studies have done little to elucidate the brain mechanisms related to the vigilance decrement. Furthermore, the tendency of these studies to treat vigilance as a unitary phenomenon has led to a neglect of important psychophysical and task variables that control the overall level of vigilance and the vigilance decrement. In fact, some papers do not even examine changes in behavioral or physiological measures over time on task, a sine qua non for appropriate assessment of vigilance. A valid functional characterization of vigilance performance is essential if such studies are to contribute to an understanding of the brain mechanisms of vigilance.

The influence of key psychophysical variables is briefly discussed in the next section. This serves as prelude to the concluding section, in which brain mechanisms are discussed in relation to the psychophysics of vigilance.

Table 11.1 Key psychophysical variables affecting vigilance performance

First-Order Factors
Sensory modality
Signal intensity
Signal duration
Background event rate
Multiple signal sources
Second-Order Factors
Signal probability
Signal regularity
Event regularity
Signal spatial uncertainty
Signal type (simultaneous or successive discrimination)

A Functional Description of Vigilance Performance

The study of vigilance, like the study of other perceptual phenomena, has profited from careful psychophysical analysis. Dember and Warm (1979) classified the psychophysical determinants of vigilance into first-order factors, which involve an immediate physical property of the stimulus, and second-order factors, in which important characteristics of the signal must be derived by the observer on the basis of experience with the task. Table 11.1 lists the most important of those factors.

First-Order Factors Key first-order factors include the sensory modality of signals and signal strength (e.g., as determined by signal intensity, duration, etc.). Perhaps the most crucial single-factor determinant of vigilance performance is the background event rate, or nonsignal stimulus rate, which has been nominated as the prepotent psychophysical factor in vigilance performance (Parasuraman et al., 1987; Warm and Jerison, 1984). Both the speed and the accuracy of signal detection vary inversely with event rate, and the vigilance decrement is often more pronounced in the context of a fast as compared to a slow event rate (Jerison and Pickett, 1964; Parasuraman, 1979).

Second-Order Factors Signal probability in vigilance experiments is typically quite low. Accordingly, one of the things that observers come to understand in vigilance experiments is that they are confronted by considerable temporal uncertainty, or uncertainty about when critical signals for detection might appear. Such uncertainty can be studied experimentally in a number of ways. One method is to vary signal density (or signal probability). Performance efficiency in vigilance tasks varies directly with signal density (Warm and Jerison, 1984). Another way to manipulate temporal uncertainty is through variations in the intervals of time between critical signals. Both the speed and the accuracy of signal detection are greater in the context of

Parasuraman, Warm, & See: Brain Systems of Vigilance

regular as compared to irregular intersignal intervals (Adams and Boulter, 1964; Warm, Dember, Murphy, and Dittmar, 1992). The intervals between neutral events that serve as carriers for critical signals in vigilance tasks also contribute to temporal uncertainty. If the interevent intervals are temporally irregular rather than regular, then temporal uncertainty is increased. Under such conditions (event asynchrony), performance is degraded in comparison to performance under conditions in which the schedule of background events is easily predictable (event synchrony; Scerbo, Warm, and Fisk, 1987).

Along with temporal uncertainty regarding critical signals and neutral events, observers in vigilance studies can also be faced with spatial uncertainty, or uncertainty as to where on the monitored display critical signals and neutral events will appear. Such uncertainty can be introduced into a vigilance task by varying the probability that signals or events will appear at different locations or by using an unpredictable sequence of display locations. Under such conditions, performance efficiency is lowered and observers come to bias their attention toward those portions of the display at which the likelihood of signal appearance is greatest (Adams and Boulter, 1964; Mouloua and Parasuraman, 1995).

Vigilance Task Taxonomy A major feature of vigilance tasks is their diversity. Not only have different sensory modalities been used, but several different stimulus dimensions have also been employed to define critical signals for detection. A key development in the psychophysics of vigilance was the insight that, despite this diversity, orderly relations can be uncovered by examining task information-processing demands, thus providing a theoretical basis for categorizing different vigilance tasks, or a taxonomy (Parasuraman and Davies, 1977). A major aspect of that taxonomy is the distinction between successive and simultaneous discrimination tasks. The former are absolute judgment tasks in which observers must compare current input with a standard retained in working memory to distinguish between signal and nonsignal events. In contrast, simultaneous tasks are comparative judgment tasks in which all of the information needed to distinguish signals from nonsignals is present in the stimuli themselves, and there is little involvement of recent memory. The taxonomy of vigilance also led to suggestions that vigilance tasks can be differentiated according to their processing resource demands (Parasuraman et al., 1987). Parasuraman and Davies (1977) proposed that, because of the memory load, successive tasks are more resource demanding than are their simultaneous cohorts. A substantial amount of research has provided empirical support for that idea (Parasuraman et al., 1987; Warm and Dember, 1998).

Brain Mechanisms and the Psychophysics of Vigilance

Although the psychophysics of vigilance has been carefully worked out, little is known about brain mechanisms associated with the functional description of vigilance performance under different task conditions. As a result, current knowledge of the neurobiology of vigilance may be context limited and, therefore, quite superficial. Given the complexities involved in studying the two questions that form the framework for the current literature on brain mechanisms and vigilance—the relationship between vigilance and brain systems regulating cortical arousal and the identification of brain regions that are involved in vigilance—one might imagine that any search for mechanisms that covary with task-determined differences in vigilance performance would be a daunting venture. Nevertheless, such studies are not only possible, but are probably essential to advance the neurobiology of vigilance. A few studies are discussed to illustrate the point that brain mechanisms of vigilance, from the cellular level to the level of global hemispheric organization, are modulated by task factors that also influence vigilance performance.

As discussed previously, a series of studies has examined the role of the basal forebrain cholinergic arousal system in vigilance (McGaughy and Sarter, 1995; Moore et al., 1992; Sarter, 1994). An important feature of that research is the development and validation of a vigilance task for rats that is sensitive not only to time on task but also to important psychophysical factors such as event rate, background noise, and signal salience. Task validation was shown, for example, by McGaughy and Sarter's finding that the vigilance decrement in the rats was greater at a high than at a low event rate (1995), as has been shown repeatedly in human studies (Jerison and Pickett, 1964; Parasuraman, 1979). Also, as discussed earlier, McGaughy and Sarter (1995) obtained evidence for cholinergic involvement in vigilance when they found that the BZR agonist CDP impaired performance on that task in both young and old rats in a dose-dependent manner. Furthermore, their finding that performance impairment interacted with signal salience and with age points to the sensitivity of the neural mechanisms (i.e., modulation of cortical release of acetylcholine) to task factors in vigilance. Unfortunately, McGaughy and Sarter (1995) did not find that the CDP-induced performance impairment increased with time on task. Such a result would have provided strong evidence for the involvement of the cholinergic system in the vigilance decrement and not just in the overall level of vigilance. Nevertheless, that study is important as it represents one of the few neurobiological studies in which the sensitivity of neural mechanisms of vigilance to task factors has been evaluated.

Examples of that type can also be found in some human studies. For instance, two task parameters have been linked to specific changes in ERP components. One study, which focused on the event rate, was described earlier, in the discussion of neural habituation theory (Parasuraman, 1985). That study showed that N100 amplitude in an auditory vigilance task was greater in the context of a slow as compared to a fast event rate and that the overall magnitude of the N100 was greater when observers were required to actively try to detect signals as opposed to when they were required to ignore the acoustic stimuli. The auditory N100 component is thought to have multiple generators in the supratemporal plane of the primary auditory cortex and the premotor areas of the frontal cortex (Näätänen, 1992). Thus, those results demonstrate the sensitivity of the N100 component and of its underlying brain generators to attentional processes in vigilance. A second study focused on the finding that supplementary olfactory stimulation can be effective in bolstering visual vigilance (Warm, Dember, and Parasuraman, 1991). Observers who were given intermittent, brief bursts of a stimulating mint odor through a modified oxygen mask detected more signals than did controls exposed to pure air bursts. That effect was associated with greater amplitude of the N160 component of the ERP; at the same time, autonomic measures of general arousal showed no stimulation-related effect (Dember, Warm, and Parasuraman, 1995). Given that the visual N160, like the auditory N100, has also been linked to attentional processes (Näätänen, 1992), these results again demonstrate the sensitivity of brain electrical measures of attentional processes to a task factor—accessory stimulation—that strongly affects vigilance.

In addition to electrophysiological changes, other studies have shown that task factors can be related to laterality effects in vigilance. Warm et al. (1976) reported that the right hemisphere may dominate in processing the temporal properties of signals in vigilance because the beneficial effects of increments in signal density are more pronounced when stimuli are presented to the left as compared to the right ear. Finally, using a secondary probe procedure in which observers had to respond to acoustic probes delivered to the right or left ear while performing a primary visual vigilance task, Davis (1988) reported that simultaneous and successive task performance may be differentially lateralized. In that study, left ear but not right ear probe detections slowed significantly over time when observers carried out a successive-type vigilance task, whereas the rate of decline in the speed of probe detections over time was similar in each ear when observers encountered the simultaneous-type task. The results were interpreted in terms of the greater load on working memory imposed by the successive task on right hemisphere systems specialized for vigilance. Irrespective of that conclusion, both studies indicate that the organization of vigilance at the global hemispheric level is also modulated by task factors.

Summary

Although research into the brain mechanisms that implement task-related changes in vigilance performance is sparse, serious pursuit of the problem is necessary for the development of a complete understanding of the neurobiology of sustained attention. In that regard, an examination of the effects of psychophysical parameters on behavioral performance and on the activation or deactivation of the LC, the basal forebrain, the frontal cortex, or other brain structures would not only enhance understanding of the functional significance of particular brain regions in vigilance, but would also clarify both the role of those multiple brain areas in vigilance performance and their interactions. The psychophysical studies described in this section indicate that vigilance involves multiple processes. The challenge for the future is to identify whether different brain systems are associated with the different processes and whether the major psychophysical factors affecting vigilance also modulate those systems.

CONCLUSIONS

This review of the extensive literature on brain systems in vigilance has been organized around two central questions. The first concerns the relationship between vigilance and brain systems that regulate cortical arousal. In answer to that question, it is clear that vigilance is distinct from arousal. A unified arousal theory is viable only for the overall level of vigilance, and not for the vigilance decrement. Fractionation of subcortical arousal systems (e.g., noradrenergic, cholinergic, dopaminergic, etc.) and examination of the effects of task factors on those systems may clarify the role of arousal in the vigilance decrement.

The second central issue concerns the brain regions that mediate vigilance and how they are functionally interrelated. In answer to that question, it is clear that the noradrenergic reticular formation and the right prefrontal cortex are involved in the overall level of vigilance, but evidence linking those areas to the vigilance decrement is weak. Studies also suggest a role for the basal forebrain cholinergic system, but again there is little evidence that that system mediates the vigilance decrement. No evidence is available pertaining to different brain regions (or components of brain networks) subserving multiple decrement processes (e.g., sensitivity decrement versus criterion shifts).

Finally, an important conclusion is that only limited information is available on the effects of task parameters on brain mechanisms of vigilance. This represents a serious shortcoming of the current research. Such information is needed in order to develop an understanding of the neurobiology of vigilance that is not context limited and therefore potentially superficial.

REFERENCES

Adams, J. A. and Boulter, L. R. (1964) Spatial and temporal uncertainty as determinants of vigilance performance. *J. Exp. Psychol.* 67: 127–131.

Allen, M. (1983) Models of hemispheric specialization. *Psychol. Rev.* 93: 73–104.

Aston-Jones, G., Chiang, C., and Alexinsky, T. (1991) Discharge of noradrenergic locus coerulus neurons in behaving rats and monkeys suggests a role in vigilance. *Prog. Brain Res.* 88: 501–520.

Aston-Jones, G., Rajkowski, J., Kubiak, P., and Alexinsky, T. (1994) Locus coeruleus neurons in monkey are selectively activated by attended cues in a vigilance task. *J. Neurosci.* 14: 4467–4480.

Belyavin, A. and Wright, N. A. (1987) Changes in electrical activity of the brain with vigilance. Electroencephalogr. Clin. Neurophysiol. 66: 137–144.

Berch, D. B. and Kanter, D. R. (1984) Individual differences. In *Sustained Attention in Human Performance*, edited by J. S. Warm, pp. 143–178. London: Wiley.

Berman, K. F. and Weinberger, D. R. (1990) Lateralization of cortical function during cognitive tasks: Regional cerebral blood flow studies of normal individuals and patients with schizophrenia. J. Neurol. Neurosurg. Psychiatry 53: 150–160.

Brouwer, W. H. and Van Wolffelaar, P. C. (1985) Sustained attention and sustained effort after closed head injury: Detection and 0.10 Hz heart rate variability in a low event rate vigilance task. *Cortex* 21: 111–119.

Buchsbaum, M. S., Nuechterlein, K. H., Haier, R. J., Wu, J., Sicotte, N., Hazlett, E., Asarnow, R., Potkin, S., and Guich, S. (1990) Glucose metabolic rate in normals and schizophrenics during the continuous performance test assessed by positron emission tomography. *Br. J. Psychiatry* 156: 216–227.

Cohen, R. M., Semple, W. E., Gross, M., and Holcomb, H. H. (1988) Functional localization of sustained attention: Comparison to sensory stimulation in the absence of instruction. *Neuropsychiatry Neuropsychology Behav. Neurol.* 1: 3–20.

Cohen, R. M., Semple, W. E., Gross, M., King, A. C., and Nordahl, T. E. (1992) Metabolic brain pattern of sustained auditory discrimination. *Exp. Brain Res.* 92: 165–172.

Craig, A. (1978) Is the vigilance decrement simply a response adjustment towards probability matching? *Hum. Fac.* 20: 441–446.

Daniel, R. (1967) Alpha and theta EEG in vigilance. *Percept. Mot. Skills* 25: 697–703.

Davies, D. R. and Krkovic, A. (1965) Skin conductance, alpha-activity, and vigilance. *Am. J. Psychol.* 78: 304–306.

Davies, D. R. and Parasuraman, R. (1977) Cortical evoked potentials and vigilance: A decision theory analysis. In *Vigilance: Theory, Operational Performance and Physiological Correlates*, edited by R. R. Mackie, pp. 285–306. New York: Plenum press.

Davies, D. R. and Parasuraman, R. (1982) *The Psychology of Vigilance*. London: Academic Press.

Davis, J. M. (1988) *Cerebral Asymmerty in Successive and Simultaneous Vigilance Tasks*. Unpublished master's thesis, University of Cincinnati.

DeArmond, S. J., Fusco, M. M., and Dewey, M. M. (1989) *Structure of the Human Brain: A Photographic Atlas* (3rd ed.). New York: Oxford University Press.

Dember, W. N. and Warm, J. S. (1979) *The Psychology of Perception* (2nd ed.). New York: Holt, Rineheart, and Winston.

Dember, W. N., Warm, J. S., and Parasuraman, R. (1995) Olfactory stimulation and sustained attention. In *Compendium of Olfactory Research*, edited by A. N. Gilbert, pp. 39–46. Dubque, IA: Kendall/Hunt.

Dencker, S. J. and Lofving, B. (1958) A psychometric study of identical twins discordant for closed head injury. *Acta Psychiatr. Neurol. Scand.* 33: 122–134.

Deutsch, G., Papanicolaou, A. C., Bourbon, W. T., and Eisenberg, H. M. (1987) Cerebral blood flow evidence of right frontal activation in attention demanding tasks. *Int. J. Neurosci.* 36: 23–28.

Dimond, S. J. (1976) Depletion of attentional capacity after total commissurotomy in man. *Brain* 99: 347–356.

Dimond, S. J. (1977) Vigilance and split-brain research. In *Vigilance: Theory, Operational Performance and Physiological Correlates*, edited by R. R. Mackie, pp. 341–355. New York: Plenum Press.

Dimond, S. J. (1979a) Performance by split-brain humans on lateralized vigilance tasks. *Cortex* 15: 43–50.

Dimond, S. J. (1979b) Tactual and auditory vigilance in split-brain man. *J. Neurol. Neurosurg. Psychiatry.* 42: 70–74.

Dimond, S. J. and Beaumont, J. G. (1971) Hemisphere function and vigilance. *Q. J. Exp. Psychol.* 23: 443–448.

Dimond, S. J. and Lazarus, J. (1974) The problem of vigilance in animal life. *Brain Behav. Evol.* 9: 60–79.

Duffy, E. (1962) *Activation and Behavior.* New York: Wiley.

Gale, A. (1977) Some EEG correlates of sustained attention. In *Vigilance: Theory, Operational Performance and Physiological Correlates,* edited by R. R. Mackie, pp. 263–283. New York: Plenum Press.

Godefroy, O., Cabaret, M., and Rousseaux, M. (1994) Vigilance and effects of fatigability, practice and motivation on simple reaction time tests in patients with lesion of the frontal lobe. *Neuropsychologia* 32: 983–990.

Green, D. M. and Swets, J. A. (1974) *Signal Detection Theory and Psychophysics.* Huntington, NY: R.E. Krieger.

Haider, M., Spong, P., and Lindsley, D. B. (1964) Attention, vigilance, and cortical evoked potentials in humans. *Science* 145: 180–182.

Hancock, P. A. (1984) Environmental stressors. In *Sustained Attention in Human Performance,* edited by J. S. Warm, pp. 103–142. London: Wiley.

Hawkins, H. L., Hillyard, S. A., Luck, S. J., Mouloua, M., Downing, C. J., and Woodward, D. P. (1990) Visual attention modulates signal detectability. *J. Exp. Psychol. Hum. Percept. Perform.* 16: 802–811.

Head, H. (1923) The conception of nervous and mental energy. II. Vigilance: A physiological state of the nervous system. *Br. J. Psychol.* 14: 126–147.

Heilman, K. M. and Van den Abell, T. (1979) Right hemisphere dominance for mediating cerebral activation. *Neuropsychologia* 17: 315–321.

Heinze, H. J., Mangun, G. R., Burchert, W., Hinrichs, H., Scholtz, M., Muntel, T., Gosel, A., Scherg, M., Johannes, S., Hundeshagen, H., Gazzaniga, M. S., and Hillyard, S. A. (1994) Combined spatial and temporal imaging of brain activity during visual selective attention in humans. *Nature* 372: 543–546.

Hoptman, M. J. and Davidson, R. (1994) How and why the two cerebral hemispheres interact. *Psychol. Bull.* 116: 195–219.

Horvath, M., Frantik, E., Kopriva, K., and Meissner, J. (1975) EEG theta activity increase coincides with performance decrement in a monotonous task. *Act. Nerv. Super. (Praha)* 18: 207–210.

Humphreys, M. S. and Revelle, W. (1984) Personality, motivation, and performance: A theory of the relationship between individual differences and information processing. *Psychol. Rev.* 91: 153–184.

Jane, J. A., Steward, O., and Gennarelli, T. A. (1985) Axonal degeneration induced by experimental noninvasive minor head injury. *J. Neurosurg.* 62: 853–858.

Jerison, H. J. (1965) Human and animal vigilance. *Percept. Mot. Skills* 21: 580–582.

Jerison, H. J. (1977) Vigilance: Biology, psychology, theory, and practice. In *Vigilance: Theory, Operational Performance and Physiological Correlates*, edited by R. R. Mackie, pp. 27–40. New York: Plenum Press.

Jerison, H. J. and Pickett, R. M. (1964) Vigilance: The importance of the elicited observing rate. *Science* 143: 970–971.

Kinomura. S., Larsson, J., Gulyas, B., and Roland, P. E. (1996) Activation by attention of the human reticular formation and thalamic intralaminar nuclei. *Science* 271: 612–515.

Koelega, H. S. (1993) Stimulant drugs and vigilance performance: A review. *Psychopharmacology* 111: 1–16.

Koelega, H. S., Verbaten, M. N., Van Leeuwen, T. H., Kenemans, J. L., Kemner, C., and Sjouw, W. (1992) Time effects on event-related brain potentials and vigilance performance. *Biol. Psychol.* 34: 59–86.

Krueger, G. P. (1989) Sustained work, fatigue, sleep loss, and performance. *Work Stress* 3: 129–141.

LaBerge, D. and Buchsbaum, M. S. (1990) Positron emission tomographic measurements of pulvinar activity during an attention task. *J. Neurosci.* 10: 613–619.

Lacey, J. I. (1967) Somatic response patterning and stress: Some revisions of activation theory. In *Psychological Stress*, edited by M. H. Appley and R. Trumbull, pp. 14–37. New York: Appleton-Century-Crofts.

Lewin, J. S., Friedman, L., Wu, D., Miller, D. A., Thompson, L. A., Klein, S. K., Wise, A. L., Hedera, P., Buckley, P., Meltzer, H., Friedland, R. P., and Duerk, J. L. (1996) Cortical localization of human sustained attention: Detection with functional MR using a visual vigilance paradigm. *J. Comput. Assist. Tomogr.* 20: 695–701.

Lindsley, D. B. (1960) Attention, consciousness, sleep, and wakefulness. In *Handbook of Physiology* (Sec. 1, Vol. 3), edited by J. Field, H. W. Magoun, and V. E. Hall, pp. 1553–1593. Baltimore, MD: Williams and Wilkins.

Loeb, M. and Alluisi, E. A. (1984) Theories of vigilance. In *Sustained Attention in Human Performance*, edited by J. S. Warm, pp. 179–205. London: Wiley.

Mackworth, J. F. (1969) *Vigilance and Habituation*. Baltimore, MD: Penguin.

Mackworth, N. H. (1950) *Researches on the Measurement of Human Performance*. Medical Research Council Special Report Series 268. London: His Majesty's Stationery Office.

Mackworth, N. H. (1957) Some factors affecting vigilance. *Adv. Sci.* 53: 389–393.

Macmillan, N. A. and Creelman, C. D. (1991) *Detection Theory: A User's Guide*. New York: Cambridge University Press.

Makeig, S. and Inlow, M. (1993) Lapses in alertness: Coherence of fluctuations in performance and EEG spectrum. *Electroencephalogr. Clin. Neurophysiol.* 86: 23–25.

Makeig, S. and Jung, T. P. (1995) Changes in alertness are a principal component of variance in the EEG spectrum. *Neuroreport* 7: 213–216.

Matthews, G., Davies, D. R., and Lees, J. L. (1990) Arousal, extraversion, and individual differences in resources. *J. Per. Soc. Psychol.* 59: 150–168.

May, P., Tiitinen, H., Sinkkonnen, J., and Näätänen, R. (1994) Long-term stimulation attenuates the transient 40-Hz response. *Neuroreport* 5: 1918–1920.

McGaughy, J. and Sarter, M. (1995) Behavioral vigilance in rats: Task validation and effects of age, amphetamine, and benzodiazapine receptor ligands. *Psychopharmacology* 117: 340–357.

Mesulam, M. M. (1981) A cortical network for directed attention and unilateral neglect. *Ann. Neurol.* 10: 309–325.

Mirsky, A. F. (1987) Behavioral and psychophysiological markers of disordered attention. *Environ. Health Perspect.* 71: 191–199.

Mirsky, A. F. and Orren, M. M. (1977) Attention. In *Neuropeptide Influences on the Brain and Behavior*, edited by L. H. Miller, pp. 233–267. New York: Raven.

Mirsky, A. F. and Rosvold, H. E. (1960) The use of psychoactive drugs as a neurophysiological tool in studies of attention in man. In *Drugs and Behavior*, edited by L. Uhr and J. G. Miller, pp. 167–178. New York: Wiley.

Moore, H., Dudchenko, P., Bruno, J. P., and Sarter, M. (1992) Toward modeling age-related changes of attentional abilities in rats: Simple and choice reaction time tasks and vigilance. *Neurobiol. Aging* 13: 759–772.

Moore, H., Sarter, M., and Bruno, J. P. (1993) Bidirectional modulation of stimulated cortical acetylcholine release by benzodiazepine receptor ligands. *Brain Res.* 596: 17–29.

Morecraft, R. J., Geula C., and Mesulam M. M. (1993) Architecture of connectivity within a cingulo-fronto-parietal neurocognitive network for directed attention. *Arch. Neurol.* 50: 279–284.

Moruzzi, G. and Magoun, H. W. (1949) Brain stem reticular formation and activation of the EEG. *Electroencephalogr. Clin. Neurophysiol.* 1: 455–473.

Mouloua, M. and Parasuraman, R. (1995) Aging and cognitive vigilance: Effects of spatial uncertainty and event rate. *Exp. Aging Res.* 21: 17–32.

Näätänen, R. (1992) *Attention and Brain Function.* Hillsdale, NJ: Lawrence Erlbaum.

Nestor, P. G., Faux, S., McCarley, R. W., Shenton, M. E., and Sands, S. F. (1990) Measurement of visual sustained attention in schizophrenia using signal detection analysis and a newly developed computerized CPT. *Schizophr. Res.* 3: 329–332.

Norman, D. A. and Bobrow, D. G. (1975) On data-limited and resource-limited processes. *Cognitive Psychol.* 7: 46–64.

Nuechterlein, K., Parasuraman, R., and Jiang, Q. (1983) Visual sustained attention: Image degradation produces rapid sensitivity decrement over time. *Science* 220: 327–329.

O'Hanlon, J. F. and Beatty, J. (1977) Concurrence of electroencephalographic and performance changes during a simulated radar watch and some implications for the arousal theory of vigilance. In *Vigilance: Theory, Operational Performance and Physiological Correlates*, edited by R. R. Mackie, pp. 189–201. New York: Plenum Press.

Ommaya, A. and Gennarelli, T. A. (1974) Cerebral concussion and traumatic unconsciousness. *Brain* 97: 633–654.

Parasuraman, R. (1979) Memory load and event rate control sensitivity decrements in sustained attention. *Science* 205: 924–927.

Parasuraman, R. (1984) The psychobiology of sustained attention. In *Sustained Attention in Human Performance*, edited by J. S. Warm, pp. 61–101. London: Wiley.

Parasuraman, R. (1985) Sustained attention: A multifactorial approach. In *Attention and Performance XI*, edited by M. I. Posner and O. S. M. Marin, pp. 493–511. Hillsdale, NJ: Lawrence Erlbaum.

Parasuraman, R. and Davies, D. R. (1976) Decision theory analysis of response latencies in vigilance. *J. Exp. Psychol. Hum. Percept. Perform.* 2: 569–582.

Parasuraman, R. and Davies, D. R. (1977) A taxonomic analysis of vigilance. In *Vigilance: Theory, Operational Performance and Physiological Correlates*, edited by R. R. Mackie, pp. 559–574. New York: Plenum Press.

Parasuraman, R., Mutter, S. A., and Molloy, R. (1991) Sustained attention following mild closed-head injury. *J. Clin. Exp. Neuropsychol.* 13: 789–811.

Parasuraman, R., Warm, J. S., and Dember, W. N. (1987) Vigilance: Taxonomy and utility. In *Ergonomics and Human Factors: Recent Research*, edited by L. S. Mark, J. S. Warm, and R. L. Huston, pp. 11–32. New York: Springer Verlag.

Pardo, J. V., Fox, P. T., and Raichle, M. E. (1991) Localization of a human system for sustained attention by positron emission tomography. *Nature* 349: 61–63.

Pennekamp, P., Bosel, R., Mecklinger, A., and Ott, H. (1994) Differences in EEG-theta for responded and omitted targets in a sustained attention task. *J. Psychophysiol.* 8: 131–141.

Posner, M. I. (1978) *Chronometric Explorations of Mind*. Hillsdale, NJ: Lawrence Erlbaum.

Posner, M. I. (1980) Orienting of attention. *Q. J. Exp. Psychol.* 32: 3–25.

Posner, M. I. and Petersen, S. E. (1990) The attention system of the human brain. *Annu. Rev. Neurosci.* 13: 25–42.

Posner, M. I. and Raichle, M. (1993) *Images of Mind*. New York: McGraw-Hill.

Povlishock, J. T., Becker, D. P., Sullivan, H. G., and Miller, J. D. (1978) Vascular permability alterations to horseradish peroxidase in experimental brain injury. *Brain Res.* 153: 223–239.

Reivich, M. and Gur, R. (1985) Cerebral metabolic effects of sensory and cognitive stimuli in normal subjects. In *Positron Emission Tomography*, edited by M. Reivich and A. Alavi, pp. 329–344. New York: Liss.

Robbins, T. W. and Everett, B. J. (1995) Arousal systems and attention. In *The Cognitive Neurosciences*, edited by M. S. Gazzaniga, pp. 703–720. Cambridge, MA: MIT Press.

Robertson, I. H., Tegner, R., Tham, K., Lo, A., and Nimmo-Smith, I. (1995) Sustained attention training for unilateral neglect: Theoretical and rehabilitation implications. *J. Clin. Exp. Neuropsychol.* 17: 416–430.

Rohrbaugh, J. W., Stapleton, J. M., Parasuraman, R., Zubovic, E. A., et al. (1987) Dose-related effects of ethanol on visual sustained attention and event-related potentials. *Alcohol* 4: 293–300.

Rosvold, H., Mirsky, A. F., Sarason, I., Bransome, E. D., Jr., and Beck, L. N. (1956) A continuous performance test of brain damage. *J. Consult. Clin. Psychol.* 20: 343–350.

Rueckert, L. and Grafman, J. (1996) Sustained attention deficits in patients with right frontal lesions. *Neuropsychologia* 34: 953–963.

Rueckert, L. M. and Levy, J. (1996) Further evidence that the callosum is involved in sustaining attention. *Neuropsychologia* 34: 927–935.

Rueckert, L. M., Sorenson, L., and Levy, J. (1994) Callosal efficiency is related to sustained attention. *Neuropsychologia* 32: 159–173.

Sarter, M. (1994) Neuronal mechanisms of the attentional dysfunctions in senile dementia and schizophrenia: Two sides of the same coin? *Psychopharmacology* 114: 539–550.

Scerbo, M. W., Warm, J. S., and Fisk, A. D. (1987) Event asynchrony and signal regularity in sustained attention. *Curr. Psychol. Res. Rev.* 5: 335–343.

See, J. E., Howe, S. R., Warm, J. S., and Dember, W. N. (1995) Meta-analysis of the sensitivity decrement in vigilance. *Psychol. Bull.* 117: 230–249.

Shaw, M. L. (1984) Division of attention among spatial locations: A fundamental difference between detection of letters and detection of luminance increments. In *Attention and Performance X*, edited by H. Bouma and D. Bouwhuis, pp. 109–121. Hillsdale, NJ: Lawrence Erlbaum.

Skinner, J. E. and Yingling, C. D. (1977) Central gating mechanisms that regulate event-related potentials and behavior: A neural model for attention. In *Attention, Voluntary Contraction, and Event-Related Cerebral Potentials*, edited by J. E. Desmedt, pp. 30–69. Basel: S. Karger.

Smith, A., and Nutt, D. (1996) Noradrenaline and attention lapses. *Nature* 380: 291.

Steriade, M. (1996) Awakening the brain. *Nature* 383: 24–25.

Steriade, M. and Llinas, R. R. (1988) The functional states of the thalamus and the associated neuronal interplay. *Physiol. Rev.* 68: 649–742.

Stickgold, R., Baker, D., Kosslyn, S., and Hobson, J. A. (1995, Mar.) On-line vigilance monitoring with the Nightcap. Paper presented at the second annual meeting of the Cognitive Neuroscience Society, San Francisco, CA.

Strauss, J., Lewis, J. L., Klorman, R., Peloquin, L. J., Perlmutter, R. A., and Salzman, L. F. (1984) Effects of methylphenidate on young adults' performance and event-related potentials in a vigilance and a paired-associates learning test. *Psychophysiology* 21: 609–621.

Teichner, W. H. (1974) The detection of a simple visual signal as a function of time on watch. *Hum. Fac.* 16: 339–353.

Valentino, D. A., Arruda, J. E., and Gold, S. M. (1993) Comparison of QEEG and response accuracy in good versus poorer performers during a vigilance task. *Int. J. Psychophysiol.* 15: 123–133.

Warburton, D. M. (1977) Stimulus selection and behavioral inhibition. In *Handbook of Psychopharmacology*, edited by L. L. Iversen, S. D. Iversen, and S. H. Snyder, pp. 385–431. New York: Plenum Press.

Warm, J. S. (ed.) (1984) *Sustained Attention in Human Performance*. London: Wiley.

Warm, J. S. and Dember, W. N. (1998) Tests of a vigilance taxonomy. In *Viewing Psychology as a Whole: The Integrative Science of William N. Dember*, edited by R. R. Hoffman, M. F. Sherrick, and J. S. Warm. Washington, DC: American Psychological Association.

Warm, J. S., Dember, W. N., Murphy, A. Z., and Dittmar, M. L. (1992) Sensing and decision-making components of the signal-regularity effect in vigilance performance. *Bull. Psychonom. Soc.* 30: 297–300.

Warm, J. S., Dember, W. N., and Parasuraman, R. (1991) Effects of olfactory stimulation on performance and stress in a visual sustained attention task. *J. Soc. Cosmet. Chemists* 42: 199–210.

Warm, J. S. and Jerison, H. J. (1984) The psychophysics of vigilance. In *Sustained Attention in Human Performance*, edited by J. S. Warm, pp. 15–59. London: Wiley.

Warm, J. S., Richter, D. O., Sprague, R. L., Porter, P. K., and Schumsky, D. A. (1980) Listening with a dual brain: Hemispheric asymmetry in sustained attention. *Bull. Psychonom. Soc.* 15: 229–232.

Warm, J. S., Schumsky, D. A., and Hawley, D. K. (1976) Ear asymmetry and temporal uncertainty in sustained attention. *Bull. Psychonom. Soc.* 7: 413–416.

Welford, A. T. (1962) Arousal, channel capacity, and decision. *Nature* 194: 365–366.

Whitehead, R. (1991) Right hemisphere processing superiority during sustained visual attention. *J. Cognitive Neurosci.* 3: 329–334.

Whyte, J., Polansky, M., Fleming, M., Coslett, H. B., and Cavallucci, C. (1995) Sustained arousal and attention after traumatic brain injury. *Neuropsychologia* 33: 797–813.

Wilkins, A. J., Shallice, T., and McCarthy, R. (1987) Frontal lesions and sustained attention. *Neuropsychologia* 25: 359–366.

Wilkinson, R. T. (1969) Sleep deprivation: Performance tests for partial and selective sleep deprivation. In *Progress in Clinical Psychology* (Vol. 7), edited by L. A. Abt and B. F. Reiss, pp. 267–279. New York: Grune and Stratton.

Wilkinson, R. T., Morlock, H. C., and Williams, H. L. (1966) Evoked cortical response during vigilance. *Psychon. Sci.* 4: 221–222.

Yokoyama, K., Jennings, R., Ackles, P., Hood, P., and Boller, F. (1987) Lack of heart rate changes during an attention-demanding task after right hemisphere lesions. *Neurology* 37: 624–630.

12 Visuospatial Attention and Parietal Function: Their Role in Object Perception

Lynn C. Robertson

ABSTRACT Studies of feature and conjunction search in normal adults and in patients with parietal lobe damage are discussed within the context of feature integration theory. The role of search in object perception and in visual awareness is also examined. The evidence from patients with unilateral and bilateral damage suggests a crucial role for both parietal lobes in explicit access of spatial information for purposes of attending to objects. These studies also indicate that feature search does not require an intact explicit spatial map, whereas conjunction search does. Illusory conjunctions are prominent and pose a real-life problem when the spatial map is impaired. The data further suggest that a major foundation of visual awareness may be the accurate computation of space from a variety of spatial maps.

It has long been known by neurologists and neuropsychologists that spatial and object deficits can occur independently of one another. Visual agnosias, defined in their classical sense as visual object recognition problems, are more often seen after damage to the temporal lobes, whereas visuospatial problems are more likely observed following damage to the parietal lobes (De Renzi, 1982).

The development of electrophysiological techniques that allow the measurement of the electrical activity of a single neuron has confirmed that dissociation in nonhuman primates (De Yoe and Van Essen, 1988; Ungerleider and Haxby, 1994). Areas along the ventral temporal pathway contain neurons that are responsive to object features such as color, brightness, and shape, whereas areas along the dorsal parietal pathway contain neurons that are responsive to spatial features necessary for localization, perception of motion, and preparation for action (Anderson, 1987; Colby, Duhamel, and Goldberg 1993a; Goodale and Milner, 1992). In addition, electrophysiological techniques have suggested the existence of a somewhat modular system for visual processing, with different areas within each pathway responding to different features. For instance, neurons in one area of the temporal lobe are more responsive to color than to other features, whereas neurons in another area are more responsive to shape (Desimone, Shein, Moran, and Ungerleider, 1985). The number of these specialized areas has been estimated at about 30, and that number seems to grow yearly (Kaas, 1989; Fellerman and Van Essen, 1991). The neuropsychological evidence collected from humans with brain injury is consistent with that modular architecture.

Although rare, several cases have been reported in which patients with focal cortical lesions have fairly isolated deficits in seeing single features such as color, motion, or shape.

It may appear surprising that the visual system basically tears the sensory input apart and sorts different features into different bins, given that there is spatial coincidence of different features from the retina through primary visual cortex and to progressively lesser extents beyond. This rendering is even harder to comprehend because our own perception of objects is that they are joined together in our visual experience; they have a shape, size, color, texture, and so forth, and they exist in a particular location. The features of an object are bound to each other to form a unique object. Each object is bound to a location and is separated from other objects either by its distinct features or by its relative location or by both. When the features of two objects are the same, as when two identical twins are pictured standing next to each other, the attribute that signals the presence of two distinct individuals is their different locations. They cannot be individuated by distinctive features, at least to the untrained eye, because they are identical. Furthermore, when two objects are different, as when two fraternal twins are pictured next to each other, either the location or the different features can signal the presence of distinct individuals. But if the visual system is modular, how does it decide which features belong to which shapes? Why is the fraternal female twin seen to be wearing the blue skirt instead of her sister's red skirt? That example presents the essence of one of the enormous problems that the visual system must solve in order to perceive unified objects and unified scenes of objects in natural settings, given evidence for a relatively modular architecture. How does the brain bind the proper features to the proper locations so that our perception of the world is at least as veridical as we need it to be?

The solution to this "binding problem" has remained elusive. This chapter focuses on evidence collected from neurological patients with spatial attentional deficits. This work is beginning to suggest ways in which the brain may solve the binding problem. At least part of the proposed solution comes from predictions made by feature integration theory (FIT), which was proposed some years ago by Treisman and Gelade (1980). That theory was developed entirely from behavioral data collected from young normal subjects before much was known about the modular architecture of the visual cortex. Perhaps the theory would have been applied to cognitive neuroscience sooner had Anne Treisman been a neurologist or if she had called her theory feature binding theory (the acronym FBT is harder to pronounce than is FIT); in any event, its relevance for the binding problem in neuropsychological research was too long ignored.

The basic tenets of FIT are that features in a display are encoded separately in individual feature maps that represent color, orientation, brightness, motion, and so forth. In multi-item arrays, these features are bound together to form individual objects through attention to their shared location. This requires the representation of a rather high level of spatial representation, or what Treisman calls the "master map of locations" (Treisman and Gelade, 1980). Although feature maps are presumed to have some location information, attention to locations in the master map (as it turns out, the map that we know and of which we are consciously aware) is required for normal feature integration. FIT further proposes that spatial attention operates as a type of filter within this map in that it temporarily inhibits features from locations outside the area attended, and thus increases the signal-to-noise ratio for features at the currently attended location relative to the background locations (Treisman, 1988).

This theory predicts that illusory conjunctions (ICs), or the improper binding of features, should appear when display durations are limited, and that ICs should be more likely when attention is diverted. Both of those predictions have been supported by evidence from studies of normal healthy subjects under controlled laboratory conditions (Prinzmetal, Presti, and Posner, 1986). When displays are brief and when spatial attention is diverted, the features of one item may be integrated inappropriately with the feature of another item (e.g., a blue T and a green O may miscombine and be perceived as a green T and a blue O).

FIT also predicts that search for a conjunction target (e.g., blue O among green Os & blue Ts) should be quite difficult, because attention needs to be deployed serially to items in the display in order to integrate the features at each location for each item or for each group of items (Wolfe, Cave, and Franzel, 1989). It follows that some location information is available to guide the search in order to avoid random selection of potential target items. Conversely, searching for a single feature (e.g., blue or O) within a display should be rapid and theoretically parallel. If the blue O is among green Ts, or even if it is among green Ts and blue Ts, a serial search is not required because the task does not require allocation of attention to locations. These predictions have also been supported by data collected from young healthy subjects (Treisman and Schmidt, 1982).

Of course, there are alternative accounts to FIT. For instance, Duncan and Humphreys (1989) proposed that conjunction search appears to be serial (reaction time increases linearly with the number of distractors or grouped distractors in the display), but that this increase could be accounted for by visual salience of the target with reference to a two-dimensional similarity scale: the similarity of the target to the distractors and the similarity of the distractors to each other. They concluded that feature search is typically fast and easy for that reason. If feature similarities are different enough in both dimensions, finding a feature target in a three-item array should take minimally less time than finding the same target in a 16-item array. Unlike the proposal of FIT that perception of conjunction and feature targets is qualitatively different (the first requiring binding and spatial attention and the second requiring neither), Duncan and Humphreys argue that the two may be qualitatively the same. Similarity is typically different for the two types of target displays, with conjunction displays producing closer similarity values than do feature displays; thus, according to Duncan & Humphreys, conjunction displays produce increased visual noise which produces slow search (although, see Treisman, 1991, where similarity is controlled and conjuction search still produces serial search patterns).

The proposition that illusory conjunction errors sometimes represent something other than erroneous binding has also been suggested, although Ashby, Prinzmetal, Ivry, and Maddox (1996) found little support for that proposition in normal subjects. Nevertheless, it should be held in mind that illusory conjunctions may represent separately seen features without the actual percept of an inappropriately bound object. For instance, a person who reports seeing a green T may actually have seen a T and the color green independently, not necessarily the two bound together in error. Note that in either case there is a binding problem, consistent with the modular architecture of the visual cortex. Both cases require some type of binding mechanism to integrate features into the whole objects that we see. Spatial attention may be required for proper binding in either case.

In cognitive psychology, the debates and discussions of limitations continue. Hundreds, and perhaps by now thousands, of articles report the effects of task and stimulus parameters on conjunction and feature search and on illusory conjunctions. In healthy normal subjects, one must go to great lengths to keep the visual system from doing accurately what it generally does so well: perceive whole objects and their spatial relations. However, in some cases when the brain has been damaged, a person may not be aware of space beyond certain borders, and in some cases those borders are defined by a single object. In the rare cases when both parietal lobes are damaged, spatial abilities can be severely impaired to the point where a person loses all practical knowledge of spatial locations and for all intents and purposes becomes functionally blind. It is interesting and important that such patients can detect simple features but have grave difficulties detecting a conjunction. Toward the end of this chapter evidence from such a patient is discussed. First findings from patients with unilateral damage and with unilateral visual neglect, where one half of space is affected, are examined.

Although the original intent of this line of research was to address questions of attentional dysfunction, the relevance of these data for FIT and the binding problem have become the focus of current investigations in collaboration with Anne Treisman. Overall, the data support the predictions of FIT, but in addition, the data demonstrate that spatial dysfunction associated with dorsal parietal damage also disrupts proper feature integration.

VISUAL SEARCH IN UNILATERAL NEGLECT

Unilateral visual neglect is a remarkable behavioral phenomenon: a person can lose visual awareness of one half of the visual world but maintain awareness of the other half. Visual neglect comes in many different forms and severities, but patients with neglect have the common problem of not responding to information that is contralateral to the side of the lesion. Also, it is well documented that the neglected space need not be defined only within head or retinal coordinates. Neglect does occur in retinal coordinates, but also in environmental and object-centered coordinates as well (Behrmann and Moscovitch, 1994; Calvanio, Petrone, and Levine, 1987; Driver and Halligan, 1994; Farah, Wong, Wallace, and Carpenter, 1990; Ladavas, 1987). It is likely that some of the differences observed among patients with neglect are due to different functional contributions associated with the different anatomical areas involved in spatial attention (Rafal and Robertson, 1995). However, the classical symptoms of neglect, defined as a spatial deficit for one half of the field, have been more closely linked to functions of the parietal lobes (Heilman and Valenstein, 1985). Electrophysiological studies with monkeys have supported the importance of parietal areas in spatial mapping as well (Anderson 1987; Anderson, Snyder, Li, and Stricanne, 1993; Colby et al., 1993a,b; Duhamel, Colby, and Goldberg, 1992).

It must be emphasized that the anatomical loci of spatial mapping is extraordinarily difficult to sort out in patients during acute stages after stroke when neglect is at its worst. It may take up to six months for neurological problems to stabilize, by which point it is more likely than not that clinical symptoms of unilateral neglect are gone. Thus, a number of experimental reports with patients concerning neuroanatomy and neglect may be somewhat misleading, because dysfunction in areas distant from the damage may be prevalent following insult to nearly any part of the same hemisphere during acute stages. One way to start to approach that problem is by testing the same patients again at a later date or by testing patients with neglect syndrome in acute stages and testing other stable patient groups based on anatomical criteria well after the acute effects have subsided. At that later stage, more subtle effects would be expected and can be observed in such measures as reaction time (RT) or signal detection.

The studies discussed in this chapter were originally conceived with those problems in mind. Patients with visual neglect were selected as subjects according to behavioral criteria and later (at least six months and up to 13 years after insult) according to anatomical criteria. Somewhat later, a patient with bilateral parietal damage was tested beginning seven months after his second stroke in 1992 and continues to be tested.

Original findings concerning visual search with patients with unilateral visual neglect were consistent with a distinction between preattentive parallel search and attentive conjunction search (for supporting evidence, see Humphreys and Riddoch, 1993). Eglin, Robertson, and Knight (1989) demonstrated that, even though these patients had moderately severe visual attention deficits that were observed clinically, they could respond rapidly to a distinct feature on the neglected side of a display. RT to find a feature on either the contralesional or ipsilesional side of a display was unaffected by the number of items.

In contrast, search for a conjunction target was slow (8.8 s on the neglected side and 2.3 s on the ipsilesional side overall). However, the most surprising result was that the rate of conjunction search was just as poor on the so-called intact, ipsilesional side of space as on the neglected side (about 300 ms per item on the ipsilesional and on the neglected side). It was as if the spatial computations of where attention should go next were performed piecemeal or slowly, first on one side and then on the other, and that the resources necessary to perform spatial computations across the visual field had been severely curtailed.

Contralesional neglect was revealed in a different measure, what we will call the contralateral delay. That is, the difference in the length of time that passed before subjects began searching the intact or neglected side of the display was extremely large. This finding is consistent with a disengagement problem of some sort or an orienting bias to an ipsilesional location that acts as the source of a spatial coordinate for spatial computations. We assume that that source would normally be located close to fixation. Initiation of a conjunction search on the neglected side could be delayed as long as 10 to 20 s. The magnitude of the delay increased as the number of distractors on the ipsilesional side increased but could not be accounted for entirely by a simple sweep from that side toward the other field. There was a bias to begin searching on the intact side, as expected, but, in addition, there was something special about the midline of the display (also coincident with body midline) that produced the contralateral delay.

The design of the original study used visual search procedures developed by Treisman and Gelade (1980), but added the factors of side of the distractors and side of the target. The side of distractors was orthogonally varied with the target side of the display and with the number of distractors on each side of the display (either 0, 10, or 19).

Figure 12.1 shows four display examples. In 12.1A, the target is on the neglected side among 19 distractors on the same side and 0 distractors on the ipsilesional side. In 12.1B, the target is on the neglected side among 19 distractors on the same side and 10 distractors on the ipsilesional side. In 12.1C, the target is on the ipsilesional side with 9 distractors on the same side and 20 distractors on the neglected side. In 12.1D, the target is on the neglected side with 19 distractors on that side and 20 distractors on the ipsilesional side. (The actual stimuli were in color. The target was a red dot with a line through it and each distractor was either a red solid dot or a blue dot with a line through it.)

The traditional procedures, in which subjects respond whether a target was present or not, could not be used. Humphreys and Riddoch (1993) have demonstrated that under such conditions patients with neglect would nearly always say "no" when the target was on the neglect side of the display. However, if the subjects knew that a target would be present in every display, they continued to search until the target was found. Their error rate

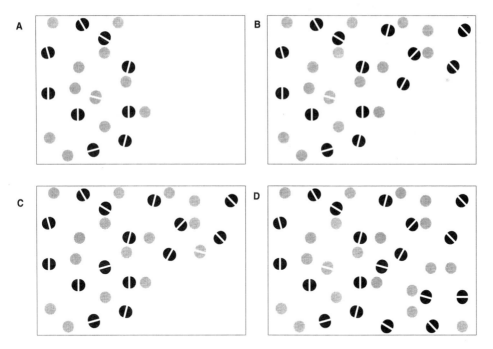

Figure 12.1 Examples of conjunction search stimuli. (A) Target and all distractors on the left; 0 distractors on the opposite side; (B) target on the left with 19 distractors on the same and 10 distractors on the opposite side; (C) target on the right with 9 distractors on the same and 20 distractors on the opposite side; (D) target on the left with 19 distractors on the same and 20 distractors on the opposite side (grey = red and black = blue).

was less than 3% under those conditions (and about 50% with the yes/no task).

A preliminary study of young healthy subjects was first run using the yes/no procedure to make sure that searching for a target in these displays would replicate other search data, and it did. The search rate was 24 ms per item for conjunction search, and the ratio of the slope for target present versus target absent trials was .54, which is very close to the 1:2 ratio for yes/no responses expected in serial search (Eglin et al., 1989).

Figure 12.2 shows the base search rate for a group of seven patients with unilateral visual neglect, calculated from conditions in which both the target and distractors were all on the ipsilesional side of the display (e.g. the mirror image of figure 12.1A for patients with right hemisphere damage). The base search rate was calculated for patients for the ipsilesional side of the displays, and right and left sides were randomly selected for each of the 12 age-matched control subjects. Both patient and control groups showed evidence of serial search (linearly increasing RTs across distractor number), but the search rate for patients was nearly 10 times that for normal age-matched control subjects.

Figure 12.3 shows the effect of opposite-side distractors (the number of distractors opposite the target side) on search functions for the patients. Data

Conjunction

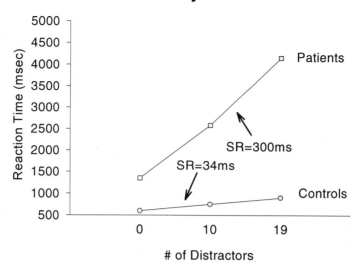

Figure 12.2 Baseline reaction time (all distractors on same side as target, 0 distractors on opposite side) for patients with unilateral visual neglect and for age-matched controls subjects. SR = search rate.

CONJUNCTION

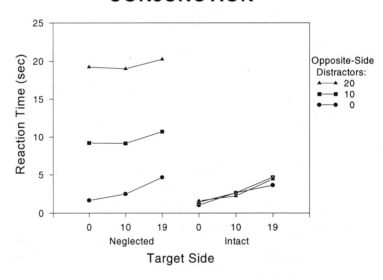

Figure 12.3 Mean reaction time for patients with unilateral visual neglect as a function of target side and distractor side. (Adapted from Eglin et al., 1989.)

from normal subjects, who showed symmetrical performance across right and left sides, are not presented. The data from patients are striking on several counts.

1. The baseline functions (no opposite-side distractors) were statistically equal. As long as there was nothing in the ipsilesional side to attract attention, search began as rapidly on the ipsilesional and neglected side of space and occurred at approximately the same slow rate (note the change in scale from figure 12.2). This finding also demonstrates that there was no primary deficit in moving the head or eyes toward the neglected side with these patients. When nothing was present to attract attention to the ipsilesional side, search began on the neglected side.

2. Distractors on the neglected side had no effect on search rate for a target on the ipsilesional side. The functions on the right of figure 12.3 lie on top of each other. This finding is not surprising, given that these patients suffered from neglect. It simply shows that when a target was present on the ipsilesional side of space, distractors on the neglected side were neglected.

3. Distractors on the ipsilesional side had huge effects on initiation of search for a target on the neglected side. It took nearly three times the base search rate of 300 ms per item to begin to search the neglected field. For example, 10 distractors on the ipsilesional side (squares) slowed response time to a left-sided target by nearly 8 s. Because patients were allowed to move their eyes and did so freely, the midline must have been defined extraretinally.

4. The effect of distractors on RT to a target on the neglected side was present for the intercept and not for the slope of the functions. Once attention was oriented to the neglected side, search occurred at nearly the same rate as it did on the ipsilesional side (although it was somewhat more variable). It was as if the subjects now realized that the previously neglected side of the display existed.

These findings were replicated in a subsequent study using small and large displays and different types of distractors and targets (Eglin, Robinson, Knight, and Brugger, 1994).

Because the patients took so long to respond, it was not possible for them to maintain fixation throughout the trial. Both control subjects and patients were allowed to move their eyes freely, following initial fixation. The relationship between the patients' eye movements and performance is unknown, but it may be the case that these eye movements allowed spatial information to be computed for the neglected side as the eyes moved, and visual search could then proceed, albeit at its overall slow pace.

Grabowecky, Robertson, and Treisman (1993) demonstrated that the magnitude of visual neglect could be changed by changes in the center of mass of a stimulus display, a change that also influences the landing position of a saccade in normals. If the center of mass defines the source of a spatial coordinate and if the spatial field is computed relative to that source, then eye movements into the neglected field may change the source and thus change the external locations over which spatial information can be computed. If spatial computations are slowed when one parietal lobe has to perform the work of two, then the pattern of data reported here would be expected.

VISUAL SEARCH IN STABLE PATIENTS WITH UNILATERAL CORTICAL LESIONS

The lesions in patients in the studies discussed previously were highly variable. Again, symptoms of neglect associated with areas outside of damaged areas seen on a magnetic resonance image (MRI) scan are not surprising in patients with recent stroke. As a result, little could be said about functional neuroanatomy associated with visual search. In a subsequent study, groups were formed based on anatomical criteria from MRI or computerized tomography (CT) evidence of a single unilateral lesion. The patient participants were all high-functioning individuals who were between 1 and 13 years post insult. None had clinical signs of unilateral neglect at the time of testing. Because they were not observed directly by us after their strokes, we were not able to test them for neglect or extinction at that time, but the charts sometimes noted evidence of these problems in acute states.

The subjects were tested with the same study design described in the previous section. The data from a group of patients with lesions centered in the dorsolateral frontal lobe, from a group with lesions centered in the parietal lobe, and from a group with lesions centered in the temporal-parietal junction are presented in figures 12.4 and 12.5. Figure 12.4 presents the data for the base search rates, which were calculated in the same way as in the previously discussed study (when no distractors were on the opposite or contralesional side of the display). Figure 12.5 presents the data from the entire factorial.

Notice that the baseline search rate for both the frontal and parietal groups were normal (42 and 50 ms), whereas the mean search rate for the temporal-parietal group was somewhat elevated (75 ms), although it was not statistically different from controls or from any other group. For patients, baseline conjunction search rates were equal for both sides of the display for all groups.

These results are consistent with full recovery of conjunction search rate in two of the three groups and with nearly complete recovery in the third (figure 12.4). Nevertheless, even for these groups there was statistical evidence of a contralateral delay, as previously observed in patients with unilateral neglect. The differences between the functions on the two sides of the figure were not as dramatic as they were for patients with neglect, but the contralateral delay was still statistically evident (figure 12.5).

However, unlike with patients with neglect, there was no special elevation at the midline of the display. The time to initiate search on the contralesional

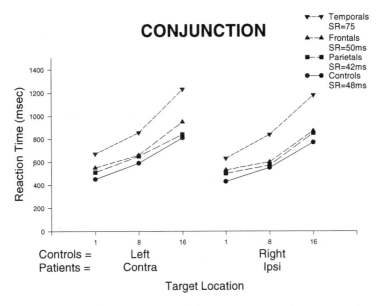

Figure 12.4 Baseline reaction time (all distractors on same side as target, 0 distracters on opposite side) for stable patients with unilateral lesions centered in the temporal-parietal junction, the dorsolateral frontal lobe, or the inferior parietal lobe, and for age-matched controls subjects. SR, search rate.

side was predicted by the base search rate, with all patients beginning to search at the most ipsilesional side of the stimulus and progressing contralesionally across the display (Eglin, Robertson, and Knight, 1991). Thus, a residual attentional bias to begin to look for targets on the side ipsilesional to the lesion remained, although the search rate itself was normal. This is also consistent with data showing that spatial cueing effects remain abnormal in these types of patients (Posner, Walker, Friedrich, and Rafal, 1984). When attention has to move in the contralesional direction to detect a target in an unexpected location, response time is slowed much more in these patients than in normal controls.

In these studies, the only group that continued to show any elevation in search time had lesions centered in the temporal-parietal junction. The overall bias of where to begin search and the search rate are dissociated, consistent with the idea that different mechanisms are responsible for the two effects. One may be primarily spatial and the other directly attentional. These results are also consistent with different contributions from various neural systems to the phenomenon of unilateral neglect (Rafal and Robertson, 1995).

VISUAL SEARCH AND ILLUSORY CONJUNCTIONS IN A PATIENT WITH BILATERAL PARIETAL DAMAGE AND BALINT'S SYNDROME

The presentation of a rare case—a patient with Balint's syndrome due to bilateral parietal lesions—afforded the opportunity to study a neurologically

Robertson: Visuospatial Attention and Parietal Function

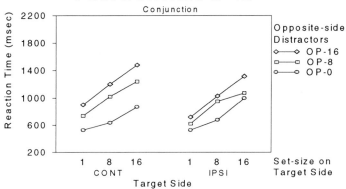

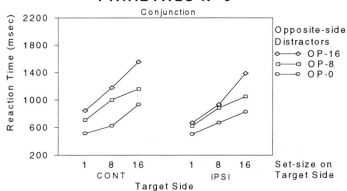

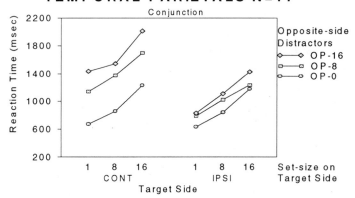

Figure 12.5 Mean reaction time for stable patients with unilateral lesions centered in temporal-parietal junction, the dorsolateral frontal lobe, or the inferior parietal lobe, and for age-matched controls as a function of target side (contralesional, ipsilesional) and distractor side. (Adapted from Eglin et al., 1991.)

stable patient who, unlike patients with unilateral lesions, did not have a second intact parietal lobe. With unilateral damage, the intact parietal lobe may compensate over time for visuospatial functions of the damaged hemisphere. The patient (RM) suffered two embolic strokes approximately seven months apart (July, 1991, and March, 1992). The resulting lesions were nearly symmetrical and were located in occipitoparietal regions (see the three-dimensional MRI reconstructed in Friedman-Hill, Robertson, and Treisman, 1995).

As a result of his second stroke, RM was left with a neuropsychological syndrome known as Balint's syndrome (sometimes called simultanagnosia or dorsal simultanagnosia). The syndrome is characterized by optic ataxia (deficit in visually guided reaching), psychic paralysis of gaze (sustained fixation in the absence of primary eye movement deficits), and peripheral inattention (Balint, 1909; Holmes, 1918; Luria, 1959). The hallmark of the syndrome appears as hyperattention to one object in a scene without conscious awareness of other objects at the same time. Formal opthalmological examination demonstrated that RM had intact visual sensation, but he had virtually no idea where things were in his environment. He could easily report the identity of a single object, whether it was very large or very small, but he could not say where it was.

Testing with this patient began in the fall of 1992, some months after his second embolic stroke. Several findings are relevant for the topic of this chapter and they can be summarized as follows.

RM had severe deficits in explicit access to spatial representations. RM made gross mistakes in spatial judgments. During initial testing, he could not discriminate right from left nor up from down except on his own body. He could report that a stimulus positioned at the top of a computer screen was at the bottom and would do so confidently. A stimulus positioned at the right of a display could be reported as on the left. This was not due to some type of spatial confusion. RM could accurately raise his right or left hand as directed and could report which of his own hands had been touched by an examiner. He had accurate information about interpersonal space in the presence of a severe deficit in locating information in visual space. This deficit was reflected in his everyday behavior and left him functionally blind. Upon initial examination he had to be escorted into the hospital and could not perform basic tasks, such as eating or dressing, without help. His visual problems improved substantially and somewhat surprisingly over a period of three years, as did his spatial abilities. Nevertheless, systematic tests of his spatial abilities showed that deficits remained apparent in the laboratory, as they did in some activities of daily life (Robertson, Treisman, Friedman-Hill and Grabowecky, 1997).

As predicted by the previous studies of patients with unilateral visual neglect as well as by FIT, RM had severe deficits in visual search for a conjunction target. Examination of RM's visual search abilities demonstrated that he could accurately and rapidly respond to a feature target in a display.

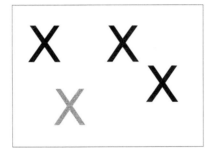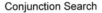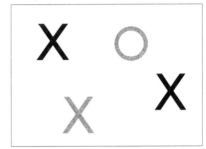

Figure 12.6 Examples of feature and conjunction search displays used when testing patient RM (grey = red, black = green). The target was a red X.

His RTs did not increase and if anything they decreased as distractors were added to the feature displays. His voice RTs were less than 1 s and he was confident in reporting whether a red X among red and green Os was present or absent in a display. Nevertheless, when he was asked to report where the feature was located, he could not do so (Grabowecky, Egly, Robertson, and Rafal, 1993).

In contrast to feature search rate, RM's ability to search for a conjunction target (a red X among green Xs and red Os) was severely impaired. In displays of only two, four, or six items (see figure 12.6), his RTs were as long as 5 s, and he was wrong nearly a quarter of the time. An important element of his mistakes is that his percentage of false alarms was higher than was his percentage of misses in conjunction search. In contrast, feature search was quite accurate, and false alarm and miss rates were approximately the same (Robertson, Treisman, Freidman-Hill, and Grabowecky, 1997).

It is intriguing to note that in a positron emission tomography (PET) study by Corbetta, Shulman, Miezin, and Petersen (1995), parietal and occipitotemporal involvement was found when normal subjects were required to attend to the conjunction of motion and color in a visual display. Ventral but not parietal areas were involved during attention to the single feature of either color or motion. In this light, it is also intriguing that RM exhibited illusory conjunctions between motion and shape as well (Bernstein and Robertson, submitted).

RM made illusory conjunctions at display times of up to 10 s (Friedman-Hill et al., 1995; Robertson et al, 1997). He did this even when he was looking directly at the item he reported. According to FIT, features of shape (X) and color (red) are conjoined by attending to spatial location. Healthy subjects make illusory conjunctions (e.g., conjoining a letter with the color of another item in the display) under conditions of limited stimulus exposure or divided attention. It did not require special conditions for RM to make illusory conjunctions, and he did so confidently while the stimulus was in full view.

Reasonably accurate spatial information is necessary to conjoin features correctly, because attention must be allocated to the location of a particular item. Given RM's spatial deficits, FIT predicts that he would make more illusory conjunctions than would normal controls. This was true, but in more dramatic ways than was at first anticipated.

In the first study, two letters, selected from O, T, or X, were presented on each trial. Each letter in a pair was either blue, red, or yellow. RM was told to report the name of the letter and its color on each trial. In RM's initial testing session, he had an IC rate of nearly 40% at an exposure time of 500 ms (unmasked) (Robertson et al., 1997). Normal subjects make virtually no conjunction errors at these display times. RM also made ICs even when he had up to 10 s to view a stimulus.

RM's IC rate improved over time as his spatial abilities improved. His rate of IC appeared consistent with the severity of his spatial deficits. Finally, it is intriguing to note that Cohen and Rafal (1991) and Arguin, Cavanagh, and Joanette (1994) reported that patients (using an elevated spatial cueing effect as an inclusion criterion) had a larger IC rate in their contralesional than in their ipsilesional visuals fields under time limited conditions. Their patients' spatial knowledge was not tested directly, but the higher rate on the contralesional side would predict that explicit access to spatial information would also be impaired.

RM appeared to have relatively intact spatial representations that he could not access (Robertson et al., 1997). Preliminary evidence suggested that spatial information was intact at subthreshold levels in RM's visual system. When the word "UP" or "DOWN" was presented in the upper on lower portion of a 10 degrees vertical rectangle with the word 2.5 degrees from the center of the rectangle, RM's voice response time to read the word (which he could do for single words) was significantly faster, by an average of about 140 ms over five sessions (range 77–197 ms), when the word was in a location consistent with its name (e.g., "UP" at the top of the rectangle) than when it was in an inconsistent location (e.g., "UP" at the bottom of the rectangle). There was either Stroop-like spatial interference from the location that was inconsistent with the meaning of the word or else there was spatial facilitation from the location that was consistent with the word meaning. Whether the data reflect facilitation or interference, some type of spatial information was coded to account for the differences.

In a different block of trials, RM was asked to report the location of the words by saying "top" or "bottom." He simply could not report the correct location any better than chance. This problem was in direct contrast to his word-naming performance. When he was to report the location of the word, he refused to venture a guess on nearly half of the 95 trials before testing was aborted. He would simply shake his head and would not respond on those trials. Of the trials in which he did guess (reluctantly), he was 51% correct, or basically at levels of chance. The same stimulus under one condition showed evidence of some type of spatial representation that under another condition could not be accessed. As his ability to report locations of objects explicitly improved over time (up to 80% correct), spatial Stroop interference continued to be tested. Although explicit spatial abilities improved substantially, the magnitude of spatial interference effects remained constant, showing that his explicit ability to localize did not increase the difference in RT between consistent and inconsistent locations.

RM showed normal exogenous cueing effects in an unpublished study performed by Egly and Rafal. They presented unpredictive cues 5 degrees to the right or left of central fixation. An asterisk appeared in either the cued or uncued box 100 ms after the brightening of the cue, and RM responded when it appeared. Catch trials with no target were included to make sure that he had to see the target before responding. RM was able to perform this task rapidly, and he showed normal RT differences between valid and invalid targets. However, when arrows were used as predictive cues in an attempt to test endogenous cueing, RM was not able to perform the task. He became confused, and it is quite possible that he was unable to interpret the cues' meaning (in fact, he appeared not to know which direction the arrows pointed). Although we do not know whether or not endogenous attention was affected in RM in a Posner cueing task, it is clear that exogenous orienting was intact, consistent with the presence of an intact attentional system that could be pulled to a cued location or to a distinct feature in a display. Coslett and Saffran (1991) reported a similar finding in another patient of this type.

SUMMARY OF FINDINGS

The evidence from patients with unilateral and bilateral damage suggests a crucial role for both parietal lobes in explicit access of spatial information for purposes of attending to objects. Over time, there was improvement in RM's explicit spatial abilities, but it was a slow and tedious process requiring extensive practice and effort, and RM had to struggle throughout. Nearly two and a half years after his second stroke, he was capable of making up/down spatial judgments with only about an 8% error rate. But spatial representations were not normal. This error rate occurred with displays that were not time limited and with stimuli that were more than 2 degrees above or below the center of the screen (locations that were nearly 5 degrees apart). Finer spatial judgments that would be easy for us still posed great difficulty for RM long after his second stroke.

These findings from patients with neglect, patients with unilateral damage without clinical signs of neglect, and a patient with bilateral parietal damage suggest the following conclusions.

1. The results support the major propositions of FIT. The detection of features appears to be a qualitatively different process than the detection of conjunctions. It seems that search for a feature does not require an explicit

spatial representation or binding, whereas search for a conjunction requires both. RM was quite accurate in detecting a feature, but even when he did, he could not say where it was. Conjunction search was impaired. Consistently, patients with unilateral neglect found features rapidly whether the object was on their contralesional or ipsilesional side, but the patients produced slopes in the order of 300 ms per item when searching for a conjunction.

2. The parietal lobes appear to be involved in representing a complex level of space that corresponds to the space that we see, attend to, and act in. Without this space, endogenous attentional control to a location is disrupted and serial search is slow.

3. Spatial information is required to properly bind features. RM's data lead directly to the prediction that the spatial representations of the dorsal parietal pathway interact with feature representations of the ventral temporal pathway to produce proper binding. If neural correlation is required in the binding process, as some have suggested (Koch and Crick, 1994; Singer and Gray, 1995), then one prediction would be that neural correlation should be found between units in targeted areas of parietal (area 7) and temporal cortex (perhaps area V4; see Luck, Chelazzi, Hillyard, and Desimone, 1997).

4. Feature integration may be a relatively late stage of processing, in the sense that it depends on a high level of spatial representation. This representation appears to be isomorphic with the natural world and it appears to define the space we perceive explicitly.

5. Spatial information below the level of awareness seems to exist in RM, and likely in patients with neglect (although this is now being tested systematically in neglect populations), but this spatial information seems to not be adequate for serial visual search. There appear to be multiple spatial maps in the brain, and each may function for different purposes (see Graziano and Gross, 1995).

Although the evidence for parietal involvement in feature binding is quite strong from our studies with patients, there are accounts of binding that do not rely on the parietal lobe. For instance, Desimone and Duncan (1995) argue that the temporal lobe is capable of binding features on its own. Electrophysiological studies have shown that there is spatial information within these cells that they argue could be adequate for feature binding. Many temporal cells respond to highly complex patterns that presumably require feature integration. However, Desimone and Duncan also mention that these responses are observed even when the animal is anesthetized. Of course, it is possible that there are representations below the surface of awareness that contain bound features in some form, and these may require spatial representations that exist below the level of awareness as well. However, if the parietal lobe functions to bring these already bound features above some threshold, then illusory conjunctions at long exposures, as we found in RM, would not be expected. When he saw the letter X it should have been bound with its proper color. If implicit conjunctions do exist, they would need to become unbound and then be reconjoined to account for RM's data.

Spatial maps that normally exist below the threshold of spatial awareness could be beneficial for a number of reasons. First, it is possible that these maps are tied to coordinates or to cortical maps that govern eye movements or to spatial maps that are retinally defined, such as in areas V1 or V2. Although in unusual situations (such as in the experimental laboratory) it might be important to explicitly know where things are located relative to our retina, it seems an inefficient way to perceive the world in which we live. Retinal spatial maps must exist in order to register the information, but the space we want to know about is the one that conforms to objects that exist in the environment. A visual system that is a slave to retinal (or even to head- or body-centered) coordinates would not be very useful for most explicit perpetual activities. A spatial representation that is reasonably iso-morphic with the three-dimensional space of the natural world must be ac-cessible for survival, and this requires computational complexity that seems to require the spatial functions of the dorsal pathway. It appears to be this spatial representation that contributes to the accurate integration of features of the objects that enter awareness.

CONCLUSIONS

It is difficult to come away from a conversation with the type of patients that I have discussed in this chapter without questioning personal assumptions about our percepts and their relationship to the physical nature of objects in the natural world. What must it be like to lose complete awareness of one half of visual space, yet not know it? What is it that supports our everyday assurance that when we look at a scene, it will look whole? What would it be like if the visual world we are used to disappeared, not by blackening as with retinal damage, but by a chaos of signals that we could not integrate? How would we interpret the experience of seeing an object but discovering that, when we reach for it, it is not there? Would we think, "Aha—Balint's syn-drome," or would we think we might be hallucinating? How would the world look if space collapsed into the one object that we could articulate at the present moment, only to be replaced abruptly and at random intervals with other objects? How would we know where to look for another object after our attention was drawn to one? How could we even be confident that another object existed?

The data discussed in the present chapter show that the consequences of a loss of conscious access to spatial representation can be harrowing (see also Coslett and Saffran, 1991; Rafal, 1996). They also offer some clues about the way normal brains may compute spatial information in order to perceive and attend to objects veridically. We have made no direct measurements of neural responses, but the data suggest a high degree of neural interaction between areas of the cortex that are responsible for veridical spatial perception (dorsal pathwells) and other areas that code features and objects and perhaps implicit spatial information (ventral pathways). It will remain for future research to determine the nature of this interaction (perhaps temporal correlations between parietal and temporal neurons). Whatever this relation turns out to be, the data from patients were predicted by FIT and, in turn, articulate the type of spatial information that is critical for the theory. Feature search does not require an intact explicit spatial map; conjunction search does. Illusory conjunctions are prominent and pose a real-life problem when the spatial map is impaired. Binding or conjunctions of features that enter awareness require a rather high level of spatial representation. The data further suggest that a major foundation for visual awareness of more than one object may be the accurate computation of space from a variety of spatial maps (for similar arguments, see Bisiach and Luzzatti, 1978; Bisiach, Luzzatti, and Perani, 1979; Rizzolatti, Riggio, and Sheliga, 1994). If this foundation fails completely, we not only lose the ability to know where things are but also how they are put together and perhaps the very basis of visual awareness itself.

ACKNOWLEDGMENTS

The work presented in this chapter was supported by the Veteran's Administration through an Associate Research Career Scientist award to the author and by research funding from the Veteran's Administration Merit Review Board and the National Science Foundation grant SBR-922221B. I wish to thank Anne Treisman for many years of collaboration in portions of this work and the graduate and postgraduate students who were fundamental for its success: Stacia Friedman-Hill, Mirjam Eglin, Robert Egly, Marcia Grabowecky, and Lori Bernstein. I would also like to thank Robert Rafal and Robert Knight for their help in screening the patients and for their informed tutorials in behavioral neurology. Last but not least, I thank the patients themselves, without which this work would not be possible.

REFERENCES

Anderson, R. A. (1987) Inferior parietal lobule function in spatial perception and visuomotor integration. In *Handbook of Physiology*, edited by V. B. Mountcastle, F. Plum, and S. R. Geiger. Bethesda, MD: American Psychological Society.

Anderson, R. A., Snyder, L. H., Li, C. S., and Stricanne, B. (1993) Coordinate transformations in the representation of spatial information. *Curr. Opin. Neurobiol.* 3: 171–176.

Arguin, M., Cavanagh, P., and Joanette, Y. (1994) Visual feature integration with an attentional deficit. *Brain Cogn.* 24: 44–56.

Ashby, F. G., Prinzmetal, W., Ivry, R., and Maddox, T. (1996) A formal theory of illusory conjunctions. *Psychol. Rev.* 103: 165–192.

Balint, R. (1909) Psychic paralysis of gaze, optic ataxia, and spatial disorder of attention (translated by M. Harvey). *Cognitive Neuropsychol.* 12: 265–281.

Behrmann, M. and Moscovitch, M. (1994) Object-centered neglect in patients with unilateral neglect: Effects of left-right coordinates of objects. *J. Cognitive Neurosci.* 6: 1–16.

Bernstein, L., and Robertson L. C. (submitted manuscrpt). Independence between illusory conjunctions of color and motion with shape following bilateral parietal lesions.

Bisiach, E. and Luzzatti, C. (1978) Unilateral neglect of representational space. *Cortex* 14: 129–133.

Bisiach, E., Luzzatti, C., and Perani, C. (1979) Unilateral neglect, representational schema and consciousness. *Brain* 102: 609–618.

Calvanio, R., Petrone, P. N., and Levine, D. N. (1987) Left visual spatial neglect is both environment-centered and body-centered. *Neurology* 37: 1179–1183.

Cohen, A. and Rafal, R. (1991) Attention and feature integration: Illusory conjunctions in a patient with a parietal lobe lesion. *Psychol. Sci.* 2: 106–110.

Colby, C. L., Duhamel, J. R., and Goldberg, M. E. (1993a) The analysis of visual space by the lateral intraparietal area of the monkey: The role of extraretinal signals. *Prog. Brain Res.* 95: 307–316.

Colby, C. L., Duhamel, J. R., and Goldberg, M. E. (1993b) Ventral intraparietal area of the macaque: Anatomic location and visual response properties. *J. Neurophysiol.* 69: 902–914.

Corbetta, M., Shulman, G. L., Miezin, F. M., and Petersen, S. E. (1995) Superior parietal cortex activation during spatial attention shifts and visual feature conjunction. *Science* 270: 802–805.

Coslett, H. B. and Saffran, E. (1991) To see but not two see. *Brain* 113: 1523–1545.

De Renzi, E. (1982) *Disorders of Space Exploration and Cognition.* Toronto: Wiley.

Desimone, R. and Duncan, J. (1995) Neural mechanisms of selective visual attention. *Annu. Rev. Neurosci.* 18: 193–222.

Desimone, R., Shein, S. J., Moran, J., and Ungerleider, L. G. (1985) Contour, color and shape analysis beyond the striate cortex. *Vis. Res.* 25: 441–452.

De Yoe, E. A. and Van Essen, D. C. (1988) Concurrent processing streams in monkey visual cortex. *Trends Neurosci.* 11: 219-226.

Driver, J. and Halligan, P. W. (1991) Can visual neglect operate in object-centered coordinates? An affirmative single case study. *Cognitive. Neuropsychol.* 8: 475–496.

Duhamel, J., Colby, C. L., and Goldberg, M. E. (1992) The updating of the representation of visual space in parietal cortex by intended eye movements. *Science* 255: 90–92.

Duncan, J. and Humphreys, G. W. (1989) Visual search and stimulus similarity. *Psychol. Rev.* 96: 433–458.

Eglin, M., Robertson, L. C., and Knight, R. T. (1989) Visual search performance in the neglect syndrome. *J. Cognitive. Neurosci.* 4: 372–381.

Eglin, M., Robertson, L. C., and Knight , R. T. (1991) Cortical substrates supporting visual search in humans. *Cereb. Cortex* 1: 262–272.

Eglin, M., Robertson, L. C., Knight, R. T., and Brugger, P. (1994) Search deficits in neglect patients are dependent on size of the visual scene. *Neuropsychology* 4: 451–463.

Farah, M. J., Wong, A. B., Wallace, M. A., and Carpenter, P. A. (1990) Frames of reference for allocating attention to space: Evidence from the neglect syndrome. *Neuropsychologia* 28: 335–347.

Fellerman, D. J. and Van Essen, D. C. (1991) Distributed hierarchical processing in the primate cortex. *Cereb. Cortex* 1: 1–47.

Friedman-Hill, S., Robertson, L. C., and Treisman, A. (1995) Parietal contributions to visual feature binding: Evidence from a patient with bilateral lesions. *Science* 269: 853–855.

Goodale, M. A. and Milner, A. D. (1992) Separate visual pathways for perception and action. *Trends Neurosci.* 15: 20–25.

Grabowecky, M., Egly, R., Robertson, L. C., and Rafal, R. (1993) Attentional control in a patient with bilateral inferior parietal lesions. *Soc. Neurosci. Abstr.* 19: 563.

Grabowecky, M., Robertson, L. C., and Treisman, A. (1993) Preattentive processes guide visual search: Evidence from patients with unilateral visual neglect. *J. Cognitive. Neurosci.* 5: 288–302.

Graziano, M. and Gross, C. G. (1995) Multiple pathways for processing visual space. In *Attention and Performance XVI*, edited by T. Inui and J. McClelland, Cambridge, MA: MIT Press.

Heilman, K. M. and Valenstein, E. (1985) *Clinical Neuropsychology.* New York: Oxford University Press.

Holmes, G. (1918) Disturbances of visual orientation. *Br. J. Opthalmol.* 2: 449–468.

Humphreys, G. W. and Riddoch, M. J. (1993) Interactive attentional system in unilateral visual neglect. In *Unilateral Neglect: Clinical and Experimental Studies*, edited by I. H. Robertson and J. C. Marshall, pp. 139–168. Hillsdale, NJ: Lawrence Erlbaum.

Kaas, J. H. (1989) Why does the brain have so many visual areas? *J. Cog. Neurosci.* 1: 121–135.

Koch, C. and Crick, F. (1994) Some further ideas regarding the neuronal basis of awareness. In *Large-Scale Neuronal Theories of the Brain*, edited by C. Koch and J. L. Davis. Cambridge: MIT Press.

Ladavas, E. (1987) Is the hemispatial deficit produced by right parietal lobe damage associated with retinal or gravitational coordinates? *Brain* 110: 167–180.

Luck, S. J., Chelazzi, L., Hillyard, S. A., and Desimone, R. (1997). Neural mechanisms of spatial selective attention in areas V1, V2, and V4 of macaque visual cortex. *J. Neurophysiol.* 77: 24–42.

Luria, A. R. (1959) Disorders of "simultaneous perception" in a case of bilateral occipitoparietal brain injury. *Brain* 83: 437–449.

Posner, M. I., Walker, J. A., Friedrich, F. A., and Rafal, R. D. (1984) Effects of parietal injury on covert orienting. *J. Neurosci.* 4: 1863–1874.

Prinzmetal, W., Presti, D. E., and Posner, M. I. (1986) Does attention affect visual feature integration? *J. Exp. Psychol. Hum. Percept. Perform.* 12: 361–369.

Rafal, R. (1996) Balint's syndrome. In *Behavioral Neurology and Neuropsychology*, edited by T. E. Feinberg and M. J. Farah. New York: McGraw-Hill.

Rafal, R. and Robertson, L. C. (1995) The neurology of visual attention. In *The Cognitive Neurosciences*, edited by M. S. Gazzaniga, pp. 625–648. Cambridge, MA: MIT Press.

Rizzolatti, G., Riggio, L., and Sheliga, B. M. (1994) Space and selective attention. In *Attention and Performance XV*, edited by C. Umilta and M. Moscovitch, Cambridge. MA: MIT Press.

Robertson, L. C., Treisman, A., Freidman-Hill, S., and Grabowecky, M. (1997) A possible connection between spatial deficits and feature binding in a patient with parietal damage. *J. Cog. Neurosci.* 9: 295–317.

Singer, W. and Gray, C. M. (1995) Visual feature integration and the temporal correlation hypothesis. *Annu. Rev. Neurosci.* 18: 555–586.

Treisman, A. (1988) Features and objects: The fourteenth Bartlett memorial lecture. *Q. J. Exp. Psychol.* 40A: 201–237.

Treisman, A. (1991) Search, similarity and integration of features between and within dimensions. *J. Exp. Psychol. Hum. Percept. Perform.* 17: 652–676.

Treisman, A. (1993) The perception of features and objects. In *Attention: Selection, Awareness, and Control*, edited by A. Baddeley, and L. Wieskrantz. Oxford: Oxford University Press.

Treisman, A. M. and Gelade, G. (1980) A feature integration theory of attention. *Cognitive Psychol.* 12: 97–136.

Treisman, A. and Schmidt, H. (1982) Illusory conjunctions in the perception of objects. *Cognitive Psychol.* 14: 107–141.

Ungerleider, L. G. and Haxby, J. (1994) What and where in the human brain. *Curr. Opin. Neurobiol.* 4: 157–165.

Ungerleider, L. G. and Mishkin, M. (1982) Two cortical visual systems. In *Analysis of Visual Behavior*, edited by J. Ingle, M. A. Goodale, and R. J. W. Mansfield, pp. 549–586. Cambridge, MA: MIT Press.

Wolfe, J. M., Cave, K. R., and Franzel, S. L. (1989) Guided search: An alternative to the feature integration model of visual search. *J. Exp. Psychol. Hum. Percept. Perform.* 15: 419–433.

13 Attention, Pattern Recognition, and Pop-Out in Visual Search

Ken Nakayama and Julian S. Joseph

ABSTRACT Theories of visual search inspired by neurophysiological investigations of early vision have postulated built-in visual primitives which determine whether visual search will occur in parallel (without attention) or whether it will require serial attentional sampling. Against this dualistic view, we argue that attention is required for all search tasks but that the spatial scale over which attention is allocated differs. Easy (often mistakenly called parallel) search can be regarded as pattern recognition, requiring attention to be distributed globally, spreading preferentially across emergent perceptual segmentations such as surfaces. Pop-out, which can accompany this easy global recognition, is a separate and distinct process, involving the automatic narrowing of attention to an odd item. Pop-out can be primed such that the deployment of attention is enhanced for repeated positions and features.

The topic of visual search has received an unusual amount of interest over the past 15 years. Several reasons explain this popularity. First, because the stimuli are plainly suprathreshold, it provides a connection to everyday life in ways that studies of early vision do not. In visual search tasks, the observer is required to find or identify a target in a multi-element array, a task not unlike the spotting of friends in a group or finding one's car in a crowded parking lot.

Second, while being complex, these displays can be varied in numerous quantifiable ways. Each display has a specific number of separate elements, with specified color, shape, and contrast at defined spacings. Thus, performance, in terms of reaction time (RT) or accuracy, can be measured in relation to these variables. What captured the most initial interest was the fact that search behavior appeared to fall into two separate classes and each was thought to exemplify a different underlying process.

The term *serial search* was attributed to cases where RTs increased with distractor number. This suggested that the observer was required to process each target one at a time by moving attention or by making saccadic eye movements. A much sought after signature to confirm this underlying hypothetical process was the 2:1 difference in RT increase for target-absent versus target-present conditions as distractor number increased. This difference was presumed to reflect the need to exhaustively sample the full display when the target was absent and, on average, to sample just half the display when the target was present.

Parallel search was deemed to occur when RTs did not increase with the number of distractors. This suggested that the underlying process was mediated by many independent detecting mechanisms, all requiring a certain amount of time but acting in parallel. The term "preattentive" (following Neisser, 1967) was used to indicate that all of these processes occurred prior to visual attention.

THEORY INSPIRED FROM THE CHARACTERISTICS OF EARLY VISION

Owing mainly to the theories of Treisman and Gelade (1980) and of Julesz (1984), visual search achieved even greater prominence. These theories promised the beginnings of a low-level, image-based explanation for visual search. Their underlying assumptions were closely related to neurophysiological ideas regarding the organization of early vision. Just as physiological descriptions of receptive fields suggested that neurons in the cortex were analyzers, specific to color, bar orientation, spatial frequency, binocular disparity, motion, and so forth, these theories of visual search suggested that there existed over the visual field feature analyzers that were arranged in a parallel array, each feature array comprising a retinotopic map. Of obvious attraction was the implicit yet ambitious linkage to the whole edifice of findings associated with the receptive fields of the visual cortex.

Although Treisman and Gelade's and Julesz's theories were inspired by neurophysiological findings, they maintained a certain distance from these results, preferring to define the characteristics of these hypothetical units a priori or to let them be characterized by the search experiments themselves. Treisman introduced the concept of feature maps, using their implied properties to explain the data from simple visual search experiments. An observer could easily find a target defined by a single unique feature—say a red target in a field of green distractors—because in the map of red features, only one locus of "red" activity would be evident and would thus "pop out." This explained the flat search functions and appeared to support the view of distributed parallel processing in early vision. Equipped with these views one could also use the presence of flat search functions as a diagnostic method to determine which features were elementary, which elements constituted the basic building blocks of perception. With more complex displays, such as Treisman's conjunctive paradigm, parallel search was not possible because the target was not unique in any simple feature map. Thus, targets had to be processed item by item.

Julesz's theory was similar, although it provided a more principled account as to why particular features pop out. Julesz postulated that there were canonical elementary particles of perception called textons. Julesz suggested that early preattentive discrimination was based on texton densities and that when densities of such textons became sufficiently inhomogeneous, then there would be a corresponding inhomogeneity in the texton map, leading to effortless selection of an item without attention.

Characteristic of both theories was the emphasis on the independence of activities in parallel channels, akin to neurons with receptive fields. The properties of the neurons themselves were deemed adequate to explain the class of visual search results in which performance did not vary with distractor number. Visual processing, therefore, proceeded more or less automatically and did not require the higher intervention of focal attention. This led to flat search functions, which in turn provided a confirming signature of an independent parallel process.

The popularity of these theories was immediate and widespread. First, they seemed to provide a satisfactory account of visual search by explaining a seemingly complex visual phenomenon in terms of something very primitive: features or textons. Second and following from this first point, the theories suggested that one might even discover new visual primitives via clever psychological experimentation. Visual search experiments by themselves might provide a powerful technique to identify new and perhaps unsuspected visual elements. Julesz's program, for example, raised the possibility that line terminators might act as basic elements.

In sum, these theories were bold and promising, accounting for complex phenomena and providing a new way to understand vision in terms of its constituents. Yet, as is occasionally the case with the most popular scientific theories, they initiated a line of research that began to undermine their own foundations. In the effort to find elementary units of vision, new stimuli were created that questioned the most basic idea, that the properties of primitive parallel array of retinotopically organized analyzers could explain these complex visual phenomena.

First, the work of Ramachandran (1988) indicated that concave depressions derived from shading easily segregated from a field of top-lit shaded spheres and could be easily detected with RT little affected by distractor number (Kleffner and Ramachandran, 1992). In a closely related study Enns and Rensink (1990) found that subjects could easily find countershaded cubes among top-lit shaded cubes. Again, set size had no appreciable effect on detection speed. Even more telling were the experiments of Wang, Cavanagh, and Green (1994), who showed that an observer could not easily detect a ⊔∣ among ⊓⊔, but that as soon as the stimuli were rotated 90 degrees, detection became much easier because the stimuli, ㄹ and 5, then looked very much like the numerals 2 and 5. A related phenomenon was shown during searches for an И among normal N distractors. Performance was excellent. Interestingly, the converse was not the case. Searching for an N among И distractors was far more difficult.

These results and others can be considered in two ways. First, Ramachandran's original results can be interpreted, as he did, by considering shaded sphere-like bulges to be yet another texton or feature. One encounters many shaded figures in the world, and perhaps it is not far-fetched to think of passive analyzers for convex shapes reproduced, distributed, and tiled over the whole visual field. The explanation, however, becomes more problematic as the list of putative textons increases. Familiar patterns like 2 and 5, as opposed to unfamiliar patterns having almost identical texton differences (simply rotated by 90 degrees), evoke very different reactions in visual search tasks. Although dense feature maps may exist for simple features such as color and orientation, it becomes much more difficult to conceive of an exhaustive set of maps for various letters, surface shapes, and so forth. Moreover, with the report of each new example of an element supporting rapid visual search, yet another map of primitives is needed, each also represented densely at different retinotopic locations and scales.

A complementary class of experiments is also relevant. He and Nakayama (1992) found that the search for a reversed *L* among normal *Ls* was easy in a multi-element search array. RT did not increase with distractor number. Thus, one could conceive of the task as being mediated at a featural level. However, performance could be severely degraded by manipulating binocular disparity such that the elements would appear to perceptually complete behind occluders, rendering them less clearly distinguishable as targets and as distractors. This indicates that even with features intact, a higher-level representation of surfaces is decisive in determining whether a visual search task can be performed easily. Analogous results were found by Suzuki and Cavanagh (1995), who showed that feature differences do not support rapid visual search when embedded in a face representation. These two experiments suggest that we only have access to higher-order representations. We do not have access to image features.

Thus, there are two sets of evidence against early vision accounts of visual search. First, the number of primitive features on the list is looming too large. Second, there is evidence that there is no response to features at all per se. For these and for other reasons, described in the following section, we argue for the need to abandon or, even more strongly, to exorcise the early vision metaphor. In its place, we suggest that easy visual search tasks be regarded as requiring a higher-order process, that of a global pattern recognition at the scale of the full search array.

ATTENTION REQUIRED FOR ALL VISUAL SEARCH TASKS

To begin anew, we first need to step back and build upon some of the major findings in perception, including those from the older Gestalt tradition and, more recently, from cognitive psychology. Phenomenological studies indicate the existence of nonlocal organizing principles that operate in vision to determine whether widely separated portions of an image are grouped together or are segregated as different units (Koffka, 1935; Kanizsa, 1979; Nakayama, He, and Shimojo, 1995). In addition, another tradition of attentional research has been spawned more recently, in the earliest days of cognitive psychology.

First, consider the properties of visual attention. One of the earliest and most obvious facts to reemerge with the birth of cognitive psychology was the inherent selectivity of attention (Broadbent, 1958). Such selection implies capacity limits and these limits were understood to vary in a graded quantitative manner (Kahneman, 1973; Sperling and Melchner, 1978). For example, it seemed reasonable to assume that with more attentional effort, performance would increase. Yet, this is not always the case.

In an important theoretical contribution, Norman and Bobrow (1975) outlined with unusual clarity a plausible relationship between many seemingly disparate domains—incoming sensory information (data), attentional effort (resources), task difficulty, and performance. Figure 13.1A depicts their postulated relationship between performance and attentional effort. Also labeled in this diagram is the customary range over which attention can be

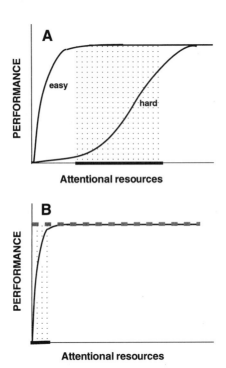

Figure 13.1 (A) Performance versus attentional resource allocation curves (redrawn from Norman and Bobrow, 1975). Note that for a hard task, added expenditures of attention improve performance. Contrast this to easy tasks in which very little attention is needed and variations of attention over the experimental range will have no effect. The thickened line on abscissa represents the range of attentional variation customarily achieved in laboratory studies of attention. (B) Comparison of two hypothetical situations in Norman and Bobrow's coordinate framework. The solid line represents a hypothetical very easy visual search task that requires only very small amounts of attention to reach asymptotic performance. The dashed line represents the hypothesized behavior of parallel search implied by early vision theories attention. The thickened line on the abscissa represents the range of attention needed to show necessity of attention on very easy search tasks.

varied in the usual laboratory experiments (denoted by the thickened line on the abscissa). From this formulation it should be clear that attention can influence performance dramatically, yet its influence occurs only within a restricted range. Above a certain level of attention (where the performance versus attention curve reaches asymptote), there is little or no effect of attention on performance. Task difficulty is also highly relevant. Added attention can improve performance of all tasks, both easy and hard, but the specific range over which this occurs differs. For example, greater attentional effort can increase performance for difficult tasks but will not have any effect on easy tasks. The latter require much less attention and cannot be further improved with greater resources or effort. In this range, Norman and Bobrow indicate that performance is data limited but not resource limited. For example, degrading the stimulus here might reduce performance, whereas reducing attention would not. One can conceive of even easier tasks in which even less attentional resources are required. Such rising curves would be shifted even further to the left, showing attentional influences on performance only for very small allocations of attention (as in the solid curve in figure 13.1B).

Norman and Bobrow's conception of attention and performance contrasts sharply with the views on visual search described in the previous section (Treisman and Gelade, 1980; Julesz, 1984). These latter theories assume two categorically distinct processes and divide visual search tasks into those that require visual attention (serial search) and a special class (parallel search) that does not. Because such theories claim that the latter processes require no attention, performance is constant in Norman and Bobrow's coordinates (refer to the dashed line in figure 13.1B). Contrast this to the presumed dependence of simple search on attention if only a very small amount of attention were necessary (represented by the rising solid curve in figure 13.1b).

From this graphic formulation, it should be clear that only the most drastic reductions of attention are capable of demonstrating the role of attention in "easy" visual search tasks. Reducing attention by arbitrarily large amounts is not enough. One needs to reduce it to the level at which its absence will have obvious and deleterious consequences. Thus, in figure 13.1B, attention needs to be reduced to the range denoted by the solid line on the abscissa. Consider an analogy with low-temperature physics. Just because temperature can be lowered dramatically, by hundreds of degrees, does not mean that all heat (kinetic energy) has been removed. In fact, almost heroic measures were required to reduce temperature to near absolute zero. Eventually, the effort succeeded and new and unexpected properties of matter were discovered— for example, superconductivity. So too with attention. We argue that the usual competing tasks in dual task studies do not consume sufficient resources and allow for small but significant amounts to be allocated elsewhere, particularly in experiments where task demands are clear. Thus, until recently we have lacked powerful methods to ensure that attention is reduced to almost zero. This technical inability seems in part to have led experimenters to conclude that attentional effort is not needed for the simplest of perceptual tasks, including pop-out tasks.

For example, Braun and Sagi (1990) argued that attention is not necessary for visual pop-out based on orientation differences. Using a dual task procedure, they varied attentional allocation between two tasks, orientation pop-out and letter discrimination, such that the letter task showed improved performance with increasing atttentional allocation to it with no corresponding decrement in performance for the pop-out task. Braun (1993) found similar results for Ramachandran's (1988) shape-from-shading array. From this Braun and colleagues drew the conclusion that attention is not required for the pop-out task. Referring to Norman and Bobrow's diagram (figure 13.1), however, note that withdrawing attentional effort from a region in which attention is not limiting will not have any effect on performance. It simply moves leftward along the curve in the region of constant performance. Thus, visual search tasks can be strongly dependent on attention but will not reveal such a dependence unless attention is sufficiently reduced. Kowler, Anderson, Dosher, and Blaser (1995) made an analogous argument against the claim that attention is not required for saccadic eye movements. In an important study employing a dual task paradigm, they showed that normal saccades required a measurable amount of attention. The programming and execution of saccades may be categorized as an easy task in Norman and Bobrow's family of curves, however. As such, it also explains why it has been so hard to actually prove the necessity of attention for saccades even though there has been much circumstantial evidence to establish this linkage (Fischer, 1987; Fischer and Weber, 1993; Mackeben and Nakayama, 1993).

Attention is also needed for even the simplest visual search tasks. Severe drops in performance can be seen in an orientation pop-out task when the demands of an additionally imposed task are very high (Joseph, Chun, and Nakayama, 1997). In this situation, a highly demanding task that proved adequate to consume required resources was used. Observers monitored a rapid serial visual presentation (RSVP) stream of letters and were required to identify a differently colored letter in the stream while performing a simultaneous task of oddball detection in an orientation pop-out task (figure 13.2). In comparison to control conditions in which performance on the pop-out task was very high using an accuracy measure, performance dropped almost to levels of chance with the addition of the RSVP letter task. The performance drop was also dependent on the asynchrony between the target letter presentation and the onset of the visual search array. Shortest lags led to the greatest interference. Subsidiary experiments indicated that the same stimuli yielded flat search functions of set size with RT as the measure, indicating that the task met the criteria of so called preattentive or parallel search. Similarly severe impairments of performance occured in a shape-from-shading oddball detection task (Joseph et al., 1996).

In a related series of studies, Rock, Linnett, Grant, and Mack (1992) and Mack, Tang, Tuma, and Kahn (1992) showed that even the simplest visual

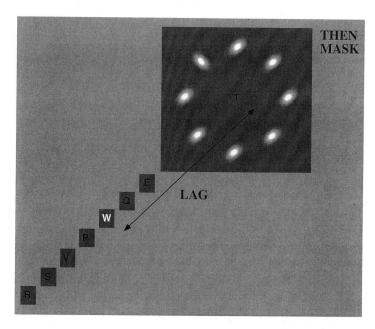

Figure 13.2 A pop-out task based on orientation differences requires visual attention. An array of oriented Gabor patches can appear with or without an orientation oddball; the task is to report whether an oddball is present. A competing task at fixation is to attend to the central region and identify the white letter in a stream of black letters. Lag refers to the time asynchrony between the presentation of the white target letter and onset of the visual search array. Oddball detection accuracy is severely impaired by the letter task. (From Joseph et al., 1997.)

tasks are compromised when attention is taken up elsewhere. They employed a clever, unconventional design in which there was only one test trial per subject. Thus, there was no reason for the unsuspecting observer to allocate attention away from the primary task on the single trial because the observer was unaware of any other task. As a consequence, performance failure in the otherwise very easy secondary task was dramatic. Rock et al. dubbed the phenomenon inattentional blindness to underscore its importance.

These studies share an important conclusion. If attention is largely removed through effective methods, either by allocating it more fully to a primary task or by not allocating it efficiently to an unexpected secondary task, the conclusion is the same: Almost all of what is considered to be conscious vision cannot occur without attention.

ATTENTION DEPLOYED TO SURFACES NOT FEATURES

Norman and Bobrow's (1975) formulation provides the basis for additional understanding about visual search, particularly when it is coupled with a more explicit description of what underlies visual task difficulty. The issue of capacity limits in attention invites an exploration of quantitative factors that might play role in visual search difficulty. What first comes to mind are the elementary notions outlined by information theory: redundancy, coding, data compression, and so forth. Stimulus coding leads to issues of perceptual organization, and it also opens the door to consideration of a greater role for perceptual and other forms of visual learning.

Norman and Bobrow also made an explicit connection between their analysis and its relationship to learning and practice. They suggested that as learning proceeds and tasks become easier, the rising portion of the performance versus attention curve should shift progressively to the left. Employing the language of information theory, we hypothesize that with extended practice information regarding the display becomes, to use Miller's (1956) phrase, chunked. Thus, in analogy to the chess master who codes the seemingly complex displays on a chessboard according to his deep knowledge of the strategy of the game, our perceptual systems expertly chunk information in visual search displays. Chunking reduces the information load on the system, and progressively less and less attention is required as chunking increases. This is the reason that the curve shifts to the left. In terms of visual search tasks, if the stimulus could become more easily codable (with fewer bits) through practice, then less attentional resources would be required to achieve the same level of performance. How is such chunking achieved in vision? Efficient coding, of course, requires redundancy and, broadly speaking, one can conceive of the code as removing much of the natural redundancy in everyday scenes (Attneave, 1954). Frequently occurring scene patterns, therefore, could be coded with fewer bits. Thus, one codes familiar faces efficiently and can spot subtle blemishes on them much more quickly than on a stranger's face.

Of course, redundancy reduction is not restricted to high-level visual patterns; it is perhaps even more relevant when considered at the mid-level organization of vision, particularly when applied to visual search tasks. Here, the whole field of perceptual psychology, including the earlier Gestalt tradition, is clearly relevant, and organizational factors spanning large retinal distances become important. Thus, similarity in color, shape, motion, and so forth all contribute to perceptual grouping, as do certain configurational patterns such as collinearity and cocurvature. Also important are processes of surface completion that either segregate or join distinct patches of images as surfaces in depth (Kanizsa, 1979; Nakayama et al., 1995).

It is likely, therefore, that efficiencies that are developed for normal scene encoding also influence visual search tasks. Visual search tasks that allow the most efficient coding of the distractors and target as separate entities are at a distinct advantage. Displays with identically colored distractors will have advantages over displays with more variegated colors because of the ability to group identical colors. This idea has been offered as an alternative to Treisman's theory because it also predicts the difficulty of finding odd targets in Treisman's conjunctive search task (Duncan and Humphreys, 1989).

It should be noted, however, that grouping is not determined by the linkage of low-level features but is a relational process determined by whether the elements conform to regularities in the world. Experiments on the spread of attention in three-dimensional space are instructive. He and Nakayama (1995) set up a binocular depth display consisting of targets at three stereoscopic depths of near, middle, and far. Observers were required to find a single odd-colored target in the array at the middle distance. The number of same-colored targets in the near and the far planes and the local slant of the individually colored target rectangles were varied. They could be slanted forward, backward, or in the same plane implied by the middle depth array. Observers performed this task easily when each of the targets in the middle depth plane were coplanar, that is, were not slanted backward or forward with respect to the middle plane (figure 13.3a,b). Thus, grouping is not de-

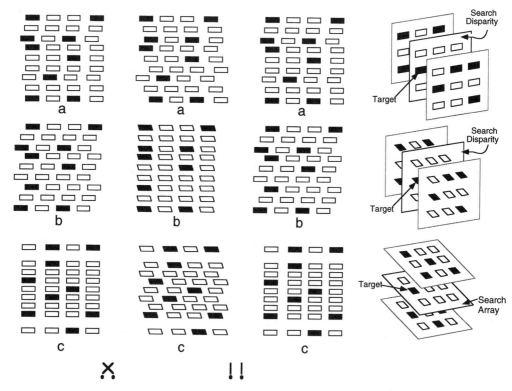

Figure 13.3 Three-dimensional search arrays showing the importance of surfaces in the deployment of attention. On the left three columns are stereograms containing elements at three distances. Left two half-images should be fused for crossed eyes, and the right two should be fused for divergent fusion. Visual search for an odd color confined to the middle distance is rapid in (a) because the elements lie in the same front parallel plane, whereas searching at the same middle distance in (b) is much more slow because the elements do not lie in that plane. Search is also easy when a subject looks for an odd target in a depth array in the middle of three horizontal stacks because elements in the middle horizontal plane are all coplanar. Because distractors of the same color as the target are also in the flanking planes, the task requires the efficient spreading of focal attention in the plane to be searched. Diagrams at right provide a pictorial description of the depth relations in the perceived display. (Redrawn with permission from He and Nakayama, 1995.)

termined by low-level cortical factors such as a common binocular disparity, as was originally hypothesized by Nakayama and Silverman (1986). Rather, the results suggest that surfaces with coplanar elements can effectively support the spread of attention to spatially distributed groups of elements. Supporting and extending this conclusion is the fact that observers were able to selectively search for targets in a set of rectangles having coplanar elements that spanned the most extreme range of binocular disparities and stereoscopic depths (see figure 13.3c). Thus, analogous to the Gestalt principle of good continuation in two dimensions, He and Nakayama (1995) showed that such a principle also operates in three dimensions, allowing coplanar elements to emerge as a surface over which selective attention can easily spread (see also Nakayama and He, 1995).

VISUAL SEARCH AS ATTENTIVE PATTERN RECOGNITION AT VARIOUS SCALES

Having argued against an early vision approach to visual search, it is worth reflecting on what we are proposing in contrast to what we are rejecting, and also commenting on what has been gained and lost. Early vision theories based their explanatory power on the elementary properties of built-in units. Lost, therefore, is the immediate hope of reducing higher-level vision to the presumed properties of single units in early cortical structures. What is gained? At worst, perhaps only the sober realization that terms like parallel processing, preattentive, features, and so forth, can no longer be used so confidently. More positively, we think our proposal opens the door for a wider range of theoretical accounts, a restructured descriptive vocabulary, and the opportunity to observe new phenomena. The remaining portion of this chapter is devoted towards those ends.

Acknowledging the severe capacity limits of visual attention, Nakayama (1990) proposed a close relationship between attention at different scales and pattern recognition. Attentional fixations, at varying loci and spatial scales, allow selected portions of the image to be matched with templates in visual memory. Due to the attentional bottleneck, the full richness of the visual scene cannot be sampled. Attentive sampling, therefore, represents a compromise between scale (the area to be sampled) and resolution (detail). Thus, a global sampling of a large portion of an image can be accomplished but only at low spatial resolution. Higher-resolution sampling can also occur but at the expense of limiting the area. Thus, to recognize the details of a scene requires narrow focusing of attention. To apply these constraints to visual search tasks, Nakayama (1990), in agreement with previous views, accepted the notion that for difficult visual search tasks, focal attention is necessary to inspect items serially. That is, each attentive fixation allows pattern recognition to occur in a restricted local area.

The divergence in thinking came mainly with the interpretation of easy search tasks, or so-called parallel search. This we also regard as pattern recognition but on a larger scale, with a concomitant loss of spatial resolution. Thus, in easy visual search, usually mistakenly called parallel search, global pattern recognition boils down to a binary decision based on a coarse sampling of the image—does the overall array correspond to one with the target present? Or does it correspond to the pattern with the target absent? As mentioned previously, this too requires attention (Joseph et al., 1996a).

POP-OUT ACCOMPANIES BUT DOES NOT ACCOUNT FOR EASY VISUAL SEARCH

As theories change, even the most basic vocabulary, apparently so descriptive at one time, can lose or change its meaning. This is true for the terms associated with visual search. If the dualistic notion of visual search with and without attention is not accepted, then the terms "preattentive vision" and "parallel processing" lose their specific referents. Thus, the term "parallel search," in particular, should be discarded. Other terms, however, cannot be so easily abandoned but need re-analysis and redefinition. One of the most commonly used terms is "pop-out." This seemingly descriptive term has very different meanings under the different theoretical perspectives.

If one adopts the early vision view of visual search, pop-out is both a phenomenological term and a mechanistic and theoretical construct. It is phenomenological because it describes the psychic fact that an odd item becomes more salient in a display. It is theoretical because it seemed to provide a mechanistic description of how, in a retinotopic array of feature or texton analyzers, only one site is active. That mechanism, in turn, played an essentially causal role in allowing simple or easy visual search to occur. According to this way of thinking, rapid search independent of distractor number occurs because of a sole active element in a parallel array of analyzers (for example, see Treisman and Gelade, 1980).

Even after rejecting the theoretical notions associated with Treisman's theory, the phenomenological term "pop-out" at first glance seems appropriate because it accompanies simple search displays. As such, we have used it earlier in this paper to denote easy visual search tasks because of the common usage of the term. Yet, this usage can also be very misleading because it is too closely tied to the notion of parallel search and glosses over the empirical characteristics of pop-out. Not being tied to an early vision conception of pop-out, we need a notion of pop-out that is more descriptive of its phenomenological characteristics. Most distinctive about the experience is the strong involuntary awareness of the odd target. In pop-out, attention is jerked suddenly to that locus. The target becomes more distinct, and fine details about its shape become more discernible. Thus, we define pop-out more descriptively as the involuntary narrowing of attention to an odd item in a field of elements.

However, it may now strike the reader that our new definition of pop-out appears to contradict our hypothesis regarding simple (easy) visual search tasks. We have argued that rapid visual search is based not on the narrowing of attention but on its opposite, a distributed spread of attention over the whole array, allowing pattern recognition at a larger scale. So how can we reconcile the spread of attention, which is required for rapid search, with its opposite, the narrowing of attention, which also accompanies it? Our view, based on the work of Bravo and Nakayama (1992), is that the two processes are distinct and occur sequentially. Pop-out occurs with the presence of an odd target but only after the global matching process required for detection. Thus, pop-out, or the narrowing of attention to the odd target, has no direct causal role in detection of the presence of a target. Thus, easy visual search tasks generally lead to two separate allocations of attention in a customary sequence: a global attentional allocation to the whole array (useful to do the rapid search task) followed by a narrowing of attention to the target (unnecessary for the same detection task).

To show that pop-out can be experimentally dissociated from visual search performance, Bravo and Nakayama (1992) employed two different tasks using the same visual search display, one requiring the global pattern match needed for visual search, the other requiring the narrowing of attention associated with pop-out. The display consisted of a set of diamonds, either red or green, and each diamond was randomly truncated, either on the right or left side (figure 13.4A). In addition, there were two types of trial

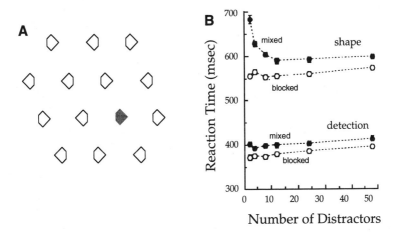

Figure 13.4 Pop-out and flat search functions do not reflect the same process. (A) Visual display for all tasks is identical, consisting of an odd-colored target (green) among distractors (red) or, vice versa, an odd red target among green distractors. In a given set of trials, target and distracter color can either stay the same for each trial (blocked) or can switch randomly from trial to trial (mixed). The two tasks are as follows. Simple search (labeled detection) consists of detecting an odd target. Pop-out task (labeled shape) requires the discrimination of the shape of the odd-colored target (whether it is truncated on the left or the right). Note the unusual relationship between distractor number and reaction time, with lower reaction times for increasing numbers of distractors. This occurs only in the mixed popout case. (Redrawn with permission from Bravo and Nakayama, 1992.)

blocks. In the blocked case, targets and distractors each had the same color from trial to trial. For example, targets would remain red and distractors would remain green within a particular block. In the mixed case, target and distractor color would reverse on a random basis from trial to trial within a block.

The first task used the usual visual search task, and subjects were asked to respond quickly as to the presence or absence of an odd-colored target. Here it should be clear that the detailed shapes of the elements were irrelevant. Not surprising, and in close agreement with the literature, search times were relatively fast and did not vary with distractor number. This result is shown in figure 13.4B as the shorter latency pair of curves denoted by the label "detection." Note that within the pair mixed trials had a small but consistently longer RT for all set sizes.

Second, to characterize pop-out and using the exact same display, the authors selected a task that required the narrow focusing of attention to the odd target. They asked observers whether the odd-colored diamond was truncated on the right or on the left. Curves labeled "shape" in figure 13.4B show that performance on this shape discrimination task was very different than simple detection performance. First, RTs were much longer. Furthermore, there was a pronounced difference between the mixed and blocked condition. In the blocked condition RTs were faster and constant across distractor number. In the mixed condition and going strongly against the usual trend for visual search tasks, slopes were negative. Increasing distractor number reduced RTs dramatically. This negative slope function has been replicated under a variety of other stimulus conditions (Bravo and Nakayama, 1992; Maljkovic and Nakayama, 1994).

Taken together, it should be clear that the behavior in the two tasks was very different. The usual visual search task had flat search functions as expected. The pop-out task, requiring a shape discrimination, can have a search function with a steep negative slope. The longer RTs for pop-out and the negative slope argue against a causal relationship between pop-out and so-called parallel search.

At this point, one might raise an objection regarding our measure of pop-out. We have assumed that the measurement of RT during shape discrimination reflects the speed of the deployment of attention to the peripheral target site. Is that warranted? We think it is because we assume that the discrimination requires focal attention. To strengthen our case, however, it would be worthwhile to have a very different indicator of attention, one that does not require visual discrimination or manual reaction. We have found such an indicator in the measurement of saccadic eye movement latencies. Earlier, we noted the need for small amounts of attention to be directed to a target prior to a saccade (Kowler et al., 1995). This leads to a simple prediction. If we measure saccadic eye movement latencies to the same visual displays, we should see the same signature that Bravo and Nakayama (1992) identified for pop-out. First, there should be flat saccadic latencies functions for cases in which the distractors and target colors remained unchanged from trial to trial. Second, saccadic latencies should be slower overall when the target and distractor colors are mixed. Most critically, saccadic latencies should also decrease with increasing distractor number. That exact pattern of results was obtained in a measurement of human saccadic eye movement latencies (McPeek and Nakayama, 1995b). This pattern of results confirms the relationship between attention and saccades and adds independent support for our distinction between pop-out and the hypothesized global pattern recognition required for easy visual search.

At this point we need to comment on the reason for the large qualitative difference between pop-out as revealed in the discrimination task and simple pattern matching as revealed in the detection task. First, the decrease in RTs with increasing distractor number in the pop-out task are predicted, at least implicitly, by several mechanistic theories of attentional deployment (Julesz, 1986; Koch and Ullman, 1985). Each theory has a slightly different emphasis, one stressing gradients of feature differences, the other, inhibitory interactions between distractors. Our own bias is that the phenomenon may be better understood at a higher level, possibly related to surface formation. At present, however, there is insufficient evidence to distinguish between these alternatives. A second, more tractable question deals with the large and consistent difference between mixed and blocked conditions. Why are RTs so much faster in the blocked condition?

PRIMING OF POP-OUT

There are several possible accounts. The most obvious explanation is the possible role of expectancy, or knowledge of the upcoming trial. In the blocked condition, observers might be expected to utilize the temporal regularities in the sequence of displays to predict what would come up on the next trial, and thereby performance would benefit. This view was quickly dispelled by Maljkovic and Nakayama (1994), who manipulated the probability of a color switch of targets and distractors, p(switch), within a block of trials. Under those circumstances, predictability was minimal when the trials were presented randomly and at a maximum when target color either remained the same on each trial or alternated on each trial. Contrary to a predictability hypothesis, RT were not lowest for maximum predictability. RT were highest when the target was completely predictable, that is, when it alternated on each trial (p(switch)=1.0). These results argue strongly against expectancy and leave only one likely alternative: priming. On each trial, it seems that some small beneficial residue of the previous trial accumulated from previous trials of the same color, such that RTs on subsequent trials of the same color will be faster.

To examine this priming in greater detail, Maljkovic and Nakayama (1994) developed a new method, memory kernel analysis, to measure the effects of a single trial over time. They looked at a sequence of many independent trials

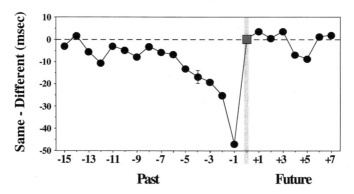

Figure 13.5 Priming of pop-out. Each point represents the influence on the current trial reaction time occasioned by the same versus different target color trials in the past (left) and future (right). Approximately 5–8 trials in the past have an influence on current trials, shortening reaction times appreciably as one compares same versus different color trials. (Reproduced with permission from Maljkovic and Nakayama, 1994.)

in which the probability of, for example, a red target among green distractors (and vice versa) was random. Then they took a given trial in the sequence, trial *n*, and analyzed it repeatedly, separately tallying RT as a function of whether on a neighboring trials, the color of the target was the same or different. They did this for essentially all preceding trials, up to fifteen. Because each trial was presented at intervals of approximately 2–3 s, they could examine the influence of events over the past 45 s. They also examined the dependence of current trials on each of next seven upcoming trials. Those trials had not yet occurred and would not be expected to influence the results. As such, they provided an estimate of the variability of the data. Because the color of the targets and distractors were randomly presented, it should be clear that the method isolated the effect of any arbitrary trial in the past because on average an equal number of intervening trials of both colors occurred; thus, the effects of those intervening trials would cancel.

Figure 13.5 plots the differences between the same-color and different-color trials for a single subject. Each point in the curve represents (whether it be the past or the future) the influence of same versus different colors on the current trial. The square symbol represents the grand mean of all the RT. Negative values indicate the speeding up of RT for same-color trials. Note that the effect is substantial: a single trial can alter the RT for the next trial by as much as 40 ms. Remarkably, single trials presented many trials earlier (over a span of 30 s) influenced behavior. The monotonically decreasing influence seen here indicates that this memory lasted for 5–8 trials, or for up to approximately 30 s. Additional experiments indicated that priming of consecutive same-color trials is cumulative and can account for the main difference in RT seen for the mixed versus blocked pop-out (shown earlier in figure 13.4B).

Maljkovic and Nakayama (1993) found that priming is involuntary and is a form of short-term implicit memory, distinguishable from explicit memory. They also showed that an analogous priming occurs for position, such that a previous deployment of attention to a given position, many trials earlier, speeds attention to that same position (Maljkovic and Nakayama, 1996). In addition, the primed position need not be in retinal coordinates but rather in the coordinates of the stimulus configuration. Finally, McPeek and Nakayama (1995a) have confirmed these results by showing a similar effect with saccadic eye movement latencies. Taken together, the results indicate that attentional deployment to an odd target is greatly influenced by past events, revealing the existence of a short-term implicit memory system.

CONCLUSIONS

Early vision theories of visual search have suggested two types of vision, one not requiring attention and responsible for "parallel" visual search, the other requiring attention and mediating more deliberate serial search. So far, we have presented three reasons to reject this early vision metaphor. First, the number of primitive features emerging is too large. With such a list, it becomes very difficult to imagine how all such patterns, including letters of the alphabet, are reproduced in all positions at all spatial scales in early cortical maps. Second, there is psychological evidence that we do not respond to elementary features at all in rapid vision, but that visual search works on a representation that is of a higher order. Visual search has no access to these putative earlier representations. Third, we have provided evidence that even the easiest, so-called parallel visual search tasks require attention.

In addition, we suggest two more reasons. Mounting evidence indicates that higher-level perceptual representations mediate most visual functions, even those traditionally thought to rely on low-level features. For example, motion perception, texture segregation, and object recognition may all be mediated by a surface level, not an image feature level (Nakayama et al., 1995). Most of this work is based on the importance of perceptual surfaces in determining whether we see image fragments as separate pieces or as connecting portions of surfaces that perceptually complete either in front of or behind occluders. Visual search is no exception, falling into line with other visual functions that depend on an intermediate surface level of representation.

Finally, we suggest a strategic reason to abandon or, even more strongly, to exorcise the early vision metaphor. It comes from a full acknowledgment of the metaphor's resilient strength, its continuing ability to define the vocabulary and, thus, even the phenomenology of visual search. Again, terms like parallel processing, preattentive vision, and so forth are powerful evocative terms that are laden with theoretical and physiological meaning at a time when such meaning should be skeptically regarded. What is needed is an alternative, more neutral vocabulary that sticks closer to the psychological facts and that opens the door to a range of new phenomena. Hopefully, we have at least partially convinced the reader that older ideas from perceptual and cognitive psychology remain alive and can form the foundation for further advances. In this regard, we have described new, unexpected facts about visual search in the second part of this chapter, relating visual search to surface representation, eye movements, and short-term memory.

How will these new psychological results be understood in terms of the rapid growth of knowledge about the brain? Most obvious is the fact that we can no longer rely on the properties of visual receptive fields to understand attention. We need an understanding of how higher-level vision (surfaces, objects, and so forth) are represented in neural circuits: a daunting challenge for the future.

ACKNOWLEDGMENTS

This work is supported in part by grants from the McKnight Foundation, Air Force Office of Scientific Research grant to K. N., and NEI grant F32-EY06531 to J. S. J. Special thanks to Marvin Chun, Charles Stromeyer, and Robert McPeek for comments on an earlier version of the manuscript.

REFERENCES

Attneave, F. (1954) Some informational aspects of visual perception. *Psychol. Rev.* 61: 183–193.

Braun, J. (1993) Shape-from-shading is independent of visual attention and may be a "texton." *Spat. Vis.* 7: 311–322.

Braun, J. and Sagi, D. (1990) Vision outside the focus of attention. *Percept. Psychophysiol.* 48: 45–58.

Braun, J. and Sagi, D. (1991) Texture-based tasks are little affected by second tasks requiring peripheral or central attentive fixation. *Perception* 20: 483–500.

Bravo, M. and Nakayama, K. (1992) The role of attention in different visual search tasks. *Percept. Psychophysiol.* 51: 465–472.

Broadbent, D. (1958) *Perception and Communication.* Oxford: Pergamon Press.

Duncan, J. and Humphreys, G. W. (1989) Visual search and stimulus similarity. *Psychol. Rev.* 96: 433–458.

Enns, J. T. and Rensink, R. A. (1990) Sensitivity to three-dimensional orientation in visual search. *Psychol. Sci.* 1: 323–326.

Fischer, B. (1987) The preparation of visually guided saccades. *Rev. Physiol. Biochem. Pharmacol.* 106: 2–35.

Fischer, B. and Weber, H. (1993) Express saccades and visual attention. *Behav. Brain Sci.* 16: 553–610.

He, Z. J. and Nakayama, K. (1992) Surface vs. features in visual search. *Nature* 359: 231–233.

He, Z. J., and Nakayama, K. (1995) Visual attention to surfaces in 3-D space. *Proc. Natl. Acad. Sci. U S A* 92: 11155–11159.

Joseph, J. S., Chun, M. M., and Nakayama, K. (1996) Attention plays a role in the perception of three-dimensional structure in shaded cube stimuli [Abstract]. *Invest. Ophthalmol. Vis. Sci.* 37: S213.

Joseph, J. S., Chun, M. M., and Nakayama, K. (1997) Attentional requirements in a "preattentive" feature search task. *Nature* 387: 805–807.

Julesz, B. (1984) Toward an axiomatic theory of preattentive vision. In *Dynamic Aspects of Neocortical Function*, edited by G. M. Edelman, W. E. Gall, and W. M. Cowan. New York: Neurosciences Research Foundation.

Julesz, B. (1986) Texton gradients: The texton theory revisited. *Biol. Cybern.* 54: 245–251.

Kahneman, D. (1973) *Attention and Effort*. Englewood Cliffs, NJ: Prentice-Hall.

Kanizsa, G. (1979) *Organization in Vision: Essays on Gestalt Perception*. New York: Praeger.

Kleffuer, D. A., and Ramachandran, V. S. (1992) On the perception of shape from shading. *Percep. Psychophys.* 52: 18–36.

Koch, C. and Ullman, S. (1985) Shifts in selective visual attention: Towards the underlying neural circuitry. *Hum. Neurobiol.* 4: 219–227.

Koffka, K. (1935) *Principles of Gestalt Psychology*. New York: Harcourt.

Kowler, E., Anderson, E., Dosher, B., and Blaser, E. (1995) The role of attention in the programming of saccades. *Vis. Res.* 35: 1897–1916.

Mack, A., Tang, B., Tuma, R., and Kahn, S. (1992) Perceptual organization and attention. *Cognitive Psychol.* 24: 475–501.

Mackeben, M. and Nakayama, K. (1993) Express attentional shifts. *Vis. Res.* 33: 85–90.

Maljkovic, V. and Nakayama, K. (1993) Priming of popout: An example of implicit short-term memory. *Soc. Neurosci. Abstr.* 19: 439.

Maljkovic, V. and Nakayama, K. (1994) Priming of popout: I. Role of features. *Mem. Cognition* 22: 657–672.

Maljkovic, V. and Nakayama, K. (1996) Priming of popout: II. Role of position. *Percept. Psychophys.* 58: 977–991.

McPeek, R. M. and Nakayama, K. (1995a) Linkage of attention and saccades in a visual search task. *Invest. Ophthalmol. Vis. Sci.* 36: S354.

McPeek, R. M. and Nakayama, K. (1995b) Repetition of target color affects saccadic latency and accuracy. Paper presented at the eighth European Conference on Eye Movements, Derby, United Kingdom.

Miller, G. A. (1956) The magical number seven, plus or minus two: Some limits on our capacity for processing information. *Psychol. Rev.* 63: 81–97

Nakayama, K. (1990) The iconic bottleneck and the tenuous link between early visual processing and perception. In *Vision: Coding and Efficiency*, edited by C. Blakemore, pp. 411–422. Cambridge, MA: Cambridge University Press.

Nakayama, K. and He, Z. J., (1995) Attention to surfaces: Beyond a Cartesian understanding of visual attention. In *Early Vision and Beyond*, edited by T. V. Papathomas. Cambridge, MA: MIT Press.

Nakayama, K., He, Z. J., and Shimojo, S. (1995) Visual surface representation: A critical link between lower-level and higher level vision. In *Visual Cognition*, edited by S. M. Kosslyn and D. N. Osherson, pp. 1–70. Cambridge, MA: MIT Press.

Nakayama, K. and Silverman, G. H. (1986) Serial and parallel processing of visual feature conjunctions. *Nature* 320: 264–265.

Neisser, U. (1967) *Cognitive Psychology.* New York: Appleton-Century-Crofts.

Norman, D. A. and Bobrow, D. G. (1975) On data-limited and resource-limited processes. *Cognitive Psychol.* 7: 44–64.

Ramachandran, V. S. (1988) Perception of shape from shading. *Nature* 331: 163–166.

Rock, I., Linnett, C. M., Grant, P., and Mack, A. (1992) Perception without attention: Results of a new method. *Cognitive Psychol.* 24: 502–534.

Sperling, G. and Melchner, J. J. (1978) The attention operating characteristic: Some examples from visual search. *Science* 202: 315–318.

Suzuki, S. and Cavanagh, P. (1995) Facial organization blocks access to low-level features: An object inferiority effect. *J. Exp. Psychol. Hum. Percept. Perform.* 21: 901–913.

Treisman, A. (1985) Preattentive processing in vision. *Comp. Vis. Graph. Image Proc.* 31: 156–177.

Treisman, A. and Gelade, G. (1980) A feature-integration theory of attention. *Cognitive Psychol.* 12: 97–136.

Wang, Q., Cavanagh, P., and Green, M. (1994) Familiarity and pop-out in visual search. *Percept. Psychophys.* 56: 495–500.

14 Attention and Visual Object Segmentation

Jon Driver and Gordon C. Baylis

ABSTRACT   The debate between space-based versus object-based accounts of visual attention is discussed. At issue is the extent to which scene segmentation can take place prior to visual selection, and whether that selection takes place within a spatial medium. Recent studies with both healthy and brain-injured persons suggest that a range of segmention processes can influence selection, leading to a variety of senses in which visual attention may be object-based. It is concluded that all these phenomena remain consistent with selection operating on a spatial array, and that different types of object-based attention must be carefully distinguished in future work on the neural substrates involved.

The last decade has seen many papers (see Kanwisher and Driver, 1992) on the issue of whether covert visual attention is directed to segmented objects, to regions of space, or perhaps to both, as we would argue. At the heart of this contemporary issue lies the old question of how much processing can take place prior to attentional selection. In the past (e.g., Broadbent, 1958), the question was posed in terms of whether or not stimulus categorization could precede attention. More recent disputes over the extent of preattentive processing concern better-specified image segmentation processes. At issue is whether or not those processes operate preattentively to allow selection of segmented objects for further attentional processing. The emerging consensus is that visual attention can indeed be object-based.

However, attention has been characterized as object-based in several subtly different ways, and the issue remains controversial. On the one hand, Baylis and Driver (1992) recently concluded that "visual attention is directed to groups derived from a preattentive segmentation of the scene according to Gestalt principles." On the other hand, in the same year, Mack, Tang, Tuma, and Kahn argued that "*no* perception of either texture segregation or Gestalt grouping" (1992, p. 488) takes place prior to attention, apparently in direct contradiction to Baylis and Driver's claim. This chapter aims to resolve such conflicts, while raising further issues.

IS THERE ANYTHING OUT THERE? NAIVE SPOTLIGHT METAPHORS FOR ATTENTION

Many theorists have likened covert visual attention to a spotlight (e.g., Posner, 1980). That metaphor can have various implications, depending on how literally one takes it. Attention might be applied to intervening positions en route between two loci, might shift at a constant rate, might "illuminate" larger areas only with a reduction in efficiency, might be impossible to split, and so on. These various spotlight properties are logically separable, and so must be separately tested. Evidence now exists to question all of them. Perhaps the most fundamental implication of the spotlight metaphor is that covert attention operates via enhancement of a restricted region in a spatial representation. Most contemporary theories acknowledge this as one means of visual selectivity. Substantial evidence for spatial enhancement certainly exists, ranging from human behavior in spatial cueing tasks (Posner, 1980) and human brain activity as indexed at the scalp (Luck and Girelli, chapter 5, this volume), to single-cell activity in behaving primates (Motter, chapter 4, this volume). However, other mechanisms of selection may also exist that are quite unlike spotlights, either because they are inhibitory (Tipper and Driver, 1988) or due to their nonspatial nature.

Moreover, the spotlight metaphor begs the very question that has traditionally concerned attention research; namely, the extent of processing prior to selection. A real spotlight needs a human operator to direct it at items of interest, as when tracking an actor across a stage. This depends on considerable perception by the operator; otherwise, an entirely blind search across the stage would result. A naive version of the spotlight metaphor might similarly characterize human vision as the blind application of tunnel vision to successive locations, in a desperate search for anything "out there."

Presumably no one would advocate such blind application of visual attention; hence, there must be some coding prior to attentional selection. A minimum of processing might be envisaged, with attention being directed to the item of highest contrast in some salience map of the input, as implied by many contemporary models of visual search (see Robertson, chapter 12, this volume). However, this immediately raises the question of how salience is computed, and how the borders of an "item" are defined (e.g., treating individual pixels as separate items would be very inefficient for most visual tasks). Object-based models typically suggest that attention is directed to the most relevant object in a fully segmented representation of the scene.

Thus, one fundamental aspect of the debate between object-based and spotlight models of attention concerns the extent of preattentive processing. A second basic issue concerns exactly what it is that is then selected by covert attention. This second question about covert attention can be illustrated by a contrast with overt shifts of attention such as eye movements. The fovea has a fixed anatomical shape and extent. Hence, eye movements can only enhance fovea-shaped regions of the scene. By contrast, covert attention may be more flexible. According to some variations on the spotlight metaphor, the hypothetical attentional beam may be narrowed or widened depending on the task (e.g., LaBerge, 1983). Such an adjustable spotlight could only select spatially contiguous regions, but some object-based models have advocated that noncontiguous regions can be selected simultaneously (e.g.,

Baylis and Driver, 1992; Driver and Baylis, 1989; McLeod, Driver, and Crisp, 1988; Pylyshyn et al., 1994). Finally, a few object-based models have argued that covert attention can be entirely nonspatial (e.g., Vecera and Farah, 1994; Humphreys, Romani, Olson, Riddoch, and Duncan, 1994). Thus, the various spotlight and object-based models have disagreed on how radically covert selection can depart from the spatial constraints that are imposed on overt orienting.

A prototypical object-based account of attention was offered informally by Neisser (1967). He suggested that visual scenes are first segmented into groups in accordance with Gestalt principles, to yield separate candidate objects. Attention is only then directed to individual objects in turn for further elaboration. Similar views have since been advocated by Kahneman (e.g., Kahneman, 1973; Kahneman and Henik, 1981; Treisman, Kahneman, and Burkell, 1983), by Duncan (1984), and by ourselves (e.g. Baylis and Driver, 1992, 1993; Driver and Baylis, 1989; Driver, Baylis, and Rafal, 1992), among others. Because all such accounts invoke Gestalt grouping, we give a brief account of this below.

ORGANIZING WHAT'S OUT THERE: GESTALT GROUPING

The Gestaltists noted that our visual experience is spontaneously organized into distinct groups and objects in a predictable manner (e.g., Rubin, 1915; Wertheimer, 1923). By phenomenal demonstration, they elucidated a number of factors that influence perceived organization. Rubin noted that the dividing contour between two regions is usually assigned to just one of them (the figure), so that the adjoining ground appears shapeless despite the common contour. Regions that are closer, smaller, surrounded, higher in contrast, convex, or symmetrical tend to become figural (see Rock, 1975). Rarely, these factors compete to yield ambiguous reversible organizations such as Rubin's faces versus vase display. Wertheimer moved beyond the assignment of single edges to consider how separate blobs are grouped together or apart phenomenally, and he identified several determining factors (figure 14.1A, B). These factors all make considerable functional sense, given that elements that share the determining properties in real-world scenes are more likely to belong to a common object. For this reason, we shall not distinguish between group-based and object-based models of attention.

Our own research has been driven by the hypothesis that many of the Gestaltists' phenomenal demonstrations may actually reflect the operation of attentional mechanisms. The subjective feeling that dividing edges belong to a figural shape but not to the adjoining ground shape may arise because when trying to attend to just the dividing edge, we tend to select instead the shape to which that edge is assigned (Baylis and Driver, 1995; Driver and Baylis, 1995, 1996a). Similarly, the subjective feeling that a column or row of dots belongs together (figure 14.1A, B) may arise because when trying to attend to a single dot, our attention tends to spread instead across the entire

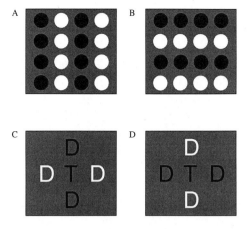

Figure 14.1 (A) Typical Gestalt demonstration, with the regularly spaced circles organized phenomenally into columns by common color. (B) Comparable circles organized into rows instead. (C) Schematic display from Baylis and Driver (1992). Participants judged the central target letter (here a *T*) while ignoring the surrounding distractors (here all *D*s). More interference was found from distractors sharing the color of the target, grouped into a column in this example. In (D) the central target is grouped by common color into a row, and the horizontally aligned distractors now interfered more than the vertical.

group in which it falls (Baylis and Driver, 1992). If so, our ability to attend selectively should be similarly constrained by Gestalt grouping when indexed by objective performance tasks.

INFLUENCES OF SEGMENTATION ON NORMAL ATTENTION

Distractor Interference with Focused Attention

A classic measure of selective attention concerns the extent to which distractors disrupt performance of a target task. Eriksen and Eriksen (1974) had participants classify target letters presented at central fixation. Distractor letters flanked each target at various separations, and could be neutral letters or letters associated with the same or opposite response to that required by the target. Slower responses in the presence of incongruent distractors were taken as evidence that those distractors were identified. The decline in such interference for more distant distractors was taken as evidence that less processing takes place outside an attentional spotlight focused on the target.

Driver and Baylis (1989) suggested that the reduced interference from more distant distractors might simply reflect a reduction in grouping between target and distractors when they were less proximate. Driver and Baylis set grouping by common motion against grouping by proximity, and found that distant distractors that moved with the target interfered more than did closer distractors in a separate motion group. They concluded that attention is directed to Gestalt groups rather than to raw locations. The dominance of motion over proximity can disappear with minor changes in stimuli and procedure (Kramer, Tham, and Yeh, 1991), presumably because when motion and proximity are pitted against each other either may predominate, depending on the exact circumstances. The precedence of motion remains a robust finding with our original displays, and subsequent studies have made a similar point for other grouping factors. Kramer and Jacobson (1991) found more interference for distractors grouped with the target by connectedness or common color. Harms and Bundesen (1983) and Baylis and Driver (1992) also observed more inteference from distractors that shared the target's color (see figure 14.1C, D), and color grouping was found capable of overriding proximity in the latter study. Finally, Baylis and Driver (1992) found that grouping of a grid of characters into rows versus columns, as determined by good continuation, could similarly affect the extent of distractor interference.

Object-Based Cueing Effects

Much of the evidence taken to indicate that covert attention operates like a spotlight has come from the spatial cueing paradigm introduced by Posner (1980). Participants judge a target that can appear at any of several known locations. Their covert attention is cued to one location in advance, either by an uninformative event there, or by an instruction about the most likely target position. Many studies find better judgments at the cued locus even though saccades towards it are prevented. This has been taken to reflect the covert focusing of an attentional spotlight upon the cued region.

However, in many such studies each possible target locus is marked by an object in which the target may appear (e.g., an outline box). With such displays, cueing effects could reflect attention to particular objects in a segmented representation of the scene, rather than to unparsed regions of space as with a strict spotlight metaphor. Egly, Driver and Rafal (1994) examined the possible contribution of object segmentation to spatial cueing effects, using displays like that in figure 14.2A. A spatially informative cue appeared at one end of a rectangle. The majority of targets for detection appeared at that cued locus (valid trials). On invalid trials, the target could appear at the opposite end of the same rectangle or the same distance away at one end of the other rectangle. Responses were slower for invalid than for valid targets within the cued rectangle, indicating the costs of a spatial attention shift within an object. However, the delay was greater still for an invalid target in the uncued rectangle, indicating a greater difficulty in shifting attention between objects than within objects over a comparable distance (or else indicating that attention tended to spread across the cued object even before the target appeared). A similar result was found when the horizontal or vertical rectangles were replaced by two rows or two columns of circles, respectively; the cue was the brief illumination of an end circle (see figure 14.2B). In this case, the cue did not point in one direction more than in any

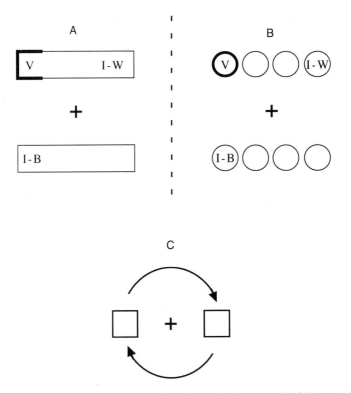

Figure 14.2 (A) Schematic display from Egly, Driver, and Rafal (1994). The ends of two rectangles mark four possible target loci equally spaced around the central fixation cross. One of these is cued by brightening one end of a rectangle (see heavy shading at top left). Valid targets appear at this location (indicated by V). Invalid targets could appear at the opposite end within the same rectangle (I-W), or a similar distance away in a different object (I-B). The two rectangles were equally likely to be vertically elongated instead, so that between-object and within-object shifts of attention were then in horizontal and vertical directions, respectively, on invalid trials. (B) Here the two rectangular objects are replaced by two groups of circles, organized into rows (as illustrated) or columns. One end of one group was cued by brightening an entire circle. (C) Schematic display from Tipper et al. (1991). Targets could appear in either box and these both moved as shown by the arrows after one box had been cued.

other, and attention would have to traverse more edges within a group than between groups on invalid trials. Thus, the object-based component of covert orienting extends to grouping by proximity as well as by connectedness, and is not due to some trivial reluctance to cross physical borders.

He and Nakayama (1995) reported related results in the three-dimensional domain. They presented participants with two stereoscopically defined rows of elements, one above and one below fixation, and cued them to expect a target in a particular row. The delay in response for invalid targets in the other row increased when the rows were placed further apart in depth on separate frontoparallel planes. This effect depends on the extent to which the two rows appear to lie on a common surface rather than merely on the difference in their disparity. Attention spreads across a common surface, as shown by the reduced validity effect when the two rows had different stereo disparities but lay on a common tilted depth plane. These results have several ramifications, but for present purposes they extend Egly, Driver, and Rafal's (1994) two-dimensional study to the three-dimensional case. Some aspects of covert orienting are evidently object-based in the sense that they operate on segmented regions of space (i.e., grouped blobs or surfaces), rather than on content-free locations in some two-dimensional or three-dimensional map.

Further spatial cueing studies have identified covert orienting mechanisms that are object-based in a somewhat different sense: the location(s) to which the mechanisms apply get updated when objects move. Tipper, Driver, and Weaver (1991) reexamined the inhibition of return (IOR) effect first observed by Posner and Cohen (1984) when spatially uninformative visual cues precede visual targets. Target detection is initially better at the cued location, but as the delay between cue and target presentation increases, this reverses, so that performance eventually becomes worst at the cued position. Posner and Cohen argued that attention is first drawn to the cued locus, and then moves on with an inhibitory bias against returning to the examined position, which might serve to prevent perseverations during search. However, inhibiting fixed locations in this way would be rather ineffective as a means for optimizing search in dynamic scenes. Tipper et al. accordingly proposed that particular *objects* rather than fixed positions may be inhibited, such that the putative inhibition follows the objects around if they move.

They used a variant of the spatial cueing task in which the two boxes marking the possible target locations could move during the trial (figure 14.2C). IOR did indeed tend to move with the cued objects, and thus can evidently be object-based in the sense that the positions to which it applies are updated as objects move. Gibson and Egeth (1994) have similarly shown that inhibited locations can be updated as an object moves, but in their case the various locations corresponded to different parts of a single object, rather than to separate objects. They used successive outline drawings that created the impression of a brick rotating in depth. Cueing one face of the brick led later to delayed responses for targets on that face, even when rotation of the brick placed the cued face in a different location.

Seminal studies by Pylyshyn and Storm (1988) and Kahneman, Treisman, and Gibbs (1992) have introduced further behavioral methods for studying how the visual system may track multiple moving objects. We can only summarize their broadest conclusions here. Pylyshyn et al. (1994) argued that several noncontiguous locations can be marked simultaneously for attentional allocation (provided they are filled by visual objects) and can be updated continuously as the objects move. Yantis (1992) suggested that such multiple tracking depends on the target elements forming a good configuration, so that the tracked locations behave like parts of a single global object (as in Gibson and Egeth, 1994). Kahneman et al. (1992) have argued on the basis of object-specific priming effects that separate object-files are set up for each segmented object. These files are updated with new information as objects change or move, to allow continuity in their perception. Tipper and colleagues' object-based IOR (figure 14.2C) could be neatly redescribed as inhibition of an object file, but the exact relationship between the object file construct and the various mechanisms of attention remains to be determined.

To summarize, cueing studies have shown that components of covert orienting can be object-based in the following three senses: they may (1) apply to different spatial regions as a function of segmentation by connectedness, proximity, or common three-dimensional surface in static displays; (2) apply to positions that are updated as an entire object moves; or (3) apply to part of an object such that the affected location in the image is updated as the view of the object changes. The latter finding raises the point that objects have intrinsic spatial structure, given by the layout of their parts relative to each other (see Baylis and Driver, 1993). This leads to more subtle versions of the object- versus space-based debate. Instead of questioning whether selection is ever spatial, we may instead ask exactly what coordinates selection operates in when it does take a spatial form. For example, spatial selection could arise in retinal, head-centered, body-centered, gravitational, or object-centered coordinates. Gibson and Egeth's (1994) findings provide an apparent example of the latter. We return to the coordinate issue later, when we consider evidence from neuropsychological deficits of attention. For the moment, the studies discussed in this section do not disprove the hypothesis that attention operates in a spatial medium (Tsal and Lavie, 1993), but they do show that this medium is not content-free; the locations that are enhanced or inhibited depend strongly on how the display is segmented.

Divided Visual Attention and Object Segmentation

Several studies have reported that divided attention is more difficult across elements of separate objects than it is for elements of a common object. However, some of the initial evidence for this can now be questioned. Treisman et al. (1983) presented a rectangular frame that either surrounded a word (with both the frame and the word either above or below fixation together) or was separated from it (with one item above and one below fixation). Participants had to read the word and judge the horizontal position of a gap in the rectangular frame. The gap remained as close to the word in the separated format as in the surrounded format, but dual-task performance was more efficient in the surrounded case. This might suggest a difficulty in dividing attention across objects (separated word and frame) versus within objects (integral word and frame). However, one could argue that there were always two objects, and that just their relative location varied. When word and frame were separated, the irrelevant contours of the frame may have provided a spatial cue that drew attention away from the word, thus impairing performance.

Duncan (1984) presented two objects, distinguished by closure and good continuation, that were always spatially superimposed; an outline box with a line struck through it. Participants had to judge one or two of the following attributes: line texture, line orientation, box height, or the location of a gap in the box. Two attributes from one object (i.e., height and gap of box, or texture and orientation of line) could be judged together almost as accurately as could one. There was a more substantial dual-task cost when participants judged one attribute from the box and one from the line. This was taken to reflect a difficulty in dividing attention across objects rather than across locations, given that the superimposed objects were in roughly the same place, and the two attributes of the box were no closer to each other than to the line attributes.

In further studies, Duncan (1993a, b) has also reported a cost for dividing attention between objects. However, in these later experiments the distinction between objects was confounded with their spatial separation, so space-based and object-based accounts were not distinguished. Moreover, Duncan's original findings (1984) have been criticized by Watt (1988) and by Baylis and Driver (1993), due to a potential problem with the box and line stimuli. The two line attributes are primarily available at high spatial frequencies, whereas the two box attributes are available at low spatial frequencies. The divided attention cost might therefore be due to diverse spatial frequencies rather than to the presence of separate objects.

To avoid this criticism, Baylis and Driver (1993) devised a way to compare one-object and two-object judgments for physically identical attributes. They used ambiguous figure and ground displays (figure 14.3A, B), analogous to Rubin's (1915) faces/vase engraving. Perceptual set was manipulated so that the two critical edges would either be assigned to a single common

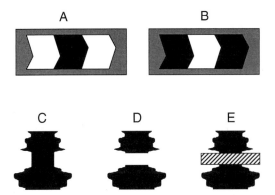

Figure 14.3 (A and B) Schematic displays from Baylis (1994). Particpants judged which of the two inner angles was lower (the left in both examples). Color instructions manipulated whether each display was seen to contain two outer figures (white in A, black in B) or one inner figure (black in A, white in B). The task was easier in the latter case. (C) Schematic display from Driver and Baylis (1995). Judgments of symmetry became harder when the same information was presented as two separate objects (D) by deleting the uninformative straight contours. Removing those same contours by occlusion instead (E) restored performance by restoring the percept of a single symmetrical object.

object (analogous to the Rubin's vase) or to two different objects (analogous to Rubin's faces). Comparing the two edges was more difficult under the two-object interpretation (also, see Baylis, 1994; Driver and Baylis, in 1995b; Gibson, 1994). This two-object cost cannot be reinterpreted in terms of stimulus factors such as diverse spatial frequencies (unlike Duncan's box-and-line stimuli) because the two-object and one-object displays were physically identical, being segmented differently only due to perceptual set. These results provide a further case of segmentation influencing attention. However, they can be reconciled with the view that attention operates in a spatial medium (Tsal and Lavie, 1993), provided that one allows that segmentation determines which spatial region will be attended. The two possible segmentations of figure 14.3A could result in different areas being attended during the edge comparison task (i.e., the outer shapes versus the central shape, with the latter distribution being more efficient).

Recently, however, Vecera and Farah (1994) have argued that object-based limits on divided attention can be entirely nonspatial. They used Duncan's (1984) stimuli and tasks, but varied whether the box and line were superimposed at fixation or separated, with one on the left and one on the right of fixation. The apparent cost of dividing attention across objects was no greater when the two objects were separated. Vecera and Farah suggested that this null effect arose because the various judgments were all based on object-centered shape representations (Marr and Nishihara, 1978). These are considered to be viewpoint independent, and thus should not code the position of shapes. Such representations have been hypothesized to arise in the visual areas of the inferotemporal lobe (IT), which are known to be involved in object recognition in humans and monkeys based on single-cell, lesion, and neuroimaging studies (see Baylis, Rolls, and Leonard, 1987; Plaut and Farah, 1991).

Vecera and Farah thus claim to have established a further sense in which attention might be object-based; it may apparently operate on spatially invariant object-centered representations when the task requires shape judgments. However, there are several reasons to doubt this conclusion. First, Hoffman and Nelson (1981) previously found that spatial separation dramatically increased the cost of dividing attention between objects in shape judgment tasks. Second, Vecera and Farah's manipulation of spatial separation was confounded with several other factors: distant objects were more eccentric, and only close objects were superimposed. Superimposition may have led to an extra difficulty in attentional selection, masking the costs of attending to more distant locations.

Third, their study used Duncan's box-and-line stimuli. As argued previously, apparent two-object costs with those stimuli may actually be due to spatial frequency differences, which presumably remain to some extent regardless of spatial separation. Finally, one can question the theoretical underpinnings of their account. Some of the judged attributes (e.g., line orientation) seem to require viewpoint-specific representations rather than

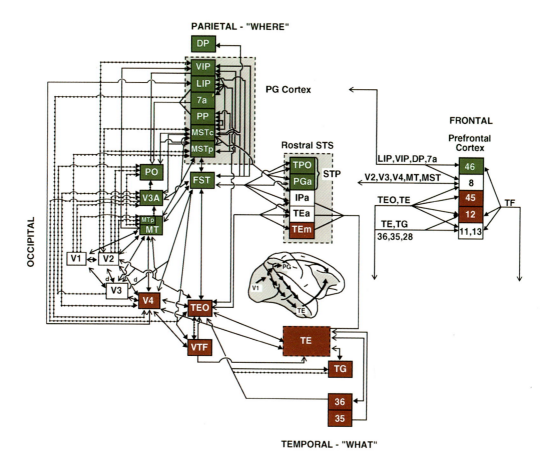

Plate 1 Visual processing pathways in monkeys derived from anatomical tract tracing methods. Heavy arrowheads indicate feedforward projections; open arrowheads indicate feedback projections. Solid lines indicate connections arising from both central and peripheral visual field representations; dotted lines indicate connections restricted to peripheral field representations. Red boxes indicate ventral pathway areas related primarily to object vision, green boxes indicate dorsal pathway areas related primarily to spatial vision, and white boxes indicate areas not clearly allied with either pathway. Shaded region on the lateral view of the brain indicates the extent of the cortex included in the diagram. (Adapted from Ungerleider, 1995.) See chapter 2. Also see table 2.1 for key to abbreviations.

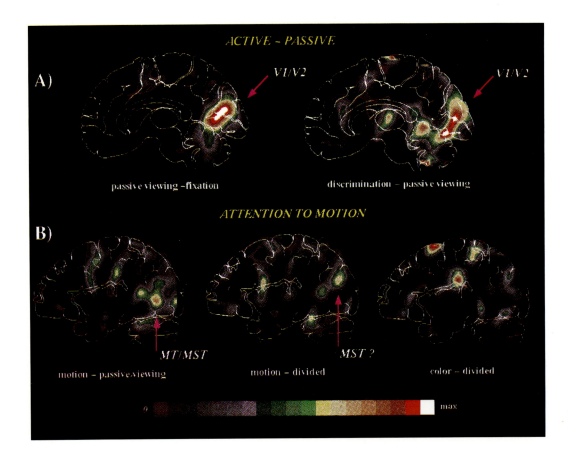

Plate 2 (A) Nonselective active-passive modulation in primary visual cortex and adjacent regions (V1/V2). Sagittal PET section 5 mm left off midline. (Left) V1/V2 activation for passive viewing of a colored moving array of objects minus viewing only a fixation point. (Right) V1/V2 modulation for discriminating threshold shape changes of the objects minus passive viewing. (B) Motion selective modulation in human homolog of middle temporal/middle superior temporal (MT/MST) area. Sagittal PET section 35 mm left off midline. (Left) MT/MST activity during threshold speed discrimination minus passive viewing. (Center) Activity when discriminating motion minus discriminating any attribute (color, shape, motion) in divided attention condition. (Right) Lack of activity during threshold color discrimination minus divided attention. See chapter 6.

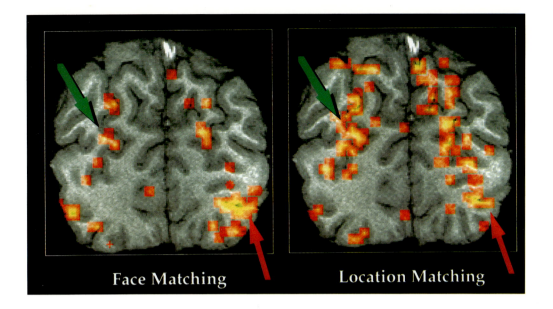

Plate 5 Differential activation of ventral and dorsal visual extrastriate areas in the occipital lobe when subjects selectively attend to the identity or location of faces. The results are from an fMRI study of an individual subject. Coronal sections are 3 cm from the occipital pole. Ventral lateral occipital areas that were more activated by face matching than by location matching are indicated with red arrows. Dorsal occipital areas that were more activated by location matching than by face matching are indicated with green arrows. (From Haxby et al., 1997.) See chapter 7.

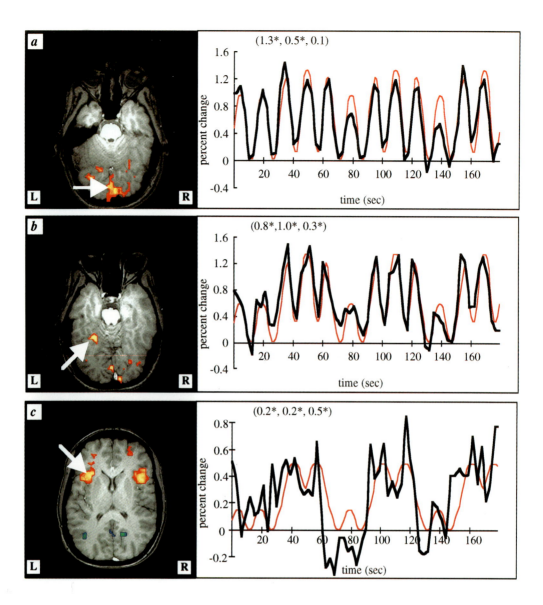

Plate 6 Two extrastriate and one prefrontal region with different patterns of response during a face working memory task. Data are from an individual subject. (a) A posterior ventral occipital area that demonstrated a mostly nonselective, transient response to visual stimuli. The weights calculated by multiple regression for the three regressors (figure 7.3) are shown in parentheses (*p < 0.05). The weighted sum of the regressors is shown in red. The obtained fMRI time series, averaged over all voxels in the region and over repeated time series, is shown in black. (b) An anterior ventral temporal area that demonstrated a more selective, still mostly transient response to faces. The sustained activity over memory delays was small, but statistically significant. (c) A prefrontal region in the inferior frontal gyrus near the anterior end of the insula that demonstrated more sustained activity over memory delays. (Adapted from Courtney et al., 1997.) See chapter 7.

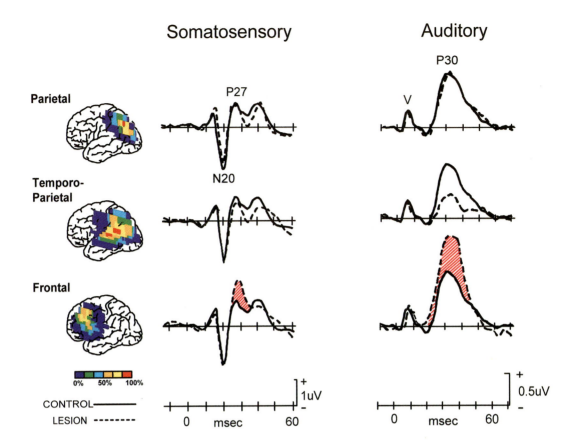

Plate 7 Primary cortical somatosensory and auditory evoked responses in control subjects (solid line) and patients (dashed line) with focal damage in lateral parietal cortex (top, n = 8), temporal-parietal junction (middle, n = 13), or in dorsolateral prefrontal cortex (bottom, n = 11). Reconstructions of the extent of damage in each patient group are shown on the left. Somatosensory potentials were elicited by square-wave pulses delivered to the median nerve at the wrist and recorded from area 3b (N20) and areas 1 and 2 (P27). Auditory evoked responses generated in the inferior colliculus (wave V) and the primary auditory cortex (P30) were elicited by clicks delivered at a rate of 13/s and a 50 dB HL intensity level. Prefrontal lesions resulted in a selective increase in the amplitudes of the P27 and P30 responses (shaded areas). See chapter 8.

PFCx - Visual Modulation

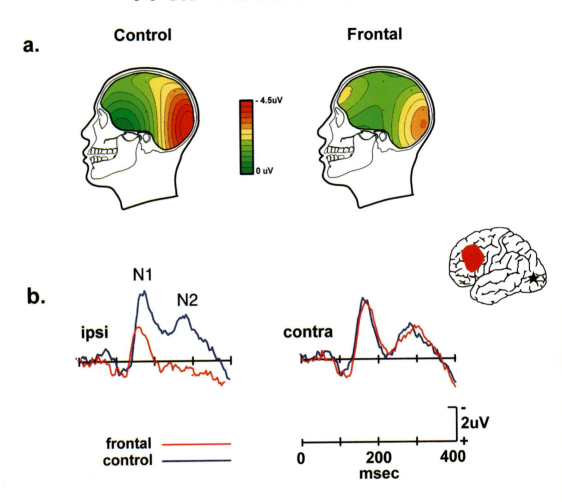

a.

Control   Frontal

- 4.5uV

0 uV

b.

N1

N2

ipsi   contra

-
2uV
+

frontal ———
control ———

0   200   400
msec

Plate 8 Prefrontal cortex modulates the visual N170 component. (a) Topographic maps display the scalp voltage distribution (in μV) of the N170 to targets. The extrastriate focus of the N170 in controls is reduced ipsilateral to prefrontal damage. (Inset) The red shading on the brain shows the area of maximum lesion overlap, and the star indicates a putative N170 generator in extrastriate cortex. (b) Group averaged ERPs for target stimuli in controls and frontal lesion patients (n = 11). Waveforms are from posterior temporal electrodes (T5/T6 in controls), ipsilateral (ipsi) and contralateral (contra) to the lesion. The N1 (N170) and N2 components are labeled. In this and subsequent figures, negative is up, stimulus onset occurs at 0 ms, and the scale is given in microvolts (μV). See chapter 8.

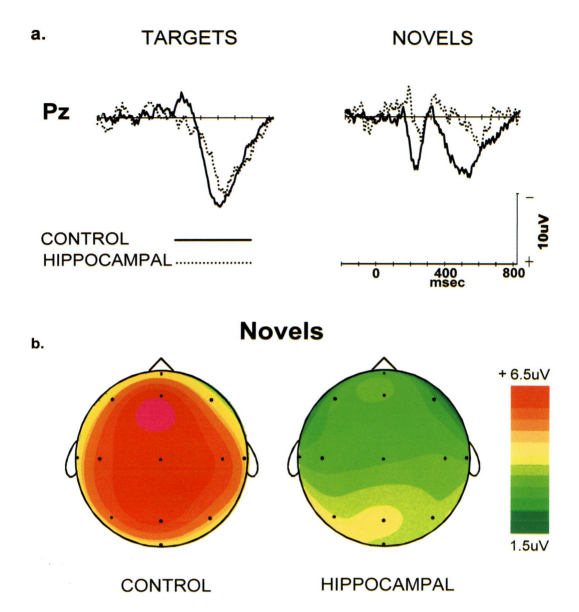

Plate 9 Visual P300 effects in patients with lesions centered in the posterior hippocampus. (a) The target P3b (left) and novelty P3a responses (right) from controls and patients. Hippocampal lesions produced reductions in the P3a while sparing the P3b. (b) Scalp voltage maps illustrate the widespread decrease in the novelty P3a after hippocampal damage. See chapter 8.

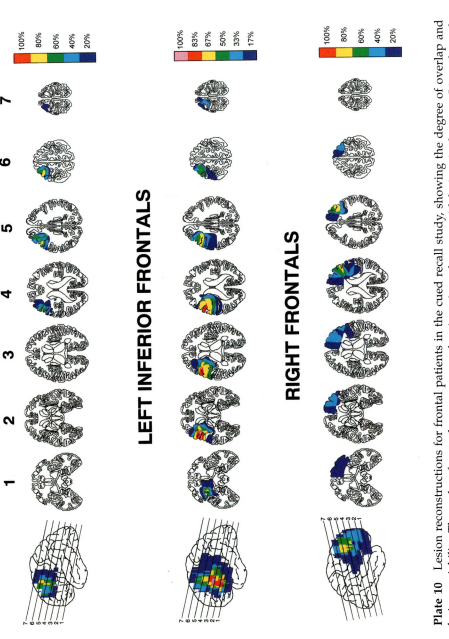

Plate 10   Lesion reconstructions for frontal patients in the cued recall study, showing the degree of overlap and lesion variability. The scale refers to the percentage of patients in each group with lesions in that area. Lines through the lateral view show the level of the axial cuts from ventral (1) to dorsal (7). (Top) Patients with left frontal lesions restricted to areas 6, 8, 9, 10, and superior 46. (Middle) Patients with left frontal lesions that included inferior areas 44, 45, and 46. (Bottom) Patients with damage to right frontal areas 6, 8, 9, 10, or 46. See chapter 8.

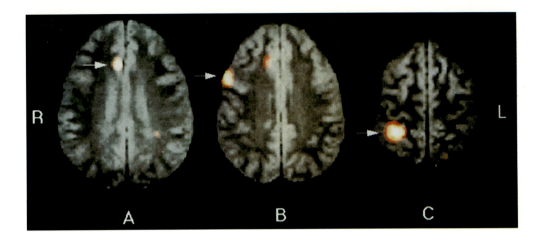

Plate 11 Areas significantly activated during the manual exploration task (Gitelman et al., 1996) as compared to the control condition. Activations in anterior cingulate, premotor cortex, and posterior parietal cortex are shown in slices A, B, and C, respectively. Note that the brain is depicted using the radiological convention with the right side of each image representing the left of the brain. R, right; L, left. See chapter 16.

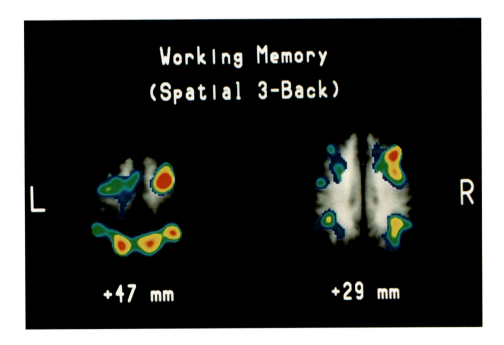

Plate 12 Areas significantly activated during the spatial working memory task of Smith et al. (1996) as compared to the control condition. Each image is superimposed on an MRI image of a composite brain. The left slice shows activation in parietal cortex, areas 7 and 40 (the lower part of the image), and in supplementary motor and premotor cortex (the top part of the image). The right slice shows activation in dorsolateral prefrontal regions (top of the image), as well as further signs of the activation in parietal regions. Note that in these images, the right of the brain is depicted in the right of the images. R, right; L, left. See chapter 16.

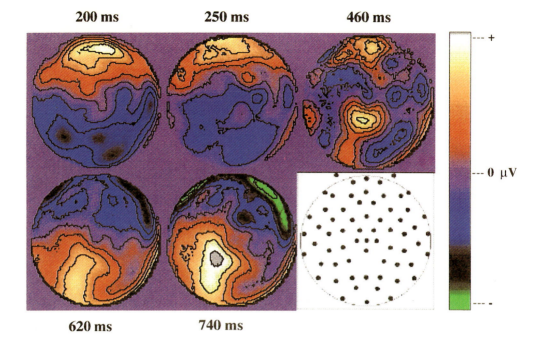

200 ms   **250 ms**   **460 ms**

620 ms   **740 ms**

Plate 13 Maps of the relative voltage differences between the generate uses and reading aloud tasks at several time slices. The colors indicate the size of the voltage differences with the bright colors indicating greater positivity in the uses task and the dark colors greater negativity in the uses task. An early frontal positivity is related to activity in the cingulate and left lateral lexical semantic areas. The later left posterior positivity is related to activity in Wernicke's area. See chapter 18.

spatially invariant object-centered representations. The common assumption that IT object recognition systems use spatially invariant representations can also be queried. Although receptive fields for cells in monkey IT are large (Plaut and Farah, 1991), they might signal stimulus position via population coding, and some IT cells are known to be viewpoint-sensitive (Oram and Perrett, 1994). Moreover, recordings from behaving monkeys (Moran and Desimone, 1985) reveal that IT activity can be spatially modulated as a function of attention, with the large receptive fields apparently shrinking around the attended object. This shows that selection can in fact operate spatially even in the very neural subsystem that Vecera and Farah propose as the site for spatially invariant selection.

Thus, the conclusions from Vecera and Farah's manipulation of spatial separation are unclear. However, several recent studies confirm that attention is less efficient to two objects than to one when the spatial extent of the display is held constant. For instance, Driver and Baylis (1995) found that judgments of symmetry were more efficient for one object (figure 14.3C) than for a comparable two-object case (figure 14.3D). The advantage for a single object held even when it was partially occluded (figure 14.3E) so that its visible components corresponded exactly to the two-object display. This suggests the importance of segmentation in depth, as with the He and Nakayama (1995) study mentioned earlier.

Taking all these results together, it seems a quite general finding that divided attention is less efficient across objects than within an object. However, this does not preclude an influence from spatial separation (Hoffman and Nelson, 1981). Moreover, the radical suggestion that object-based limits on divided attention are spatially invariant (Vecera and Farah, 1994) does not seem well supported at present. In closing, it should be acknowledged that there may be some specific exceptions to the general rule that attention cannot be efficiently divided across distinct objects. In particular, Braun and colleagues (e.g., Braun and Sagi, 1991; Braun, chapter 15, this volume) have reported that detection or localization for unique texture elements can be combined with a central form discrimination task without dual-task decrement, even though the separate texture and form targets presumably appear as quite separate objects. We return to the case of texture segregation later.

Segmentation and Visual Search

Much attentional theorizing has been based on the visual search task. For the present purposes, we note only that visual search depends strongly on how the display is segmented. For instance, a target is more detectable among nontargets if the latter form a separate good continuation group (Prinzmetal and Banks, 1977). Conjunction search for shape and color becomes more efficient when the items are spatially organized into groups of common color or shape (Treisman, 1982). Attention can also be restricted to items on one surface in stereoscopic depth (Nakayama and Silverman, 1986; He and

Nakayama, 1995) or to one motion group (McLeod et al., 1988) during various conjunction tasks. Such exclusion of spatially intermingled items seems problematic for the spotlight metaphor. Finally, search is affected by similarity between nontargets, as well as by similarity between target and nontargets. In general, search is less efficient when nontargets are heterogenous. This is thought to occur because heterogenous nontargets form a less coherent group than homogenous nontargets, and are thus harder to reject en masse (Duncan and Humphreys, 1989).

Yantis and colleagues have adapted the visual search task to examine which stimulus properties capture attention. Yantis and Jonides (1984) found that items with sudden onset tended to be examined first during an apparently serial scan, whereas items with other unique properties (e.g., color) apparently were not. They concluded that visual transients capture attention. However, further studies (e.g., Yantis, 1993) have suggested that the critical factor is whether an item is segmented as a new object, distinct from the other items. For instance, motion per se apparently does not capture attention, but motion that newly segments an object from a background that it was previously grouped together with does lead to attention capture.

Treisman's (1982) feature integration theory was initially based on visual seach data, which suggested that spatial attention integrates visual features coded by otherwise separate modules. Several studies have since found that segmentation strongly constrains feature conjunction so that miscombinations of presented features (so-called illusory conjunctions) are less likely between separate objects or groups than within them (Baylis, Driver, and McLeod, 1992; Prinzmetal, 1995). To the extent that feature conjunction depends on the distribution of attention (see Nakayama and Joseph, chapter 13, this volume), this implies that attention tends to be applied to individual segmented groups rather than being divided across them.

Attention and the Figure-Ground Assignment of Dividing Edges

This review has so far taken us a long way from the original insights of the Gestaltists with which the chapter began. Rubin (1915) noted phenomenally that the dividing contour between two regions appears to belong to a figural shape on just one side, with the adjoining region appearing as a shapeless background. We hypothesize that this phenomenal experience arises because attention automatically spreads across the figural shape to which the dividing edge is assigned by bottom-up segmentation processes. In other words, when we try to attend just the dividing edge, we select instead the entire shape to which it belongs, providing another sense in which visual attention can be object-based.

We recently tested this hypothesis in a series of edge-matching studies (Driver and Baylis, 1996). Edges were presented in rapid succession for comparison (e.g., figure 14.4A followed by 14.4B or 14.4C). Viewers were unable to prevent figure-ground segmentation for the critical edges and showed

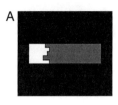

figure-shape probe   ground-shape probe

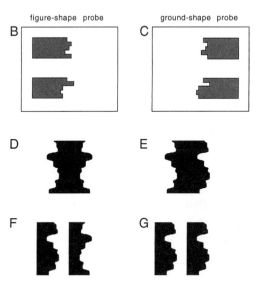

Figure 14.4 (A) Schematic display from Driver and Baylis (1996). A jagged edge divides a rectangle into a small bright figure against a darker ground. This edge had to be compared to those on two shapes presented 500 ms later, with participant selecting which of the two probe shapes had the matching edge (the upper one in both examples). The probe shapes where either blocked out as for the preceding figure (B) or as for the preceding ground (C). The task was easier in the former case, despite the reversal in contrast polarity for the edge itself. (D) Schematic display from Baylis and Driver (1995) for judgment of symmetry, which is easier than detection of translation between edges, as in (E). Reversing figure-ground assignment for one of the two edges made symmetry much harder to detect (F) but made translation easier to detect (G).

better performance when two successive edges had a corresponding assignment (figure 14.4B after 14.4A) rather than a reversed assignment (figure 14.4C after 14.4A), even after hundreds of trials in which the reversed assignment could be equally anticipated. Evidently, matching performance was based on figural shapes rather than on the raw edges themselves. We concluded that attention cannot be restricted to relevant edges but spreads instead across the segmented figural shapes to which the edges are assigned.

A similar conclusion was drawn from a study of symmetry and repetition detection by Baylis and Driver (1995). Detection of symmetry between two otherwise random edges (figure 14.4D) became dramatically harder when figure-ground assignment was reversed for just one of them (figure 14.4F). Conversely, detection of contour repetition (figure 14.4E), which is usually harder than symmetry detection (figure 14.4D), became much easier after the same manipulation (figure 14.4G). The difficulty of symmetry detection in displays like figure 14.4F persisted even when that format could be reliably anticipated and even though only the curved contours were relevant to the prescribed task. Once again, attention could not be restricted to just the relevant edges and applied instead to segmented figural shapes.

Interim Summary of Normal Evidence, and a Possible Challenge

A number of subtly different issues have been covered, and the conclusions so far can be summarized as follows. When people attempt to focus attention on a target at a known location, distractors that are grouped with the target interfere more than do comparable distractors that are not so grouped. When a target is expected at a cued location, attention spreads more rapidly to invalid locations in the same object, group, or surface than it spreads to other locations at a comparable distance. Moreover, the inhibitory aftereffects of uninformative cues can be object-based in the sense that they follow objects or their parts around as they move. Divided attention is often less efficient across objects than within objects, although spatial separation can also be a limiting factor. Visual search is powerfully influenced by segmentation processes and the same applies to feature integration. Finally, when attempting to judge just edges, people end up selecting the figural shapes to which those edges are automatically assigned.

Although these conclusions cover several distinct issues, they all seem broadly consistent with Neisser's (1967) view that segmentation processes can precede attention so that coherent groups in filled positions, rather than raw locations in a content-free representation of space, can then be selected for further analysis. This general position has been challenged by Mack et al. (1992), who claim that no grouping or segregation processes operate prior to attention. They presented standard texture or grouping displays with the addition of a large superimposed cross. Participants had to judge which arm of the cross was longer, but after the third display were asked surprise questions about the background grouping or texture elements. Responses across subjects were at chance for this one critical trial. Mack et al. took this to mean that the background organization was not extracted by the visual system when unattended.

How can this be reconciled with the findings reviewed previously? Mack et al. only address this for the case of visual search, noting that although pop-out in visual search is often held to index preattentive processing, in fact the entire area of the search display is relevant to the viewer who intends to detect a target within it. Hence, parallel search may index processing under *diffuse* attention, rather than under true inattention. This point might also apply to some of the evidence discussed previously. However, note that the studies on distractor interference involved focused attention: targets appeared at a known and fixed central location, with any interference measured from peripheral distractors at irrelevant locations. Hence, there was no reason for attention to be diffuse, and yet effects of distractor grouping were still found. Thus, we would maintain that grouping can take place outside focused attention. Nevertheless, Mack and colleagues' point about the possibility of diffuse attention in many paradigms remains well taken, and future research might usefully test the extent of grouping under conditions of true inattention.

Unfortunately, Mack and colleagues' own method for administering such tests seems problematic. Their experiments relied on explicit retrospective reports following a surprise question about a previously ignored stimulus. This is well known to be an unreliable index of the extent of initial processing. Classic studies of auditory attention (see Broadbent, 1958) found that subjects could report little about an ignored message when asked surprise questions, and this was initially taken to indicate little processing. However, subsequent studies found evidence for substantial processing when indexed by more indirect and on-line methods. Likewise, in vision, poor explicit memory for unattended objects (Rock and Gutman, 1981) contrasts with the considerable processing revealed by indirect on-line measures, such as negative priming (Tipper and Driver, 1988). Future work should employ indirect on-line methods to assess the full extent of grouping under inattention, to determine whether a similar contrast arises between considerable implicit processing versus the poor explicit memory for grouping found by Mack et al. (1992).

INFLUENCES OF SEGMENTATION ON PATHOLOGICAL ATTENTION

Neglect, Extinction, and Balint's Syndrome

The possible role of segmentation processes in three neuropsychological deficits of attention (each described more fully by Rafal, chapter 22, this volume) is now examined. Neglect is a common deficit after unilateral brain injury, in which patients fail to acknowledge or respond appropriately to events toward the contralesional side of space. In extinction, such a deficit may be apparent only for events that compete with a simultaneous event further towards the ipsilesional side. Both these deficits are prevalent after right parietal damage, though they can be found in some form after various unilateral lesions. They are increasingly characterized as attentional disorders, because explanations of the contralesional deficit in terms of peripheral input or output losses can often be ruled out. Finally, Balint's syndrome is associated with bilateral posterior lesions, with the occipitoparietal border particularly implicated. As with neglect, Balint's syndrome is probably a multicomponent disorder, involving dysfunction in several processes due to the fairly large lesion; indeed, the syndrome is increasingly regarded as involving bilateral neglect. The classic triad of symptoms involves problems with deliberate saccades, misreaching under visual guidance, and a tendency for attention to get locked onto particular stimuli.

Neglect and extinction are ostensibly spatial deficits. Although both can take various forms, in every case events towards one side are disadvantaged. Several accounts of neglect and extinction have been put forward in terms of an attentional spotlight that is biased towards the ipsilesional side (Kinsbourne, 1993) or that has difficulty disengaging from that side (Posner, Walkerm, Friedrich, and Rafal, 1984) following the unilateral lesion. At first glance, then, these deficits seem to be consistent with purely space-based models of normal attention. However, more recent studies have shown that neglect and extinction can be dramatically affected by segmentation processes. As with normal attention, this had led to a variety of senses in which pathological attention can be object-based.

Figure-Based Neglect

When copying drawings, neglect patients often omit details towards the contralesional side. If asked to copy a scene containing several objects in a row, many patients neglect the contralesional side of every object in their copy, but produce details on the ipsilesional side of each object even for those that fall well to the contralesional side of the original page (Gainotti, Messerli, and Tissot, 1972). One interpretation of this tendency is that figure-ground segmentation processes initially parse the scene into candidate objects, or distinct blobs. This might proceed normally for both contralesional and ipsilesional objects, with the ipsilesional bias only arising at a subsequent spatially selective stage of attending to individual components within each figure in turn, to copy them in detail. Such an account would fit models of normal function in which segmentation precedes attention (e.g., Neisser, 1967) and likewise precedes pathologically biased attention.

However, there are difficulties interpreting copying evidence, because the task is temporally extended and allows patients to move their eyes and body. Driver et al. (1992) therefore examined whether figure-ground segmentation would influence neglect in a more controlled task. They presented figure-ground displays in which a horizontal rectangle was divided by a random jagged contour towards its left (figure 14.5A) or right end (figure 14.5B). The smaller of the two resulting areas was somewhat brighter, and was therefore seen as a figure by normal observers, with the dividing jagged contour appearing to belong just to it. The task for a right parietal patient with left neglect was to fixate the center of each rectangle and compare the jagged dividing edge with another jagged edge that appeared 500 ms later in total isolation (see bottom of figure 14.5A or 14.5B) at the center of the otherwise empty black screen. Note that this edge-matching task is very like that used with normal subjects to study figure-ground segmentation and attention (see figure 14.4A–C). The only difference was the use of centered isolated edges as probes to avoid any neglect within the probes themselves.

We tested how the patient's matching performance varied as a function of whether the small bright figure was on the left or right of the original dis-

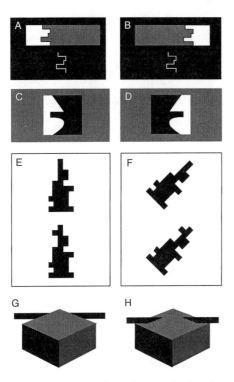

Figure 14.5 (A and B) Schematic displays from Driver et al. (1992) Their left-neglect patient had to compare the jagged edge from each figure-ground display (top half of A and B) to the isolated central edge presented 500 ms later (bottom half), while fixating centrally throughout. Performance was better for when the edge originally shown in the contralesional left visual field (A), as that edge falls to the right of the perceived figure. Similarly, left-neglect patients were better at recognizing figures when their defining edges fell to the right of the figure (as in C, which depicts a white table lamp) than when the figure appeared on the right with the edge to its left (as in D). (E) Typical display from Driver and Halligan (1991); left-neglect patients tended to miss the slight difference on the left of the two shapes and continue to do so even when the shapes were tilted (F) so that the difference fell to the right of the patient. (G and H) Displays from Mattingley et al. (1997). Patients with left extinction had to detect the presence or absence of black bars on the left and right (both are present in each illustration). Failures to detect the left bar in the presence of the right bar were frequent with displays like (H) but were reduced for displays like (G) where the two bars form a single occluded object.

play. The purely space-based prediction would be for poorer performance following displays like figure 14.5A, where the critical jagged edge fell towards the patient's contralesional (and thus neglected) side. However, in this situation the edge also fell towards the ipsilesional side of the shape that would be considered as the figure for a normal observer (i.e., on the right of the small bright shape; see figure 14.5A), whereas it fell to the left of this figure in figure 14.5B. Thus, if the patient could segment figure from ground in both ipsilesional and contralesional visual fields, with his neglect subsequently applying to the contralesional side of any figure, his performance should be poorer when judging contours that originally fell to his good ipsilesional side, because these contours fell on the contralesional side of the figure. The results clearly supported this figure-based prediction. Further evidence consistent with figure-based neglect has since been reported for other cases of neglect after right parietal damage, in a drawing task for reversible figure-ground displays (Marshall and Halligan, 1994). In subsequent work, using meaningful shapes, we similarly found that left neglect could impair recognition of shapes to the right of a dividing edge (e.g., figure 14.5D) compared with recognition of shapes to the left of that edge (figure 14.5C). In other words, the central edge suffered when assigned to the left of a figure (as in figure 14.5D). These studies show that neglect can be object-based in the sense that it applies to the contralesional side of segmented figures. They also confirm our conclusion, drawn earlier from normal evidence, that when people attempt to select just edges, their attention operates instead on the shape to which those edges are assigned.

Axis-Based Neglect

Driver and colleagues' (1992) results show that neglect can apply to segmented figures, but what provides the divide between the relatively spared and impaired sides of such figures? One possibility stems from work on normal shape perception, in which it has been argued that the visual system describes shapes relative to their principal axis of elongation or symmetry (e.g., Marr and Nishihara, 1978). This possibility was tested by Driver and Halligan (1991), who presented their left neglect patient with displays comprising two elongated nonsense shapes, one above the other, and required her to judge whether the shapes were the same or different. Any difference was minor, and appeared either on just the right or just the left. As would be expected, the left-neglect patient tended to miss differences only on the left of upright shapes (see figure 14.5E). This deficit might arise in various coordinates, because the neglected differences fell to the left of the patient and of the page, as well as to the left of each shape's principal axis. The more informative data came from displays in which both shapes were tilted 45 degrees (see figure 14.5F). Differences on the left side of each shape then fell to the right of the patient and page, and yet continued to be neglected. This pattern suggests that neglect can apply to the contralesional side of the extracted principal axis for segmented shapes. We have replicated this result with other patients, and Driver, Baylis, Goodrich, and Rafal (1994) observed axis-based neglect in a further task that ruled out any explanation in terms of biased eye movement patterns.

Intrinsic Handedness and Object-Centered Neglect

The results discussed in the preceding section might be summarized as showing that neglect can apply to the left of segmented figures, with principal axes providing the divide between left and right sides for each shape. But consider this question: what determines the side of the axis that will be treated as being on the left? Marr and Nishihara (1978) originally invoked principal axes for the derivation of viewpoint-independent representations, in which left and right do not refer to where things fall relative to the viewer, but only to the intrinsic handedness of shapes (e.g., to the difference in shape between left hands and right hands, which is maintained regardless of viewpoint). By contrast, the type of neglect discussed in the preceding section must apply to viewer-centered representations, in the sense that the layout of information is still coded relative to the perceiver in terms of what counts as leftward. The shapes in figures 14.5E and F are meaningless and unfamiliar, and so do not have any intrinsic left or right side. Instead, which side is left and which is right is determined solely by the current viewpoint. For example, if figure 14.5E and 14.5F were viewed from behind the page, then the differences would fall on the right rather than on left of each shape.

Other researchers have examined whether neglect can be object-based in the different sense of applying to one intrinsic side of a familiar object, so that the same information is neglected regardless of the current viewpoint. Farah, Brunn, Wong, Wallace, and Carpenter (1990) found no such pattern when drawings of familiar objects with conventional uprights were tilted 90 degrees. However, Behrmann and Moscovitch (1994) found just such an effect with tilted asymmetric letters, and likewise for Caramazza and Hillis (1990) with various formats of letter strings (e.g., tilted or mirror reversed). We suspect that asymmetric letters and words may be atypical visual shapes, in that only they require an assignment of intrinsic handedness for correct recognition (e.g., a *b* becomes a *d* in mirror-image format).

Tracking of Moving Object Position in Neglect

A study of neglect by Behrmann and Tipper (1994) adapted the normal procedure of Tipper et al. (1991) described earlier (figure 14.2C). Left neglect patients were shown two circles connected by a horizontal line (i.e., a barbell) and were required to detect targets, which could appear in either circle. As expected, the patients were slower to detect targets on the left. However, if the entire barbell visibly rotated through 180 degrees, then performance became poorer for targets in the circle that had moved to the right of the display (and had previously been on the left). This suggests that the positions to which neglect applies can be updated as stimuli move, but the initial published data on this phenomenon (Berhmann and Tipper, 1994) may arise because the patients tracked the right circle with pursuit eye movements as it moved, and then merely responded more quickly to fixated targets. Future work may rule out this trivial explanation.

Segmentation and Extinction

Thus far we have only discussed evidence for object-based influences on neglect. Extinction is often regarded as a more primitive spatial phenomenon, in which patients can detect isolated events toward either the contralesional or ipsilesional side but miss contralesional stimuli presented simultaneously with a competing ipsilesional event (Baylis, Driver, and Rafal, 1993). In some respects, this can be thought of as a limit on dividing attention. It has long been known that normal subjects are likely to miss one of two brief simultaneous targets, even under conditions in which they can monitor either of two streams for an occasional single target (Duncan, 1980). Extinction might thus be viewed as a pathological exaggeration of the normal difficulty with two simultaneous targets that is so severe that it can prevent detection even for quite salient events, and which is spatially specific such that the most contralesional event invariably suffers in a competitive situation.

As discussed previously, normal divided attention can be substantially influenced by segmentation processes, and is more difficult across two distinct objects or groups. Recent studies have found that the same is true of extinction. Driver, Mattingley, Rorden, and Davis (1997) reported that extinction between two simultaneous circles was eliminated when the two were linked by a horizontal line to form a single barbell. Ward, Goodrich, and Driver (1994) similarly found that more subtle grouping principles, such as good continuation, could reduce extinction by linking the two events into one global object, so that they became allies rather than competitors for selection. Mattingley, Davis and Driver (1997) have since found that even three-dimensional grouping factors can influence extinction, reducing it when the two events that must be detected appear as parts of a single occluded object (as for the two black bars in figure 14.5G, but not for figure 14.5H). Thus, as described earlier for normal attention, pathological attention seems to be influenced by depth interpretations in addition to purely two-dimensional segmentation factors. Top-down influences can also contribute when familiar stimuli are employed. Extinction between two letter strings is reduced when they form a familiar compound word (Behrmann, Moscovitch, Black, and Mozer, 1990) just as neglect may be reduced for words compared with unfamiliar strings (Farah, Wallace, and Vecera, 1993). Thus, the effective segmentation can depend on prior learning for particular strings.

Possible Hemispheric Differences in Object-Based Attention

Egly, Driver, and Rafal's (1994) adaptation of the cueing technique for measuring normal spatial shifts of attention both within objects and between objects was previoulsy described (see figure 14.2A). This measure was also used with right- and left-parietal patients. As expected (compare Posner et al., 1984), the right hemisphere patients were particularly impaired for contralesional targets after an ipsilesional cue. This spatial abnormality was superimposed on a quite normal influence from the distinction between objects. However, the left-parietal group showed a further abnormality. Their difficulty with contralesional targets after an ipsilesional cue was exacerbated when a shift of attention between separate objects was required.

This extra impairment was surprising, given that right hemisphere neglect patients are typically more impaired clinically than are left hemisphere patients, for various reasons (see Rafal, chapter 22, this volume). However, subsequent evidence supports left hemisphere specialization for shifts of attention between objects. Egly, Rafal, Driver, and Starrveveld (1994) found that the between-object cost was apparent only in the right visual field of a split-brain patient. Humphreys and Riddoch (1995) studied a patient with bilateral damage who tended to neglect the left half of individual objects (consistent with his right hemisphere damage) but also tended to neglect entire objects that appeared on the right (consistent with impairment of left hemisphere mechanisms for shifting between objects). This pattern was found across several tasks. When he read a word (i.e., treating the string as a single object), letters on the left were neglected, but when he named each letter in the word (treating the string as several distinct objects), right letters were missed.

The possibility of hemispheric asymmetries could be tested further by applying the various neuroimaging techniques described in other chapters of this volume (such as positron emission tomography or functional magnetic resonance imaging) to healthy people as they carry out comparable within- or between-object covert orienting tasks. The suggested specialization of the left hemisphere for between-object shifts may relate to Robertson's observations (chapter 12, this volume) concerning hemispheric specialization for global versus local stimulus properties, and also to Kosslyn and colleagues' (1989) hypothesis that the left hemisphere specializes in coding categorical spatial properties (e.g., the distinction between separate objects) rather than metrical spatial properties (e.g., the precise distance between the objects). Finally, left hemisphere specialization for between-object shifts might explain why combined left and right hemisphere lesions produce the drastic restriction of attention found in Balint's syndrome.

Segmentation and Balint's Syndrome

One of the defining symptoms of Balint's syndrome is a difficulty in attending to more than one object at a time (simultanagnosia). This is usually apparent from patients' phenomenal reports, and can apply even to spatially superimposed stimuli (e.g., the patient may report seeing the clinician's eyes yet not his or her spectacles, or vice versa). The deficit can also be documented more formally. For instance, Driver et al. (1997) reported a Balint's syndrome patient who could detect both of two simultaneous circles only when they were connected to form a single barbell (also, see Luria, 1959). The same study found a similar pattern in the performance of unilateral extinction patients, the only difference being that in the Balint's case one could not predict which of the two unconnected circles would be missed. As in extinction, the difficulty with multiple objects can also be modulated by the familiarity of a configuration. Baylis, Driver, Baylis, and Rafal (1994) reported a Balint's case who could read familiar whole words (thus taking in all the letters) even though he was unable to identify all the component letters when he treated them as individual objects.

Humphreys et al. (1994) studied two bilateral patients who could read words or name pictures when the stimuli were presented in isolation; when the patients were presented with simultaneous pictures and words, however, they could only name the pictures. This inattention to the word in the presence of a picture was quite insensitive to spatial factors. For instance, it persisted regardless of whether the simultaneous picture and word were superimposed or separated, and it was found even when the word was foveal. Humphreys et al. concluded that the deficit was entirely nonspatial and was due instead to competition between abstract pictorial and verbal representations. However, it remains possible that the competitive advantage for pictures was driven by lower-level properties such as their greater size, complexity, and contrast (or closure, as the authors note). Moreover, the pathologically biased attentional competition might still operate within a spatial medium, contrary to the authors' conclusion that it was entirely nonspatial. This could be tested by examining whether subsequent probe stimuli are detected more reliably at the location of the detected picture than at the location of the undetected word.

It is relatively easy to explain the lateral biases in attention that emerge following unilateral brain injury in neglect and extinction. These biases may arise because each hemisphere tends to induce competing tendencies for orienting in the contralateral direction when activated (Kinsbourne, 1993). This competition should become pathologically biased in favor of the ipsilesional direction after a unilateral lesion. However, it is harder to explain in such terms the drastic attentional impairments of Balint's syndrome following bilateral injury. The difficulty in becoming aware of more than one object at a time may relate to a left hemisphere problem in shifting between objects, together with a narrowed attentional focus consequent on right hemisphere damage. Alternatively, simultanagnosia may reflect a fundamental restriction in the capacity available for representing multiple stimuli when the parietal lobe is damaged. This may also apply to a lesser extent after unilateral lesions, but might tend to be overlooked due to the more obvious lateral bias.

CONCLUSIONS

Both the normal and the neuropsychological evidence indicate that visual attention can be object-based in a number of ways. We suspect that in future work it will be important to distinguish these different types of object-based attention instead of conflating them under a single "object-centered" heading. The boundary conditions for each type and the specific neural mechanisms that are involved may well differ. Nonetheless, it is clear that many segmentation processes influence the distribution of normal and pathological attention and that these influences might all operate within a spatial medium.

The numerous findings of segmentation effects on neglect, extinction, and Balint's syndrome are broadly consistent with a suspected extrastriate or ventral site for the effective segmentation processes (Driver, 1995, 1996), given that most patients with these attentional deficits have lesions restricted primarily to more dorsal visual areas, which would not be expected to directly disrupt segmentation processes.

Future Directions

Many questions remain. Some of these concern the specific neural areas involved in the various segmentation processes that influence attention. Progress on this will surely come from the various neuroimaging techniques that have recently been introduced for the study of brain activity in normal humans. Surprisingly little is known about how segmentation processes operate at the level of single neurons in behaving primates; nonetheless, the study of object-based coding at this level has already begun promisingly (Olsen and Gettner, 1995).

Finally, in much of our discussion we have assumed that object segmentation precedes attention whenever influences of segmentation are found. However, it is possible that the relationship between processes of segmentation and of spatial selection is one of interactive activation (Farah et al., 1993; Humphreys and Riddoch, 1993), with each able to mutually influence the other, rather than a strictly sequential arrangement with all segmentation fully preceding selection. This particular issue should be resolvable via those neuroimaging techniques that can reveal the exact time course of internal processing events.

REFERENCES

Baylis, G. C. (1994) Visual attention and objects: Two-object cost with equal convexity. *J. Exp. Psychol. Hum. Percept. Perform.* 20: 208–212.

Baylis, G. C. and Driver, J. (1992) Visual parsing and response competition: The effects of grouping. *Percept. Psychophys.* 51: 145–162.

Baylis, G. C. and Driver, J. (1993) Visual attention and objects. *J. Exp. Psychol. Hum. Percept. Perform.* 3: 451–470.

Baylis, G. C. and Driver, J. (1995) Obligatory edge assignment in vision: the role of figure and part segmentation in symmetry selection. *J. Exp. Psychol. Hum. Percept. Perform.* 21: 1323–1342.

Baylis, G. C., Driver, J., Baylis, L., and Rafal, R. D. (1994) Reading of letters and words in a patient with Balint's syndrome. *Neuropsychologia* 32: 1273–1286.

Baylis, G. C., Driver, J., and McLeod, P. (1992) Movement and proximity constrain conjunction errors of colour and form. *Perception* 21: 201–218.

Baylis, G. C., Driver, J., and Rafal, R. (1993) Visual extinction and stimulus repetition. *J. Cognitive Neurosci.* 5: 453–466.

Baylis, G. C., Rolls, E. T., and Leonard, C. M. (1987) Functional subdivisions of the temporal lobe neocortex. *J. Neurosci.* 7: 330–342.

Behrmann, M. and Moscovitch, M. (1994) Object-centered neglect in patients with unilateral neglect. *J. Cognitive Neurosci.* 6: 1–16.

Behrmann, M., Moscovitch, M., Black, S. E., and Mozer, M. (1990) Perceptual and conceptual mechanisms in neglect. *Brain* 113: 1163–1183.

Behrmann, M. and Tipper, S. P. (1994) Object-based attentional mechanisms. In *Attention and Performance XV*, edited by C. Umiltà, and M. Moscovitch. Cambridge, MA: MIT Press.

Braun, J. and Sagi, D. (1991) Texture-based tasks are little affected by a second task which requires peripheral or central attentive fixation. *Perception* 20: 483–500.

Broadbent, D. E. (1958) *Perception and communication.* London: Pergamon Press.

Caramazza, A. and Hillis, A. E. (1990) Internal spatial representation of written words: Evidence from unilateral neglect. *Nature* 346: 267–279.

Driver, J. (1995) Object segmentation and visual neglect. *Behav. Brain Res.* 71: 135–146.

Driver, J. (1996) What can extinction and neglect reveal about the level of "preattentive" processing. In *Convergent Methods in the Study of Attention*, edited by A. F. Kramer, M. G. H. Coles, and G. D. Logan. Washington, DC: APA Press.

Driver, J. and Baylis, G. C. (1989) Movement and visual attention: The spotlight metaphor breaks down. *J. Exp. Psychol. Hum. Percept. Perform.* 15: 448–456.

Driver, J. and Baylis, G. C. (1995) One-sided edge-assignment in vision: 2. Part decomposition, shape description and attention to objects. *Curr. Dir. Psychol. Sci.* 4: 201–206.

Driver, J. and Baylis, G. C. (1996) Figure-ground segmentation and edge-assignment in short-term visual matching. *Cognitive Psychol.* 31: 248–306.

Driver, J., Baylis, G. C., Goodrich, S. J., and Rafal, R. D. (1994) Axis-based neglect of visual shapes. *Neuropsychologia* 32: 1353–1365.

Driver, J., Baylis, G. C., and Rafal, R. D. (1992) Preserved figure-ground segregation and symmetry perception in visual neglect. *Nature* 360: 73–75.

Driver, J. and Halligan, P. W. (1991) Can visual neglect operate in object-centerd coordinates? An affirmative single-case study. *Cognitive Neuropsychol.* 8: 475–496.

Driver, J., Mattingley, J. B., Rorden, C., and Davis, G. (1997). Extinction as a paradigm measure of attentional bias and restricted capacity following brain injury. In *Parietal Lobe Contributions to Orientation in 3D Space*, edited by R. Thier and H.-O. Karanth, pp. 401–429. Berlin: Springer-Verlag.

Duncan, J. (1980) The locus of interference in the perception of simultaneous stimuli. *Psychol. Rev.* 87: 272–300.

Duncan, J. (1984) Selective attention and the organization of visual information. *J. Exp. Psychol. Gen.* 113: 501–517.

Duncan, J. (1993a) Coordination of what and where in visual attention. *Perception* 22: 1261–1270.

Duncan, J. (1993b) Similarity between concurrent visual discriminations: Dimensions and objects. *Percept. Psychophys.* 54: 425–430.

Duncan, J. and Humphreys, G. W. (1989) Visual search and stimulus similarity. *Psychol. Rev.* 96: 443–458.

Egly, R., Driver, J., and Rafal, R. (1994) Shifting visual attention between objects and locations: Normality and pathology. *J. Exp. Psychol. Gen.* 123: 161–177.

Egly, R., Rafal, R., Driver, J., and Starrveveld, Y. (1994) Covert orienting in the split-brain reveals hemispheric specialization for object-based attention. *Psychol. Sci.* 5: 380–383.

Eriksen, B. A. and Eriksen, C. W. (1974) Effects of noise letters on identification of a target letter in a nonsearch task. *Percept. Psychophys.* 16: 143–149.

Farah, M. J., Brunn, J. L., Wong, A. B., Wallace, M., and Carpenter, P. A. (1990) Frames of reference for allocation of spatial attention. *Neuropsychologia* 28: 335–347.

Farah, M. J., Wallace, M. A. and Vecera, S. P. (1993) What and where in visual attention. In *Unilateral Neglect*, edited by I. H. Robertson, and J. C. Marshall. Hillsdale, NJ: Lawrence Erlbaum.

Gainotti, G., Messerli, P., and Tissot, T. (1972) Qualitative analysis of unilateral spatial neglect in relation to laterality of cerebral lesion. *J. Neurol. Neurosurg. Psychiatry* 35: 545–550.

Gibson, B. (1994) Visual attention and objects: One versus two, or convex versus concave? *J. Exp. Psychol. Hum. Percept. Perform.* 20: 203–207.

Gibson, B. and Egeth, H. (1994) Inhibition of return to object-based and environment-based location. *Percept. Psychophys.* 55: 323–339.

Harms, L. and Bundesen, C. (1983) Color segregation and selective attention in a nonsearch task. *Percept. Psychophys.* 33: 11–19.

He, Z. J. and Nakayama, K. (1995) Visual attention to surfaces in 3–dimensional space. *Proc. Natl. Acad. Sci.* 92: 11155–11159.

Hoffman, J. E. and Nelson, B. (1981) Spatial selectivity in visual search. *Percept. Psychophys.* 30: 283–290.

Humphreys, G. W. and Riddoch, M. J. (1993) Interactive attentional systems and unilateral visual neglect. In *Unilateral Neglect*, edited by I. H. Robertson and J. C. Marshall. Hillsdale, NJ: Lawrence Erlbaum.

Humphreys, G. W. and Riddoch, M. J. (1995) Separate coding of space within and between perceptual objects. *Cognitive Neuropsychol.* 12: 283–312.

Humphreys, G. W., Romani, C., Olson, A., Riddoch, M., and Duncan, J. (1994) Nonspatial extinction following lesions of the parietal lobes in humans. *Nature* 372: 357–359.

Kahneman, D. (1973) *Attention and Effort.* Englewood Cliffs, NJ: Prentice-Hall.

Kahneman, D. and Henik, A. (1981) Perceptual organization and attention. In *Perceptual Grouping and Atention*, edited by M. Kubovy, and J. R. Pomerantz. Hillsdale, NJ: Lawrence Erlbaum.

Kahneman, D., Treisman, A., and Gibbs, B. (1992) The reviewing of object files. *Cognitive Psychol.* 24: 175–219.

Kanwisher, N. G. and Driver, J. (1992) Objects, attributes and visual attention: Which, what and where. *Curr. Dir. Psychol. Sci.* 1: 26–31.

Kinsbourne, M. (1993) Orientational bias model of unilateral neglect. In *Unilateral Neglect*, edited by I. H. Robertson and J. C. Marshall. Hillsdale, NJ: Lawrence Erlbaum.

Kosslyn, S. M., Koenig, O., Barett, A., Cave, C. B., Tang, J., and Gabrielli, J. D. E. (1989) Hemispheric specialization for categorical and coordinate relations. *J. Exp. Psychol. Hum. Percept. Perform.* 15: 723–735.

Kramer, A. F. and Jacobson, A. (1991) Perceptual organization and focused attention. *Percept. Psychophys.* 50: 267–284.

Kramer, A. F., Tham, M. P., and Yeh, Y. Y. (1991) Movement and focused attention. *Percept. Psychophys.* 50: 537–546.

LaBerge, D. (1983) Spatial extent of attention to letters and words. *J. Exp. Psychol. Hum. Percept. Perform.* 9: 371–380.

Luria, A. R. (1959) Disorders of "simultaneous perception" in a case of bilateral occipitoparietal brain injury. *Brain* 83: 437–449.

Mack, A., Tang, B., Tuma, R., and Kahn, S. (1992) Perceptual organization and attention. *Cognitive Psychol.* 24: 475–501.

Marr, D. and Nishihara, H. K. (1978) Representation and recognition of the spatial organisation of three-dimensional shapes. *Proc. Soc. Lond.* B200: 269–294.

Marshall, J. C. and Halligan, P. W. (1994) The yin and yang of visuo-spatial neglect: A case study. *Neuropsychologia* 32: 1037.

Mattingley, J. B., Davis, G., and Driver, J. (1997) Preattentive filling-in of visual surfaces in parietal extinction. *Science* 275: 671–674.

McLeod, P., Driver, J., and Crisp, J. (1988) Visual search for a conjunction of movement and form is parallel. *Nature* 332: 154–155.

Moran, J. and Desimone, R. (1985) Selective attention gates processing in the extrastriate cortex. *Science* 229: 782–784.

Nakayama, K. and Silverman, G. (1986) Serial and parallel processing of visual feature conjunctions. *Nature* 320: 264–265.

Neisser, U. (1967) *Cognitive Psychology.* New York: Appleton-Century-Crofts.

Olsen, C. R. and Gettner, S. N. (1995) Object-centered direction selectivity in macaque supplementary eye field. *Science* 269: 985–988.

Oram, M. W. and Perrett, D. I. (1994) Responses of anterior superior temporal polysensory (STPa) neurons to "biological motion." *J. Cognitive Neurosci.* 6: 99–116.

Plaut, D. and Farah, M. J. (1991) Visual object representation: Interpreting neurophysiological data within a computatonal framework. *J. Cognitive Neurosci.* 2: 320–343.

Posner, M. I. (1980) Orienting of attention. *Q. J. Exp. Psychol.* 32: 3–26.

Posner, M. I. and Cohen, Y. (1984) Components of visual orienting. In *Attention and Performance X*, edited by H. Bouma and D. Bouwhuis. Hillsdale, NJ: Lawrence Erlbaum.

Posner, M. I., Walkerm, J. A., Friedrich, F. J., and Rafal, R. D. (1984) Effects of parietal injury on covert orienting of attention. *J. Neurosci.* 4: 1863–1974.

Prinzmetal, W. (1995) Visual feature integration in a world of visual objects. *Curr. Dir. Psychol. Sci.* 4: 90–94.

Prinzmetal, W. and Banks, W. P. (1977) Good continuation affects visual detection. *Percept. Psychophys.* 21: 389–395.

Pylyshyn, Z., Burkell, J., Fisher, B., Sears, C., Schmidt, W., and Trick, L. (1994) Multiple parallel access in visual attention. *Can. J. Psychol.* 48: 260–283.

Pylyshyn, Z. and Storm, R. W. (1988) Tracking multiple independent targets. *Spat. Vis.* 3: 179–197.

Rock, I. (1975) *An Introduction to Perception.* Cambridge, MA: MIT Press.

Rock, I. and Gutman, D. (1981) The effect of inattention on form perception. *J. Exp. Psychol. Hum. Percept. Perform.* 7: 275–285.

Rubin, E. (1915) *Visuell Wahrgenommene Figuren.* Copenhagen: Glydendalske.

Tipper, S. P. and Driver, J. (1988) Negative priming between pictures and words in a selective attention task. *Mem. Cognition* 16: 64–70.

Tipper, S. P., Driver, J., and Weaver, B. (1991) Object-centerd inhibition of return of visual attention. *Q. J. Exp. Psychol.* 43A: 289–298.

Treisman, A. (1982) Perceptual grouping and attention in visual search for features and for objects. *J. Exp. Psychol. Human. Percept. Perform.* 8: 194–214.

Treisman, A., Kahneman, D., and Burkell, J. (1983) Perceptual objects and the cost of filtering. *Percept. Psychophys.* 33: 527–532.

Tsal, Y. and Lavie, N. (1993) Location dominance in attending to color and shape. *J. Exp. Psychol. Hum. Percept. Perform.* 19: 131–139.

Vecera, S. and Farah, M. J. (1994) Does visual attention select objects or locations? *J. Exp. Psychol. Gen.* 123: 146–160.

Ward, R., Goodrich, S., and Driver, J. (1994) Grouping reduces visual extinction. *Vis. Cognition* 1: 101–129.

Watt, R. J. (1988) *Visual Processing.* Hillsdale, NJ: Lawrence Erlbaum.

Wertheimer, M. (1923) Untersuchen zu lehre von der Gestalt. *Psychologische Forschung* 1: 47–58.

Yantis, S. (1992) Multielement visual tracking: Attention and perceptual organization. *Cognitive Psychol.* 24: 295–340.

Yantis, S. (1993) Stimulus-driven attentional capture. *Curr. Dir. Psychol. Sci.* 2: 156–161.

Yantis, S. and Jonides, J. (1984) Abrupt visual onsets and visual attention. *J. Exp. Psychol. Hum. Percept. Perform.* 10: 601–621.

15   Divided Attention: Narrowing the Gap between Brain and Behavior

Jochen Braun

ABSTRACT   Psychophysical experiments in which attention is divided between different parts of a visual scene have made crucial contributions to the understanding of attention. This chapter reviews a number of noteworthy studies from the last two decades in which attention was divided with the help of either cueing or dual task paradigms. Special emphasis is given to recent dual task experiments that suggest that parallel attentional mechanisms contribute directly to visual experience.

Over the last decade, research on visual attention has made startling progress on a number of fronts. One exciting development is the discovery that visual attention modulates neural responses in many parts of visual cortex (reviewed by Desimone and Duncan, 1995; Maunsell, 1995). As a result, visual attention has ceased to be exclusively a concern of cognitive psychology and has entered the purview of neurobiology. Another source of excitement is the realization that there are two kinds of attentional processes—serial and parallel (for reviews, see Julesz, 1991; Treisman, 1993)—and that this duality accounts for a wide range of psychophysical observations. Given the bewildering variety of approaches used to study attention, any classification, even a relatively coarse one, that associates psychophysical findings with specific attentional processes is a godsend. The distinction between serial and parallel attentional processes has proven especially helpful in this respect.

This chapter focuses on the human psychophysics of divided attention, that is, on situations in which the observer attends to one part of the visual scene but also discriminates visual information in another part. As will become clear, paradigms of this sort afford insights into the nature of visual attention that are not easily attained by other paradigms. One important case in point is the time course with which attention shifts from one stimulus to another. Another is the quantitation of attentional requirements, including the demonstration that some visual tasks require essentially complete—that is, focused—attention. Yet another case in point is the investigation of vision outside the focus of attention. These and many related issues are settled by experiments in which attention is divided.

This review concentrates on psychophysical studies that measure attentional effects in terms of visual sensitivity (d') (Green and Swets, 1966) rather than reaction time. Measurements of d' not only distinguish sensory from nonsensory (e.g., memory and motor) components of a visual task, but also greatly facilitate comparisons with neurophysiology. Studies of the neural basis of attention typically investigate how activity levels (i.e., firing rates) of visual cortical neurons change with the behavioral relevance of a visual stimulus. Activity levels of feature-selective neurons have been shown to correlate, at least in some cases, with d' (e.g., Britten, Shadlen, Newsome, and Movshon, 1992; Salzman and Newsome, 1994). Accordingly, attentional changes in d' are likely to reflect changes in neuronal activity levels somewhere in the visual system.

This chapter begins with a brief synopsis of visual search and visual texture segregation. Studies of attention in awake, behaving monkeys are then summarized. This permits examination of some gratifying correlations between psychophysical and physiological studies of attention. Next, psychophysical studies in which the disposition of attention was manipulated by cueing are described, followed by studies in which observers divided attention evenly between two visual tasks of equal importance. Both kinds of studies show that different types of visual sensitivity differ greatly in the extent to which they depend on attention. A further section is devoted to studies in which observers focused attention on a primary task but also carried out a secondary task elsewhere in the visual field. It is concluded that certain types of visual sensitivity are essentially independent of attention and that observers enjoy significant visual capabilities outside the attentional focus. The final section discusses implications of these findings for visual attention and for the supporting neural mechanisms.

VISUAL SEARCH AND VISUAL TEXTURE SEGREGATION

Visual attention is often studied with the closely related paradigms of visual search (Treisman and Gelade, 1980) and visual texture segregation (Julesz, 1981). In a visual scene containing many discrete stimuli, there may be certain stimuli that are readily detected among the others and for which detection times do not (or only slowly) increase with the total number of stimuli (this phenomenon is called pop-out or parallel search). There may also be certain other stimuli that are more difficult to detect and for which detection times increase rapidly with the total number of stimuli (a phenomenon called scrutiny or serial search). An influential theory holds that visual search is serial if no single feature (color, shape, motion, etc.) but only a combination of features distinguishes target from nontarget stimuli (a phenomenon known as conjunction search; Treisman, 1991, 1993). However, convincing alternative accounts have been offered as well (Duncan and Humphreys, 1989, 1992; Wolfe, 1994). Essentially, visual search appears to be serial if (1) target and nontarget stimuli exhibit highly similar features or if (2) featural differences among nontargets are large enough to obscure any differences between target and nontargets.

These results are extended by studies of visual texture segregation (Julesz, 1991). Whether singularities or discontinuities of visual texture segregate effortlessly or are perceived only with serial scrutiny depends critically on the spatial separation between textural elements. Specifically, visual textures do not segregate effortlessly when textural elements are spaced too far apart (Sagi and Julesz, 1987; Sagi, 1990; Nothdurft, 1991; Bravo and Nakayama, 1992). These observations motivate computational models of visual texture processing that quantitatively account for human performance on the basis of surround inhibition within a two-dimensional array of feature-selective filters (Koch and Ullman, 1985; Malik and Perona, 1990; Rubenstein and Sagi, 1990; Watt, 1991). Within a certain spatial range, similar visual features mask each other, and this effect is compounded in a dense visual texture. Locally unique features are not masked in this way and thus segregate effortlessly.

Following widespread usage, a stimulus that is detected seemingly effort-lessly is referred to as a pop-out stimulus (Treisman and Gelade, 1980). One essential characteristic of a pop-out stimulus is that it possesses a feature (color, shape, motion, etc.) that is locally unique in that it is not found among other stimuli nearby. Another requirement for pop-out is that the rest of the visual field be relatively quiet, in other words, that there be only a few prominent stimuli with locally unique features in the entire field of view. Interactions between multiple prominent stimuli are poorly understood, but are often described in terms of a competition for visual saliency or for pop-out (Koch and Ullman, 1985; Desimone and Duncan, 1995).

ATTENTIONAL MODULATION OF VISUAL CORTICAL RESPONSES

Feature-Specific Surround Inhibition

Over the last several decades, much has been learned about the neural mech-anisms underlying vision. It has been established that the visual world is multiply represented by approximately 30 visual cortical areas, and that neu-rons in those areas encode a wide variety of visual information (Felleman and Van Essen, 1990; Van Essen and Gallant, 1994). Much of this informa-tion was obtained with localized visual stimuli such as bars, edges, or gra-tings. Only recently have more complex stimuli been studied (Allman, Miezin, and McGuinness, 1985), and very little indeed is known about the response of visual cortex to natural visual scenes (Gallant, Connor, and Van Essen, 1994). This more recent work has made it clear that visual cortical re-sponses do not summate linearly; in other words, the neuronal response to a complex visual scene is not simply the sum of the neuronal responses to each component of the scene (Maunsell, 1995).

Although nonlinear interactions between stimuli inside and outside the classical receptive field (cRF) of visual cortical neurons are far from under-stood, an important component of those interactions appears to be inhibition between similar stimuli. In area V1, the response of 80% of orientation-selective neurons to a bar of the preferred orientation is suppressed when similarly oriented bars are presented nearby (Knierim and Van Essen, 1992; Press, Knierim, and Van Essen, 1994). In the middle temporal area (MT), the response of 40% of direction-selective neurons to dots moving in the preferred direction is suppressed when nearby dots move in the same direction (Allman et al., 1985). In area V4, the response of most cells to a stimulus of preferred wavelength or shape is suppressed when stimuli of similar wavelength or shape are present in the surrounding visual field (Desimone, Schein, Moran, and Ungerleider, 1985).

As a result of this inhibition from outside the cRF, the visual cortical response to a given stimulus is attenuated when similar stimuli are present nearby in the visual field (figure 15.1a). It is generally agreed that this interaction contributes to the psychophysical phenomenon of pop-out (Desimone and Duncan, 1995; Koch and Ullman, 1985; Nakayama, 1991; Robinson and Petersen, 1992). In effect, stimuli that are odd or unusual in some way—that is, stimuli with a feature not shared by surrounding stimuli—acquire greater intensity, and that heightened intensity contributes to visual saliency and pop-out.

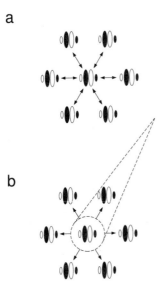

a

b

Figure 15.1 Feature-specific surround inhibition in visual cortex and its hypothetical suppression by attention. (a) Classical receptive fields of neurons selective for vertical orientation, with reciprocal inhibition between the central neuron and six surrounding neurons. Due to this inhibition, the center response is suppressed when central and surrounding receptive fields contain similar (vertical) stimuli. (b) Attention may isolate the central neuron by suppressing inhibition received by, but not inhibition originating from, the central neuron. In this case, the center response is strong even when central and surrounding receptive fields contain similar (vertical) stimuli.

Attentional Effects

A second broad conclusion from studies of the neural mechanisms of vision is that attention modulates visual responses at almost all cortical levels (Desimone and Duncan, 1995; Maunsell, 1995). Of particular interest are response modulations in visual cortical areas of the so-called temporal pathway (areas V2, V3, and V4, and inferotemporal areas; Desimone and Ungerleider, 1989; Felleman and Van Essen, 1990). Neurons in these areas appear to represent features of visual objects (e.g., color and shape), and inferotemporal areas have been implicated in visual recognition and memory (Miller, Li, and Desimone, 1991, 1993; Ungerleider, 1995). In these areas, visual responses to a stimulus are stronger (in up to half of the neurons) when the stimulus is relevant to behavior (i.e., when the animal is carrying out a visual task with respect to the stimulus) than when the stimulus is merely viewed passively (Chelazzi, Miller, Duncan, and Desimone, 1993; Haenny, Maunsell, and Schiller, 1988; Maunsell, 1995; Moran and Desimone, 1985; Motter, 1994; Spitzer, Desimone, and Moran, 1988). Apparently, visual attention enhances neuronal responses to stimuli that are relevant to behavior. Functional brain-imaging studies suggest that attention has a similar effect on visual responses in human observers (Ungerleider, 1995).

A puzzling aspect of these results is that attentional effects are often rather small (typically a 20% to 50% change in firing rate), although on occasion more robust effects are observed as well (Maunsell, 1995). It is quite possible, however, that the experiments carried out so far have not revealed the true extent of attentional influences. There is increasing evidence that the displays used in typical single-neuron studies (i.e., one isolated stimulus in an otherwise empty visual field) are particularly ill-suited to reveal attentional effects (Motter, 1993; Reynolds, Chelazzi, Luck, and Desimone, 1994; Reynolds, Nicholas, Chelazzi, and Desimone, 1995). Focusing attention on one of several stimuli seems to yield much more robust effects (Moran and Desimone, 1985; Motter, 1993). In fact, with dense arrays of many similar stimuli, attentional modulation of visual responses can be demonstrated even in area V1 (Motter, 1993; Press et al., 1994).

The apparent connection between attentional effects and the presence of competing stimuli has not escaped notice (Desimone and Duncan, 1995; Motter, 1993). It seems possible that attention modulates visual responses mostly indirectly, by suppressing surround inhibition at the attended location. This would allow attention to "protect" (Reynolds et al., 1995) the response to attended stimuli from the inhibitory influence of nearby unattended stimuli and would explain why, in the absence of nearby stimuli, attention has so little effect. However, an attentional suppression of surround inhibition may not be the whole story. Some physiological observations suggest that attention strengthens, rather than weakens, inhibition from attended to unattended locations (Desimone, 1992; Moran and Desimone,

1985; Niebur and Koch, chapter 9, this volume). Although it remains to be seen how these various effects can be reconciled, one obvious possibility is that attention suppresses inhibition in one direction only, namely, from unattended to attended locations (figure 15.1b).

CUEING EXPERIMENTS

Although it has long been recognized that visual performance is strongly influenced by attention (Helmholtz, 1850/1962; James, 1890/1981), quantitative measurements of those effects had to await the development of signal detection theory (Green and Swets, 1966; Macmillan and Creelman, 1991). Under certain assumptions about the statistical distribution of signal and noise, it is possible to disambiguate the extent to which a change in visual performance (fraction of correct responses in a visual task) is due to a change of the signal-to-noise level (sensitivity, or d', effects) or due to change in the propensity of the observer to report one outcome rather than another (criterion, or β, effects). d' can be computed not only from an observer's responses in distinguishing stimulus A from stimulus B, but also from repeated measurements of neuronal activity in response to stimulus A or B (e.g., Salzman and Newsome, 1994). For this reason, d' is especially useful for comparing psychophysics and neurophysiology.

One way to manipulate the distribution of attention across the visual field is visual cueing (Posner, Snyder, and Davidson, 1980). In this paradigm, an observer is asked to discriminate (or simply detect) a stimulus that appears at one of several possible locations. Typically 100 ms to 1 s prior to the appearance of the stimulus, a cue indicates a location that, in most trials, is the location at which the stimulus is about to appear. Observers avail themselves of this information and attend more to cued than to uncued locations. One can then compare visual sensitivity when the stimulus appears at the cued (more attended) location and when it (unexpectedly) appears at an uncued (less attended) location. Typically, cueing effects are maximal at the cued location and decrease with increasing distance from that location.

In experiments of this type, d' for some visual tasks, notably the discrimination of simple shapes, is significantly larger at cued than at uncued locations (Bashinski and Bacharach, 1980; Downing, 1988; Mueller and Findlay, 1987; Shaw, 1984). Depending on the value of d' without any cue, cueing can increase d' anywhere from 0.2 to 2.0 (e.g., Mueller and Findlay, 1987; Downing, 1988). However, there also are visual tasks in which d' is much less sensitive to cueing. For example, for the detection of a sudden luminance increment in an otherwise unchanged display, some studies report no cueing effect whatsoever (Mueller and Findlay, 1987; Shaw, 1984), whereas others report only a small effect (Downing, 1988; Hawkins et al., 1990; Mueller and Humphreys, 1991; see also Kinchla, 1992). The interpretation of these different results is complicated by the fact that the displays contained, in addition

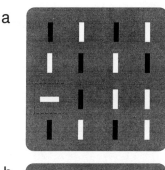

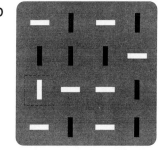

Figure 15.2 Displays (schematic) used in a cueing experiment by Nakayama and Mackeben (1989). A cue (dashed-line box) indicates the location of the target (in the actual display, the cue is displayed prior to the display of the array of target and nontargets). Observers report the color of the target. (a) When the target is defined by a unique (horizontal) orientation, cueing has little or no effect on performance. (b) When the target is defined by a unique combination of orientation and color (white and vertical), cueing dramatically improves performance. (After Nakayama and Mackeben, 1989.)

to cue and target, other prominent stimuli (e.g., bright boxes around all possible target positions) that may have obscured the luminance increment and interfered with its pop-out.

A study that avoided competition for pop-out between the target and other prominent stimuli was conducted by Nakayama and Mackeben (1989). Observers discriminated the color (black or white) of an odd target bar in a dense array of horizontal or vertical black or white bars. When the target bar was defined by a unique orientation and was embedded in a relatively quiet display with bars of uniform orientation (figure 15.2a), the presence of a cue at the target position had little or no effect on discrimination performance. When the target was defined by a unique combination of orientation and color and was embedded in a relatively noisy display with bars of both orientations (figure 15.2b), cueing enhanced performance dramatically. These observations provide further (and more direct) support for one of the main inferences from visual search experiments: sensitivity for a unique feature in an otherwise uniform display is much less dependent on attention than is sensitivity for other types of targets. The second important result of Nakayama and Mackeben's study is that cueing effects depend strongly on the relative timing of cue and target. Cueing is most effective for cue lead times between approximately 50 ms and 200 ms, but a smaller effect persists for at least 500 ms. It is rather surprising that the cueing effect increases transiently, rather than monotonically, with cue lead time, and the authors interpret this result in terms of transient and sustained components of attention. Apparently, the initial shift of attention to the target is time-locked to the cue and cannot be delayed voluntarily. Subsequent shifts of attention to the target seem to be less effective than the initial one, perhaps because of the so-called inhibition of return (e.g., Gibson and Egeth, 1994; Pratt and Abrams, 1995).

SYMMETRICAL DUAL TASK EXPERIMENTS

Another way to manipulate the distribution of attention across the visual field is to pose two concurrent visual tasks. If visual persistence is limited by masking, then the observer is prevented from performing the tasks sequentially and is forced to divide attention between them. Appropriate instructions can influence whether attention is evenly divided or favors one task over the other. A valuable guide to the subtleties of dual task methodology has been compiled by Sperling and Dosher (1986). This section discusses dual task experiments that are symmetrical in the sense that attention is evenly divided between two visual tasks of equal importance to the observer.

Dual-Task Interference and its Origin

A classic dual task experiment of this type was carried out by Sperling and Melchner (1978). A series of arrays of letters were presented, at a rate of four arrays per second, with one critical array embedded in the middle of the series. The critical array contained one target numeral at one of four inside-array locations and another target numeral at one of four outside-array locations (figure 15.3). Observers had to separately report the identity and location of each numeral (and also rate their confidence in the accuracy of their reports). Inside and outside characters and arrays were of different size, so that both component tasks presented comparable difficulty. (In some blocks of trials, observers reported only outside targets and ignored inside targets, whereas in other blocks they did the reverse; this established performance rates when attention was focused on only one task.) Instructions were varied so that observers divided attention evenly in some blocks of trials and favored the inside or outside numeral in other blocks of trials. Results were reported in the format of an attention-operating characteristic (Sperling and Dosher, 1986). The two tasks proved to be mutually exclusive in that average concurrent performance was only slightly better than half the average isolated performance (the outcome obtained when observers performed only one task in each trial). It follows that the detection of a numeral among letters requires full

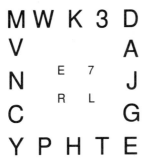

Figure 15.3 Display used in a classic dual task study by Sperling and Melchner (1978). An array with 16 outside and 4 inside characters contains a large (outside) and a small (inside) numeral target. Observers attempt to independently detect and identify both numeral targets. The difference in size ensures that performance is comparable when either numeral is detected in isolation. When both numerals are detected, average performance decreases by a factor of approximately two, demonstrating that only one numeral can be detected at a time. (After Sperling and Melchner, 1978.)

attention and precludes the performance of a similar task elsewhere in the display.

An important concern in dual task studies is the processing stage at which the two tasks interfere. Maintaining and acting upon two sets of behavioral goals raises problems over and above the need to discriminate two visual stimuli (Allport, 1980; Duncan, 1980). Dual task interference at this "executive" level is known as the psychological refractory period (Pashler, 1994). Much of this higher-level interference can be avoided by allowing observers enough time to respond to each task in turn. In addition, interference at the level of visual processing can be exacerbated by visual masking (which limits the time available for visual processing). In other words, the behavioral situation can be designed to favor interference at the level of processes that are time-locked to stimulus presentation (e.g., visual attention).

Persuasive evidence that interference between two discrimination tasks arises at the level of visual processing comes from Duncan (1984). Two superimposed objects (or figures, in the sense of Gestalt psychology; Wertheimer, 1923) were presented briefly, with the shape of each object possessing two features that varied independently (figure 15.4). In some blocks of trials, observers discriminated two features of the same object, ignoring the other object, while in other blocks of trials they discriminated one feature of each object, ignoring the other feature of each object. Note that in both cases observers had to maintain and act upon two sets of behavioral goals. For purposes of comparison, observers discriminated one feature of one object in yet other blocks of trials. Interference between dual discriminations occurred only when the discriminated features belonged to different objects. When the discriminated features belonged to the same object, concurrent performance was comparable to isolated performance. The most

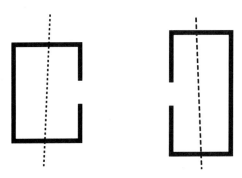

Figure 15.4 Two example displays used by Duncan (1984). Two objects appear, each with two independently varying features: a box of small or large size and with a gap on the left or right side, and a line of clock- or counterclockwise tilt that is either dashed or dotted. Observers can concurrently discriminate two features of the same object, but not two features from two different objects. This shows that dual task interference arises at a visual level of processing. (After Duncan, 1984.)

likely interpretation of this outcome is that interference arises at the level of visual attention: observers can attend to features of one object but not features of two different objects (even when the two objects occupy the same region of space).

Experiments of this type suggest that the attentional enhancement of sensitivity is most pronounced for a single visual object and weakens rapidly when other visual objects become equally relevant to the observer. This agrees with the impression gained introspectively that attention is most effective when focused on a single stimulus or visual location. The need to focus attention to attain maximal sensitivity also explains, of course, why visual performance is often serial, that is, why the discrimination of additional stimuli often requires additional viewing time.

Dividing and Shifting Attention

It is not self-evident that attention can be literally divided between simultaneously presented stimuli. In many studies of divided attention, it is unclear whether observers simply devote attention to one task on some trials and to another task on other trials (a phenomenon known as mixed strategy; Sperling and Dosher, 1986), or whether they truly devote partial attention to both tasks during each and every trial (pure strategy). When a contingency analysis of the observer's success or failure in both tasks is performed (i.e., when the conditional probabilities of success on one task given the success, or failure, on the other are compared) it is usually found, however, that observers adopt an largely pure attentional strategy (Bonnel, Possamai, and Schmitt, 1992; Bonnel and Miller, 1994; Braun and Julesz, 1997; Sperling and Dosher, 1986). The remaining possibility, that attention switches very rapidly between tasks during a single trial, is difficult to rule out but seems unlikely from a neural point of view. In fact, the one study that has been undertaken to address this issue found no evidence for rapid switching (Miller and Bonnel, 1994).

Timing of Shifts of Attention

A related issue is the time for which attention must focus on one stimulus before it may shift to another. An upper bound estimate of attentional dwell time has recently been reported by Duncan, Ward, and Shapiro (1994). Two stimuli (letters or digits) were presented at varying (but distant) locations, each followed after 45–60 ms by a visual mask. One stimulus appeared first and the other followed after a delay of up to 900 ms. The observer's task was to identify both stimuli. The two tasks interfered (i.e., concurrent performance was below isolated performance) as long as the delay between objects was 450 ms or less, with maximal interference at a delay of 200 ms. Essentially the same outcome has been obtained in other studies (Braun and Julesz, 1997; Julesz and Braun, 1992). Duncan and his colleagues concluded that attentional dwell time can be as high as several hundred milliseconds. However, this value neglects any time that may be required for attention to shift from one object and to another, and thus should be considered an upper bound.

Significantly shorter attentional dwell times were obtained when two stimuli were presented simultaneously rather than sequentially (Braun and Sagi, 1991). Using brief presentation times and visual masking, a given level of letter discrimination performance was found to require 45–60 ms more presentation time when the observer had to first discriminate another letter. (The order in which letters were discriminated was manipulated via appropriate instructions.) By this measure, attentional dwell times are comparable to presentation times (typically 40–80 ms for letter discrimination), which is consistent with the idea that visual attention operates during the persistence time of the stimulus, rather than later, when the stimulus has already been committed to visual memory. The reasons for the discrepancy between successive and simultaneous stimulus presentation are unclear. Perhaps attentional shift times are substantially smaller when the second stimulus is already present while attention still dwells on the first. This not only provides more time to prepare the shift, but also avoids potentially disruptive visual onsets.

That sequential presentation can hinder, rather than help, the concurrent discrimination of letter shapes is clear also from recent work of Julesz and colleagues (Hung, Wilder, Curry, and Julesz, 1995; Saarinen and Julesz, 1991). When four numerals were presented either simultaneously or in rapid succession (each followed by a mask), observers identified these numerals more often than expected from levels of chance. Identification rates decrease with increasing presentation rate (50 ms, 30 ms, and 16 ms per numeral), but

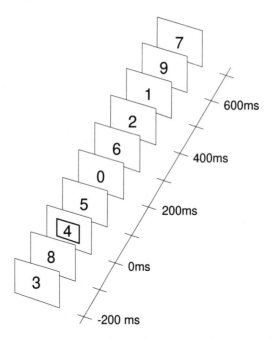

Figure 15.5 Illustration of the experiment by Sperling and Weichselgartner (1987). Numerals are presented in rapid sequence, and one critical numeral is highlighted by the presence of a frame around it. Observers attempt to recall the four earliest numerals simultaneous with, or subsequent to, recall of the critical numeral. Recall frequency exhibits a distinctly bimodal distribution, implicating two distinct attentional processes. (After Weichselgartner and Sperling, 1987.)

remain significant even at the fastest rate (4% correct at 16 ms per numeral). The great surprise is that this trend reversed abruptly when all numerals were presented simultaneously ($\approx$30% correct at 0 ms per numeral), suggesting that attention can much more readily be divided between simultaneous than between sequential stimuli.

A particularly intriguing study of the dynamics of attention was carried out by Sperling and Weichselgartner (1987). A series of numerals was presented at rates of up to 12.5 numerals per second, and one critical numeral near the middle of the series was highlighted, an effect achieved either through brightening the numeral or by drawing a frame around it (figure 15.5). Observers were asked to identify numerals that occurred immediately after the critical one. Recall was distributed bimodally, in that the vast majority of recalled numerals had been presented either 0–100 ms (first glimpse) or 300–400 ms after the critical numeral (second glimpse). Further experiments revealed fundamental differences between the attentional mechanisms underlying each period of recall: the first period appeared to be due to a "fast, effortless, automatic process that records the cue and neighboring events," whereas the second period of recall seemed to be mediated by a "slower, effortful, and controlled process." Although not often cited, this study provides strong evidence that attention is not a unitary process but comprises two partially concurrent mechanisms that operate independently of each other.

Lack of Dual Task Interference

Bonnel and colleagues reported a series of dual task experiments involving line-length discrimination (Bonnel and Miller, 1994; Bonnel et al., 1987) as well as luminance detection (Bonnel, Stein, and Bertucci, 1992). The outcome for line-length discrimination resembled that obtained with letter or shape discrimination (see the discussion in the previous section), namely, substantial interference between tasks. No interference was encountered, however, between independent detections of two luminance increments. An intermediate outcome was obtained for two independent discriminations of luminance increments or decrements (Bonnel et al., 1992), a finding that the authors attributed to altered task requirements (discrimination versus detection) rather than to altered physical stimulation (decrements versus increments). Unfortunately, they did not investigate two independent detections of luminance decrements, which would have settled the issue. (Bashinski and Bacharach, [1980] found attentional effects on d' for luminance decrements.)

Lack of dual task interference has also been observed in the independent detection of two pop-out targets (Braun, 1993; Braun and Sagi, 1990). In these studies, up to two target stimuli were embedded in a dense array of background stimuli, and the entire array was presented only briefly before being masked. Target stimuli differed from background stimuli either in orientation (Braun and Sagi, 1990) or in direction of shading (Braun, 1993). Observers independently reported the presence or absence of a target in the top and bottom halves of the array. Performance was the same whether two targets or only one target was detected (and the other target ignored), demonstrating that two pop-out targets can be detected in parallel.

When two tasks fail to interfere, relatively little can be concluded about attention. Lack of interference leaves open the possibility that both tasks require significant, though less than complete, attention. This ambiguity can be avoided in asymmetrical dual task experiments, in which one task requires complete, that is, focused, attention.

ASYMMETRICAL DUAL TASK EXPERIMENTS

In asymmetrical dual task experiments, instructions favor one task over the other and induce a highly unequal distribution of attention. Ideally, the primary task (the one favored by instructions) is so demanding that optimal performance is reached only when attention is completely focused on that task. In such a situation, primary task performance can be used to monitor the distribution of attention.

Detecting Pop-Out Outside the Focus of Attention

All experimental paradigms mentioned thus far agree that not all tasks require visual attention in equal measure. In particular, pop-out targets appear to be a privileged kind of visual stimulus, the detection of which requires relatively little attention. However, it remains unclear whether pop-out requires so little attention that a stimulus can be detected even when attention focuses elsewhere in the visual field. In other words, it remains possible that "when attention is narrowly focused elsewhere, pop-out no longer occurs" (Treisman, 1993).

Braun and Julesz (1997) addressed this issue with an asymmetrical dual task experiment. Attention was focused on a primary letter task that involved discriminating five randomly rotated letters (Ts or Ls) near the center of the display. This task was particularly demanding and left little or no attention available for secondary tasks. To document this fact, an attention-operating characteristic (Sperling and Dosher, 1986) was established for a situation in which the letter task was performed concurrently with one particular secondary task (probe task) (figure 15.6a). The results showed that performance of the letter task did not leave enough attention available to measurably benefit the probe task (i.e., probe task performance did not differ significantly from levels of chance). Having characterized the attentional requirements of the letter task in this way, the authors combined the letter task with the detection of a pop-out, specifically, the detection of a uniquely oriented peripheral stimulus embedded in a dense array of background stimuli (figure 15.6b). Sensitivity for this detection task varied greatly with the ori-

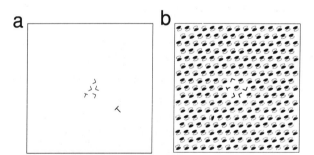

Figure 15.6 Illustration of the displays used by Braun and Julesz (1997). In both displays, a combination of five Ts and/or Ls appear near the center, and observers discriminate whether these are the same or whether one letter is different (primary task). (a) As a secondary task, observers identify a single peripheral letter (probe task). Although by itself the secondary task is relatively "fast and effortless," it cannot be performed in the dual task situation. (b) Gabor elements (represented by black and white ellipses) of identical orientation form a dense background for a single uniquely oriented Gabor element (Gabor target). As a secondary task, observers report whether the Gabor target occurs in the top or bottom half of the display. By itself, this task can be relatively "slow and effortful," but it is nevertheless performed well in the dual task situation. (After Braun and Julesz, 1997.)

entation difference between target and background stimuli. For the largest orientation differences investigated (45 degrees), pop-out was indeed "fast and effortless" ($d' \approx 1.8$ at 80 ms presentation time) for isolated performance of the detection task. For the smallest orientation differences investigated (15 degrees), however, detection of the uniquely oriented stimulus was more appropriately described as "slow and effortful" ($d' \approx 0.3$ at 225 ms presentation time). The results of performing letter and detection tasks concurrently could not have been more clear: there was little or no dual task interference and, most surprisingly, this outcome did not change as the difficulty of the detection increased.

One implication of this result is that being fast and effortless or slow and effortful does not predict the extent to which a visual task depends on attention. Compare the relatively effortful detection tasks with the relatively effortless probe task just discussed (isolated performance of $d' \approx 1.4$ at a presentation time of 140 ms). It seems that one has to be very cautious about judging attentional requirements purely on the basis of sensitivity or presentation time. However, the main conclusion from this study is that pop-out and attentional focus are essentially independent of each other. Focusing attention elsewhere in the visual field does not noticeably impede pop-out, and vice versa. The most straightforward interpretation of this result is that pop-out occurs outside the focus of attention. A more roundabout interpretation postulates a residual amount of attention that remains available throughout the field of view even when attention is narrowly focused, and attributes the detection of pop-out to this residual amount of attention (ambient attention). Whichever interpretation one prefers, the fact remains that pop-out enters visual experience directly, that is, without noticeable disturbance of the attentional focus. This shows that parallel attentional processes contribute directly to visual experience, operating side by side with serial attentional processes. This finding conflicts with hierarchical models of attention, according to which parallel processes contribute only indirectly to visual experience, namely, by drawing serial attention to any location that pops out (Duncan and Humphreys, 1992; Nakayama, 1991; Neisser, 1967; Treisman, 1993; Wolfe, 1994).

The possibility of probing visual sensitivity outside the focus of attention opens some virgin territory for behavioral experimentation. Cueing experiments permit the comparison of relatively more or relatively less attended locations, but they cannot ensure the highly unequal allocation of attention that can be attained in a dual task situation. Note, however, that this territory is not so virginal from the point of view of neurophysiology, where it has for some time been possible to compare visual responses in attended and unattended parts of the visual field.

Perception without attention has also been investigated by Rock and colleagues (Mack, Tang, Tuma, Kahn, and Rock, 1992; Rock, Linnett, Grant, and Mack, 1992). Although those authors also used a dual task paradigm, absence of attention was ensured less by the demanding nature of the primary

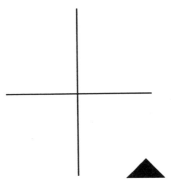

Figure 15.7 Display used by Rock et al. (1992). Observers discriminate the aspect ratio of the cross figure (here, the cross is higher than it is wide) when another stimulus appears unexpectedly (e.g., black triangle). Although observers are often unaware of the unexpected stimulus, its presence, position, and color is sometimes correctly reported. (After Rock et al., 1992.)

task than by the fact that the observer did not expect the target stimulus of the secondary task. (To ensure unexpectedness, only one critical trial was conducted with every observer.) The primary task consisted of judging the aspect ratio of a cross figure, and the secondary task involved reporting the presence, position, shape, color, or perceptual grouping of one or more unexpected stimuli (figure 15.7). The results suggested that neither texture segregation nor perceptual grouping were discriminable when the relevant stimuli were not expected by the observer, but that the presence, position, and color of unexpected stimuli were discriminable to some extent.

These results are difficult to compare with those from other dual task experiments in which the observer strives to maximize performance on both tasks (so that his success can be measured by an attention-operating characteristic). Nevertheless, it seems clear that unattended and unexpected stimuli are perceived even more poorly than are unattended but expected ones. In many cases, observers reported being not even aware of the unexpected stimulus. The extent to which a stimulus must be anticipated by the observer in order to reach awareness remains a fascinating area for future work.

Stimulus Competition Outside the Focus of Attention

As discussed previously, feature-specific surround inhibition at several levels of the visual system results in pop-out. In effect, visual stimuli enter a competition in which only the most odd or unusual stimuli prevail to become visually salient (Desimone and Duncan, 1995; Koch and Ullman, 1985). Asymmetrical dual task experiments can be used to compare stimulus competition outside and inside the attended part of the visual field. This can help to clarify the relationship between stimulus competition and attention, which is of considerable interest in view of the variety of neurophysiological evidence that exists on this point.

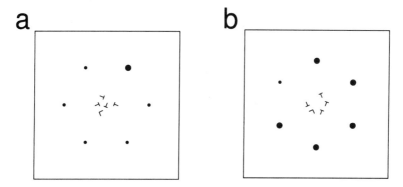

Figure 15.8 Illustration of an experiment by Braun (1994). In addition to the combination of five *T*s and *L*s posing the primary task, there are six peripheral stimuli, one of which is unique in 50% of trials. The unique stimulus is defined by either size (as shown), luminance, chromaticity, or pattern. As a secondary task, observers report the presence or absence of a unique peripheral stimulus. (a) When the secondary task involves a larger (more intense) target among smaller (less intense) distractors, it is performed well even in the dual task situation. (b) When the secondary task involves a smaller (less intense) target among larger (more intense) distractors, dual task performance is at levels near chance. This suggests that competition between prominent stimuli is more severe "outside" the focus of attention. (After Braun 1994.)

A series of experiments of this type have explored situations in which several prominent stimuli are present in the periphery of the display (Braun, 1994; Braun and Koch, 1995). Control experiments showed that, as long as a peripheral stimulus remained the only stimulus outside the attentional focus, it remained detectable in the dual task situation. The aim of the main experiment was to determine whether peripheral stimuli would remain detectable in combination with other peripheral stimuli in the dual task situation. Visual displays were modeled after a study with nonhuman primates (Schiller and Lee, 1991) in order to compare results from invasive and noninvasive techniques (see below). One peripheral stimulus served as the target of a detection task, and the others served as distractors (figure 15:8). Target and distractors differed with respect to either size, luminance, chromaticity, or pattern and, as a result, also differed in their respective stimulus intensity. (Although intensity is a function of the physical stimulus, it can also be quantified psychophysically, for example by measuring the detectability d' of a stimulus in an otherwise empty display.) Two types of detections were distinguished: more-intense target among less-intense distractors, and less-intense target among more-intense distractors. Competition is expected to favor detection of a more-intense target, which should pop out among less-intense distractors. The result was that, without the inclusion of the letter task, both types of detection tasks were performed comparably well. With the inclusion of the letter task, detection of a more-intense target was performed well but detection of a less-intense target was near levels of chance. Accordingly, the detection of a more-intense target behaved like the detection of a single pop-out target in the dual task situation, whereas the detection of a less-intense target behaved like the discrimination of a single letter. It is tempting to interpret this outcome in terms of an attentional suppression of stimulus competition: inside the attended region competition is weak and sensitivity to both types of targets is comparable, whereas, outside the attended region competition is strong and sensitivity to less-intense targets collapses.

Using essentially the same visual displays, very similar effects on visual sensitivity for more- or less-intense targets were obtained following a lesion in visual cortical area V4 of macaque monkeys (Schiller and Lee, 1991). Why should a lesion alter visual sensitivities in the same way as the imposition of a concurrent task? One possibility is that a lesion of area V4 disrupts the normal operation of attention. In the absence of attention, competition between stimuli may be strong and sensitivity to less-intense targets among more-intense distractors may collapse, whereas sensitivity to more-intense targets among less-intense distractors may remain.

Feature Discrimination Outside the Focus of Attention

The subjective experience of observers outside the focus of attention is of evident interest. Observers report being fully aware of pop-out targets outside the attentional focus (Braun, 1994; Braun and Julesz, 1997), which suggests that simple features of such stimuli may be discriminable. Results discussed earlier make clear, of course, that complex features such as letter identity will not be discriminable outside the attentional focus.

The discrimination of simple features outside the attentional focus was studied by Braun and Julesz (1997). A second aim was to study the perception of more than one pop-out target outside the focus of attention. In one experiment, two peripheral targets of chromatic hue popped out among an array of stimuli of neutral hue (figure 15.9a). Each target assumed one of two hues (total of four hues) and observers independently discriminated the hue of both targets. (To ensure that responses truly reflected a judgment of hue, hues were calibrated to render the target not only equally luminous but also equally detectable in the background array.) Sensitivity for hue discrimination was essentially the same with and without the concurrent letter task. This echoes the outcome of comparable cueing experiments (Nakayama and Mackeben, 1989) and demonstrates hue discrimination outside the attentional focus.

Similar results were obtained when observers discriminated both color and orientation of two pop-out targets (figure 15.9b). Although the discrimination of two targets involved four independent binary discriminations, observers performed comparably well with and without the concurrent letter task. Note that color and orientation not only had to be correctly perceived, but also had to be associated with the correct target, a requirement that shows that observers were individually aware of both targets and their features.

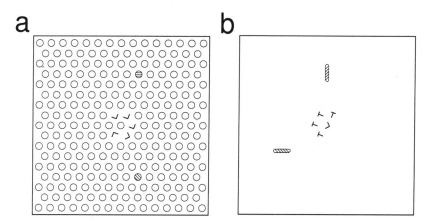

Figure 15.9 Displays used by Braun and Julesz (1997). Five *T*s or *L*s appear near the center (primary task). (a) As a first type of secondary task, observers independently discriminate the respective hues of two peripheral targets (represented here by hatching). Each target assumes one of two hues (chosen to be equally luminous and equally detectable). (b) As a second type of secondary task, observers independently discriminate the respective colors (represented by hatching) and orientations of two peripheral targets. Each target assumes one of four colors and one of two orientations. In both displays, secondary tasks are performed well in the dual task situation, and observers report being visually aware of the discriminated information. This shows that parallel attentional processes contribute directly to visual experience. (After Braun and Julesz, 1997.)

These findings show that observers enjoy a significant ability to discriminate visual information outside the attentional focus. This ability appears to involve conscious vision and seems to be based on normal visual awareness of the discriminated information. Thus, it would appear that parallel attentional mechanisms contribute certain types of information to the observer's visual experience, among them the presence, location, color, and orientation of stimuli that pop out from the visual scene.

CONCLUSIONS

A number of crucial advances in our understanding of attention are the fruit of divided attention experiments. For example, cueing experiments show that attention enhances visual sensitivity d', which implies that attention modulates relatively early stages of visual processing, a conclusion that is gaining increasing support from neurophysiological evidence. Divided attention experiments provide most of the information that is currently available about attentional dynamics (dwell times and shift times). However, it must be admitted that understanding of this topic remains seriously incomplete and that important issues, such as the discrepancy between sequential and simultaneous displays, remain to be worked out. Both cueing and divided attention experiments show that different types of visual sensitivity are differentially affected by attention and, in particular, that pop-out targets constitute a privileged class of stimuli that place little demand on attention.

The impressive track record of divided attention experiments is evidently due to the success of this paradigm in manipulating the allocation of attention across the visual field. The direct manipulation of attention by a cue or by a second visual task seems to be more effective and seems to lead to more consistent results than does the indirect manipulations of attention that are attempted by other paradigms (e.g., visual search or priming).

A comparatively recent development are dual-task experiments that show that the perception of pop-out is largely independent of attentional focus. The straightforward interpretation of these results is that serial and parallel attentional mechanisms can operate side by side and can contribute independently to visual experience. This would imply a revision of the widely accepted view that a unitary attentional process has exclusive control over access to visual awareness. Instead, it would suggest that serial and parallel attentional processes simultaneously and independently bring to visual awareness information from inside and outside the attentional focus. The existence of serial and parallel attentional processes (i.e., focal attention and pop-out) is, of course, well accepted, but previously the two types of processes were not considered to be independent. In fact, positive evidence for their independence, such as the bimodal distribution of recall observed by Sperling and Weichselgartner (1987), has been largely ignored.

What distinguishes visual information that is perceived independently of—that is, outside—the attentional focus? The short answer seems to be selection by parallel processes such as surround inhibition and global competition. One indication of this is the apparent limitation to features that are processed in parallel (e.g., position, color, orientation) (Julesz, 1991; Nakayama, 1991; Treisman, 1993). Features not processed in parallel are also not discriminated outside the attentional focus (e.g., letter identity). The second indication is the evident limitation to stimuli that pop out from the visual scene. Stimuli that pop out usually possess a locally unique feature that is not shared by surrounding stimuli. When several stimuli are prominent in this way, pop-out seems to be determined by a global competition among prominent stimuli, which seems to intensify outside the focus of attention. The current answer to the question of how many stimuli can pop out simultaneously is at least two.

The notion that parallel processes select the information that is perceived outside the attentional focus is attractive because it accords well with neurophysiological findings. Feature-specific surround inhibition enhances neuronal responses to stimuli with locally unique features. Global competition, for which there is some evidence in inferotemporal cortex (Miller et al., 1993; Sato, 1995), may further inhibit neuronal responses to all but a few stimuli in the visual field (Desimone and Duncan, 1995; Koch and Ullman, 1985). In the end, only the most prominent stimuli in the visual field may elicit a strong neuronal response—those that are visually salient and pop out—whereas all others may elicit little or no response. Accordingly, visual experience outside the focus of attention may be limited simply by the strength of the neuronal response after surround inhibition and global competition have taken effect. Inside the attended part of the scene, inhibition received by attended stimuli seems to be suppressed, whereas inhibition originating from attended stimuli may be left intact or may even be enhanced. Thus, attended stimuli always elicit a strong response, even when other parts of the visual scene are more prominent.

Hopefully, this review has made clear that experiments on divided attention indeed go far towards bridging the gap between psychophysics and neurophysiology. Two areas in which more work is desirable are attentional dynamics (shift times and dwell times) and parallel attentional mechanisms. On the latter subject, quantitative computational modeling of surround inhibition and global competition in natural images would probably prove helpful. Interactions between the various parts of a visual scene may well be too complex to yield to an entirely qualitative analysis, and a quantitative model of these interactions would greatly facilitate both psychophysical and neurophysiological experiments on attention.

ACKNOWLEDGMENTS

Support from the National Science Foundation (Integrative Biology and Neuroscience, and the Engineering Research Center for Neuromorphic Engineering) and from the Office of Naval Research is gratefully acknowledged. In addition, I would like to thank Christof Koch and Pietro Perona for continued encouragement and support.

REFERENCES

Allman, J. M., Miezin F., and McGuinness, E. (1985) Direction- and velocity-specific responses from beyond the classical receptive field in the middle temporal area (MT). *Perception* 14: 105–126.

Allport, D. A. (1980) Attention and performance. In *Cognitive Psychology: New Directions*, edited by G. Claxton. London: Routledge and Kegan Paul.

Bashinski, H. S. and Bacharach, V. R. (1980) Enhancement of perceptual sensitivity as the result of selectively attending to spatial locations. *Percept. Psychophys.* 28: 241–248.

Bonnel, A. M. and Miller, J. (1994) Attentional effects on concurrent psychophysical discriminations: Investigations of a sample size model. *Percept. Psychophys.* 55: 125–247.

Bonnel, A. M., Possamai, C. A., and Schmitt, M. (1987) Early modulations of visual input: A study of attentional strategies. *Q. J. Exp. Psychol.* 39A: 757–776.

Bonnel, A. M., Stein, J. F., and Bertucci, P. (1992) Does attention modulate the perception of luminance changes? *Q. J. Exp. Psychol.* 44A: 601–626.

Braun, J. (1993) Shape-from-shading is independent of visual attention and may be a "texton." *Spat. Vis.* 7: 311–322.

Braun, J. (1994) Visual search among items of different salience: Removal of visual attention mimics a lesion in extrastriate area V4. *J. Neurosci.* 14: 554–567.

Braun, J. and Julesz, B. (1997) Withdrawing attention at little cost: Detection and discrimination tasks. *Percep. Psychophys.*, in press.

Braun, J. and Koch, C. (1995) Stimulus competition and non-attentive selection: interactions between motion and orientation contrasts. *Invest. Ophthalmol. Vis. Sci.* (Suppl.): 36.

Braun, J. and Sagi, D. (1990) Vision outside the focus of attention. *Percept. Psychophys.* 48: 45–58.

Braun, J. and Sagi, D. (1991) Texture-based tasks are little affected by a second task which requires peripheral or central attentive fixation. *Perception* 20: 483–500.

Bravo, M. J. and Nakayama, K. (1992) The role of attention in different visual-search tasks. *Percept. Psychophys.* 51: 465–472.

Britten, K. H., Shadlen, M. N., Newsome, W. T., and Movshon, J. A. (1992) The analysis of visual motion: A comparison of neuronal and psychophysical performance. *J. Neurosci.* 12: 4745–4765.

Cheal, M. and Lyon, D. R. (1994) Attention in visual search: Multiple search classes. *Q. J. Exp. Psychol.* 47A: 49–69.

Chelazzi, L., Miller, E. K., Duncan, J., and Desimone, R. (1993) A neural basis for visual search in inferior temporal cortex. *Nature* 363: 345–347.

Desimone, R. (1992) Neural circuits for visual attention in the primate brain. In *Neural Networks for Vision and Image Processing*, edited by G. Carpenter, and S. Grossberg, pp. 343–364. Cambridge: MIT Press.

Desimone, R. and Duncan, J. (1995) Neural mechanisms of selective visual attention. *Annu. Rev. Neurosci.* 18: 193–222.

Desimone, R., Schein, S. G., Moran, J., and Ungerleider, L. G. (1985) Contour, color and shape analysis beyond the striate cortex. *Vis. Res.* 25: 441–452.

Desimone, R. and Ungerleider, L. G. (1989) Neural mechanisms of visual processing in monkeys. In *Handbook of Neuropsychology* (Vol. 2), edited by F. Boller, and J. Grafman, pp. 267–299. Amsterdam: Elsevier.

Downing, C. (1988) Expectancy and visual-spatial attention: Effects on perceptual quality. *J. Exp. Psychol. Hum. Percept. Perform.* 14: 188–202.

Duncan, J. (1980) The demonstration of capacity limitation. *Cognitive Psychol.* 12: 75–96.

Duncan, J. (1984) Selective attention and the organization of visual information. *J. Exp. Psychol. Gen.* 113: 501–517.

Duncan, J. and Humphreys, G. (1989) Visual search and stimulus similarity. *Psychol. Rev.* 96: 433–458.

Duncan, J. and Humphreys, G. (1992) Beyond the search surface: Visual search and attentional engagement. *J. Exp. Psychol. Hum. Percept. Perform.* 18: 578–588.

Duncan, J., Ward, R., and Shapiro, K. (1994) Direct measurement of attentional dwell time in human vision. *Nature* 369: 313–315.

Felleman, D. J. and Van Essen, D. C. (1990) Distributed hierarchical processing in the primate cerebral cortex. *Cereb. Cortex* 1: 1–47.

Gallant, J. L., Connor, E. and Van Essen, D. C. (1994) Responses of visual cortical neurons in a monkey freely viewing natural scenes. *Soc. Neurosci. Abstr.* 20: 838.

Gibson, B. S. and Egeth, H. (1994) Inhibition and disinhibition of return—Evidence from temporal-order judgments. *Percept. Psychophys.* 56: 669–680.

Green, D. M. and Swets, J. A. (1966) *Signal Detection Theory and Psychophysics*. New York: Wiley.

Haenny, P. E., Maunsell, J. H. R., and Schiller, P. H. (1988) State dependent activity in monkey visual cortex: 2. Retinal and extraretinal factors in V4. *Exp. Brain Res.* 69: 245–259.

Hawkins, H. L., Hillyard, S. A., Luck, S. J., Mouloua, M., Downing, C. J., and Woodward, D. P. (1990) Visual attention modulates signal detectability. *J. Exp. Psychol. Hum. Percept. Perform.* 16: 802–811.

Helmholtz, H. (1962) *Handbuch der Physiologischen Optik*. New York: Dover. (Original work published 1850.)

Hung, G., Wilder, J., Curry, R., and Julesz, B. (1995) Simultaneous better than sequential for brief presentations. *J. Opt. Soc. Amer.* 12A: 441–449.

James, W. (1981) *The Principles of Psychology*. Cambridge, MA: Harvard University Press. (Original work published 1890.)

Julesz, B. (1981) Textons, the elements of texture perception and their interactions. *Nature* 290: 91–97.

Julesz, B. (1991) Early vision and focal attention. *Rev. Mod. Phys.* 63: 735–772.

Julesz, B. and Braun, J. (1992, Oct.) Early vision: Dichotomous or continuous? Paper presented at annual meeting of the Psychonomic Society, St. Louis, MO.

Kinchla, R. A. (1992) Attention. *Annu. Rev. Psychol.* 43: 711–742.

Knierim, J. J. and Van Essen, D. C. (1992) Neuronal responses to static texture patterns in area V1 of the alert macaque monkey. *J. Neurophysiol.* 67: 961–980.

Koch, C. and Ullman, S. (1985) Shifts in selective visual attention: Towards the underlying neural circuitry. *Hum. Neurobiol.* 4: 219–227.

Mack, A., Tang, B., Tuma, R., Kahn, S., and Rock, I. (1992) Perceptual organization and attention. *Cognitive Psychol.* 24: 475–501.

Macmillan, N. A. and Creelman, C. D. (1991) *Detection Theory: A User's Guide*. Cambridge, MA: Cambridge University Press.

Malik, J. and Perona, P. (1990) Preattentive texture discrimination with early vision mechanisms. *J. Opt. Soc. Am.* 7: 923–932.

Maunsell, J. H. R. (1995) The brain's visual world—Representation of visual targets in cerebral cortex. *Science* 270: 764–769.

Miller, E. K., Gochin, P. M., and Gross, C. G. (1993) Suppression of visual responses of neurons in inferior temporal cortex of the awake macaque by addition of a second stimulus. *Brain Res.* 616: 25–29.

Miller, E. K., Li, L., and Desimone, R. (1991) A neural mechanism for working and recognition in inferior temporal cortex. *Science* 254: 1377–1379.

Miller, E. K., Li, L., and Desimone, R. (1993) Activity of neurons in anterior inferior temporal cortex during a short-term memory task. *J. Neurosci.* 13: 1460–1478.

Miller, J. and Bonnel, A. M. (1994) Switching or sharing in dual-task line-length discrimination. *Percept. Psychophys.* 56: 431–446.

Moran, J. and Desimone, R. (1985) Selective attention gates visual processing in the extrastriate cortex. *Science* 229: 782–784.

Motter, B. C. (1993) Focal attention produces spatially selective processing in visual cortical areas V1, V2 and V4 in the presence of competing stimuli. *J. Neurophysiol.* 70: 909–919.

Motter, B. C. (1994) Neural correlates of attentive selection for color or luminance in extrastriate area V4. *J. Neurosci.* 14: 2178–2189.

Mueller, H. J. and Findlay, J. (1987) Sensitivity and criterion effects in the spatial cueing of visual attention. *Percept. Psychophys.* 42: 383–399.

Mueller, H. J. and Humphreys, G. W. (1991) Luminance-increment detection: Capacity-limited or not? *J. Exp. Psychol. Hum. Percept. Perform.* 17: 107–124.

Nakayama, K. (1991) The iconic bottleneck and the tenuous link between early visual processing and perception. In *Vision: Coding and Efficiency,* edited by C. Blakemore, pp. 411–422. Cambridge: Cambridge University Press.

Nakayama, K. and Mackeben, M. (1989) Sustained and transient components of focal visual attention. *Vis. Res.* 29: 1631–1647.

Nothdurft, H. C. (1991) Texture segmentation and pop-out from orientation contrast. *Vis. Res.* 31: 1073–1078.

Pashler, H. (1994) Dual-task interference in simple tasks—Data and theory. *Psychology* 116: 220–244.

Posner, M. I., Snyder, C. R. R., and Davidson, B. J. (1980) Attention and the detection of signals. *J. Exp. Psychol. Gen.* 109: 160–174.

Pratt, J. and Abrams, R. A. (1995) Inhibition of return to successively cued spatial locations. *J. Exp. Psychol. Hum. Percept. Perform.* 21: 1343–1353.

Press, W. A., Knierim, J. J., and Van Essen, D. C. (1994) Neuronal correlates of attention to texture patterns in macaque striate cortex. *Soc. Neurosci. Abstr.* 20: 838.

Reynolds, J., Chelazzi, L., Luck, S., and Desimone, R. (1994) Sensory interactions and effects of selective spatial attention in macaque area V2. *Soc. Neurosci. Abstr.* 20: 1054.

Reynolds, J., Nicholas, J., Chelazzi, L., and Desimone, R. (1995) Spatial attention protects macaque V2 and V4 cells from the influence of non-attended stimuli. *Soc. Neurosci. Abstr.* 21: 1759.

Robinson, D. L. and Petersen, S. E. (1992) The pulvinar and visual salience. *Trends Neurosci.* 15: 127–132.

Rock, I., Linnett, C. M., Grant, P., and Mack, A. (1992) Perception without attention: Results of a new method. *Cognitive Psychol.* 24: 502–534.

Rubenstein, B. S. and Sagi, D. (1990) Spatial variability as a limiting factor in texture-discrimination tasks: Implications for performance asymmetries. *J. Opt. Soc. Am.* 7A: 1632–1642.

Saarinen, J. and Julesz, B. (1991) The speed of attentional shifts in the visual field. *Proc. Natl. Acad. Sci.* 88: 1812–1814.

Sagi, D. (1990) Detection of an orientation singularity in gabor textures: Effect of signal density and spatial frequency. *Vis. Res.* 30: 1377–1390.

Sagi, D. and Julesz, B. (1987) Short-range limitation on detection of feature differences. *Spat. Vis.* 1: 39–49.

Salzman, C. D. and Newsome, W. T. (1994) Neural mechanisms for forming a perceptual decision. *Science* 264: 231–237.

Sato, T. (1995) Interactions between two different visual stimuli in the receptive fields of inferior temporal neurons in macaques during matching behaviors. *Exp. Brain Res.* 105: 209–219.

Schiller, P. H. and Lee, K. (1991) The role of primate extrastriate area V4 in vision. *Science* 251: 1251–1253.

Shaw, M. L. (1984) Division of attention among spatial locations: A fundamental difference between detection of letters and detection of luminance increments. In *Attention and Performance X*, edited by H. Bouma, and D. G. Bouwhuis, Hillsdale, NJ: pp. 109–121. Lawrence Erlbaum.

Sperling, G. and Dosher, E. (1986) Strategy and optimization in human information processing. In *Handbook of Perception and Performance*, edited by K. Boff, L. Kaufman, and J. Thomas, 1–65. New York: Wiley.

Sperling, G. and Melchner, M. J. (1978) The attention operating characteristic: Some examples from visual search. *Science* 202: 315–318.

Sperling, G. and Weichselgartner, E. (1987) Dynamics of automatic and controlled visual attention. *Science* 238: 778–780.

Spitzer, H., Desimone, R., and Moran, J. (1988) Increased attention enhances both behavioral and neuronal performance. *Science* 240: 338–340.

Treisman, A. (1991) Search, similarity, and integration of features between and within dimensions. *J. Exp. Psychol. Hum. Percept. Perform.* 17: 652–676.

Treisman, A. (1993) The perception of features and objects. In *Attention: Selection, Awareness, and Control*, edited by A. Baddeley, and L. Weiskrantz, pp. 1–36. Oxford: Clarendon Press.

Treisman, A. and Gelade, G. (1980) A feature integration theory of attention. *Cognitve Psychol.* 12: 97–136.

Ungerleider, L. G. (1995) Functional brain imaging studies of cortical mechanisms for memory. *Science* 270: 769–775.

Van Essen, D. C. and Gallant, J. L. (1994) Neural mechanisms of form and motion processing in the primate visual system. *Neuron* 13: 1–10.

Watt, R. (1991) Seeing texture. *J. Cognitive Neurosci.* 1: 137–139.

Wertheimer, M. (1923) Untersuchungen zur Lehre von der Gestalt. *Psychologische Forschung* 4: 301–350.

Wolfe, J. M. (1994) Guided search 2.0: A revised model of visual search. *Psychon. Bull. Rev.* 1: 202–238.

16 Spatial Working Memory and Spatial Selective Attention

Edward Awh and John Jonides

ABSTRACT   Spatial working memory has been previously dissociated from other working memory systems, but there has been relatively little previous research on the specific subcomponents of spatial working memory. This chapter reviews neuroanatomical evidence that is relevant to a specific model of spatial working memory in which covert shifts of spatial selective attention are hypothesized to mediate the on-line maintenance of location-specific representations.

Consider this simple memory task. A single dot appears somewhere in the visual field, marking a location. That location must be stored in memory for several seconds, after which time another dot appears. The subject's task is to decide whether the location of the second dot is identical to that of the first. What processes are involved in performance of this task? A simple analysis suggests that the observer must first encode the location of the memorandum, then store that location in short-term or working memory for a brief period, and then compare the stored memory representation against the probe dot that appears thereafter. Of those three processes, what is involved in storage? If spatial working memory is at all similar to verbal working memory, there are two components (Awh et al., 1996). One is a set of processes required for the storage of a memory representation of the dot's location. The other is a rehearsal process required to somehow refresh that representation with some fidelity in expectation of the upcoming retrieval test. But what is the specific nature of that putative rehearsal process?

Decades of research on spatial selective attention have left little doubt that observers make faster and more accurate responses to stimuli that fall in expected rather than in unexpected locations. More recently, there have been compelling demonstrations of location-specific attentional modulation of early sensory processing, which might account for such expectancy effects (see Mangun, Hansen, and Hillyard, 1987). In other words, spatial selective attention may cause enhanced processing in the specific cortical regions that process an attended region of space. The central thesis of this chapter is that the interaction of spatial attention and early visual processing may mediate the rehearsal of information in spatial working memory. Simply put, keeping the representation of a location active in memory recruits the same mechanisms that are involved in selectively attending to that location. Awh, Smith, and Jonides (1995) have provided a measure of behavioral evidence that renders this hypothesis plausible. They showed that the requirement to retain a location in working memory resulted in a side benefit. When an intervening choice reaction time stimulus was presented during the retention interval, faster responses were observed for stimuli that fell in memorized locations. This is just as it should be if, as a strategy for remembering, subjects allocate their attention to the target location.

If there is a close parallel between spatial selective attention and spatial working memory processes, then the neuroanatomical sites that participate in tasks of the two types should show a strong overlap. This issue is examined first in an in-depth review of the neuroanatomical basis for tasks that require subjects to engage spatial selective attention versus those that require subjects to engage spatial working memory. The evidence comes from a variety of sources, including studies of the behavior of single cells, the effects of lesions in humans, and neuroimaging of humans. To anticipate the conclusions, there is a striking concordance among the various techniques in support of the hypothesis that spatial attention and spatial working memory are mediated by very similar cortical circuits.

THE NEURAL BASIS OF SPATIAL SELECTIVE ATTENTION

An influential theory of the neural processes involved in spatial attention was proposed by Mesulam (1981, 1990). One essential claim of his theory is that attentional processes are mediated by the activation of a network that includes four primary brain regions: (1) a frontal component (the dorsolateral, or premotor, prefrontal cortex) provides a spatial map for the coordination of exploratory motor processes, (2) a posterior parietal component coordinates the formation of a spatial representation of extrapersonal space, (3) processes of the anterior cingulate gyrus provide a spatial map of motivational valence, and (4) a subcortical reticular component modulates the overall arousal and vigilance necessary for attentional processing.

Mesulam asserted that the components of this network mediate two qualitatively different types of attentional processing. One is tonic in nature and involves regulation of the overall threshold that stimuli must exceed in order to reach consciousness. The reticular component is claimed to mediate that process. The other type is described as phasic and involves the selection (i.e., location-specific enhancement) of items that will receive the benefits of attentional resources from the multiple items that reach threshold. The frontal, parietal, and cingulate components of the network are claimed to subserve that type of attentional processing. Within those areas, Mesulam acknowledged that there is relatively sparse evidence supporting the putative role of the cingulate in motivational valence. Rather, the majority of neuroscientific studies of spatial attention place emphasis on the frontal and parietal components of attentional processing, and thus only those components are examined here.

The four components of Mesulam's model could be said to comprise the *source* of attentional modulation (Posner and Petersen, 1990). The *site* of the effects, however, is likely to be quite different. The beneficial effects of attention may occur at the level of early sensory processing or during later postperceptual processing stages (for a review, see Yantis and Johnston, 1990). Because a growing body of evidence suggests the presence of sensory effects (e.g., Mangun et al., 1987), studies of extrastriate and striate participation in spatial selective attention are also examined.

Evidence from Unit Recording

Prefrontal Regions   There is an extensive literature demonstrating the participation of prefrontal brain regions in directed visual attention (for a review, see Fuster, 1984). A typical finding is that selected populations of prefrontal neurons show enhanced responses to behaviorally relevant (i.e., attention-attracting) stimuli. For instance, Kodaka, Mikami, and Kubota (1994) identified neurons in the prefrontal cortex of monkeys that showed significant increases in response to extrafoveal stimuli when they were behaviorally relevant compared to when they were not. Mikami, Ito, and Kubota (1982) also identified a relatively small group of neurons whose response patterns were diagnostic of whether extrafoveal attention was required even before the stimuli appeared. The firing patterns of those neurons were modulated during the period in which relevant stimuli were expected in peripheral space, a result that suggests a prefrontal mechanism that mediates the tonic engagement of spatial selective attention.

Of course, one might ask of these and other studies that involve responses to relevant and irrelevant stimuli whether the changes in neural activity reflect attentional modulation of sensory processing or response-related processing. An elegant dissociation of those processing components was provided by di Pellegrino and Wise (1993a, 1993b), who examined attention-related neurons in both the dorsolateral prefrontal and dorsal premotor areas. Each trial of their experimental task was comprised of the following events. First, one of eight possible lights was illuminated in the periphery (the prime stimulus, or PS1). Next, zero to four of the remaining lights were illuminated, and the monkey was trained to not respond to these distractors. When the prime stimulus was illuminated again (PS2), the monkeys were trained to respond in one of two ways. In one case, the direction of a limb movement was determined by the location of the prime stimulus (compatible condition). In the other case, the direction of the limb movement was fixed, and the reoccurrence of the prime stimulus served only to trigger the movement (incompatible condition). This design allows comparison of responses to attended (PS1 and PS2) and unattended (distractor) stimuli. In addition, the compatible and incompatible conditions constituted a manipulation of the response-related significance of PS1 and PS2 that also controlled for the sensory and attentional aspects of the tasks.

Prefrontal neurons were analyzed in terms of their phasic responses to the onset of PS1, PS2, and the distractor stimuli (di Pellegrino and Wise, 1993a). Those observations were consistent with those of Kodaka et al. (1994), who demonstrated enhanced neuronal responses to behaviorally relevant stimuli. Likewise, di Pellegrino and Wise found groups of neurons in both the dorsolateral and premotor parts of prefrontal cortex that showed location-specific, enhanced modulation of responses to PS1 and PS2 relative to those for spatially identical distractor stimuli. An additional analysis of tonic neuronal responses (di Pellegrino and Wise, 1993b) provided further evidence of attentional processing. Cells were identified in both prefrontal and premotor cortex with sustained higher rates of discharge throughout the delay period between PS1 offset and PS2 onset, a result that suggests their participation in the tonic maintenance of directed spatial attention.

In addition, an analysis of tonic responses as a function of compatibility (i.e., the response-related significance of PS1 and PS2) suggested an interesting dissociation of prefrontal and premotor function. Modulations of these attentional responses as a function of compatibility were more prevalent for the premotor neurons—the responses of which tended to decrease in the incompatible condition—than for the prefrontal neurons, a result that suggests that the premotor area is more heavily involved in response-related attentional processing. It is noteworthy that di Pellegrino and Wise (1993a) distinguished between two strategies that the monkeys could use in the performance of these tasks: (1) they might direct attention toward the location of the primary stimulus and respond when another stimulus appeared in the attended region, or (2) they might memorize the location of the prime stimulus and respond whenever a stimulus was detected at the remembered location. The model of spatial working memory proposed here suggests that those two processes may be one and the same.

Parietal Regions Initial studies of the responses of neurons in the parietal cortex for attentional tasks focused on the eye movement–related responses of these neurons. Lynch, Mountcastle, Talbot, and Yin (1977) studied the activity of neurons in area 7 of parietal cortex in monkeys during tasks that required ocular fixation and tracking of visual targets. They found that most neurons in that area were activated during the ocular activities, but only when the stimuli that the animals were observing were behaviorally relevant. When the identical eye movements occurred spontaneously or during casual inspection of the environment, the parietal neurons did not respond, results that suggest a role for attention in describing the behavior of those neurons.

Bushnell, Goldberg, and Robinson (1981) went a step beyond the study of Lynch et al. (1977) by dissociating the putative attentional function of parietal neurons from their role in emitting a response. They measured the responses of parietal neurons in area 7 during several tasks that called for a variety of responses—some ocular and some manual. They replicated previous findings that a significant portion of those neurons responded in a spatially specific manner just before saccades to relevant behavioral targets. Beyond this, they found a strikingly similar profile of responses in the same populations of cells when the animals performed a peripheral attention task that did not require ocular responses. Furthermore, animals were trained on attentional tasks that required hand-reach responses (but no ocular responses), and location-specific enhancement of responses to attended stimuli was again observed—within the same neuronal population that had shown those effects during the saccade task. The results provide good support for response-independent mediation of spatial selective attention by cells in parietal cortex.

Extrastriate Regions   Some of the first evidence from unit recordings about attentional modulation of early visual processing comes from a study by Moran and Desimone (1985). They recorded activations of cells in the extrastriate cortex (area V4) of monkeys during a task that required focal direction of attention. At the start of each trial, two stimuli were presented simultaneously in separate locations within the receptive field of the recorded neuron. The visual characteristics of the stimuli were controlled such that one was effective in eliciting a response from the cell, whereas the other was not. The monkeys had been trained to attend to one of the stimulated locations. Five hundred ms later, a second pair of stimuli appeared and the animals had to indicate whether the stimulus at the attended location matched the initial attended stimulus. Comparing across trials, the experimenters were able to observe neuronal responses to spatially identical attended and unattended stimuli. They found that when an effective stimulus in the cell's receptive field was attended, the cell responded well. However, when the animal attended to an ineffective stimulus, the response was greatly reduced, despite the presence of an effective stimulus within the receptive field. Thus, the cell's responsiveness was determined by the attended stimulus. The authors suggested that this result may indicate a shrinking of the receptive field of the cell around the attended region.

Notice that the attentional effect depended on a number of factors. First, obtaining a good response from a cell required not only directed spatial attention, but also the presence of an effective stimulus at the attended location. This contrasts with the attentional effects obtained in frontal and parietal cortex, where simple spots of light were adequate to drive the cells' responses. Second, because there were always two stimuli, the observed attentional modulation was dependent on the presence of competing stimuli within the cell's receptive field. The investigators provided direct support for that interpretation by showing that when effective stimuli were presented alone within the receptive field, they always elicited a positive response, regardless of whether they were attended. The authors concluded from this result that attention did not serve so much to enhance neuronal responses as to suppress a neuron's response to unattended stimuli within its receptive field.

Using a very different paradigm, Fischer and Boch (1981) had previously shown that extrastriate neuronal responses were enhanced just prior to saccadic eye movements to peripheral stimuli. Moreover, a follow-up study (Fischer and Boch, 1985) suggested that those enhancements were dissociable from response-related or visuosensory aspects of the task. They recorded neuronal responses within the prelunate gyrus (area V4) of monkeys during four conditions. During the fixation task, the monkeys fixated a central point and pressed a key to indicate its presence. After a variable period, the spot dimmed and the monkeys had to release the key within 700 ms to get a water reward. Stimuli occurred peripherally as well, but the animals were required to ignore them. During the saccade task, the central fixation point was extinguished simultaneously with the appearance of a peripheral spot. In this case, the monkeys made a saccade to the peripheral stimulus and responded manually when they detected its dimming. The first two tasks allowed a comparison of responses to peripheral stimuli that were either ignored or were the target of a saccade. A delayed saccade task was similar to the saccade task, except that the offset of fixation occurred 1 s after the onset of the peripheral target stimulus, and the dimming always occurred at fixation. In that task, the monkeys maintained fixation and detected the dimming at the central location; then they executed a saccade to the peripheral stimulus when the central spot was extinguished. The fourth task, the suppressed saccade task, was a modified version of the delayed saccade task in which the offset of the central fixation was only temporary. If the offset were short enough (about 400–600 ms), the animals tended to not execute the saccade to the peripheral target. Tasks 3 and 4 allowed observation of neuronal responses to identical series of stimulus events, with and without eye movements.

The results of the fixation and saccade tasks replicated Fischer and Boch's earlier findings: neuronal responses to the onset of peripheral stimuli were enhanced in a spatially specific manner when the fixation point was extinguished, and a saccade to the peripheral stimulus was triggered (in 74% of cells tested). Although this enhancement could have been driven by a direction of attention to the peripheral stimulus, it is also possible that the increased response was due simply to the onset of the peripheral target (regardless of whether attention was directed to its location). The results of the delayed saccade task suggest that this explanation is unlikely, however. Recall that the peripheral stimulus appeared before the offset of the fixation point, during a period in which the monkey was still motivated to attend centrally. Although there was an initial increase in response when the peripheral stimulus appeared, it was transient and activation quickly returned to baseline. However, after the offset of the fixation point, the response to the peripheral stimulus was enhanced again until the saccade occurred (in 76% of the cells tested). These results show a clear dissociation of enhanced neuronal responses and the onset of the peripheral stimulus. Finally, the results of the suppressed saccade task are crucial. Although the first three experiments suggest that the enhancement was not related to stimulus onset alone, there was still a confounding of neuronal enhancement and the execution of a sac-cade. The results of the suppressed saccade task show that even when the monkey did not choose to make a saccade to the peripheral stimulus, there was a reliable enhancement of the response to the peripheral stimulus after the offset of the central fixation dot (in 80% of cases without eye move-ments). In addition, further control experiments provided evidence that the offset of the fixation point was not the causal factor in those enhancements. A reasonable interpretation of the results is that the offset of the central fixation point directly preceded a redirection of visual attention to the peripheral target, which caused enhanced extrastriate responses to the at-tended stimulus.

Striate Regions   Although the studies reported here demonstrate atten-tional influences on extrastriate processing, similar effects are elusive in the earliest processing areas (V1 and V2). For example, Moran and Desimone (1985) tested V1 neurons in the same paradigm described in the preceding section and failed to observe similar attentional modulation (also, see Mohler and Wurtz, 1977).

One possibility is that attentional effects within striate cortex are depen-dent on specific testing conditions, perhaps different from those required in extrastriate studies. Evidence supporting this possibility comes from a study by Motter (1993; also, see chapter 4, this volume). He recorded the responses of cells in areas V1, V2, and V4 during a focal attention task. Two tasks were employed. The first was used to assess the baseline response of those neu-rons to visual stimulation. At the start of each trial, the monkeys fixated a central spot and depressed a key. While they maintained fixation and held down the key, peripheral stimuli were presented that the monkey had been trained to ignore. Then a small bar was superimposed on the fixation target. The onset of the bar was the monkey's signal to release the key and depress either a right or left key (within 600 ms) to indicate the orientation of the bar. The task allowed measurement of responses to unattended peripheral stimuli as well as identification of the optimal orientations and receptive fields of the tested cells. The second task required responses to the peripheral stimuli and manipulated whether the relevant stimulus was attended or not. Once again, the monkeys fixated centrally and depressed a key. Then, an array of small dot cues was presented in the periphery. Each dot marked the potential location of a relevant behavioral stimulus. After a variable period of time, all but one of the dots were extinguished. The remaining dot marked the position of the relevant stimulus in an array that appeared 200–400 ms later. The number of stimuli in the array varied from three to eight in 85% of the trials, and was restricted to a single stimulus in 15% of the trials. Manip-ulation of the location of the final dot allowed comparison of neuronal responses when attention was directed toward or away from the cell's receptive field.

In 35% of the area V1 neurons tested, there was a spatially specific modulation of responses to stimuli depending on whether attention was directed toward or away from the neuron's receptive field. The same effect was observed in 39% and 45% of the cells tested in areas V2 and V4, respectively. Attentional effects were observed in all three cortical areas tested, but there were important qualitative differences among the areas. The effects observed in areas V1 and V2 interacted strongly with the nature of the receptive field stimulus. In both of those regions the attentional effects were usually limited to stimuli near the optimal orientation of the tested cell. By contrast, the effects in area V4 typically extended over a broader range of orientations, sometimes including all of the tested values. Also, the nature of the attentional modulation differed among the cortical areas. In area V1 and V2, 70% of the neurons showed enhanced responses when attention was directed toward the receptive field. However, in area V4, the effect of attention was more evenly split between enhancement (58%) and suppression of neuronal responses. Furthermore, while the variation of array size from three to eight stimuli had little effect on the responses of area V1 and V2 neurons, area V4 neurons usually showed significant attentional effects in the trials with larger arrays. Finally, in all three areas, the attentional effects were partially dependent on the presence of competing stimuli. Approximately 67% of attention-sensitive cells in each area failed to demonstrate the effects when the array contained only a single stimulus.

Summary of Evidence from Unit Recordings   The unit recording studies of spatial selective attention reveal a network of cortical sites that is generally consistent with the model proposed by Mesulam. There are prefrontal areas whose activations are directly correlated with motor-related attentional processing. In addition, the dorsolateral prefrontal cortex is implicated in the tonic maintenance of directed spatial attention, independent of response activities. Studies of neuronal responses in parietal cortex also suggest that it has a direct role in the control of spatial attention, independent of any specific response modality. Finally, there is compelling evidence that processing within striate and extrastriate regions is directly modulated by spatial attention, although that effect occurs only under relatively specific experimental conditions.

It should be noted that the appropriate homology between nonhuman primate and human cortical areas is an unresolved issue. For instance, Brodmann identified the inferior parietal lobe in humans as areas 39 and 40, but he found no architectonic equivalent to those regions in the monkey. Instead, Brodmann designated the inferior parietal region in monkeys as area 7, and it has been argued that this region may be homologous to area 7 (superior parietal) in humans (see Mesulam, 1981). As we shall see when we review studies of imaging, that hypothesis is in accord with the evidence from human neuroimaging studies that consistently associate area 7 activations with shifts of spatial attention, as well as with human lesion evidence that relates superior parietal damage to visual extinction (e.g., Posner, Walker, Friedrich, and Rafal, 1984; Vallar, 1993). Nevertheless, the syndrome that is classically associated with impaired spatial attention is hemineglect, and here it is the inferior parietal region that is the most consistent site of lesion overlap (Vallar, 1993). In line with this, it has been pointed out that the cytoarchitecture of human areas 39 and 40 is most similar to area 7 in monkeys (see Mesulam, 1981). Clearly, the issue of the human homolog to the monkey inferior parietal lobe is unresolved. Hence, caution is required when using nonhuman primate evidence to make inferences about functional localization in humans.

Evidence from Studies of Human Lesions

This discussion of human lesion studies is abbreviated because numerous general reviews can be consulted about this topic (e.g., Vallar, 1993; DeRenzi, 1982). Some of the earliest evidence from human lesions regarding spatial attention focused on the role of the parietal cortex, particularly in the right hemisphere (for a review, see Weinstein and Friedland, 1977). There is also ample evidence suggesting that right frontal regions are important for directed attention (for a review, see Foster, Eskes, and Stuss, 1994). However, although both areas are implicated, studies that include patient populations with frontal or parietal lesions indicate that attentional deficits are most prevalent in parietal cortex (e.g., Vallar and Perani, 1987). Finally, there are also reports associating attentional deficits and subcortical lesions. These data implicate posterior and medial thalamic areas as well as the basal ganglia in processes of spatial attention (for a review of the neural correlates of hemineglect, see Vallar, 1993). Overall, the data from human lesions are generally consistent with those from unit recordings in animals in implicating frontal and parietal sites in attentional processes. A point of divergence is the oft-cited importance of right hemisphere lesions in disrupting attentional processing in humans.

Distinct attentional disorders result from lesions of the inferior and superior areas of parietal cortex. In particular, right *inferior* parietal lesions are the most frequent correlate of hemineglect, which may be defined as the failure to explore the contralesional side of space, although elementary sensorimotor processing remains intact. But *superior* parietal lesions are instead associated with symptoms such as visual extinction (Vallar, 1993). Extinction differs from neglect in that subjects can perceive isolated stimuli in the contralesional field, but perception is impaired when an accompanying stimulus appears on the normal side. Thus, although it appears that both the superior and inferior aspects of parietal cortex are important for intact attentional processing, the specific roles of each region may be functionally dissociable.

One might ask whether the deficits studied in humans reflect damage to the same selective attention mechanism that was under study in the unit recording experiments. Although the paradigms rely on very different methodologies, of course, there are reasons to believe that they may indeed tap the same functional network. First, both paradigms implicate a frontal-parietal attentional network. Second, the effects of frontal and parietal lesions in humans have been studied using attentional spotlight paradigms. These tasks are more directly comparable to the single-cell studies that are the typical clinical assessments of neglect. Posner et al. (1984) showed that patients with parietal damage had difficulty with a spatial precueing task in which the brightening of one of two peripheral boxes informed subjects of the most likely location of a target for detection. When an invalid precue appeared in the ipsilesional visual field, subjects had great difficulty responding to the contralesional targets. Both right and left parietal patients showed this extinctionlike reaction time pattern, but it was more pronounced in the right parietal group. Posner et al. suggested that their results reflected impairment of a disengagement mechanism that must be initiated before shifts of spatial attention can occur. Alivisatos and Milner (1989) also used a spatial precueing experiment to examine the effects of unilateral frontal lobectomy. Their subjects performed a choice reaction time task and were given precues regarding the location of the impending stimulus. Patients with unilateral damage showed significantly less benefit from the spatial precues (relative to a neutral, uninformative condition) than did either normal subjects or control subjects with temporal lobectomies. It appears, then, that the evidence from human lesions is in good agreement with the data from recordings of cells in infrahuman animals. Both sets of studies implicate frontal and parietal mechanisms in a way that is consistent with the putative network proposed by Mesulam (1981).

Evidence from Human Neuroimaging

Studies of spatial selective attention using neuroimaging techniques are discussed next. Such studies are an important source of converging evidence because they allow whole-brain assessments of the neural substrate of spatial selective attention in normal human populations. The dependence of most neuroimaging studies on the subtraction methodology (Fox, Mintun, Reiman, and Raichle, 1988) is an important consideration. This technique associates discrete cortical areas with specific cognitive functions on the basis of differential activations between an experimental and a control condition. Consequently, the interpretation of the activated areas in any particular study must be considered in the context of the specific subtraction that was employed.

Using positron emission tomography (PET), Corbetta, Miezin, Shulman, and Petersen (1993) examined activations related to spatial selective attention. The primary experimental task required subjects to track the onset of a series of peripheral targets. During each trial, subjects fixated centrally while a series of targets was illuminated. Eighty percent of the time each stimulus appeared in a predictable location relative to the last one, allowing subjects to shift attention toward the locations of the ensuing targets, which appeared either on the left or right of fixation. Behavioral testing demonstrated that subjects were reliably faster to respond to validly cued targets, a result that shows that subjects were shifting attention to the cued locations as planned.

In order to determine the brain regions activated by the attentional components of the task, activations when subjects had to shift attention were compared with activations in a central detection task. During that task, subjects detected the onset of a central target while randomly flashed peripheral targets were to be ignored. The central detection task was intended to control for the peripheral sensory stimulation and the response-related processing found in the shifting task. (Because subjects had an intended central focus of attention, the irrelevant peripheral stimuli were unlikely to attract attention automatically; Yantis and Jonides, 1990.) Subjects were also scanned during passive viewing of a similar display (random peripheral locations were stimulated). Both the shifting task and the passive viewing task might cause shifts of visual attention; however, only the shifting condition should have activated brain regions that coordinate motor-related attentional processing, given that subjects were not making responses to attended stimuli in the passive viewing condition.

Subtraction of activations in the central detection task from those in the shifting task revealed significant changes in superior parietal cortex, superior frontal cortex, inferior frontal cortex, and anterior cingulate cortex (area 24). Note that, although superior parietal and superior frontal sites are a common theme in neuroimaging studies of selective attention (as we shall see in the section on imaging studies of working memory), the foci reported by Corbetta et al. are significantly anterior to those that are commonly observed. The sites of frontal and parietal activation were contralateral to the field of visual presentation, with the exception of bilateral parietal responses to right visual field stimulation. The superior frontal responses were absent in the passive viewing task relative to the central detection task. Two main differences between the shifting and passive conditions might explain the difference in effect with respect to the frontal responses: (1) those regions may mediate motor-related attentional processing, or (2) frontal regions may be more important for voluntary shifts of attention (rather than for the automatic shifts that might have been elicited in the passive viewing task). The fact that the parietal activations were present in both the shifting and passive viewing conditions suggests that that region is generally involved in the shifting of spatial attention, whether it is voluntary or automatic.

The Corbetta et al. (1993) experiment was designed to reveal effects of attention that one might call phasic in character. That is, subjects were required to shift their attention from one location to another. By contrast, Heinze et al. (1994) used both PET and event-related potential (ERP) techniques to observe brain responses during the tonic maintenance of attention. Subjects attended to the right or left side of a bilateral stimulus array, and they made judgments about stimuli appearing on the attended side. Each condition involved attention to only a single location, with no shifts of attention required. When a condition that required only passive viewing was subtracted from the conditions involving unilateral attention, PET revealed contralateral activation in the fusiform gyrus of extrastriate visual cortex in the attentional conditions, a result that suggests a location-specific enhancement of visual response to the bilateral stimulus array. In addition, the subtraction of the passive viewing condition from that in which subjects had to attend to the left revealed activation in anterior cingulate cortex and left superior frontal cortex (supplementary motor area 6), whereas subtraction of the passive viewing condition from the attend-right condition revealed a further site of activation in the thalamus.

The ERP recordings confirmed the early attentional modulations in extrastriate cortex by revealing signals of significantly larger amplitude at latencies of 80–130 ms; the ERP effects were also localized to occipital cortex contralateral to the attended side. Thus, both the timing and localization of the attentional responses suggest enhancement of early visual processing by the tonic allocation of spatial selective attention. The lack of parietal activation in these conditions is consistent with the notion that superior parietal cortex is involved in shifting attention rather than in tonically maintaining it on a single location (see Petersen, Corbetta, Miezin, and Shulman, 1994).

Duncan et al. (1996) have also used neuroimaging to examine the brain regions involved in spatial directed attention. Subjects made visual discriminations of either the orientation or displacement (or both) of peripheral stimuli. When PET activations related to simple detection of the same stimuli were subtracted from those in the discrimination conditions, a network of activations was observed in bilateral superior parietal cortex, right lateral frontal cortex, right occipital-temporal-parietal junction, anterior cingulate, left motor/premotor cortex, basal ganglia, pulvinar, and bilateral cerebellum.

Presumably, the discrimination conditions required relatively more allocation of attention to the periphery than did the detection condition, and they therefore should have activated the areas that mediate spatial selective attention. However, these activations reflect not only the relatively higher peripheral attention demands of the discrimination tasks, but also the processing of orientation and displacement information. In order to pinpoint the activations related to spatial attention, the investigators examined the relative increases in activation between detection, judgments of orientation or displacement, and judgments of both orientation and displacement. The rationale was that each increase in processing demands would be accompanied by a corresponding increase in attentional processing; thus, areas that showed monotonic increases in activation across the three conditions respectively are likely to play a role in spatial attention. By contrast, this pattern of results would not be expected in the areas related to stimulus presentation or the discrimination of specific stimulus characteristics.

The bilateral superior parietal focus showed the monotonic increases associated with attentional processing. Although the type of discrimination did not affect the level of activity in that region, the number of peripheral discriminations was a key factor. This region showed greater activation in all single-discrimination conditions than in the control condition, and showed the greatest activation in the task that required concurrent judgments of orientation and displacement. The authors pointed out that this result mirrors that of Bushnell et al. (1981), in which area 7 parietal responses were enhanced by attention, regardless of the specific task performed. The same pattern of increased activation during dual discriminations was observed in left premotor and nearby lateral prefrontal cortex, but in no other regions. The results suggest that superior parietal regions and left premotor and lateral prefrontal areas participate directly in the allocation of spatial attention to peripheral locations.

Vandenberghe et al. (1996) applied PET measurements to a paradigm similar to that of Duncan et al. (1996). Subjects in the study of Vandenberghe et al. made either detection or orientation-discrimination responses for stimuli that were presented either centrally or peripherally, with or without accompanying distractor stimuli. Subtraction of the activations in the detection conditions from those in the conditions requiring orientation discriminations showed relative increases in superior parietal lobule (bilaterally), right supplementary motor cortex, left premotor cortex, anterior cingulate, inferior occipital cortex (bilaterally), and right putamen. In right and medial superior parietal regions, the difference between discrimination and detection was greater when peripheral as opposed to central stimuli were presented; in fact, there was no significant difference in the activation of those regions between detection and orientation judgments with central stimuli. It is possible that the superior parietal cortex is particularly important when attention must be shifted peripherally; this would be consistent with the Corbetta et al. (1993) finding that detection of centrally appearing targets did not cause greater superior parietal responses than passive viewing of a similar stimulus display. Vandenberghe et al. argued against this possibility by pointing out that detection of peripheral targets in their experiment resulted in smaller superior parietal responses than did detection of central targets. However, tasks involving only detection of stimuli in fixed, predictable locations may be inappropriate for testing such a hypothesis because they may require only limited allocation of directed spatial attention.

The bilateral increases in inferior occipital cortex may reflect attentional enhancement of visual responses or, alternatively, the effects of making orientation judgments. There are two arguments for the former. The activation differences between orientation and detection judgments were greater with central than with peripheral stimulus presentations. It is unclear why this interaction would occur if these activations were driven by orientation processing, given that the peripheral presentations probably entailed more difficult discriminations. Indeed, performance accuracy with the peripheral stimuli was 6% lower than accuracy with central presentations. Also, the sites of extrastriate enhancement in this study are remarkably similar to those localized in the Heinze et al. (1994) experiment, in which response selection characteristics were completely matched. Overall, then, this study implicates a network of regions in selective attention that includes frontal and superior parietal regions, and also provides evidence of attention-enhanced extrastriate responses.

Until recently, neuroimaging studies have focused on spatial attention to visual displays. However, a study by Gitelman et al. (1996) employed PET to study spatial attention during a manual exploration task. The experimental task required subjects to move a computer mouse over a surface in their right hemispace as they searched for hidden targets. Auditory feedback informed subjects when the mouse had entered a target region. Activations in that condition were compared to those in a control condition during which subjects moved the mouse in a spiral pattern (again in their right hemispace), but without any search objective. Thus, the exploratory task placed higher demands on the processes of spatial attention, whereas the control task recruited similar motoric and perceptual processing.

Subtraction of the control from the experimental activations (depicted in figure 16.1 and color plate 11) revealed four signficant sites of activation in the right hemisphere: premotor cortex (area 6), posterior parietal cortex (at the border of areas 7 and 40), anterior cingulate cortex (area 24), and a sub-cortical activation that included the head of the right caudate nucleus. These data suggest that the neural network mediating directed spatial attention is not tied to a single input modality. The cortical sites activated by the manual exploration of space agree well with the network model proposed by Mesulam, as well as with other studies that utilized visual displays.

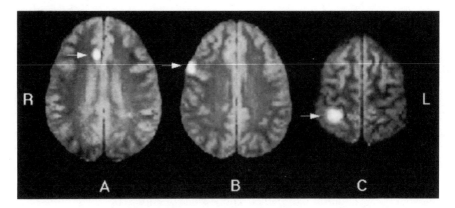

Figure 16.1 Areas significantly activated during the manual exploration task (Gitelman et al., 1996) as compared to during the condition. Activations in anterior cingulate, premotor cortex, and posterior parietal cortex are shown in slices (A), (B), and (C) respectively. Note that the brain is depicted using the radiological convention in which the right side of each image represents the left of the brain. R, right; L, left. See plate 11 for color version.

Varieties of Attention

The results also indicate a marked right hemisphere dominance for spatial attention. This finding is consistent with a broad array of human lesion evidence (Vallar, 1993), and it is also reflected in some of the neuroimaging studies reviewed here. In particular, right hemispheric dominance (as indicated by reported z-scores and the relative frequency of right hemisphere activations) was also observed in the Corbetta et al. (1993), and Duncan et al. (unpublished manuscript) studies. Further striking evidence in favor of right hemispheric dominance comes from an experiment by Spiers et al. (1990). Forty-eight epileptic patients underwent unilateral suppression of hemispheric function by sodium amobarbital. The results showed that disruption of scanning and contralateral neglect occurred after right but not left hemisphere suppression. As we shall see in the next major section, the possibility of right hemisphere dominance in spatial attention is in accord with similar findings during neuroimaging of spatial working memory.

Despite the use of widely varying experimental paradigms, the neuroimaging studies reviewed here consistently implicate a frontal-parietal network of activations in the control of spatial selective attention. The superior parietal activations are directly correlated with the requirement of shifting attention. The frontal responses are less reliable, and the specific localization of these responses is more variable. Although all studies included frontal activations around Brodmann's area 6, the specific focus varied between the inferior and superior aspect of that region (i.e., between premotor and supplementary motor areas). Also, some conditions entailing allocation of spatial attention failed to activate any part of area 6. Finally, while unit recording studies consistently implicated dorsolateral prefrontal regions in spatial selective attention, the neuroimaging studies included no evidence of such activations.

Although only two of the five reviewed studies showed evidence of attentionally enhanced visual responses, there is an underlying consistency in these data. In particular, the rate of stimulus presentation was predictive of whether modulations of visual responses were observed. The interstimulus intervals employed by Heinze et al. and Vandenberghe et al. averaged 300 ms and 550 ms, respectively, and both studies included evidence of enhanced visual responses. On the other hand, the Corbetta et al. and Duncan et al. studies had much longer average interstimulus intervals (1500 ms and 1656 ms, respectively), and no visual enhancement was observed in these studies. Finally, the study by Gitelman et al. involved no visual presentations at all, and no activation was observed in visual cortex. It is possible that faster presentation rates drive visual responses more effectively, and are therefore more likely to reveal modulations of these responses.

Another possibility—perhaps directly related to the rate of stimulus presentation—is that the tasks were more difficult in the studies that demonstrated enhanced visual processing. The average behavioral accuracy in the Vandenberghe et al. and Heinze et al. studies (where attention-enhanced visual responses were observed) was only 79% and 57%, respectively. By contrast, the average accuracy in the Duncan et al. study was 87%, and the Corbetta et al. task resulted in near-ceiling performance levels, and no attentional enhancement of visual response was observed in these studies. The report by Gitelman et al. did not include behavioral measures of performance.

THE NEURAL BASIS OF SPATIAL WORKING MEMORY

The neuroanatomical evidence regarding spatial working memory is examined next. The bulk of evidence regarding this memory system has been generated through unit recording and lesion studies in nonhuman primates, and, more recently, through neuroimaging studies of humans. Having considered the network of cortical sites that mediates spatial selective attention, evidence about spatial working memory can be reviewed with an eye toward the possible correspondence between attention and memory.

Evidence from Nonhuman Primates

Spatial memory is a long-standing topic of research with nonhuman primates, and there are numerous reviews of this research (for in-depth reviews, see Fuster, 1995; Goldman-Rakic, 1987; Ungerleider 1995).

A prototypical paradigm for spatial working memory studies has been the delayed response task. Trials begin with a cue that indicates a location to be remembered for several seconds, after which a response based on that spatial memory is required. Both lesion studies and single-unit recordings have consistently shown that the regions surrounding the principal sulcus in monkeys (putatively homologous to the dorsolateral prefrontal cortex in humans) are of primary importance in the performance of these tasks (Goldman-Rakic, 1987). More recent studies have also implicated regions of the parietal cortex in spatial working memory. Chafee, Funahashi, and Goldman-Rakic (1989) observed neuronal responses in posterior parietal cortex during performance of an oculomotor delayed response task. They found that 28% of the tested neurons showed sustained activations during the delay period of the memory task. Those response patterns mirror those that have been observed in neurons of the dorsolateral prefrontal cortex (for a review, see Fuster, 1984), and suggest that parietal cortex is also directly involved in short-term maintenance of spatial information.

The extensive connectivity between the frontal and parietal regions is well known (e.g., Petrides and Pandya, 1984) and suggests that those areas are central nodes in a highly interactive network mediating spatial cognition (Goldman-Rakic, 1987; Fuster, 1995). A compelling picture of frontal-parietal interactions has emerged, in which parietal cortex serves as a receiving area of sensory information and calculates spatial coordinates that are transmitted to prefrontal regions. The prefrontal regions, through extensive reciprocal connections with parietal regions, mediate the continued activation of posterior sensory representation.

Recently, direct tests of the interaction between prefrontal and parietal regions have been carried out. Goldman-Rakic and Chafee (1994) observed neuronal responses in posterior parietal cortex during performance of an oculomotor delayed response task. Those measurements were carried out before, during, and after the dorsolateral prefrontal cortex was cryogenically suppressed. They found that the responses of most parietal cells (previously demonstrated to play a role in spatial memory) were significantly reduced during prefrontal cooling. Their results support the notion that prefrontal cortex mediates posterior parietal memory activations through reciprocal feedback connections.

Evidence from Human Neuroimaging

Studies in humans using neuroimaging measurements of brain activity also provide support for the role of parietal and prefrontal structures in spatial working memory. They suggest a role for occipital structures as well, a role that has not been investigated in studies of animal models. It has been suggested that these studies can be grouped into two classes based on the type of task that has been used and the resulting pattern of brain activations (a distinction first articulated by Owen, Evans, and Petrides, 1996). One type of task requires subjects to store spatial information during a retention interval and then to retrieve all or part of that information. The second type requires not only storage, but also some manipulation or monitoring of that information to satisfy task requirements. Thus, the two types of task share encoding, storage, and possibly retrieval processes, but the second type also includes processes responsible for the manipulation of spatial information. Let us examine tasks of the two types, and we shall see that they share many parts of a working memory circuit but differ in the nature of prefrontal activation.

Storage Tasks   Jonides et al. (1993) used PET to measure brain activations during a spatial working memory task that required storage and retrieval of three spatial locations. Each trial of the memory task began with three target dots appearing on the circumference of an imaginary circle surrounding a fixation point. A 3 s delay followed, after which a probe circle appeared on the screen. The task was to indicate whether the probe surrounded the location of one of the previously presented dots. The activations in the memory task were compared to those in a control task that involved nearly identical stimulus presentations, but the target dots and the probe circle were presented simultaneously after the delay interval. Thus, the control task involved similar stimulus presentations and responses, but it did not require active maintenance of information about spatial locations in memory.

The memory task caused significantly higher activations than the control task in four right hemisphere regions: a ventral prefrontal region (area 47), premotor cortex (area 6), inferior parietal cortex (area 40), and extrastriate cortex (area 19). The field of view of the PET camera in the experiment was somewhat restricted in that the most superior aspects of posterior cortex were not clearly observable. Thus, there was no opportunity to observe activations in superior parietal cortex (area 7), an area that we have cited as central to spatial attentional processes. Nevertheless, the study does provide evidence of a frontal-parietal circuit involved in spatial working memory in humans. In addition, the study reported activations in extrastriate cortex, consistent with the idea that early visual circuits may be involved in spatial working memory as well.

That pattern of activations was echoed in an experiment by Courtney, Ungerleider, Keil, and Haxby (1996), who also used PET to observe brain regions activated by working memory for spatial locations. During each spatial memory trial, subjects saw an array of 24 irregularly positioned boxes. Three faces appeared, one at a time, for 1500 ms, each in three separate boxes. A 500 ms delay followed, after which a single probe face (faces were used as stimuli to compare these results to those from a face memory task) was presented. Subjects had to indicate whether the probe occupied one of the memorized locations. This task was compared to a control task, in which subjects simply indicated when the fourth stimulus in the sequence appeared by pressing the right or left response button.

Two subtractions were reported. Comparison of the memory activations to those in the control task revealed memory-related activations in right and left superior parietal cortex (area 7), and right occipital cortex (area 19). The activations in the location memory condition were also directly compared with those in a face memory condition in which subjects had to match the probe against the target faces on the basis of identity, not location. The location memory condition showed relatively higher activations in right and left supplementary motor cortex (area 6), in right and left superior and inferior parietal cortex (areas 7 and 40, respectively), in left extrastriate cortex (area 19), and in striate cortex (area 17). The data of Courtney et al. (1996) suggest a more bilateral role of memory structures in a spatial storage task than do the data of Jonides et al. (1993). Nevertheless, there is good agreement between the studies about the involvement of structures in superior posterior prefrontal cortex, in extrastriate cortex, and in posterior parietal cortex. The data of Courtney et al. (1996) also implicated area 7 of parietal cortex, consistent with the proposed relationship between processing in spatial working memory and shifts of spatial attention.

Perhaps the most wide-ranging of the studies of spatial working memory is that by Owen et al. (1996). They took PET measurements of brain activations during the performance of several varieties of spatial working memory tasks intended to tap either simple storage or storage and monitoring processes. In one spatial span storage task (the spatial span task), eight red circles were presented in random locations on a screen. Subsequently, a sequence of five of the circles changed from red to blue and then back to red at the rate of 500 ms each. Immediately after the fifth circle turned back to red, subjects were required to touch each of the five circles in any order they wished. In the other fixed spatial sequence storage task, eight randomly positioned red circles were presented. Subjects simply had to touch the circles in a well-learned fixed sequence. When each circle was touched, it turned blue for 500 ms and then returned to red to indicate that the next circle in the sequence should be touched. Both of these conditions were compared to a baseline control condition in which eight red circles were presented in random locations, except for one centrally located one. Subjects monitored the central circle, which turned from red to blue once per second; they had to touch the circle each time it changed colors. This task was intended to involve similar perceptual and response requirements as the experimental tasks.

The two storage tasks of Owen et al. (1996) resulted in activations in right ventrolateral prefrontal cortex (area 47), in bilateral premotor cortex (area 6) for the spatial span task only, in bilateral superior parietal cortex (area 7), and in bilateral occipital cortex. That pattern of results is very similar to that of Jonides et al. (1993), and it accords well with some of the activations found in the study by Courtney et al. (1996) as well. The bulk of the evidence from these three experiments (from different laboratories and with different tasks) is in good agreement about the nodes involved in a circuit concerned with the storage of spatial information in working memory. These nodes include premotor cortex, inferior frontal cortex, superior parietal cortex, posterior parietal cortex, and occipital cortex. Furthermore, it appears that right hemisphere structures in these areas are more activated during spatial working memory than are those in the left hemisphere.

Storage and Manipulation Tasks Going beyond tasks that require just storage of spatial information, Smith, Jonides, and Koeppe (1996) used PET to observe brain activations during the performance of a continuous spatial working memory task. Subjects saw a series of single stimuli appear in various locations around the circumference of an imaginary circle. (The task used letter stimuli to facilitate comparison with a verbal memory task used in another condition of the experiment, but we shall ignore the verbal nature of the stimuli and treat them simply as markers for location.) The task was to indicate whether or not each stimulus occupied the same location as the stimulus presented three items back in the sequence. This is a demanding task, for which subjects must maintain three spatial locations in working memory at any moment to be successful, and the memory load is continuous because each older location is replaced by a newer location as the sequence continues. It is clear that the task requires more than just storage of the relevant locations. For instance, the temporal order of the relevant locations must be preserved in order to facilitate the item-by-item updating of the current memory set.

Activations in the spatial memory condition were compared to those in a control condition that required subjects to monitor a similar sequence of stimuli presented in various locations; in this case, subjects were required to discriminate only whether each stimulus occupied one of three unchanging

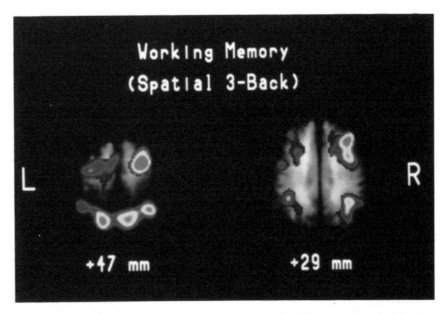

Figure 16.2 Areas significantly activated during the spatial working memory task of Smith et al. (1996) as compared to during the control condition. Each image is superimposed on an MRI image of a composite brain. The left slice shows activation in parietal cortex, areas 7 and 40 (the lower part of the image), and in supplementary motor and premotor cortex (the top part of the image). The right slice shows activation in dorsolateral prefrontal regions (top of the image), as well as further signs of the activation in parietal regions. Note that in these images, the right of the brain is depicted in the right of the images. R, right; L, left. See plate 12 for color version.

locations that had been committed to long-term memory before the beginning of the sequence. Thus, the need for working memory in the control condition was minimal. Subtraction of the activations in the control condition from those in the spatial memory condition (depicted in figure 16.2 and color plate 12) revealed a bilateral pattern of activation (with right hemisphere dominance) in dorsolateral prefrontal cortex (areas 9, 10, and 46), in supplementary motor area, and in superior and inferior parietal cortex (areas 7 and 40, respectively). In addition, a unilateral right hemisphere activation was observed in premotor cortex (area 6). The activations in this experiment bear a striking similarity to those found by Jonides et al. (1993), by Courtney et al. (1996), and by Owen et al. in their storage tasks (1996), with one exception: the continuous working memory task of Smith et al. (1996) recruited activations in dorsolateral prefrontal cortex, an area that was not activated in the pure storage tasks.

Owen et al. (1996) included three tasks in their experiment that, by their analysis, also involved more than just the storage of spatial information. In the first, each trial started with the sequential presentation of three blue circles (for 250 ms each) in random locations of a blank screen. After a 3 s delay, eight red circles were simultaneously presented on the screen, and the task was to touch the three red circles that matched the memorized locations.

Owen et al. (1996) asserted that this task involved not only the storage of spatial information but also involved processes necessary to pick the locations out from among a number of distractors. In a second task, a random arrangement of eight red circles was presented on the screen, and subjects searched through the array by touching individual circles until one of them turned blue. After the blue circle changed back into a red one, the subjects were instructed to continue searching for the new target, while avoiding touching the circles that had already turned blue. This task is similar to that of McCarthy et al. (1994), which is discussed next. Subjects were explicitly instructed not to use any systematic spatial strategies, but to search in a random fashion. The task also involved more than mere storage because subjects had to devise search strategies to sample the locations that had not already been selected in the display. The third task was similar to the second except that an array of 12 instead of 8 circles was presented.

All three of the tasks generated very similar patterns of activation; each task resulted in bilateral activations in superior parietal cortex (area 7) and in occipital cortex. In addition, there were sites of activation in right inferior parietal cortex (area 40) in all tasks, in left ventrolateral prefrontal cortex (area 47) in tasks 2 and 3, in right premotor activation (area 6) in tasks 1 and 3, in left premotor cortex (area 6) in all tasks, and in anterior cingulate cortex (area 32) in tasks 2 and 3. Except for the site in anterior cingulate, the activations are consistent with the tasks described previously that involve storage alone. In addition, however, Owen et al. (1996) found activations in dorsolateral prefrontal cortex in their three tasks, consistent with a role for that area in manipulation of stored spatial information. The nature of the manipulation involved in the three tasks appears quite different, and there is no clear account of how they share similarities; nevertheless, by the account of Owen et al. (1996), all the tasks involved a sort of monitoring function that might recruit dorsolateral prefrontal processes.

The role of dorsolateral prefrontal structures in spatial working memory tasks has also been investigated by McCarthy et al. (1994) using functional magnetic resonance imaging (fMRI). They required subjects to monitor a sequence of stimuli that appeared in a set of haphazard locations. Subjects were required to respond whenever the current stimulus appeared in a location that had already been occupied. In order to perform accurately, subjects had to keep in memory the set of previously stimulated locations. Activations in the memory condition were compared to a baseline of activation with no task requirements. Two additional control tasks were also included, both of which required peripheral attention to the locations of visually identical stimuli but did not require memory of those stimuli.

The window of view in this experiment was restricted to a single anterior coronal slice that included only parts of areas 9, 46, 23, and 47. Thus, the posterior areas (in parietal and occipital cortex) that may have been activated by the spatial memory task were not observed. Comparison of the memory task to the baseline condition revealed significantly higher activations in mid-dorsolateral prefrontal cortex (area 46) and in the cingulate gyrus (area 23). The activations in area 46 were bilateral but dominant in the right hemisphere. The results are consistent with the second and third spatial monitoring tasks of Owen et al. (1996) described previously, who also found activations in dorsolateral prefrontal cortex. In addition, however, the control tasks used by McCarthy et al. (1994) showed activations in dorsolateral prefrontal cortex, in the same region activated in the memory task. This is consistent with the possibility that the memory and control tasks in the experiment had overlapping functional profiles; perhaps both tasks required allocation of peripheral attention.

Summary of Neuroimaging Experiments Data from the set of neuroimaging experiments on spatial working memory agree well. This can be seen by inspecting table 16.1, which lists the various experiments and notes the areas of activation found in each. The table reveals that only a small number of sites of activation have been found in spatial working memory experiments. The sites include inferior prefrontal, premotor, supplementary motor, superior parietal, posterior parietal, and occipital areas in cortex. In addition, when the task involves more than just storage of information, there is evidence of dorsolateral prefrontal activation as well.

To summarize the information in the table, the studies by Jonides et al. (1993) and Courtney et al. (1996) used tasks that could be described as pure storage tasks; accordingly, the prefrontal activations in those tasks were restricted to premotor and ventrolateral prefrontal cortex. By contrast, due to the continuous nature of the memory task used by Smith et al. (1996), constant updating of the memory set was required; the presentation of each new stimulus necessitated dropping the first item in memory and adding a new one (while preserving the temporal order of the memorized items). Thus, this task required significant manipulation of the items in spatial working memory, and the results show that there were strong bilateral activations in dorsolateral prefrontal cortex.

The interpretation of the task by McCarthy et al. (1994) is somewhat less clear. Although that task did require updating spatial memory as new items were presented (and added to the list of memorized positions), it may be that this type of manipulation is qualitatively different from the temporal ordering required in the continuous task of Smith et al. (1996). Likewise, the interpretation of the dorsolateral prefrontal activations noted by Owen et al. (1996) in their spatial monitoring tasks also assumes that these tasks share some processes in common with the very different continuous working memory task of Smith et al. (1996).

However this issue resolves itself, there is at least clear unanimity about the remaining areas of activation, and it is these that are most germane to the hypothesis under discussion in this review. Four areas in particular were activated in at least three of the four studies reported: bilateral superior parietal

Table 16.1 Activations across five neuroimaging studies of spatial working memory

	Dorsolateral Prefrontal	Ventral Prefrontal	Superior Area 6	Superior Parietal	Inferior Parietal	Early Visual Regions	Anterior Cingulate
				Pure Storage Tasks			
Jonides et al. (1993)							
Spatial memory		R	R		R	R	
Courtney et al. (1996)†							
Location memory—control				R & L		R	
Location memory—face memory			R & L	R & L	R & L	L & midline	
Owen et al. (1996)							
Fixed array		R	R & L	R & L		R & L	midline
Fixed span		R		R & L		R & L	
				Tasks Requiring Manipulation			
Smith et al. (1996)							
3-back task	R & L		R & L	R & L	R & L		
Owen et al. (1996)							
Spatial monitoring I	R		R & L	R & L	R	R & L	
Spatial monitoring II	R	L	L	R & L	R	R & L	midline
Spatial monitoring III	R	L	R & L	R & L	R	R & L	midline
McCarthy et al. (1994)							
Memory vs. baseline	R & L						midline

Note: This table displays every region significantly activated by these spatial working memory tasks, with the following exceptions: Owen et al. also observed significant activations in sensorimotor cortex (during the spatial montoring I task) and in precuneous (in the spatial monitoring III and fixed span tasks). However, to our knowledge, these activations have not appeared in any other studies of spatial working memory. R = right; L = left; shaded regions were outside of that experiment's field of view.
† The Courtney et al. subtractions listed here are drawn from a single spatial memory condition.

cortex (area 7) in three of three studies where it was observable; right inferior parietal cortex (area 40) in all studies and bilaterally in two studies; superior frontal cortex (area 6) in all studies and bilaterally in three studies; extrastriate cortex in three of four studies. Note that the experiment by McCarthy et al. (1994) could not be included in this summary due to the restricted field of view of their fMRI camera. However, when their experiment is considered, three of five studies showed activation of dorsolateral prefrontal cortex (areas 9, 10, and 46) and of anterior cingulate cortex (area 32). It is interesting to note that with the single exception of the experiment by Courtney et al., every spatial working memory study reported here showed a striking right hemisphere dominance. Right hemisphere dominance is defined here as greater right hemisphere activation than left (as judged by the reported z-values) for any bilateral area of activation, as well as a larger incidence of unilateral activations in the right hemisphere. This feature of the spatial working memory evidence is in line with similar observations in the literature regarding spatial selective attention.

These studies show that a frontal-parietal circuit is a prominent feature of the neuroanatomical substrate of spatial working memory. The specific sites of activation in frontal cortex are variable (again reminiscent of the selective attention evidence) and may reflect current imprecision in understanding the functional categories subserved by this part of the brain. Activations in superior and inferior parietal cortex, however, are quite robust; it seems clear that at least two sites in parietal cortex are essential nodes in the network subserving spatial working memory. Finally, activations in extrastriate cortex are abundant in these studies and may reflect enhanced visual responses during the memory conditions. Interestingly, these extrastriate activations seem to be more prevalent in spatial memory conditions (three of four studies) than in the spatial selective attention studies reviewed previously (two of four studies). One possibility is that the memory tasks constituted a more challenging load on the selective attention system, causing a greater allocation of attentional resources. We have already seen that the incidence of visual activations within neuroimaging work on selective attention varies directly with task difficulty. The relative prevalence of visual enhancements in enhancement in the spatial memory conditions over enhancement in the spatial attention conditions may reflect differences in task difficulty—and thus in the degree of attentional allocation—rather than an underlying functional difference.

CONCLUSIONS

This review of the literature concerned with the anatomical substrates of spatial selective attention and spatial working memory was motivated by a simple hypothesis: that spatial selective attention may be recruited in the service of spatial working memory. In the form of an analogy, this hypothesis amounts to the claim that there is a rehearsal process involved in spatial working memory, similar to the role that rehearsal is claimed to have for verbal working memory. For spatial working memory, the assumption is that processes involved in spatial selective attention operate during the retention interval of a spatial working memory task to allocate attention in turn to each location that must be retained, keeping the representation of that location activated in memory. According to this hypothesis, there should be some overlap in the brain circuitry that is activated during spatial attention and during spatial working memory tasks.

This review suggests that there is overlap. The major nodes in each processing network lie in frontal and parietal regions. There is also considerable evidence of enhanced extrastriate responses to attended or memorized locations. Whether there are two overlapping circuits or a unitary memory and attention circuit is unclear. Although it is apparent that there is a core set of brain regions that are reliably activated by both spatial memory and by attention paradigms, there are possible exceptions. Multiple neuroimaging experiments have identified inferior parietal (area 40) and dorsolateral prefrontal areas in spatial working memory experiments; but those areas have not been activated in studies of spatial selective attention (with the possible exception of the study by Gitelman et al., 1996, which reports a posterior parietal area at the border of area 7 and 40). Thus, it is possible that the circuitry subserving spatial selective attention comprises a subset of the overall spatial working memory network. For example, it may be that processes of spatial attention are responsible for a rehearsal function in spatial working memory, but that additional processes are involved in memory tasks (such as creating the code that represents the spatial array) that are not shared with spatial selective attention tasks. Of course, the activation differences between memory and attention tasks may be in part an artifact of the specific paradigms that have been employed in tests of working memory and selective attention. For instance, as already discussed, there may have been differences in task difficulty between the memory and attention experiments. Other potentially relevant differences include faster stimulus presentation rates and the consistent presence of landmarks (by which subjects guided their attentional shifts) in the selective attention tasks. Future within-study analyses of the relationship between working memory and attention may provide clearer leads about the effects of these task factors. Nevertheless, the overall pattern of results suggests a similarity in neuroanatomical substrates between attention and spatial working memory that goes beyond mere artifact.

In addition to similar neuroanatomical substrates, it can be argued that there is functional correspondence between the roles suggested for the individual areas within these networks. The attentional literature has converged upon a role for the superior parietal cortex in formation of high-level spatial representations required by shifts of attention, whereas the prefrontal regions have been implicated in the tonic maintenance of directed spatial attention. Similarly, spatial working memory paradigms have suggested a role for prefrontal cortex in the tonic activation of posterior parietal sensory representations. Although this highly interactive relationship between the frontal and parietal regions has been interpreted as the cortical instantiation of spatial working memory (Fuster, 1995; Ungerleider, 1995), we suggest that another label—spatial selective attention—may also provide a fruitful means of interpreting this phenomenon. Thus, the major conclusion of this review is that the neuroanatomical correspondence between spatial working memory and spatial selective attention is a direct reflection of an underlying functional correspondence. Future investigations may help to reveal the full extent of the correspondence.

ACKNOWLEDGMENTS

The authors are indebted to Patricia Reuter-Lorenz and to Edward E. Smith for very helpful comments and advice during the preparation of this manuscript. Thanks also to Rik Vandenberghe and John Duncan for making available previously unpublished manuscripts. The preparation of this manuscript was supported in part by a grant from the Office of Naval Research and in part by a grant from the National Institute on Aging.

REFERENCES

Alivisatos, B. and Milner, B. (1989) Effects of frontal or temporal lobectomy on the use of advance information in a choice reaction time task. *Neuropsychologia* 27: 495–503.

Awh, E., Jonides, J., Smith, E. E., Schumacher, E. H., Koeppe, R. A., and Katz, S. (1996) Dissociation of storage and rehearsal in verbal working memory: Evidence from PET. *Psychol. Sci.* 7: 25–31.

Awh, E., Smith, E. E., and Jonides, J. (1995) Human rehearsal processes and the frontal lobes: PET evidence. In *Structure and Functions of the Human Prefrontal Cortex*, edited by J. Grafman, K. Holyoak, and F. Boller, pp. 97–119. New York: New York Academy of Sciences.

Bushnell, M. C., Goldberg, M. E., and Robinson, D. L. (1981) Behavioral enhancement of visual responses in monkey cerebral cortex. I. Modulation in posterior parietal cortex related to selective visual attention. *J. Neurophysiol.* 46: 755–772.

Chafee, M., Funahashi, S., and Goldman-Rakic, P. S. (1989) Unit activity in the primate posterior parietal cortex during an oculomotor delayed-response task. *Soc. Neurosci. Abstr.* 15: 786.

Corbetta, M., Miezin, F., Shulman, G. L., and Petersen, S. E. (1993) A PET study of visuospatial attention. *J. Neurosci.* 13: 1202–1226.

Courtney, S. M., Ungerleider, L. G., Keil, K., and Haxby, J. V. (1996) Object and spatial visual working memory activate separate neural systems in human cortex. *Cereb. Cortex* 6: 39–49.

Daffner, K., Ahern, G., Weintraub, S., and Mesulam, M. M. (1990) Dissociated neglect behavior following sequential strokes to the right hemisphere. *Ann. Neurol.* 28: 97–101.

De Renzi, E. (1982) *Disorders of Space Exploration and Cognition*. Chichester, England: Wiley.

di Pellegrino, G., and Wise, S. P. (1993a) Effects of attention on visuomotor activity in the premotor and prefrontal cortex of a primate. *Somatosens. Mot. Res.* 10: 245–262.

di Pellegrino, G., and Wise, S. P. (1993b) Visuospatial versus visuomotor activity in the premotor and prefrontal cortex of a primate. *J. Neurosci.* 13: 1227–1243.

Duncan, J., Orban, G. A., Vandenberghe, R., Ward, R., Dupont, P., Bormans, G., and Mortelmans, L. (1996) Distinct regions of the human parietal lobe active in spatial discrimination and directed attention. Unpublished manuscript.

Fischer, B. and Boch, R. (1981) Enhanced activation of neurons in prelunate cortex before visually guided saccades of trained rhesus monkeys. *Exp. Brain Res.* 44: 129–137.

Fischer, B. and Boch, R. (1985) Peripheral attention versus central fixation: Modulation of the visual activity of prelunate cortical cells of the rhesus monkey. *Brain Res.* 345: 111–123.

Foster, J. K., Eskes, G. A., and Stuss, D. T. (1994) The cognitive neuropsychology of attention: A frontal lobe perspective. *Cognitive Neuropsychol.* 11: 133–147.

Fox, P. T., Mintun, M. A., Reiman, E. M., and Raichle, M. E. (1988) Enhanced detection of focal brain responses using intersubject averaging and change-distribution analysis of subtracted PET images. *J. Cereb. Blood Flow Metab.* 8: 642–653.

Fuster, J. M. (1984) Behavioral electrophysiology of the prefrontal cortex. *Trends Neurosci.* 7: 408–414.

Fuster, J. M. (1995) *Memory in the Cerebral Cortex.* Cambridge, MA: MIT Press.

Gitelman, D. R., Alpert, N. M., Kosslyn, S., Daffner, K., Scinto, L., Thompson, W., Mesulam, M. M. (1996) Functional imaging of human right hemispheric activation for exploratory movements. *Ann. Neurol.* 39: 174–179.

Goldman-Rakic, P. S. (1987) Circuitry of primate prefrontal cortex and regulation of behavior by representational memory. In *Handbook of Physiology* (Vol. 5), edited by V. B. Mountcastle, pp. 373–417. Washington, DC: American Physiological Society.

Goldman-Rakic, P. S. and Chafee, M. (1994) Feedback processing in prefronto-parietal circuits during memory-guided saccades. *Soc. Neurosci. Abstr.* 20: 808.

Heinze, H. J., Mangun, G. R., Burchert, W., Hinrichs, H., Scholz, M., Münte, T. F., Gös, A., Scherg, M., Johannes, S., Hundeshagen, H., Gazzaniga, M. S. and Hillyard, S. A. (1994) Combined temporal imaging of brain activity during visual selective attention in humans. *Nature* 372: 543–546.

Jonides, J., Smith, E. E., Koeppe R. A., Awh, E. S., Minoshima, S., and Mintun, M. A. (1993) Spatial working memory in humans as revealed by PET. *Nature* 363: 623–625.

Kodaka, Y., Mikami, A., and Kubota, K. (1994) Attention to a visual stimulus enhances neuronal responses in monkey prefrontal cortex. *Soc. Neurosci. Abstr.* 20: 986.

Lynch, J. C., Mountcastle, V. B., Talbot, W. H., and Yin, T. C. T. (1977) Parietal lobe mechanisms for directed visual attention. *J. Neurophysiol.* 40: 362–389.

Mangun, G. R., Hansen, J. C., and Hillyard, S. A. (1987) The spatial orienting of attention: Sensory facilitation or response bias? In *Current Trends in Event-Related Potential Research*, edited by R. Johnson, Jr., J. W. Rohrbaugh, and R. Parasuraman, pp. 118–124. Amsterdam: Elsevier.

McCarthy, G., Blamire, A. M., Puce, A., Nobre, A. C., Bloch, G., Hyder, F., Goldman-Rakic, P. S., and Shulman, R. G. (1994) Functional magnetic resonance imaging of human prefrontal cortex activation during a spatial working memory task. *Proc. Natl. Acad. Sci. USA* 91: 8690–8694.

Mesulam, M. M. (1981) A cortical network for directed attention and unilateral neglect. *Ann. Neurol.* 10: 309–325.

Mesulam, M. M. (1990) Large-scale neurocognitive networks and distributed processing for attention, language, and memory. *Ann. Neurol.* 28: 597–613.

Mikami, A., Ito, S., and Kubota, K. (1982) Modifications of neuron activities of the dorsolateral prefrontal cortex during extrafoveal attention. *Behav. Brain Res.* 5: 219–223.

Mohler, C. W. and Wurtz, R. H. (1977) Role of striate cortex and superior colliculus in visual guidance of saccadic eye movements in monkeys. *J. Neurophysiol.* 40: 74–94.

Moran, J. and Desimone, R. (1985) Selective attention gates visual processing in the extrastriate cortex. *Science* 229: 782–784.

Motter, B. C. (1993) Focal attention produces spatially selective processing in visual cortical areas V1, V2, and V4 in the presence of competing stimuli. *J. Neurophysiol.* 70: 909–919.

Owen, A. M., Evans, A. C., and Petrides, M. (1996) Evidence for a two-stage model of spatial working memory processing within the lateral frontal cortex: A positron emission tomography study. *Cereb. Cortex* 6: 31–38.

Petersen, S. E., Corbetta, M., Miezin, F. M., and Shudman, G. L. (1994) PET studies of parietal involvement in spatial attention: Comparison of different task types. *Can. J. Psychol.* 48: 319–338.

Petrides, M. and Pandya, D. N. (1984) Projections to the frontal cortex from the posterior parietal region in the rhesus monkey. *J. Comp. Neurol.* 228: 105–116.

Posner, M. I. and Petersen, S. E. (1990) The attention system of the human brain. *Annu. Rev. Neurosci.* 13: 25–42.

Posner, M. I., Walker, J. A., Friedrich, F. A., and Rafal, R. D. (1984) How do the parietal lobes direct covert attention? *Neuropsychologia* 25: 135–145.

Smith, E. E., Jonides, J., and Koeppe, R. A. (1996) Dissociating verbal and spatial working memory using PET. *Cereb. Cortex* 6: 11–20.

Spiers, P. A., Schomer, D. L., Blume, H. W., Kleefield, J., O'Reilly, G., Weintraub, S., Osborne-Shaefer, P., Mesulam, M. M. (1990) Visual neglect during intracarotid amobarbital testing. *Neurology* 40: 1600–6100.

Ungerleider, L. G. (1995) Functional brain imaging studies of cortical mechanisms for memory. *Science* 270: 769–775.

Vallar, G. (1993) The anatomical basis of spatial neglect in humans. In *Unilateral Neglect: Clinical and Experimental Studies*, edited by I. H. Robertson and J. C. Marshall. East Sussex, United Kingdom: Lawrence Erlbaum.

Vallar, G. and Perani, D. (1986) The anatomy of unilateral neglect after right-hemisphere stroke lesions. A clinical/CT-scan correlation study in man. *Neuropsychologia* 24: 609–622.

Vallar, G. and Perani, D. (1987) The anatomy of spatial neglect in humans. In *Neurophysiological and Neuropsychological Aspects of Spatial Neglect*, edited by M. Jeannerod, pp. 235–258. Amsterdam: Elsevier.

Vandenberghe, R., Dupont, P., De Bruyn, B., Bormans, G., Mortelmans, L. and Orban, G. (1996) The influence of stimulus location on the brain activation pattern in stimulus detection and in orientation discrimination: A PET experiment. *Brain* 119: 1263–1276.

Weinstein, E. A. and Friedland, R. D. (Eds.) (1977) *Hemi-Inattention and Hemisphere Specialization* (Advances in Neurology No. 18). New York: Raven Press.

Yantis, S. and Johnston, J. C. (1990) On the locus of visual selection: Evidence from focused attention tasks. *J. Exp. Psychol. Hum. Percept. Perform.* 16: 135–149.

Yantis, S. and Jonides, J. (1990) Abrupt visual onsets and selective attention: Voluntary versus automatic allocation. *J. Exp. Psychol. Hum. Percept. Perform.* 16: 121–134.

17 Attention and Language

Ira Fischler

ABSTRACT Language coordinates form with meaning. This chapter examines how the various components of language are engaged and coordinated by the attentive brain. Emphasis is placed on perceptual and conceptual processing of single words and to recent evidence from neuroimaging and electrophysiology regarding the localization and real-time dynamics of those processes. The relation of attentional systems for language to those for other cognitive skills is discussed.

Attention and language are two of the most widely studied aspects of human cognitive skills. One might therefore expect a tradition of research exploring how these basic elements of cognition stand together, with studies of how language directs and controls what we attend to (see Logan, 1995), and, conversely, of how different aspects of language make different demands on our various attentional skills and abilities. Indeed, the seminal work on attention in the 1950s asked a simple question to which there is an increasingly complex answer: Is an unattended word understood?

Yet within the study of attention, language has often been more a convenient vehicle for stimulus delivery and response than it has been the target of analysis. Similarly, in studies of language comprehension and production, whether through speech or through reading and writing, there has been limited concern with issues of attentional direction, engagement, or effort. The assumption has been that for the skilled, native user of a language it is the content of language—what is being talked about or read about—that is the focus of attention, whereas the process remains in the automatic twilight of effortless skill.

But with the explosion of brain-mapping methods presented in this volume, and with increased interest in how complex cognitive functions map onto neural systems, a cognitive neuroscience of attention and language appears to be forming. Researchers utilizing the new imaging methods such as functional magnetic resonance imaging (fMRI) and positron emission tomography (PET) are beginning to explore cognitive functions of a higher order than vision and pattern recognition (e.g., McCarthy, Blamire, Rothman, Gruetter, and Shulman, 1993; Posner, Petersen, Fox, and Raichle, 1988). Neuropsychologists are becoming more interested in attentional aspects of language disorders and aphasias (e.g., Shuren, Smith Hammond, Maher, Rothi, and Heilman, 1995), in the brain mechanisms that selectively engage language systems (e.g., Nadeau and Crosson, 1997), and the possible interaction of attention and knowledge systems in degenerative disorders (Parasuraman and Martin, 1994). Event-related brain potentials (ERPs) are being used to map the time course of activation of components of word knowledge (e.g., Nobre and McCarthy, 1994) and to study how attention and effort influence those processes (e.g., Bentin, Kutas, and Hillyard, 1995; Raney, 1993).

After briefly sketching a conceptual model of language, this chapter will focus on recent efforts to explore both the functional neuroanatomy of language skills and how those systems are engaged by attentional mechanisms. Although there is increasing interest in the cognitive neuroscience of syntax (for examples from the ERP literature, see Osterhout, 1994, and Friederici, 1995), the processing of the form and meaning of individual words will be emphasized here.

COMPONENTS OF LANGUAGE

As with most broad constructs, the particular skills and codes that are subsumed under the label "language" are breathtakingly diverse. There is sensory encoding of the sound of the speaker's voice or the visual features of print; the phonological categories of speech sounds that let us distinguish "ban" from "pan" in English; the lexical representation in our "mental dictionary" that distinguishes words from nonwords and that may include knowledge of the roles words play in sentences; orthographic knowledge of how a word is spelled; the semantic knowledge that informs us of the meaning of what we hear or read; syntactic rules and conventions that determine the allowable sequence of words and other morphemes; prosodic information about the sound envelope of an utterance that lets us distinguish a question from a demand; and other pragmatic knowledge about the conventions of conversation that tell us when to listen and when to speak and when we have been insulted. When we speak, many of those codes are engaged in reverse: we start with an intended meaning, choose words and structure, and end with articulatory commands and gestural accompaniments that must be translated into motor activity so that we can say what we mean.

Most contemporary models of language skill take an information-processing approach in positing that the various codes are reflected in different, identifiable stages of processing. Some stages may be discrete and sequential, whereas others may occur concurrently; some may occur with little attention or effort, and others may require substantial concentration and engagement. As will be discussed later, neuropsychological models of language parallel this approach and assume some degree of localization of the various functions and codes. The model shown in figure 17.1, based on

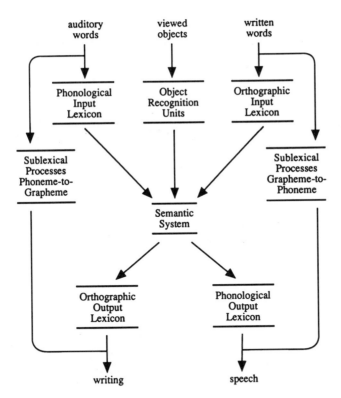

Figure 17.1 Some of the subcomponents of a cognitive system for understanding and producing words, with auditory, visual, and pictorial input, and spoken and written output. (After Ellis and Young, 1988.)

one presented by Ellis and Young (1988), is typical, illustrating the routes a word can take from sensory input to various sublexical, lexical, and semantic analyses, and out to speech and writing.

CHALLENGES TO THE FUNCTIONAL LOCALIZATION OF LANGUAGE

Given the diversity of the component processes and the newness of many of the cognitive neuroscience techniques documented in this volume, it may not be surprising that there are frequent cases of inconsistent findings about which language functions are supported by what regions of the brain. For example, using dense-array electroencephalographic (EEG) recording, Nobre and McCarthy (1994) reported a family of topographically diverse ERPs to words and wordlike strings, including a reduction in a late negative component (N400) when a word was preceded by a semantically related word (compare Kutas and Hillyard, 1980), whereas Curran, Tucker, Kutas, and Posner (1993) found little evidence of any priming-related components in the N400 region. Using PET measures of regional cerebral blood flow (rCBF), Petersen,

Fox, Snyder, and Raichle (1990) found evidence for a left frontal locus of lexical-semantic knowledge about words, whereas Howard et al. (1992), using similar PET methods, found more temporal than frontal activity for a task requiring lexical analysis.

Uncertainty about localization of language is not a new problem. Patterns of aphasia that may result from strokes and from other trauma, for example, can show substantial variability in the association between neural structure and language function (see Benson, 1993). Electrical stimulation of the cortex during surgery shows similar diversity in the areas that disrupt naming (Ojemann, 1994).

Some of the puzzling results are certainly due to methodological differences between laboratories using the new techniques. More relevant to this paper is that subtle (or not so subtle) differences in the tasks that subjects are given can create substantial changes in the topographical pattern of activation. Cherktow and Bub (1994) reviewed how interpretation of PET regional activity can be clouded by vague links between alleged processing components and tasks, by questionable assumptions about pure insertion of stages between two tasks when the subtractive method is used to isolate component processes, and by apparently innocuous variations such as the duration, rate, or sequencing of verbal stimuli (see Fox and Raichle, 1984). For example, in trying to reconcile differences in localization of language areas between those reported by Howard et al. (1992) and by Petersen et al. (1990), Price et al. (1994) found that, with other factors held constant, both the reliability and topography of active PET regions could be dramatically affected by a change of stimulus duration from 150 ms to 1 s. They suggested that the longer duration eased demands on working memory.

The effects of task variables on patterns of brain activity show that, in a broad sense, attentional factors must be considered in any study of language and localization. Attentional focus on certain codes or processes will produce more extensive, longer, or more widespread activity in the brain areas involved in those processes. These effects can be quite localized. Corbetta, Miezin, Dobmeyer, and Shulman (1990) showed how attention to specific attributes of a visual stimulus (e.g., color, form, or movement) increased PET activity in the corresponding cortical regions known to process those attributes. Much of the work to be reviewed here takes this selective engagement approach to activating and localizing language functions.

With this framework in mind, studies of activation of language function in which language competes with other processes for access to a limited-capacity executive attentional system are first discussed. Aspects of the functional neuroanatomy of several more specific language skills will then be considered, focusing on perceptual and conceptual processing of words, in which attention to particular codes or levels is varied by the nature of the task or of the materials. Finally, the role of practice and automaticity in the issue of localization of those language functions will be considered.

LANGUAGE AND RESOURCE ALLOCATION

A view of attention as a limited resource that can be allocated to various cognitive tasks (Kahneman, 1973) motivates several recent models of how language processes may be engaged and protected from other potentially competing processes. Traditionally, subcortical activating systems in the thalamus, with its rich and diverse connectivity to the cortex, have been considered a likely site for selective engagement of specific cortical functions. In vision, structures within the thalamus have been associated with selective attention to features of objects in particular locations of space (see LaBerge, 1995). Nadeau and Crosson (1997) have suggested a similar activating role in language processing for the anterior thalamus—as part of a circuit including the frontal cortex language areas, inferior thalamic peduncle, nucleus reticularis, and the centromedian nucleus—for effortful generative tasks involving lexical-semantic knowledge. Patients with lesions to the anterior thalamus have been shown to be selectively impaired in naming tasks given semantic input, that is, pictures or auditory definitions (Raymer, Moberg, Crosson, Nadeau, and Gonzalez Rothi, 1992).

PET evidence during tasks involving a high degree of attentional effort and control has implicated the anterior cingulate gyrus in the medial frontal lobe as a cortical locus of a central executive attention mechanism (see Posner and DiGirolamo, chapter 18, this volume). This area appears active in a number of effortful language tasks. Compared to a passive listening baseline, the anterior cingulate gyrus was one of several areas selectively engaged when subjects had to generate verbs for visually presented nouns (Petersen et al., 1990; compare McLaughlin et al., 1992), or when they had to shadow (repeat as quickly as possible) an auditory message (Petersen, Fox, Posner, Mintun, and Raichle, 1989). Because the same area is involved in tasks requiring the direction of visual attention to particular locations in space (Posner, Inhoff, Friedrich, and Rafal, 1987), Posner and others have pointed to the cingulate gyrus as part of a common system for executive attention (compare Fuentes, Carmona, Agis, and Catena, 1994).

Further evidence supporting the notion of a common attentional system for language and spatial tasks was provided by Petry, Crosson, Gonzalez Rothi, Bauer, and Schauer (1994). Patients with left hemisphere damage and with documented aphasia were given Posner's test of covert orienting of visual attention (COVAT), in which a central cue directs attention to one side of visual space as the likely location of a subsequent target. These patients were particularly slow when a target was presented in the right visual field following a cue to attend to the left; their performance was similar to that of patients with unilateral neglect (see Posner, et al. 1987). Interestingly, the degree of impairment in this specific cueing effect was correlated with six of seven measures of language impairment obtained from standard aphasia test batteries.

Petry et al. (1996) also found evidence for a common system for visual and lexical-semantic engagement. In a dual task version of the Posner COVAT task, subjects saw a word followed by the lateral cue. Merely having to name the central word prior to responding to the lateral target reduced and delayed the attentional effects normally seen for valid versus invalid visual cues. Generating a semantic associate to the central word greatly increased the interference.

Some recent ERP data from our own laboratory (Fischler, Howland, Sikkema, and Besson, 1996), using a divided attention task, supports the role for a frontal attentional system in tasks combining visual and verbal demands. During half of the blocks of a recognition memory task for pairs of words, participants concurrently monitored an auditory list of digits for the occasional occurrence of three consecutive odd digits. During other blocks, recognition memory was the only task. Figure 17.2 shows ERPs in the word pairs under full (solid lines) and divided (dotted lines) attention conditions. Beginning shortly after the presentation of the first word, and extending through about 600 ms after the second word, the ERPs in the divided attention condition were more negative than in the full attention condition. The attentional effects were earlier and much larger for the frontal locations than for the parietal locations.

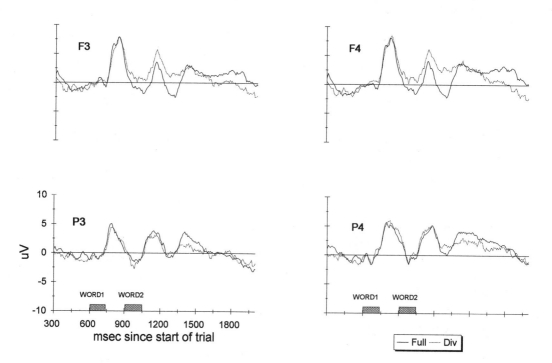

Figure 17.2 ERPs to pairs of words during a recognition memory task. F3 and F4 are frontal locations and P3 and P4 are parietal locations, over the left and right hemispheres, respectively. The solid lines are the ERPs to word pairs under full attention blocks; the dotted lines are the ERPs to words pairs under divided attention conditions.

ACTIVATION OF PHONOLOGICAL CODES FOR WORDS

This section examines more specific aspects of language processing, the functional neuroanatomy of these aspects, and the role of attention in engagement of those systems. We focus first on what Anderson (1995) refers to as perceptual aspects of words, in particular their phonological representation. Because the elicitation of these codes is commonly thought to be relatively automatic or obligatory given the appropriate sensory input (see Carr, 1992), many studies of phonology and orthography simply present words or pseudowords (orthographically or phonologically legal nonwords) or both, and require subjects to passively look or listen; areas of activation are then compared to those obtained with nonlinguistic control materials. For the most part, results of imaging studies using passive tasks support the classic view of two left hemisphere regions being particularly important in the representation, maintenance, and production of phonological codes: the posterior portion of the left superior temporal gyrus, or Wernicke's area, and the dorsolateral portion of the left inferior frontal gyrus, or Broca's area (Geschwind, 1965). There remains, however, considerable controversy about the role those areas play in particular aspects of language processing (compare Ojemann, 1994; Benson, 1993; Kolb and Wishaw, 1990, pp. 580–581).

In one study (Price et al., 1992), subjects passively listened to spoken words that varied in presentation rate. PET analyses of rCBF indicated increases in activity in the primary auditory cortex and in the middle region of the left superior temporal gyrus bilaterally; the increases were sensitive to presentation rate. In contrast, activity in Wernicke's area was restricted to the left hemisphere and was insensitive to presentation rate. Both the asymmetry and rate invariance of the response in Wernicke's area suggested to Price et al. that the sensory input had been transformed into a more specifically linguistic code for further processing in Wernicke's region.

Most studies vary both the stimuli and the task to selectively activate systems involved in phonological processing. For example, Demonet, Price, Wise, and Frackowiak (1994) presented phoneme pairs, used a pure tone discrimination as a baseline control task, and varied both the difficulty of the phoneme discrimination (with /b/ as a target and either /p/ or /d/ as distractors) and whether the task required a sequential decision about phoneme pairs (e.g., /b/ preceded by /d/). Demonet and colleagues had previously shown (Demonet et al., 1992) that the sequential, difficult task activated both Wernicke's and Broca's regions of the left hemisphere. In the 1994 study, for the easy discrimination task, both sequential and nonsequential versions of the task activated the middle portion of the left superior temporal gyrus, a result that implicates early stages of phonological processing common to other auditory language tasks. In contrast, the difficult discrimination task was associated with increases of activity in the left fusiform gyrus for the nonsequential task, which the authors interpreted as signs of a strategy of translating the phoneme to a graphemic or orthographical representation in face of the difficult phonemic discrimination. The difficult, sequential task was the only condition to replicate the previously reported activity in the frontal area corresponding to Broca's, which the authors took as evidence for that region's involvement in maintenance and rehearsal of phonological and articulatory codes.

Other imaging and ERP studies have supported the notion that the left temporal region is involved in the representation of phonological codes that must be "assembled" from visually presented words according to correspondences between graphemes and phonemes (compare Posner and Carr, 1992). Visually presented words and pseudowords activate regions around Wernicke's area when the task encourages this assemblage; so, for example, visually presented lists of words and pseudowords were associated with an N280 component of the ERP over the posterior left temporal region when subjects monitored the list for target words from a semantic category (Nobre and McCarthy, 1994). The frontal regions of the system are activated when the task requires fine-grained analysis or production of particular sequences of sounds, as during speech production or rehearsal. Thus, Broca's area was active in tasks requiring discrimination of consonant sequences but not of vowels (Fiez et al., 1995), matching of consonants in rapidly presented syllable pairs (Zattore, Evans, Myer, and Gjedde, 1992), rhyme generation (Shaywitz et al., 1995), and covert rehearsal (Hinke, Hu, Stillman, and Kim, 1993; Paulesu, Frith, and Frackowiak, 1993).

ACTIVATION OF LEXICAL AND SEMANTIC CODES FOR WORDS

The ability to represent the phonemic or orthographical pattern that corresponds to a word is the means of communication: the goal is to communicate information, and the semantic representation of the concepts that a word stands for is the heart of language. It is no coincidence that "semantics" is located in the middle of the language model of figure 17.1.

Often, discussions about the localization of lexical and semantic levels of representation are collapsed into the notion of lexical-semantic networks, and perhaps not surprisingly are traditionally described as diffuse or widespread. In many tasks, as well, it is difficult to distinguish these two aspects of language. However, on logical, behavioral, and neuropsychological grounds, we can distinguish among these, and might expect attentional engagement of lexical and semantic processes to be separable. Damasio and Damasio (1992), for example, argue for the importance of neural convergence zones that mediate lexical and conceptual representations and that can be very selectively impaired (see Localization of Semantic Knowledge).

The semantic priming paradigm, in which the speed or accuracy of responses to a word is facilitated by prior presentation of a semantically related word, has been useful in distinguishing lexical and semantic knowledge. Certain aphasic patients, for example, may be impaired in lexical retrieval but show intact semantic priming (see Milberg, Blumstein, Katz, and

Gershberg, 1995). Distracting attention from the lexical level by having normal subjects perform a letter-matching task on the prime word eliminates the semantic priming effect on a lexical decision but preserves lexical access—as evidenced by a significant repetition priming effect for word but not for nonword targets (Besner, Smith, and MacLeod, 1990). Similarly, Posner, Sandson, Dhawan, and Shulman (1989) found that engaging attention through a shadowing task eliminated the semantic priming effect but did not reduce the amount of repetition priming. As in the Besner et al. (1990) study, Posner et al. (1989) found no repetition priming for nonword stimuli, a result that implies that lexical access to visual word forms was automatic and did not require the engagement of the frontal executive attentional network (see the previous discussion).

Lexical Knowledge and Access

Within the lexical level, there is some agreement that, rather than a single amodal lexicon, different lexicons exist that correspond to the different modes of input and output (see figure 17.1; also, see Posner and Carr, 1992). Attempts to localize these have met with mixed success. For visual word forms, for example, Petersen et al. (1990) identified a region in the left medial extrastriate cortex as a visual word-form center, because it appeared to be selectively activated by words and pseudowords and not by random letter strings. Howard et al. (1992), however, compared performance when words were read aloud to performance in a control condition in which the word "crime" was spoken when a false-font string was shown; they reported activity in the posterior portion of the left middle temporal gyrus. Others have associated lexical access with more anterior portions of the left temporal lobe (Damasio, 1990). Nobre and McCarthy (1995), using intracranial electrodes, found large negative field potentials within the anterior portion of the left medial temporal lobe for visual words presented in isolation but not for orthographically illegal nonwords, consistent with their earlier findings with scalp ERPs (Nobre and McCarthy, 1994).

For the auditory input lexicon, regions in and around the classic Wernicke's area in the posterior portions of the left superior and middle temporal gyrus are most often implicated (e.g., Zattore et al., 1992).

Localization of Semantic Knowledge

Neural systems that represent the meaning of words have proved particularly challenging to isolate anatomically, which has led some to conclude that semantic knowledge is by its nature diffusely represented, probably by the sort of distributed processing systems that have played a large role in recent models of memory and cognition in cognitive science. Even when the pattern of impairment due to lesions seems to necessitate a very localist model of semantic memory, the cell assemblies representing that knowledge may be part of a distributed network (e.g., Small, Hart, Nguyen, and Gordon, 1995).

Some of the most intriguing recent cases of impairments of semantic memory involve dissociations between specific classes of words. Some dissociations have been shown to be artifacts of word frequency (e.g., King and Kutas, 1995) or of the visual complexity of objects to be named. Other cases appear to be genuine impairments of lexical or semantic knowledge. These cases include a double dissociation between nouns and verbs, with some patients selectively impaired in processing the former, and some the latter (e.g., Damasio and Tranel, 1993; Hillis and Caramazza, 1995), even when the perceptual code is identical (e.g., a patient who cannot generate the word "comb" in response to its definition, and then will say it is used to "comb the hair"). Damasio (e.g., 1990) has argued that such dissociations are related to lesions of frontal (action-related) versus temporal (sensory feature–related) lobes. Others have claimed that closed-class words that serve grammatical functions, such as "but" and "of," are more associated with left frontal areas than are the open-class content words—nouns, most verbs, and adjectives. Neville, Mills, and Lawson (1992), for example, reported a left anterior N280 component (compare Nobre and McCarthy, 1994) that was larger for closed-class words (but, compare King and Kutas, 1995).

Similarly, there are cases of semantically bounded dissociations among nouns referring to particular concept types. One frequently cited example is the contrast between natural categories (e.g., living things) and artificial categories (e.g., tools) (e.g., Sacchett and Humphreys, 1992). As with the dissociation between nouns and verbs, this may be related to a basic distinction between concepts defined more by sensory features, such as living things, and concepts that are defined more by their function. Damasio and Damasio (1992) describe cases of patients who dissociate the ability to generate or comprehend proper nouns versus common nouns, and suggest that the mediation of more specific classes occurs toward the anterior and lateral portions of the left temporal lobes, whereas the mediation of more general classes occurs toward the posterior and medial portions. There are cases of yet more specific impairments, such as in the comprehension of words referring to vegetables, garden objects, or medical terms (e.g., see Moberg, Crosson, Boone, and Gonzalez Rothi, 1992). Attentional factors may be involved in at least some of these semantically bounded disorders. The patient in the Moberg et al. study, B. C., had sustained a hemorrhagic lesion of the left thalamus, including portions of the pulvinar and centromedian nucleus. I have already discussed the possible role of corticothalamic circuits in the selective engagement of linguistic processes. B. C. was selectively impaired in his ability to retrieve words referring to terms related to his medical condition or to items found in the hospital, when he was given definitions. The restriction of the impairment to concepts that presumably were frequently activated in his immediate environment might suggest a problem with what we might call active domains of meaning. Intriguingly, another patient with a selective impairment to concepts involving vegetables was an avid gardener. One possible mechanism for this peculiar pattern might be inappropriate or excessive inhibition of what normally should be activation of frequently accessed concepts.

This odd speculation about the possible costs of recent attention to semantic domains raises the more general issue about how semantic knowledge is selectively engaged by attentional mechanisms, and it is to that broader topic that this chapter now turns.

Attention and Meaning

Attention to semantic aspects of words is one of the most powerful determinants of subsequent memory; when attention is directed to perceptual attributes of words, such as their spelling or case, explicit memory is substantially impaired (e.g., Craik and Tulving, 1975). A number of PET studies have varied whether semantic or other attributes of stimuli are attended to. Although task parameters vary widely across studies, there is, in broad terms at least, some agreement about which regions are involved in effortful attention to semantic information: the inferior portions of the left frontal lobes, usually somewhat anterior to but at times including Broca's area (e.g., Petersen et al. 1990), and the middle or posterior portions of the left temporal lobes, particularly the superior area. Using the fMRI technique, McCarthy et al. (1993) also found enhanced activity in the left inferior frontal lobe during a verb generation task compared to activity during a variety of nonsemantic control tasks. One or both of these regions have shown significant PET activity during a variety of semantic tasks, including during a semantic feature-matching task to auditory word pairs (Demonet et al., 1992, who also saw activity in the left supramarginal and angular gyri), during semantic categorization, category association, and verb generation (Wise et al., 1991), and during lexical decision making (Frith, Friston, Liddle, and Frackowiak, 1991).

Others have used dense-array ERP recordings to track the time course of the regions activated in PET studies of word processing. For example, Posner and Raichle (1994, p. 145) report a study of word processing in which the decision involved either a visual feature or a semantic category. The semantic categorization task was associated with an enhanced negativity over left frontal sites beginning around 300 ms after word onset. In a dense-array ERP replication of the Petersen et al. (1990) PET study of verb generation versus reading aloud, Snyder, Abdullaev, Posner, and Raichle (1995) reported ERP components corresponding to the left frontal and temporal areas of activity that were associated with the verb generation task discussed previously. Interestingly, the frontal activity was in a latency range (about 200 ms after presentation of the word) consistent with the other ERP studies of the initial stages of lexical and semantic processing; the parietotemporal activity, however, was quite late, with a maximum amplitude around 700 ms. It seems likely that the lateness of the latter component reflects the need in the verb generation task to suppress or inhibit more automatic associations (e.g., "nail" in response to "hammer") and produce a novel but semantically appropriate response, which apparently requires coordinated circuits in the inferior frontal and posterior temporal regions.

The semantic priming paradigm, with either sentences or single words as primes, has been frequently used in studies of ERPs and semantic processing of words (see Van Petten, 1993; Nobre and McCarthy, 1994). As was described previously, the N400 component elicited by words in isolation can be attenuated or eliminated by predictive semantic contexts. It is thought that the semantic context reduces the extent of semantic processing needed to comprehend the word in that context (see Fischler and Raney, 1991).

The N400 priming effect has most often been maximal in central and parietal locations, with a bilateral distribution frequently somewhat larger on the right than on the left sites. It has been distinguished from an earlier negativity that appears to be more frontal and left maximal. Several recent studies using newer methods of referencing, larger arrays, and calibration with areas of activity revealed through PET or fMRI have examined the topography of the semantic priming effect in ERPs. Using a 50-site montage, Nobre and McCarthy (1994) found that content words in the absence of semantic context elicited early negativities (N330) at frontotemporal and midline anterior sites and a subsequent more posterior negativity (N380) whose distribution for words in lists versus sentences was different. Both components were attenuated by appropriate associative or sentence contexts (compare Curran et al., 1993).

Attention to the meaning of context and target words appears to be an important determinant of the presence or size of the N400 priming effect in these studies. Tasks that require nonlexical decisions—for example, vowel or consonant matching (Besson, Fischler, Boaz, and Raney, 1992) or case matching (Chwilla, Brown, and Hagoort, 1995)—or that reduce the expectancy that related pairs will be shown (Holcomb, 1988) reduce or eliminate the semantic priming effect on the N400. Presenting prime words in an unattended spatial location, either auditorally in an unattended ear (Bentin et al., 1995) or visually to the left or right of fixation (McCarthy and Nobre, 1993) similarly eliminates the semantic priming effect in the ERPs.

Even within the semantic level of processing, directing attention to the semantic relation enhances the priming effect on ERPs. Figure 17.3 shows the ERPs for words following related versus unrelated prime words during the study phase of our memory and distraction task described previously (Fischler et al., 1995). The left panel depicts ERPs when subjects decided if the pair of words were semantically related; the right panel depicts ERPs when they matched pairs based on a semantic feature of animateness. Attention to the association produced a greater difference between the related and unrelated target words in the N400 region.

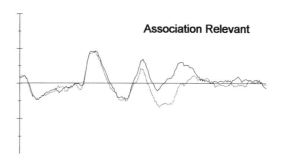

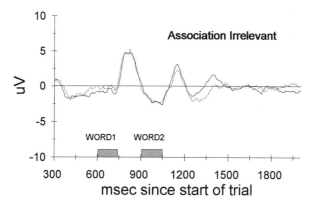

Figure 17.3 ERPs to pairs of words. (Top) Participants decide if the second word pair is an associate of the first (association relevant condition). (Bottom) Participants decide if the second word matches the first on the semantic feature of animateness (association irrelevant task). The solid lines are the ERPs to related word pairs; the dotted lines are the ERPs to unrelated word pairs.

Word Meaning, Attention, and the Right Hemisphere

The vast majority of studies reviewed here implicate the left cerebral hemisphere in language. There is, however, reasonable evidence that the right hemisphere has at least some knowledge of word form and meaning (e.g., Kolb and Wishaw, 1990, p. 589). Others have suggested that the right hemisphere's lexical knowledge is more diffuse than that of the left hemisphere. Nakagawa (1991) visually presented prime words centrally, followed by a related or unrelated target word to the left or right hemisphere. Under full attention conditions, presentation of a target word to the left hemisphere produced priming only for strong, primary associates, whereas priming of right hemisphere targets was broader and extended to weaker associates. Under a dual task divided attention condition, in contrast, this asymmetry disappeared, and both left and right fields showed the broader pattern of priming.

PRACTICE, AUTOMATICITY, AND THE ATTENTIVE BRAIN

It is thought that well-learned, practiced skills or responses to stimuli can become automatic—not just faster and more accurate, but dealt with in a qualitatively different way than are more effortful or unfamiliar tasks. Evidence for automatic and attentional components of semantic priming suggests that different brain regions may be involved in activation of habitual associations than are involved in activations requiring novel, contextually appropriate responses. Raichle et al. (1994) demonstrated such a dissociation in the verb generation task. Prior to the PET session, subjects practiced generating verbs for the same set of nouns presented repeatedly. With less than 15 minutes of total practice, the regions of activity associated with the verb generation task was transformed. In particular, the left inferior prefrontal and left posterior temporal cortices, as well as the bilateral anterior cingulate gyrus, were no more active than in a condition in which the presented words were simply read aloud. In contrast, the bilateral insular cortex, an area that had been apparently inhibited by the novel verb generation task, was again active with the practiced associations. Interestingly, Cherktow et al. (1992) reported that when patients with Alzheimer's disease passively viewed or heard words, the anterior cingulate gyrus was activated, as if this previously effortless and automatic task had come to require focal attention.

It is worth noting that the practiced tasks produced not just different, but significantly fewer and smaller, areas of activity, compared with activity generated by the unfamiliar and effortful conditions. A similar point has been made about localization of language functions by Kolb and Wishaw (1990, p. 571), based on lesion and stimulation findings. In the semantic priming literature, there are also cases in which, under conditions that produce evidence for automatic semantic priming (presenting the prime word under brief, masked conditions such that the prime word cannot be identified), the N400 effect is eliminated (Brown and Hagoort, 1993; compare Bentin et al., 1995).

The implication is that many of the skills related to language, the activation of which may be more like automatic pattern-matching of input to highly accessible memories (compare Logan, 1992), may be relatively silent to current methods of imaging brain structure and activation. The challenge will be to determine if this silence is due to reduced intensity of activation in areas that subserve particular codes and processes, to reduced intensity of attentional systems that engage those areas, or to qualitative shifts from areas where activity is more detectable to those where activity is less detectable, for whatever reason (e.g., for declarative versus proceduralized knowledge). Studies that track different stages of acquisition of language skills, such as might be involved for novice versus more skilled bilinguals (see Kroll and Sholl, 1992) will, from this perspective, provide a critical complement to the study of language in the expert speaker.

CONCLUSIONS

Despite the complex and multidimensional nature of human language skill, we have seen how the components of this skill, their functional neuro-anatomy and their selective engagement in real time, can be segmented and understood. The emerging work in cognitive neuroscience reviewed here—by combining the theoretical and experimental precision of information-processing models, the spatial precision of PET and, increasingly, fMRI work, and the fine temporal resolution of electrophysiological activity—has begun mapping out the real-time brain processes involved in language comprehension and production.

There are many uncertainties, some dealing with the dimensions along which language should be fractionated, some dealing with the assumptions made about tasks used to isolate language components, and some dealing with obtaining a clean signal from the noise inherent in many of the emerging imaging techniques. Nonetheless, we have seen how many of the findings discussed here can be interpreted within an increasingly coherent and detailed model of how the brain represents and creates meaning through language, and how these systems are selectively engaged as attention is allocated to the various tasks of understanding and producing language.

ACKNOWLEDGMENTS

I have benefited greatly from discussions with colleagues at the Center for Neuropsychological Studies and at the Brain Institute at the University of Florida. Preparation of the chapter was supported by the Center for the Study of Attention and Emotion at the University of Florida and by grant P50-MH52384 from the National Institutes of Health. I am grateful to Mireille Besson, Bruce Crosson, and Steve Nadeau for comments on an earlier version of this paper.

REFERENCES

Anderson, J. R. (1995) *Cognitive Psychology and its Implications* (4th ed.) New York: W. H. Freeman.

Benson, D. F. (1993) Aphasia. In *Clinical Neuropsychology* (3rd ed.), edited by K. M. Heilman and E. Valenstein, pp. 17–36. New York: Oxford University Press.

Bentin, S., Kutas, M., and Hillyard, S. A. (1995) Semantic processing and memory for attended and unattended words in dichotic listening: Behavioral and electrophysiological evidence. *J. Exp. Psychol. Hum. Percept. Perform.* 21: 54–67.

Besner, D., Smith, M. C., and MacLeod, C. M. (1990) Visual word recognition: A dissociation of lexical and semantic processing. *J. Exp. Psychol. Learn. Mem. Cogn.* 16: 862–869.

Besson, M., Fischler, I., Boaz, T., and Raney, G. (1992) Effects of automatic associative activation on explicit and implicit memory tests. *J. Exp. Psychol. Learn. Mem. Cogn.* 18: 89–105.

Brown, C. and Hagoort, P. (1993) The processing nature of the N400: Evidence from masked priming. *J. Cognitive Neurosci.* 5: 34–44.

Carr, T. H. (1992) Automaticity and cognitive anatomy: Is word recognition "automatic"? *Am. J. Psychol.* 105: 201–237.

Cherktow, H. and Bub, D. (1994) Functional activation and cognition: The ^{15}O PET subtraction method. In *Localization and Neuroimaging in Neuropsychology*, edited by A. Kertesz, pp. 151–184. San Diego, CA: Academic Press.

Cherktow, H., Hamel, E., Bub, D., Meyer, E., Wisbord, S., Evans, A., and D'Antono, B. (1992) Increased activation of anterior cingulate region in dementia of the Alzheimer's type. *Neurology* 42 (Suppl. 3): 316.

Chwilla, D. J., Brown, C. M., and Hagoort, P. (1995) The N400 as a function of the level of processing. *Psychophysiology* 32: 274–285.

Corbetta, M., Miezin, F. M., Dobmeyer, S., and Shulman, G. L. (1990) Attentional modulation of neural processing of shape, color, and velocity in humans. *Science* 248: 1556–1559.

Craik, F. I. and Tulving, E. (1975) Depth of processing and the retention of words in episodic memory. *J. Exp. Psychol. Gen.* 104: 268–294.

Curran, T., Tucker, D. M., Kutas, M., and Posner, M. I. (1993) Topography of the N400: Brain electrical activity reflecting semantic expectancy. *Electroencephalogr. Clin. Neurophysiol.* 88: 188–209.

Damasio, A. R. (1990) Category-related recognition defects as a clue to the neural substrates of knowledge. *Trends Neurosci.* 13: 95–98.

Damasio, A. R. and Damasio, H. (1992) Brain and language. *Sci. Am.* 267: 88–95.

Damasio, A. R. and Tranel, D. (1993) Nouns and verbs are retrieved with differently distributed neural systems. *Proc. Natl. Acad. Sci. U S A* 90: 4957–4960.

Demonet, J. F., Chollet, F., Ramsey, S., Cardebat, D., Nespoulous, J. L., Wise, R., Rascol, A., and Frackowiak, R. (1992) The anatomy of phonological and semantic processing in normal subjects. *Brain* 115: 1753–1768.

Demonet, J. F., Price, C., Wise, R., and Frackowiak, R. S. J. (1994) A PET study of cognitive strategies in normal subjects during language tasks. *Brain* 117: 671–682.

Ellis, A. W. and Young, A. W. (1988) *Human Cognitive Neuropsychology*. Hillsdale, NJ: Lawrence Erlbaum.

Fiez, J. A., Raichle, M. E., Miezin, F. M., Petersen, S. E., Tallal, P., and Katz, W. F. (1995) PET studies of auditory and phonological processing effects of stimulus characteristics and task demands. *J. Cognitive Neurosci.* 7: 357–375.

Fischler, I., Howland, B., Sikkema, R., and Besson, M. (1996) Attention, semantic priming and memory for word pairs: An ERP analysis. Unpublished manuscript.

Fischler, I. and Raney, G. E. (1991) Language by eye: Behavioral and psychophysiological approaches to reading. In *Handbook of Cognitive Psychophysiology: Central and Autonomic Nervous System Approaches*, edited by J. R. Jennings and M. G. H. Coles, pp. 511–574. Chichester, England: Wiley and Sons.

Fox, P. T. and Raichle, M. E. (1984) Stimulus rate dependence of regional cerebral blood flow in human striate cortex, demonstrated by PET. *J. Neurophysiol.* 51: 1109–1120.

Friederici, A. (1995) The time course of syntactic activation during language processing: A model based on neuropyschological and neurophysiological data. *Brain Lang.* 50: 259–281.

Frith, C. D., Friston, J. K., Liddle, P. F., and Frackowiak, R. S. J. (1991) A PET study of word finding. *Neuropsychologia* 29: 1137–1148.

Fuentes, L. J., Carmona, E., Agis, I. F., and Catena, A. (1994) The role of the anterior attentional system in semantic processing of both foveal and parafoveal words. *J. Cognitive Neurosci.* 6: 17–25.

Geschwind, N. (1965) Disconnexion syndromes in animals and man. *Brain* 88: 585–644.

Hillis, A. E. and Caramazza, A. (1995) Representation of grammatical categories of words in the brain. *J. Cognitive Neurosci.* 7: 396–407.

Hinke, R. M., Hu, X., Stillman, A. E., and Kim, S. (1993) Functional magnetic resonance imaging of Broca's area during internal speech. *Neuroreport* 4: 675–678.

Holcomb, P. J. (1988) Automatic and attentional processing: An event-related brain potential analysis of semantic priming. *Brain Lang.* 35: 66–85.

Howard, D., Patterson, K., Wise, R., Brown, W. D., Friston, K., Weiller, C., and Frackowiak, R. (1992) The cortical localization of the lexicons. *Brain* 115: 1769–1782.

Kahneman, D. (1973) *Attention and Effort.* Englewood Cliffs, NJ: Prentice-Hall.

King, J. W. and Kutas, M. (1995, March) A brain potential whose latency indexes the length and frequency of words. Paper presented at the annual meeting of the Cognitive Neuroscience Society, San Francisco.

Kolb, B. and Whishaw, I. Q. (1990) *Fundamentals of Human Neuropsychology* (3rd ed.). New York: W. H. Freeman.

Kroll, J. F. and Sholl, A. (1992) Lexical and conceptual memory in fluent and nonfluent bilinguals. In *Cognitive Processing in Bilinguals,* edited by R. J. Harris, pp. 191–204. Amsterdam: North-Holland.

Kutas, M. and Hillyard, S. A. (1980) Reading senseless sentences: Brain potentials reflect semantic incongruity. *Science* 207: 203–205.

LaBerge, D. (1995) *Attentional Processing: The Brain's Art of Mindfulness.* Cambridge, MA: Harvard University Press.

Logan, G. D. (1992) Attention and preattention in theories of automaticity. *Am. J. Psychol.* 105: 317–339.

Logan, G. D. (1995) Linguistic and conceptual control of visual spatial attention. *Cognitive Psychol.* 28: 103–174.

McCarthy, G., Blamire, A. M., Rothman, D., Gruetter, R., and Shulman, R. G. (1993) Echo-planar magnetic resonance imaging studies of frontal cortex activation during word generation in humans. *Proc. Natl. Acad. Sci.* 90: 4954–4956.

McCarthy, G. and Nobre, A. C. (1993) Modulation of semantic processing by spatial selective attention. *Electroencephalogr. Clin. Neurophysiol.* 88: 210–219.

McLaughlin, T., Steinberg, B., Christensen, B., Law, I., Parving, A., and Friberg, L. (1992) Potential language and attentional networks revealed through factor analysis of rCBF data measured with SPECT. *J. Cereb. Blood Flow Metab.* 12: 535–545.

Milberg, W., Blumstein, S. E., Katz, D., and Gershberg, F. (1995) Semantic facilitation in aphasia: Effects of time and expectancy. *J. Cognitive. Neurosci.* 7: 33–50.

Moberg, P. J., Crosson, B., Boone, J. R., and Gonzalez Rothi, L. J. (1992) Category-specific naming deficit after dominant thalamic and capsular hemorrhage. *J. Clin. Exp. Neuropsychol.* 14: 34.

Nadeau, S. E. and Crosson, B. (1997) Subcortical aphasia. *Brain Lang.* 58: 355–402.

Nakagawa, A. (1991) Role of anterior and posterior attention networks in hemisphere asymmetries during lexical decisions. *J. Cognitive Neurosci.* 3: 313–321.

Neville, H. J., Mills, D. L., and Lawson, D. S. (1992) Fractionating language: Different neural subsystems with different sensitive periods. *Cereb. Cortex* 2: 244–258.

Nobre, A. C. and McCarthy, G. (1994) Language-related ERPs: Scalp distributions and modulation by word type and semantic priming. *J. Cognitive Neurosci.* 6: 233–255.

Nobre, A. C. and McCarthy, G. (1995) Language-related field potentials in the anterior-medial temporal-lobe. 2. Effects of word type and semantic priming. *J. Neurosci.* 15: 1090–1098.

Ojemann, G. A. (1994) Cortical stimulation and recording in language. In *Localization and Neuroimaging in Neuropsychology*, edited by A. Kertesz, pp. 35–55. San Diego, CA: Academic Press.

Osterhout, L. (1994) Event related brain potentials as tools for comprehending language comprehension. In *Perspectives on Sentence Processing*, edited by C. J. Clifton, L. Frazier, and K. Rayner, pp. 15–44. Hillsdale, NJ: Lawrence Erlbaum.

Parasuraman, R. and Martin, A. (1994) Cognition in Alzheimer's disease: Disorders of attention and semantic knowledge. *Curr. Opin. Neurobiol.* 4: 237–244.

Paulesu, E., Frith, C. D., and Frackowiak, R. S. (1993) The neural correlates of the verbal component of working memory. *Nature* 362: 342–345.

Petersen, S. E., Fox, P. T., Posner, M., I., Mintun, M., and Raichle, M. E. (1989) Positron emission tomographic studies of the processing of single words. *J. Cognitive Neurosci.* 1: 153–170.

Petersen, S. E., Fox, P. T., Snyder, A., and Raichle, M. E. (1990) Activation of extrastriate and frontal cortical activity by words and word-like stimuli. *Science* 249: 1041–1044.

Petry, M., Crosson, B., Fischler, I., Gonzalez Rothi, L. J., Fennell, E., Bauer, R., and Agresti, A. (1996) The effect of language on visual spatial attention: Implications for theories of selective attention. Paper presented at the meeting of the International Neuropsychological Society, Chicago.

Petry, M. C., Crosson, B., Gonzalez Rothi, L. J., Bauer, R. M., and Schauer, C. A. (1994) Selective attention and aphasia in adults: Preliminary findings. *Neuropsychologia* 32: 1397–1408.

Posner, M. I. and Carr, T. H. (1992) Lexical access and the brain: Anatomical constraints on models of word recognition. *Am. J. Psychol.* 105: 1–26.

Posner, M. I., Inhoff, A. W., Friedrich, F. J., and Rafal, R. D. (1987) Isolating attentional systems: A cognitive-anatomical analysis. *Psychobiology* 15: 107–121.

Posner, M. I., Petersen, S. E., Fox, P. T., and Raichle, M. E. (1988) Localization of cognitive operations in the human brain. *Science* 240: 1627–1631.

Posner, M. I. and Raichle, M. E. (1994) *Images of Mind.* New York: Scientific American Library.

Posner, M. I., Sandson, J., Dhawan, M., and Shulman, G. L. (1989) Is word recognition automatic? A cognitive-anatomical approach. *J. Cognitive Neurosci.* 1: 50–60.

Price, C., Wise, R., Ramsay, S., Friston, K., Howard, D., Patterson, K., and Frackowiak, R. (1992) Regional response differences within the human auditory cortex when listening to words. *Neurosci. Lett.* 146: 179–182.

Price, C. J., Wise, R. J. S., Watson, J. D. G., Patterson, K., Howard, D., and Frackowiak, R. S. J. (1994) Brain activity during reading. *Brain* 117: 1255–1269.

Raichle, M. E., Fiez, J. A., Videen, T. O., Macleod, A. M. K., Pardo, J. V., Fox, P. T., and Petersen, S. E. (1994) Practice-related changes in human brain functional-anatomy during nonmotor learning. *Cereb. Cortex* 4: 8–26.

Raney, G. E. (1993) Monitoring changes in cognitive load during reading: An event-related brain potential and reaction time analysis. *J. Exp. Psychol. Learn. Mem. Cogn.* 19: 51–69.

Raymer, A. M., Moberg, P. J., Crosson, B., Nadeau, S. E., and Gonzalez Rothi, L. J. (1992) Lexical deficits in two cases of thalamic lesion. *J. Clin. Exp. Neuropsychol.* 14: 33–34.

Sacchett, C. and Humphreys, G. W. (1992) Calling a squirrel a squirrel but a canoe a wigwam: A category-specific deficit for artefactual objects and body parts. *Cognitive Neuropsychol.* 9: 73–86.

Shaywitz, B. A., Shaywitz, S. E., Pugh, K. R., Constable, R. T., Skudlarski, P., Fulbright, R. K., Bronen, R. A., Fletcher, J. M., Shankweiler, D. P., Katz, L., and Gore, J. C. (1995) Sex-differences in the functional-organization of the brain for language. *Nature* 373: 607–609.

Shuren, J. E., Smith Hammond, C., Maher, L. M., Rothi, L. J. G., and Heilman, K. M. (1995) Attention and anosagnosia: The case of a jargonaphasic patient with unawareness of language deficit. *Neurology* 45: 376–378.

Small, S. L., Hart, J., Nguyen, T., and Gordon, B. (1995) Distributed representations of semantic knowledge in the brain. *Brain* 118: 441–453.

Snyder, A. Z., Abdullaev, Y. G., Posner, M. I., and Raichle, M. E. (1995) Scalp electrical potentials reflect regional cerebral blood-flow responses during processing of written words. *Proc. Natl. Acad. Sci. USA* 92: 1689–1693.

Van Petten, C. (1993) A comparison of lexical and sentence-level context effects in event-related potentials. *Lang. Cognitive Proc.* 8: 485–531.

Wise, R., Chollet, F., Hadar, U., Friston, K., Hoffner, E., and Frackowiak, R. (1991) Distribution of cortical neural networks involved in word comprehension and word retrieval. *Brain* 114: 1803–1817.

Zattore, R. J., Evans, A. C., Meyer, E., and Gjedde, A. (1992) Lateralization of phonetic and pitch discrimination in speech processing. *Science* 360: 339–340.

18 Executive Attention: Conflict, Target Detection, and Cognitive Control

Michael I. Posner and Gregory J. DiGirolamo

ABSTRACT According to cognitive models, executive attention is required when tasks involve planning, error detection, novelty, difficult processing, or conflict. These are situations in which it becomes impossible to process more than one target event at a time, and neuroimaging studies have found activation in frontal midline areas. The anatomy and time course of executive control is examined in the rapid generation of novel word meanings and in Stroop conflict tasks. Evidence relating this higher-level attention network to psychopathology and to cognitive development is reviewed, and states that might serve to dissociate components of the executive network are discussed.

All normal individuals have a strong subjective feeling of intentional or voluntary control of their behavior. Asking people about goals or intentions is probably the single most predictive indicator of their behavior during problem solving (Newell and Simon, 1972). The importance of intentions and goals is illustrated by observations of patients with frontal lesions (Duncan, 1995) or mental disorders (Frith, 1992), either of which cause disruption in the central control over behavior or the subjective feelings of such control. Despite these indices of central control, it has not been easy to specify exactly the functions or mechanisms of executive control (or executive attention).

This chapter first reviews efforts to develop a cognitive model of executive control and considers how experimental methods can be used to explore conditions in which executive attention operates. In the second section, neuroimaging studies that employ those cognitive methods to explore the anatomy and circuitry of executive attention are examined. The third section considers evidence from lesion, schizophrenia, and developmental studies that provide further tests of which areas are involved in executive attention. Finally, future opportunities for dissociating components of executive function are considered.

It has always been hard to define executive attention precisely because the term has been used in many ways. We try to avoid these difficulties by using a specific model of higher-level control to specify when executive attention is a necessary aspect of information processing. Moreover, we believe some progress is being made in identifying components that might provide further analysis of the mechanisms that together constitute executive attention.

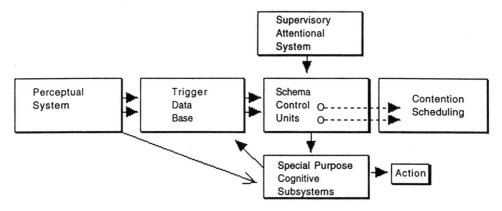

Figure 18.1 The Norman-Shallice model of attention. (Adapted from Norman and Shallice, 1986.)

THE NORMAN-SHALLICE MODEL OF EXECUTIVE CONTROL

Norman and Shallice (1980, 1986) proposed one representative model of executive control that assumes multiple, isolable subsystems of cognitive processing. These multiple subsystems interact to coordinate goals and actions (see, Allport, 1980a, 1980b) and are controlled by two qualitatively different mechanisms. The first level of control operates via contention scheduling, which uses schemas or condition-to-action statements to coordinate well-learned behaviors and thoughts (compare Newell and Simon, 1972). Once a schema is selected, it remains active until it reaches its goal or it is inhibited by a competitive schema or by higher-level control.

The contention-scheduling mechanism corresponds to routine selection. When the situation is novel or highly competitive (i.e., when it requires executive control), a supervisory attentional system intervenes and provides additional inhibition or activation to the appropriate schema for the situation (see figure 18.1). The supervisory system has access to the overall representation of the environment and the goals of the person, unlike the contention-scheduling mechanism, which involves only competition among subsystems.

Norman and Shallice (1980, 1986) argued that the executive control of the supervisory system is necessary for five types of behaviors or situations in which the routine or automatic processes (Shallice, 1994) of the contention-scheduling mechanisms are inadequate: (1) planning or decision making, (2) error correction, (3) novel or not well-learned responses, (4) conditions judged difficult or dangerous, and (5) overcoming habitual responses.

We also suggest that executive control operates only in certain situations or during portions of tasks when these executive functions are necessary. Executive control operations are necessary when routine functions (subsystems) are insufficient for the task at hand, or when subsystems must be overridden due to environmental or goal changes. Executive control is not a continuous and universal process present in every cognitive activity, though these cognitive operations may play an important part in the unification of thought and action (see, Allport, 1980a, 1980b). We further suggest that executive control operations are dissociable from other cognitive operations in a task (see Rogers and Monsell, 1995). This chapter will examine the evidence on the brain systems involved in situations calling for executive control.

MEANS OF CONTROL

In the Norman-Shallice model, contention scheduling works via local inhibition of competing schemas. In a recent review of the neuroscience literature, Desimone and Duncan (1995) also argued that visual sub-processing systems perform selection via a local competition in which the receptive fields are viewed as critical resources for which stimuli are competing. Desimone and Duncan believe that the competition for these sub-processing systems is resolved via inhibition in the local neural circuit. In addition, Desimone and Duncan proposed that the competition can be biased by a top-down mechanism that selects objects that are important to the current behavior or goal. Several studies have found preferential increases of neuronal activity (Motter, 1993; Spitzer, Desimone, and Moran, 1988), or of blood flow (Corbetta, Miezin, Dobmeyer, Shulman, and Petersen, 1991), for selected features or locations. Scalp electrical recording has demonstrated both increases of electrical activity from selected events and decreases from competing events compared to a neutral condition (Luck, Heinze, Mangun, and Hillyard, 1990). Like the supervisory system mechanism of the Norman-Shallice model, competition for control of behavior appears to be resolved at local sites by the relative amplification of the selected competitor.

INTERFERENCE BETWEEN TARGETS

In order to understand the mechanisms of supervisory control it is necessary to have reliable experimental techniques for causing executive control to be employed. A well-established principle of cognitive psychology is that there will be interference whenever two tasks require access to the same underlying systems. Interference between tasks that use quite separate input and output pathways has been taken as a method for the measurement of central attentional control.

Early work in attention presented subjects with two separate streams of information, one to each ear, and required subjects to rivet their attention to one stream by repeating it back (shadowing) (Broadbent 1958, 1973). Most information from the nonshadowed ear is lost. In a basic experiment of that era, Treisman and Geffen (1967) asked subjects to tap a key whenever they heard the word "tap". When it occurred in the attended ear they tapped the key nearly 100% of the time but when it occurred in the unattended ear they almost never did. On the other hand, it has been shown that significant events presented in the unattended ear, or visually, during shadowing can still produce priming or galvanic skin response (Corteen and Wood, 1972; Corteen and Dunn, 1974; Dawson and Schell, 1982; Posner, Sandson, Dhawan, and Shulman, 1989).

When the requirement to shadow one of the two messages was relaxed (Duncan, 1980; Ostry, Moray, and Marks, 1976; Shiffrin, McKay, and Shaffer, 1977) and instead subjects were required to monitor 1 or many channels, accuracy of detection of the target remained very high regardless of the number of channels. In opposition to the shadowing results, subjects appeared to have nearly unlimited capacity to monitor incoming messages. A theoretical account by Duncan (1980) helped to reconcile the shadowing and monitoring studies. He showed that attention could be summoned to one of several input channels with very great effectiveness, but when a target occurred on one channel, processing of targets on any other channel dropped dramatically. Even when if subjects only thought a target had been present and made a false report, performance on simultaneous signals greatly deteriorated (Ostry et al., 1976). Thus, major interference is found among items selected for focal attention (targets).

That important insight continues to be rediscovered in various domains. When events are presented in rapid succession (Raymond, Shapiro, and Arnell, 1995; Shapiro, Raymond, and Arnell, 1994), attending to one target appears to reduce the ability to detect a second target for 0.5 s (the attentional blink). Although in the attentional blink experiments there is a stream of information presented at a rapid rate, studies of the psychological refractory period indicate that, even in self-paced tasks, if attention is given to the processing of one signal, new signals that appear prior to the response are delayed (Pashler, 1993; Pashler and Johnston, 1989).

Some of these ideas have been applied to paradigms that require subjects to switch between successive tasks, a paradigm that is more in line with what might be the function of an executive mechanism (Allport, Styles, and Hsieh, 1994; Rogers and Monsell, 1995; Spector and Biederman, 1976). In this paradigm subjects perform one task (e.g., naming ink colors) and then switch to a different task (naming the value of a digit). The switch might be signaled by a change of stimulus or by a change in task with the stimulus, remaining the same. Irrespective of the nature of the task, subjects appear to be slower on the first trial following a switch even when the task is paced so that no new event is presented until after the previous event has been responded to (Rogers and Monsell, 1995). Thus, there is a clear cost in switching between tasks. However, it is less clear that the cost is due to an operation involved in switching set; rather, there appears to be some residue of having done one task that makes processing the new task more difficult.

Overall these results show that the difficulty in processing simultaneous or successive targets extends across a wide range of tasks. Apparently, having to commit attention to an event interferes with processing other events at this level irrespective of the similarity between the two tasks. That observation supports the idea of some kind of central process that is common to a wide range of targets. The problem remains of how to define the meaning of targets? It is simple if the experimenter identifies some event for special processing, as when a key press must be made to detect, discriminate, identify, or classify a stimulus. However, events may serve as targets because they automatically force processing. This may happen when a transient visual onset stimulus forces orienting (Yantis and Jonides, 1990), or when a distractor with a competing classification is placed close to a target (Eriksen and Eriksen, 1974). Often, the tendency to read the name of a visual word interferes with other more arbitrary responses to that word such as identifying the ink color (known as the Stroop effect) or providing associations such as its use or its superordinate category. The next section uses these target interference effects to explore the anatomy of executive attention.

IMAGING EXECUTIVE FUNCTION

Anatomy

Several studies have shown that tasks requiring supervisory control are severely affected by lesions of the frontal lobes (Duncan, Burgess, and Emslie, 1995; Shallice, 1988 Shallice and Burgess, 1991a, 1991b). However, the tasks used in those studies were quite complex, with many components, and the frontal lobes are a large part of the brain. Studies using neuroimaging methods may provide better localization of supervisory functions.

The methods of neuroimaging, in particular positron emission tomography (PET) (see Corbetta, chapter 6, this volume), allow examination of brain anatomy during task performance. Many studies involving the detection of targets or the resolution of conflict among targets have found activation in a midline frontal area called the anterior cingulate. Studies using two of these tasks, the generate-uses task (see Petersen, Fox, Posner, Mintun, and Raichle, 1988, 1989; Posner, Petersen, Fox, and Raichle, 1988) and the Stroop task (Stroop, 1935; for a review, see MacLeod, 1991), are examined in some detail.

The generate-uses task involves an experimental condition in which subjects are required to provide the use of a familiar visually or auditorily presented word and a control task in which the subject merely reads or says aloud the word name. Blocks of 40 trials were used during which blood flow measurements were averaged (Petersen, Fox, Posner, Mintun, and Raichle, 1988). The subtraction of the control condition from the experimental condition revealed three cortical areas of activation. There were activations in the anterior cingulate and in two left lateral areas, one in a frontal area anterior to Broca's area and one in Wernicke's area. The lateral areas were near classical language areas. The midline area seemed more likely to be related to attention to the task.

What happens when subjects practice generating the same use over and over again? The Norman-Shallice model would predict that, following practice, a schema would be formed that would trigger when the stimulus was presented, and the supervisory system would not be necessary. Raichle et al. (1994) had subjects perform the generate-uses task while undergoing PET scans and found the expected activation of the anterior cingulate during the experimental condition compared to when subjects were required merely to repeat the word aloud. In addition, Raichle et al. had subjects practice the same list repeatedly, generating the same appropriate use for each word until the list was highly learned. Following the extended practice, subjects again were scanned. This time, the anterior cingulate and the left lateral activation were gone; instead, there was increased activation in the anterior insula, activation similar to that found when subjects read the words aloud. Following the practice, Raichle et al. had subjects generate a use for a new, unpracticed list. Again, the anterior cingulate and left lateral areas were active. Thus, the anterior cingulate is active when the supervisory system is necessary for appropriate behavior, according to the Norman-Shallice model, and the anterior cingulate is inactive when the supervisory system should be inactive and the contention-scheduling mechanisms are active. However, in the studies just reviewed, the cingulate was not alone; the lateral activations behaved in a similar manner. This could be because attention increased the lateral activations, and when attention was reduced they fell below significant threshold.

The Stroop task involves the naming of the color of ink of a word that can be congruent (i.e., match the color of the ink it is printed in; e.g., the word "RED" in red ink); neutral (i.e., noncolor related; e.g., the word "LOT" in red ink); or incongruent (i.e., a mismatch of the word with the color of ink the word is printed in; e.g., the word "RED" in blue ink). One computational breakdown of the Stroop task can be outlined as follows: (1) remember instructions to vocalize the ink color, (2) attend to the visually presented stimulus, (3) determine the ink color of the word, (4) inhibit the naming of the word, and (5) make the appropriate response (being careful to not name the color word presented). Anterior cingulate activation is confirmed by five separate Stroop (or Stroop-like) studies (see Bench, Frich, Grasby, Friston, Paulesu, Frackowiak, and Dolan, 1993; Carter, Mintun, and Cohen, 1995; George et al., 1994; Pardo, Pardo, Janer, and Raichle, 1990; Taylor, Kornblum, Minoshima, Oliver, and Koeppe, 1994), although the specifics of the studies may account for the varied locations of the activations (figure 18.2).

The first Stroop PET study was conducted by Pardo and his colleagues (1990) as a means of testing the neural areas specifically involved in selective attention and cognitive control. Each subject always began with the congruent condition and then went on to the incongruent condition at the next scan. The resulting imaging data was obtained by subtracting the congruent condition from the incongruent condition. The anterior cingulate was active in three areas on the right medial portion and in one area in the left inferior sulcus. The averaging necessary for the PET methodology requires that ex-

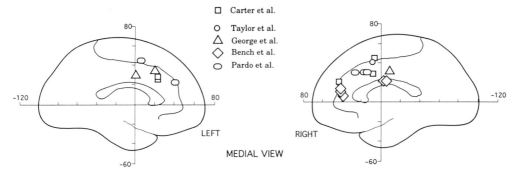

Figure 18.2 Activation of anterior cingulate in five Stroop or Stroop-like studies.

periments be blocked in one task of the same condition for 40 s followed by a brief rest, and the next condition of the task for another 40 s. The resulting paradigm is problematic for the Stroop task, as one cannot know if in the congruent condition the subject is deciphering the ink color or merely reading the word. Pardo and his colleagues always had the subjects perform the congruent condition first. Because the subjects' first exposure to the task was the congruent condition, there was no necessity or attentional set (see Perret, 1973) to name the ink color.

Given the computational similarity of the congruent and incongruent conditions (as was discussed previously), it is surprising that activation of the anterior cingulate was detected using the subtraction that Pardo et al. employed. Bench et al. (1993) attempted to replicate the Pardo et al. (1990) findings using the PET methodology. Unlike Pardo et al., Bench and his colleagues used a faster presentation rate and three conditions: (1) naming the ink color of colored crosses; (2) naming the ink color of neutral words ("front," "back," "top," and "down"); and (3) naming the ink color of incongruent color word names. In the subtraction of the neutral words from the incongruent condition, there was no activation of the anterior cingulate. Bench and his colleagues were so surprised by that finding that they conducted another study using the exact paradigm of Pardo et al. (1990); the subtraction of congruent condition data from incongruent condition data produced no significant areas of activation anywhere in the brain. If one compares the computational processes in the congruent and incongruent condition, both require inhibition of the competing color word in order to respond to the ink color; thus, the same processes are occurring in different degrees in the two conditions. Bench et al. (1993) reported an increase in activity in the right anterior cingulate during both the congruent and incongruent conditions in comparison to activity during the crosses condition. That finding suggests that the effort to name the ink color and avoid the word can influence both the congruent and incongruent conditions in the same way. Bench and his colleagues also concluded that the frequency of stimulus presentation greatly affected the activation of the anterior cingulate in that more stimuli and a faster pace increased the blood flow to the cingulate. That result suggests that, as attentional demands are increased in making a faster judgment, the anterior cingulate also increases its role in the task.

In yet another PET study of the Stroop effect, George et al. (1994) used three conditions: (1) number symbols in (#) colored ink; (2) incongruent color words in colored ink; and (3) emotional words in colored ink ("sad," "grief," "misery," and "bleak"). Unlike the previous studies, George and his colleagues had subjects name the ink colors of words in lists with the stimuli presentation being self-paced. They found increased activation in the left midcingulate, the left anterior cingulate, and the right midcingulate. George et al. (1994) interpreted these results by suggesting that different portions of the cingulate were involved in different computational tasks. The studies that were self-paced and that emphasized the response selection seemed to show a left midcingulate activation; in contrast, in studies that were externally paced, the right anterior cingulate seemed to be active.

The commentary of George et al. on self- versus externally paced stimulus presentation receives support from a Stroop-like study by Taylor et al. (1994). In that study, subjects were taught to respond to single letters with another single letter; that is, in the congruent condition, subjects saw the letter *J* and responded by saying "jay"; *J* in the incongruent condition, subjects saw the letter *J* and responded by saying a different letter that they had been taught corresponded to *J* "F," for example). Taylor et al. found activation of the left cingulate sulcus in a subtraction of congruent from incongruent conditions. It is important to note that in the Taylor et al. study, the incongruent task involved a different computation than the congruent task. The congruent task was computationally simple: the stimulus appeared and the subject named it; there was no degree of incompatibility with this task. In the incongruent condition, the subject had to keep from naming the letter presented and instead name the different letter that the subject was taught corresponded to that stimulus.

Another recent Stroop PET study sought to investigate the role of the anterior cingulate computations in both the congruent and incongruent conditions. To control for strategy, Carter et al. (1995) used a block design with separate congruent and incongruent conditions, each containing neutral words on 50% of the trials. All of the trials of the neutral block were noncolor words in colored ink. Carter et al. found bilateral anterior cingulate activation in both the incongruent and congruent conditions when a 100% neutral block was subtracted from each condition. Moreover, the right anterior cingulate was active when the congruent condition was subtracted from the incongruent condition. These results suggest that the anterior cingulate performs the same attentional control process in all conditions, but to varying degrees. To complete correctly any of these blocks, the subject had to both inhibit reading the word and select the appropriate ink color. The difficulty of the task varied as the irrelevant dimension (the word) more closely corresponded to the relevant dimension (the ink color) (see Klein, 1964).

The Norman-Shallice model (1980, 1986) suggests five situations in which the supervisory system would be necessary for appropriate behavior or successful execution of a task or goal. The first of those situations is circumstances involving internally planned, or voluntary, actions. Using PET, Passingham and his colleagues (Colebatch, Cunningham, Deiber, Frackowiak, and Passingham, 1991; Deiber et al., 1991) have shown significantly increased activation in the anterior cingulate during voluntary, planned arm and hand movements when compared to activation during resting, during learned sequence movements, and during fixed sequence movements. Two other situations in which the Norman-Shallice model holds the supervisory system to be necessary are situations that require overcoming habitual responses and situations in which responses are not well learned or else contain novel sequences of actions. Those factors fit the generate use and Stroop tasks. Another situation in which the Norman-Shallice model necessitates supervisory system involvement is in error correction or detection (troubleshooting); studies involving error detection will be considered in the next section.

Circuitry

In order for a brain area to perform a supervisory function it must influence widely distributed parts of the brain in which computations related to the task are performed (Posner and Raichle, 1994). Anatomical studies suggest that the anterior cingulate, like many brain regions, has close contact with many other cortical areas (Goldman-Rakic, 1988). The cingulate's connections to lateral frontal areas involved in word recognition and to posterior parietal areas involved in orienting are particularly strong.

Recently, efforts have been made to trace the dynamics of those interactions by use of event related potentials (ERPs) (for reviews of ERP methods, see Näätänen, 1992; Rugg and Coles, 1995). Although it is a difficult task to determine the neural generator from the scalp distribution of ERPs, if the generator is known from PET or functional magnetic resonance imaging (fMRI) studies, it is much easier to evaluate whether the scalp distribution could come from that generator (for an example of this methodology, see Heinze et al., 1994). The algorithms to relate a generator to the scalp distribution (Scherg, 1989) work best when fewer generators are involved. This method assumes that the scalp ERP arises from the summation of some number of sources within the brain (dipoles) of different locations, orientations, strengths, and time courses. Using a best-fit method, those sources are modeled until the solution of the model most closely matches the empirically obtained scalp electrical data. Thus, in complex tasks, it is important to use a subtraction that isolates only a small number of brain areas.

One effort to do so is in the localization of a scalp negativity that follows making an error (Dehaene, Posner, and Tucker, 1994; Gehring, Gross, Coles, Meyer, and Donchin, 1993). When subjects were aware of making an error in speeded tasks they showed a very strong negativity following the key press in a localized area over the mid-frontal scalp. Further analysis using the brain electrical source analysis (BESA) algorithm (Scherg and Berg, 1993) showed that the error negativity most likely came from the anterior cingulate. Errors can be either slips (i.e., incorrect execution of a motor program) or mistakes (i.e., selection of an inappropriate intention). The Norman-Shallice model would predict supervisory system involvement in the recognition of an execution of an incorrect motor program, but not if the contention scheduling had selected what was thought to be an appropriate response. Dehaene, et al. (1994) have shown that error negativity follows a slip, when the person knows the error, but does not follow a mistake, when the person is unaware of the error (Tucker, Liotti, Potts, Russell, and Posner, 1994).

Studies that subtract the repeat words task from the generate uses task using ERPs have provided a means of integrating the anatomy found by PET with a specific time course (Snyder, Abdullaev, Posner, and Raichle, 1995). Figure 18.3 (see color plate 13) shows scalp potential maps of electrical differences between the two tasks. The figure shows increased positivity of the generate use task over the repeat word task that occurs very early over frontal sites and much later over left posterior sites.

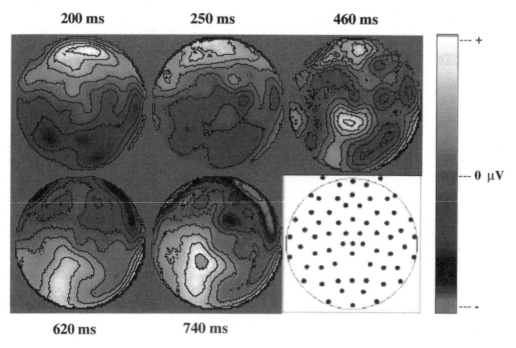

Figure 18.3 Maps of the relative voltage differences between the generate used and reading aloud tasks at several time slices. The colors (see plate 13) indicate the size of the voltage differences with the bright colors indicating greater positivity in the uses task and the dark colors greater negativity in the uses task. An early frontal positivity is related to activity in the cingulate and left lateral lexical semantic areas. The later left posterior positivity is related to activity in Wernicke's area.

Using BESA, it was possible to show that the early frontal activity could be fit best by a midline generator (presumably anterior cingulate) starting about 170 ms after the visual presentation of the word. That activation was presumably related to focal attention. The cingulate activation stayed present and was joined after 50 ms by a left frontal activation. At about 650 ms a single generator was found, presumably related to Wernicke's area activation. Abdullaev and Posner (1997) took a further step in replicating the PET results. They had subjects generate uses for the same list of words several times. As in the PET data, the left frontal and cingulate activations (as localized by the BESA methodology) tended to go away following practice, but the activations were restored when a new list was presented or when subjects were required to generate a new use for the practiced words.

Functions

These experiments suggest that the anterior cingulate is active during tasks that require some thought and is reduced or disappears as tasks become routine, as in the case of reading words aloud or following practice with generating the uses for the same words.

What is the cingulate activation actually doing? According to our analysis, the cingulate and other midline frontal areas are involved in producing the local amplification in neural activity that accompanies top-down selection of items. It is easiest to understand this function in the domain of word processing. It is well known from cognitive studies that a target word is processed more efficiently following the presentation of a related prime word (Posner, 1978). A portion of the improvement occurs automatically because the prime word activates a pathway shared with the target. However, another portion of the activation is top-down because the attention to the prime leads the subject to expect a particular type of target. If the prime is masked or of low validity, the improvement in the processing of the target will be mostly automatic; however, if the prime is of high validity or if subjects are instructed to use the prime to think of another category, top-down effects dominate. If the target is ambiguous (e.g., "palm"), the prime (e.g., "tree") can lead to a single conscious interpretation that fits with both prime and target (for a review, see Simpson, 1984). We believe that the cingulate, in conjunction with other midline areas, is responsible for those top-down effects, in that it provides a boost in activation to items associated with the expectation.

Anatomically, we see the cingulate in contact with areas of the left lateral and posterior cortex that seem to be involved in understanding the meaning of a given target word. Indeed, the time course of activation of the cingulate (170 ms) and the left lateral frontal (220 ms) cortex found during the generate use task supports our speculation that attention interacts with the semantic activation pattern (Snyder et al., 1995).

Primes presented to the right visual field (left hemisphere) produce rapid activation of close semantic associates, whereas primes presented to the left visual field (right hemisphere) act more slowly and activate more remote associations. Interference with attention to the visual input by use of a dual task, such as shadowing reduces the semantic priming and produces a pattern of activation like that found for right hemisphere primes irrespective of the visual field the prime is actually presented in (Nakagawa, 1991). This finding provides evidence for the specific role of attentional control in semantic activation.

In addition, we believe that the cingulate and associated structures play a role in the voluntary reactivation of brain areas that are activated automatically by visual input. For example, feature analysis of visual input appears to involve a right extrastriate area. If subjects are instructed to examine a feature of same stimulus (e.g., look in a word for a letter with a thick stroke), the same extrastriate brain regions that are initially activated by stimulus presentation are reactivated, but much later in time (Posner and Raichle, 1994, pp. 137–140). We believe that the cingulate is important for voluntary reactivation of these extrastriate regions to complete the feature detection task. We also believe that the cingulate network is involved when elements of thought have to be reordered in time. By increasing the level of activation (amplification) of brain areas that carry out specific computations, one can change the time course of the organization of the component operations (Posner and Raichle, 1994, pp. 145–148).

LESIONS, SCHIZOPHRENIA, AND DEVELOPMENT

Lesions of the frontal lobe often produce disorganized or incoherent behavior (Duncan et al., 1995; Shallice and Burgess, 1991a,b). In neuropsychology, the dysexecutive syndrome that follows closed head injury, stroke, or degenerative disorders of frontal structures involves the loss of the ability to plan coherently, to solve problems, or to organize the routines of daily life. Patients suffering from this syndrome have difficulty with problem-solving tasks such as the Tower of Hanoi task, in which planning ahead is an important component.

There has been some controversy about the importance of cingulate involvement in the loss of executive function. Large lesions of the frontal midline produced by strokes can have devastating effects on human behavior. Damasio (1994), who has studied many of these patients, has written:

Before leaving the subject of human brain lesions, I would like to propose there is a particular region in the human brain where the systems concerned with emotion, attention and working memory interact so intimately that they constitute the source for the energy for both external action (movement) and internal action (thought, animation, reasoning). This fountain head region is the anterior cingulate cortex, another piece of the limbic puzzle. (p. 71)

This observation comes from patients who show akinetic mutism following strokes in the general area of the cingulate. These patients can orient to events but initiate little in the way of spontaneous behavior. One woman studied by Damasio (1994) recovered and when Damasio asked her what was going on during the period of time when she suffered from the brain injury and why she hadn't initiated any behavior or communication, she said, "I really had nothing to say" (p. 73). The fact that there can be recovery after a brief period of akinetic mutism suggests that there is considerable distribution of executive function both within the cingulate and in other structures related to it. There is a history of work with cats and monkeys involving lesions of the cingulate (Kennard, 1954, 1955; Ward, 1948) that has produced results similar to Damasio's studies. Both cats and monkeys with extensive anterior cingulate lesions show the same lack of initiation of voluntary behavior or movement.

However, as more discrete cingulate lesions have been used to treat patients with pain or anxiety, there has been little evidence of the gross loss of conscious control reported in the studies cited previously (Corkin, Twitchell, and Sullivan, 1979; Ballantine, Levy, Dagi, and Giriunas, 1977; Oschner, personal communication). Perhaps this relates to the various areas of the cingulate that might be involved in higher-order attention, as illustrated by figure 18.2. In order to see any deficits in surgical patients it has been necessary to study the specific tasks that have shown consistent activation of the anterior cingulate during imaging (Janer and Pardo, 1991). Janer and Pardo (1991) tested a 34-year-old, right-handed, college-educated female one week before and two weeks after bilateral anterior cingulotomy along with 10 control subjects on the following three cognitive tasks: (1) semantic monitoring task (decide whether a word names a dangerous animal), (2) generate uses task, and (3) Stroop task.

As one would expect, the patient showed an overall increase in reaction times following her surgery. She showed no significant increase in reaction times postoperation when the semantic monitoring task involved no animals, but when nondangerous animals (e.g., cat) were presented she showed impairment following the cingulotomy and also made more errors for nondangerous animals than did normal control subjects.

The data from the verb generation task also revealed a significant difference between the control subjects and the patient following her cingulotomy. The control subjects in their second testing showed an improvement in naming a use for the noun; in contrast, the patient showed an increased reaction time for naming a use for the noun following the cingulotomy.

Another difference between the patient and the control subjects was that the latter were able to detect their errors, sometimes even before they reached the output stage. The patient never made any pre-output hesitations symptomatic of detecting errors. Control subjects made 32 hesitation errors during their second testing; the patient never made a hesitation error following her cingulotomy. The patient never detected an impending mistake in her performance even though she made more errors than the control subjects. Again, the cingulotomy patient showed differences from the control subjects on a task for which ERP data has implicated the anterior cingulate (Dehaene et al., 1994).

Janer and Pardo also tested their patient and control subjects on a Stroop task, using the same methodology as that used in the PET study done by Pardo and his colleagues (1990). Both congruent and incongruent conditions of the classical Stroop task were used. Both the control subjects and the patient performed faster in the congruent condition than in the incongruent condition during both times of testing. The control subjects performed faster on the second testing of both the congruent and the incongruent conditions. The patient performed equally at both times of testing in the incongruent condition. However, the patient showed a significant deficit in congruent condition performance following the cingulotomy. That result proves difficult to reconcile with cingulate involvement in conflict situations. There is, however, an interpretation of the Stroop task that might explain a deficit in the congruent condition following cingulotomy. Both the incongruent and the congruent condition require the same selective attentional mechanisms, but to different degrees. In the congruent task, the subject had to selectively attend to the color of the ink. Because word naming can be an automatic process (Posner and Snyder, 1975), the word naming in both conditions should have occured and would have slowed processing. Hence, the patient's difficulty in naming the ink color in the congruent condition might support a deficit in selective attention, which was suggested by her performance in the other tasks. Nevertheless, we are faced with the problem that the patient did not show a deficit in her performance of the incongruent condition following her cingulotomy. The results with this single patient clearly require further investigation of cingulate operations.

Schizophrenia

Some recent analyses of schizophrenia are based on ideas of dysregulation of the anterior cingulate (Early, Posner, Reiman, and Raichle, 1989a, 1989b). This view began with observations that patients suffering from the early positive symptoms of schizophrenia had difficulty directing attention toward the right visual field (Posner, Early, Reiman, Pardo, and Dhawan, 1988). This finding has now been confirmed by others (Maruff, Currie, Hay, McArthur-Jackson, and Malone, 1995).

The same schizophrenic patients had difficulties in dealing with a single word made to conflict with a spatial location in a Stroop-like task. This result, and other language-related difficulties in schizophrenics, suggested to us that the deficit was arising in the anterior cingulate, given that the anterior cingulate, and other midline areas, serves to exercise control over both language and shifts of spatial attention. We were also able to relate our specific findings with more general deficits in schizophrenic thought, such as the tendency to attribute aspects of their thoughts to others and the difficulty in producing coherent sentences.

These early studies did not provide as much evidence as one would like, but more recent evidence has continued to suggest that the cingulate (see, Dolan et al., 1995), in conjunction with basal ganglia and lateral frontal cortex, might be central to the positive symptoms of schizophrenia. Benes (1993) reported analysis of the cingulate following the death of patients who suffered from schizophrenia. Figure 18.4 points out her view of the central role for the cingulate and also presents a cellular model in which the GABA input to the pyramidal cells is affected in the schizophrenic patients. Benes suggested that decreased inhibitory inputs and increased excitatory inputs reduces regulatory firing of the pyramidal neurons in the anterior cingulate.

Our previous work (Early et al., 1989a, 1989b) showed how many of the disorders found in schizophrenic patients could arise from dysregulation of the control processes of executive attention (see also Frith, 1992). This dysregulation would be expected as the result of the cellular abnormalities that Benes has outlined.

Development

Supervisory control has been frequently invoked in the study of working memory (Baddeley, 1986). When subjects explicitly recall events they draw upon supervisory mechanisms to search memory. In recent years a distinction between such explicit recall mechanisms and implicit memory has become important, and one domain in which it has been examined is in the learning of spatial sequences. For example, Curran and Keele (1993) have studied the learning of a fixed sequence of spatial positions by normal subjects. They distinguished between unambiguous associations, in which each stimulus always implied the next location, and context-dependent associations, in which the nature of the association depended upon context. These adult studies (Curran and Keele, 1993) indicated that unambiguous associations could be learned, presumably implicitly, even when attention was diverted by a secondary task, but context-dependent associations could not be learned without focal attention. Recent PET data of these tasks suggest that implicit learning of the sequences involves mostly subcortical areas, but explicit learning involves higher cortical areas (Grafton, Hazelton, and Ivry, 1995).

Clohessy (1994) reported that 4- and 10-month-old infants could learn simple sequences of unambiguous association, which they indicated by correct eye movements in anticipation of the next event in the sequence. The studies of 4- and 10-month-old infants also employed a complex sequence in which one of the associations was context dependent or ambiguous. In that sequence, infants were shown a sequence in which the target moved from monitor 1 to monitor 2 and then, after returning to 1, moved to monitor 3 (i.e., $1 \rightarrow 2 \rightarrow 1 \rightarrow 3$). Thus, the association of the location that followed

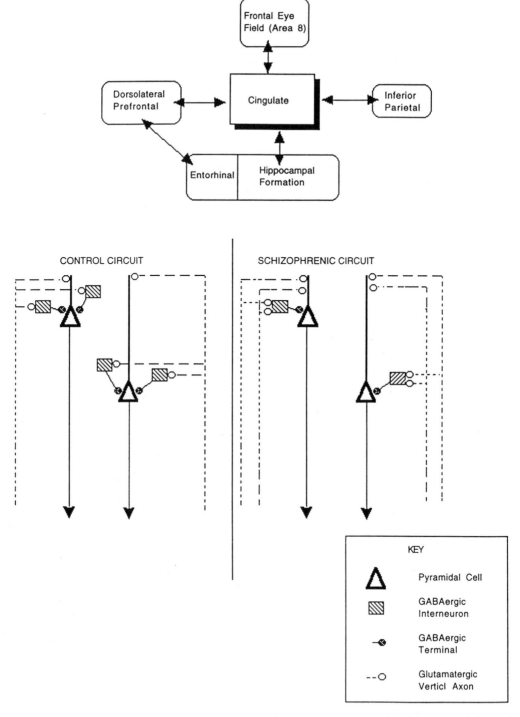

Figure 18.4 The upper diagram displays cingulate connections to areas implicated in the psychopathology of schizophrenia including areas active in attention, working memory, and emotion. The lower figure shows a schematic of anterior cingulate pyramidal neurons in layers II and III in normal control subjects (left) and in patients with schizophrenia (right). The schizophrenic circuit shows less inhibitory connections (GABAergic interneurons) to the neurons and more excitatory connections (glutamatergic axons) to their dendrites. (Adapted from Benes, 1993.)

monitor 1 was dependent upon where in the sequence the task was. The ability to learn ambiguous associations could then serve as a marker task for the development of the more complex forms of attention related to executive control by anterior, midline structures. Clohessy found that infants of 4 and 10 months learned to correctly anticipate the unambiguous returns to position 1 but showed no evidence of learning the context-dependent association.

By 18 months, infants are showing many signs of higher-level attentional control. This includes the "language explosion," emergence of multiple word utterances, the ability to sort and classify objects, and evidence of self-recognition (Meltzoff, 1990). There was clear evidence that the 18-month-old infants learned the context-dependent association (Posner, Rothbart, Thomas-Thrapp, and Gerardi, in press). Some infants showed by their correct anticipation that they had learned the skill very well and others showed little evidence of learning. This finding suggests that infants of that age are only beginning to acquire the ability to learn context-dependent sequencing, which would make it worthwhile to observe how this form of learning develops in somewhat older infants.

Posner et al. (in press) were also able to show some links between the learning by infants at that age and aspects of their language performance in daily life. A significant correlation was found between their laboratory performance in sequence learning and parental reports of the number of words the infant used. Although this link needs to be replicated and extended, it does provide tentative support for the development of higher-level supervisory attention systems in importance of both the learning of complex sequences and in the control of language during the second year of life.

CONCLUSIONS

The results summarized in this chapter describe areas of the brain that appear to be active during the functions described by Norman and Shallice, and requiring a degree of supervisory behavior or executive control. It is important to dissociate the components of executive control so as to provide a more analytic treatment at both the cognitive and anatomical levels. In this section we consider some current efforts that might yield dissociations of the components of executive function.

A basis for dissociating conscious experience from feelings of control arises in REM sleep (Hobson, 1989). Dreaming is clearly conscious experience, but except in the rare case of "lucid dreaming" this form of conscious behavior is not accompanied by feelings of control. Although the specific brain areas involved are unknown, REM sleep is known to involve the reduction or loss of the catecholamines, norepinephrine, and serotonin.

A number of recent theories have sought to determine the cognitive deficit arising from a loss of basal ganglia function. One way to characterize the deficit is to suppose that the basal ganglia are important for switching the organism between sets. Thus Parkinson's disease patients can show either a difficulty in turning on motor behavior or a similar reduction in the ability to shift task set (Hayes, Davidson, Keele, and Rafal, 1995). The basal ganglia are the source of dopamine input to the anterior cingulate, and thus the two frontal structures have a very close relationship. Moreover, studies of visual attention have provided rather specific hypotheses of how subcortical structure and cortical structures are coordinated in the act of orienting (Posner and Dehaene, 1994), which could serve as a model for more anterior systems.

Lateral frontal areas appear to be involved in holding information that is not currently present in front of the mind. Thus, monkey (Wilson, Scalaidhe, and Goldman-Rakic, 1993) and human data (Jonides, Smith, Koeppe, and Awh, 1993) point to the involvement of lateral frontal cortex in working memory. The close connection between executive function and temporary representations has played a prominent role in theories of working memory (Baddeley, 1986), and the close anatomical connections between the anterior cingulate and lateral areas of the frontal cortex may be the basis of that connection. Some places where this might occur are outlined below.

An important aspect of coherent behavior is possession of a set of goals (goal tree) that can control current behavior (Carbonnell, 1981). Recently, Duncan (1986, 1995) has argued that goal neglect, in which subjects are less able to order and implement a set of instructed goals, can arise from frontal lesions. It is likely that the orbitofrontal area may be of central importance to this executive function.

The analysis of executive function as a unified aspect of attention has progressed substantially in terms of both cognitive criteria and brain function. The prospect of further dissociation of some of these functions and their identification with particular structures lies largely in the future. Of course, executive control raises the problem of the homunculus; but, as Attneave (1959) first suggested, progress is made by dissociating operations from the overall homunculus one component at a time. As this efforts proceeds, it may be possible to understand to what extent executive attention is best thought of as a unitary system or as a more distributed system.

ACKNOWLEDGMENTS

This research was supported by the Office of Naval Research contract 0014-89-J3013 and by the James S. McDonnell Foundation and Pew Memorial Trusts through the support of the Center for the Cognitive Neuroscience of Attention.

REFERENCES

Abdullaev, Y. G. and Posner, M. I. (1997) Time course of activating brain areas in generating verbal associations. *Psychol. Sci.* 8: 56–59.

Allport, D. A. (1980a) Attention and performance. In *Cognitive Psychology*, edited by G. Claxton, pp. 112–153. London: Routledge and Kegan Paul.

Allport, D. A. (1980b) Patterns and actions: Cognitive mechanisms are content-specific. In *Cognitive Psychology*, edited by G. Claxton, pp. 26–64. London: Routledge and Kegan Paul.

Allport, D. A., Styles, E., and Hsieh, S. (1994) Shifting intentional set: Exploring the dynamic control of tasks. In *Attention and Performance XV: Conscious and Nonconscious Information Processing*, edited by C. Umilta and M. Moscovitch, pp. 421–452. Cambridge, MA: MIT Press.

Attneave, F. (1959) In defense of the homunculi. In *Sensory Communication: Contributions to the Symposium on Principles of Sensory Communication*, edited by W. A. Rosenblith, pp. 777–782. Cambridge, MA: MIT Press.

Baddeley, A. D. (1986) *Working Memory*. Oxford: Clarendon Press.

Ballantine, H. T., Levy, B. S., Dagi, T. F., and Giriunas, I. B. (1977) Cingulotomy for psychiatric illness: Report of 13 years' experience. In *Neurosurgical Treatment in Psychiatry, Pain, and Epilepsy*, edited by W. H. Sweet, S. Obrador, and J. G. Martin-Rodriguez, pp. 333–353. Baltimore: University Park.

Bench, C. J., Frith, C. D., Grasby, P. M., Friston, K. J., Paulesu, E., Frackowiak, R. S. J., and Dolan, R. J. (1993) Investigations of the functional anatomy of attention using the Stroop test. *Neuropsychologia* 31: 907–922.

Benes, F. M. (1993) Relationship of cingulate cortex to schizophrenia and other psychiatric disorders. In *Neurobiology of Cingulate Cortex and Limbic Thalamus*, edited by B. A. Vogt and M. Gabriel, pp. 581–605. New York: Birkhauser.

Broadbent, D. E. (1958) *Perception and Communication*. London: Plenum Press.

Broadbent, D. E. (1973) *Decision and Stress*. New York: Academic Press.

Carbonnell, J. (1981) *Subjective Understanding of Belief Systems*. Ann Arbor, MI: University of Michigan Press.

Carter, C. S., Mintun, M., and Cohen, J. D. (1995) Interference and facilitation effects during selective attention: An H_2 ^{15}O PET study of stroop task performance. *Neuroimage* 2: 264–272.

Clohessy, A. B. (1994) Visual anticipation and sequence learning in four and ten-month-old infants and adults. Unpublished doctoral dissertation. University of Oregon.

Colebatch, J. M., Cunningham, V. J., Deiber, M. P., Frackowiak, R. S. J., and Passingham, R. E. (1991) Regional cerebral blood flow during unilateral arm and hand movements in human volunteers. *J. Neurophysiol.* 65: 1392–1401.

Corbetta, M., Miezin, F. M., Dobmeyer, S., Shulman, G. L., and Petersen, S. E. (1991) Selective and divided attention during visual discrimination of shape, color, and speed: Functional anatomy by positron emission tomography. *J. Neurosci.* 11: 2383–2402.

Corkin, S., Twitchell, T. E., and Sullivan, E. V. (1979) Safety and efficacy of cingulotomy for pain and psychiatric disorders. In *Modern Concepts in Psychiatric Surgery*, edited by E. R. Hitchcock, H. T. Ballantine, and B. A. Meyerson, pp. 129–163. Amsterdam: Elsevier.

Corteen, R. S. and Dunn, D. (1974) Shock-associated words in nonattended message: A test for momentary awareness. *J. Exp. Psychol.* 102: 1143–1144.

Corteen, R. S. and Wood, B. (1972) Autonomic response for shock associated words in an unattended channel. *J. Exp. Psychol.* 94: 308–313.

Curran, T. and Keele, S. W. (1993) Attentional and nonattentional forms of sequence learning. *J. Exp. Psychol. Learn. Mem. Cogn.* 19: 189–202.

Damasio, A. R. (1994) *Descartes' Error: Emotion, Reason, and the Human Brain*. New York: G. P. Putnam.

Dawson, M. E. and Schell, A. M. (1982) Electrodermal responses to attended and unattended significant stimuli during dichotic listening. *J. Exp. Psychol. Hum. Percept. Perform.* 8: 315–324.

Dehaene, S., Posner, M. I., and Tucker, D. M. (1994) Localization of a neural system for error detection and compensation. *Psychol. Sci.* 5: 303–305.

Deiber, M. P., Passingham, R. E., Colebach, J. G., Friston, K. J., Nixon, P. D., and Frackowiak, R. S. J. (1991) Cortical areas and the selection of movement: A study with positron emission tomography. *Exp. Brain Res.* 84: 393–402.

Desimone, R. and Duncan, J. (1995) Neural mechanisms of selective attention. *Annu. Rev. Neurosci.* 18: 193–222.

Dolan, R. J., Fletcher, P., Frith, C. D., Friston, K. J., Frackowiak, R. S. J., and Grasby, P. M. (1995) Dopaminergic modulation of impaired cognitive activation in the anterior cingulate cortex in schizophrenia. *Science* 378: 180–182.

Duncan, J. (1980) The locus of interference in the perception of simultaneous stimuli. *Psychol. Rev.* 87: 272–300.

Duncan, J. (1986) Disorganization of behavior after frontal lobe damage. Cognitive *Neuropsychol.* 3: 271–290.

Duncan, J. (1995) Attention, intelligence and frontal lobes. In *The Cognitive Neurosciences*, edited by M. S. Gazzaniga, pp. 721–733. Cambridge: MIT Press.

Duncan, J., Burgess, P., and Emslie, H. (1995) Fluid intelligence after frontal lobe lesion. *Neuropsychologia* 33: 261–268.

Early, T. S., Posner, M. I., Reiman, E. M., and Raichle, M. E. (1989a) Hyperactivity of the left striato-pallidal projection. Part I: Lower level theory. *Psychiatr. Dev.* 2: 85–108.

Early, T. S., Posner, M. I., Reiman, E. M. and Raichle, M. E. (1989b) Left striato-pallidal hyperactivity in schizophrenia. Part II: Phenomenology and thought disorders. *Psychiatr. Dev.* 2: 109–121.

Eriksen, B. A. and Eriksen, C. W. (1974) Effects of noise letters upon identification of a target letter in a nonsearch task. *Percept. Psychophys.* 16: 143–149.

Frith, C. D. (1992) *The Cognitive Neuropsychology of Schizophrenia*. Hillsdale, NJ: Lawrence Erlbaum.

Gehring, W. J., Gross, B., Coles, M. G. H., Meyer, D. E. and Donchin, E. (1993) A neural system for error detection and compensation. *Psychol. Sci.* 4: 385–390.

George, M. S., Ketter, T. A., Parekh, P. I., Rosinsky, N., Ring, H., Casey, B. J., Trimble, M. R., Horwitz, B., Herscovitch, P., and Post, R. M. (1994) Regional brain activity when selecting response despite interference: An H_2 ^{15}O PET study of the Stroop and an emotional Stroop. *Hum. Brain Map.* 1: 194–209.

Goldman-Rakic, P. S. (1988) Topography of cognition: Parallel distributed networks in primate association cortex. *Annu. Rev. Neurosci.* 11: 137–156.

Grafton, S. T., Hazelton, E. and Ivry, R. (1995) Functional mapping of sequence learning in normal humans. *J. Cognitive Neurosci.* 7: 497–510.

Hayes, A, Davidson, M., Keele, S. W., and Rafal, R. (1995, April) Toward a functional analysis of the basal ganglia. Paper presented at the 2nd annual meeting of the Cognitive Neuroscience Society, San Francisco.

Heinze, H. J., Mangun, G. R., Burchert, W., Hinrichs, H., Scholtz, M., Muntel, T. F., Gosel, A., Scherg, M., Johannes, S., Hundeshagen, H., Gazzaniga, M. S., and Hillyard, S. A. (1994) Combined spatial and temporal imaging of brain activity during visual selective attention in humans. *Nature* 372: 543–546.

Hobson, J. A. (1989) *Sleep*. New York: Scientific American Library.

Janer, K. W. and Pardo, J. V. (1991) Deficits in selective attention following bilateral anterior cingulotomy. *J. Cognitive Neurosci*. 3: 231–241.

Jonides, J., Smith, E. E., Koeppe, R. A., and Awh, E. (1993) Spatial working memory in humans as revealed by PET. *Nature* 363: 623–625.

Kennard, M. A. (1954) Effect of bilateral ablation of cingulate area on behavior of cats. *J. Neurophysiol*. 18: 159–169.

Kennard, M. A. (1955) The cingulate gyrus in relation to consciousness. *J. Nerv. Ment. Dis*. 121: 34–39.

Klein, G. S. (1964) Semantic power measured through interference of words with color-naming. *Am. J. Psychol*. 77: 576–588.

Luck, S. J., Heinze, H. J., Mangun, G. R., and Hillyard, S. A. (1990) Visual event-related potentials index focused attention within bilateral stimulus arrays. II. Functional dissociations of P1 and N1 components. *Electroencephalogr. Clin. Neurophysiol*. 75: 528–542.

MacLeod, C. M. (1991) Half a century of research on the Stroop effect: An integrative review. *Psychol. Bull*. 109: 163–209.

Maruff, P., Currie, J., Hay, D., McArthur-Jackson, C. and Malone, V. (1995) Asymmetries in the cover orienting of visual spatial attention in schizophrenia. *Neuropsychologia* 31: 1205–1223.

Meltzoff, A. N. (1990) Towards a developmental cognitive science. In *The Development and Neural Bases of Higher Cognitive Functions*, edited by A. Diamond, pp. 1–37. New York: New York Academy of Sciences.

Motter, B. C. (1993) Focal attention produces spatially selective processing in visual cortical areas V1, V2, and V4 in the presence of competing stimuli. *J. Neurophysiol*. 70: 909–919.

Näätänen, R. (1992) *Attention and Brain Function*. Hillsdale, NJ: Lawrence Erlbaum.

Nakagawa, A. (1991) Role of anterior and posterior attention networks in hemispheric asymmetries during lexical decisions. *J. Cognitive Neurosci*. 3: 313–321.

Newell, A., and Simon, H. A. (1972) *Human Problem Solving*. Engelwood Cliffs, NJ: Prentice-Hall.

Norman, D. A., and Shallice, T. (1980) *Attention to Action: Willed and Automatic Control of Behavior* (Technical Report No. 99). La Jolla, CA: Center for Human Information Processing.

Norman, D. A., and Shallice, T. (1986) Attention to action: Willed and automatic control of behavior. In *Consciousness and Self-Regulation*, edited by R. J., Davidson, G. E. Schwartz, and D. Shapiro, pp. 1–18. New York: Plenum Press.

Ostry, D., Moray, N., and Marks, J. (1976) Attention practice and semantic targets. *J. Exp. Psychol. Hum. Percept. Perform*. 2: 326–336.

Pardo, J. V., Pardo, P. J., Janer, K. W., and Raichle, M. E. (1990) The anterior cingulate cortex mediates processing selection in the Stroop attentional conflict paradigm. *Proc. Natl. Acad. Sci. USA* 87: 256–259.

Pashler, H. (1993) Dual-task interference and elementary psychological mechanisms. In *Attention and Performance XIV: Synergies in Experimental Psychology, Artificial Intelligence, and Cognitive Neuroscience*, edited by D. E. Meyer and S. Kornblum, pp. 245–264. Cambridge, MA: MIT Press.

Pashler, H., and Johnston, J. C. (1989) Chronometric evidence of central postponement in temporally overlapping tasks. *Q. J. Exp. Psychol.* 41A: 19–45.

Perret, E. (1973) The left frontal lobe of man and the suppression of habitual responses in verbal categorical behavior. *Neuropsychologia* 12: 323–330.

Petersen, S. E., Fox, P. T., Posner, M. I., Mintun, M., and Raichle, M. E. (1988) Positron emission tomography studies of the cortical anatomy of single-word processing. *Nature* 331: 585–588.

Petersen, S. E., Fox, P. T., Posner, M. I., Mintun, M. A., and Raichle, M. E. (1989) Positron emission tomography studies of the processing of single words *J. Cognitive Neurosci.* 1: 153–170.

Posner, M. I. (1978) *Chronometric Explorations of Mind.* Hillsdale, NJ: Lawrence Erlbaum.

Posner, M. I., and Dehaene, S. (1994) Attentional networks. *Trends Neurosci.* 17: 75–79.

Posner, M. I., Early, T. S., Reiman, E., Pardo, P. J., and Dhawan, M. (1988) Asymmetries in hemispheric control of attention in schizophrenia. *Arch. Gen. Psychiatry* 45: 814–821.

Posner, M. I., Petersen, S. E., Fox, P. T., and Raichle, M. E. (1988) Localization of cognitive operations in the human brain. *Science* 240: 1627–1631.

Posner, M. I., and Raichle, M. E. (1994) *Images of Mind.* New York: Scientific American Library.

Posner, M. I., Rothbart, M. K., Thomas-Thrapp, L., and Gerardi, G. (in press) Development of orienting to locations and objects. In *Visual Attention,* edited by R. Wright. New York: Oxford University Press.

Posner, M. I., Sandson, J., Dhawan, M., and Shulman, G. L. (1989) Is word recognition automatic? A cognitive anatomical approach. *J. Cognitive Neurosci.* 1: 50–60.

Posner, M. I., and Snyder, C. R. (1975) Facilitation and inhibition in the processing of signals. In *Attention and Performance V,* edited by P. M. A. Rabbit and S. Dornic, pp. 669–682 New York: Academic Press.

Raichle, M. E., Fiez, J. A., Videen, T. O., MacLeod, A. M. K., Pardo, J. V., Fox, P. T., and Petersen, S. E. (1994) Practice-related changes in human brain functional anatomy during nonmotor learning. *Cereb. Cortex* 4: 8–26.

Raymond, J., Shapiro, K. L., and Arnell, K. M. (1995) Similarity and the attentional blink. *J. Exp. Psychol. Hum. Percept. Perform.* 21: 653–662.

Rogers, R. D., and Monsell, S. (1995) Costs of a predictable switch between simple cognitive tasks. *J. Exp. Psychol. Gen.* 124: 207–221.

Rugg, M. D., and Coles, M. G. H. (Eds.) (1995) *Electrophysiology of Mind.* Oxford: Oxford University Press.

Scherg, M., (1989) Fundamentals of dipole source analysis. In *Auditory Evoked Magnetic Fields and Potentials: Advances in Audiology,* edited by F. Granooli, and G. L. Romani. pp. 1–30. Karger: Basal.

Shallice, T. (1988) *From Neuropsychology to Mental Structure.* New York: Cambridge University Press.

Shallice, T. (1994) Multiple levels of control processes. In *Attention and Performance XV: Conscious and Nonconscious Information Processing,* edited by C. Umilta and M. Moscovitch, pp. 395–420. Cambridge, MA: MIT Press.

Shallice, T. and Burgess, P. W. (1991a) Deficits in strategy applications following frontal lobe damage in man. *Brain* 114: 727–741.

Shallice, T. and Burgess, P. W. (1991b) Higher-order cognitive impairments and frontal lobe lesions in man. In *Frontal Lobe Function and Injury,* edited by H. S. Levin, H. M. Eisenberg, and A. L. Benton, pp. 125–138. New York: Oxford University Press.

Shallice, T., Burgess, P., Schon, F., and Baxter, D. (1989) The origins of utilization behavior. *Brain* 112: 1587–1598.

Shapiro, K. L., Raymond, J. E., and Arnell, K. M. (1994) Attention to visual pattern information produces the attentional blink in rapid serial visual presentation. *J. Exp. Psychol. Hum. Percept. Perform.* 20: 357–371.

Shiffrin, R. M., McKay, D. P. O., and Shaffer, W. O. (1977) Attending to 49 positions at once. *J. Exp. Psychol. Hum. Percept. Perform.* 2: 14–22.

Simpson, G. B. (1984) Lexical ambiguity and its role in models of word recognition. *Psychol. Bull.* 96: 316–340.

Snyder, A., Abdullaev, Y. G., Posner, M. I., and Raichle, M. E. (1995) Scalp electrical potentials reflect regional cerebral blood flow responses during processing of written words. *Proc. Natl. Acad. Sci. USA* 92: 1689–1693.

Spector, A. and Biederman, I. (1976) Mental set and mental shift revisited. *Am. J. Psychol.* 89: 669–679.

Spitzer, H. R., Desimone, R., and Moran, J. (1988) Increased attention enhances both behavioral and neuronal performance. *Science* 240: 338–340.

Stroop, J. R. (1935) Studies of interference in serial verbal reactions. *J. Exp. Psychol.* 18: 643–662.

Taylor, S. F., Kornblum, S., Minoshima, S., Oliver, L. M., and Koeppe, R. A. (1994) Changes in medial cortical blood flow with a stimulus-response compatibility task. *Neuropsychologia* 32: 249–255.

Treisman, A. M. and Geffen, G. (1967) Selective attention: Perception or response? *Q. J. Exp. Psychol.* 19: 1–18.

Tucker, D. M., Liotti, M., Potts, G. F., Russell, G. S., and Posner, M. I. (1994) Spatiotemporal analysis of brain electrical fields. *Hum. Brain Map.* 1: 134–152.

Ward, A. A., Jr. (1948) The anterior cingulate gyrus and personality. In *The Frontal Lobes*, edited by Association for Research in Nervous and Mental Disease, pp. 438–445. Baltimore: Williams and Wilkins.

Wilson, F. A. W., Scalaidhe, S. P. O., and Goldman-Rakic, P. S. (1993) Dissociation of object and spatial processing domains in the primate prefrontal cortex. *Science* 260: 1955–1958.

Yantis, S. and Jonides, J. (1990) Abrupt visual onsets and selective attention: Voluntary versus automatic allocation. *J. Exp. Psychol. Hum. Percept. Perform.* 16: 121–134.

IV Development and Pathologies of Attention

19 Developing an Attentive Brain

Mark H. Johnson

ABSTRACT Evidence from cognitive neuroscience studies of visual attention in infants and in children is reviewed. Developments in overt orienting to peripheral stimuli in infants have been associated with the onset of functioning in several brain oculomotor pathways. Specifically, the development of those pathways allows for the ability to (1) inhibit automatic saccades, (2) generate anticipatory saccades, and (3) tolerate delays before a planned saccade. Attempts to study covert orienting in infants have involved observation of the effects of brief peripheral cues and measurements of heart rate–defined periods of sustained attention. These studies indicate that by about four months of age infants are capable of covert shifts of attention. Developments in covert attention that continue into childhood are also described. Finally, the role of attention in cognitive development is outlined, including the predictive value of infant attention for later development.

Two reciprocal but complementary issues regarding attention and development are discussed in this chapter. The first concerns what has been learned about visual attention from a developmental cognitive neuroscience approach. The neurodevelopmental approach involves a number of methods for studying the postnatal emergence of neural systems and the dissociation of hierarchically arranged systems. The hierarchical arrangement of neural systems is more difficult to study with neuropsychological investigations of adult attention (see Johnson and Gilmore, 1996). The second issue concerns the important role of attention during development in facilitating the specializations of neurocognitive processing that are observed in adults. A number of authors have speculated on the crucial role that attentional systems play in biasing the input to plastic cortical circuits and in the onset of regulation of behavior.

The chapter is split into three sections. The first two sections review much of what has been learned about attention from the neurodevelopmental approach. The first of these sections reviews overt shifts of attention and the second covert attentional processes. These sections focus mainly on research with infants, because it is during that early period of postnatal life that the brain develops most rapidly, a situation that makes comparison to cognitive changes easier at that early period than it is later in development. A further reason for the focus on infancy is that this is when attention plays the most critical role in guiding experience. The third section of the chapter illustrates

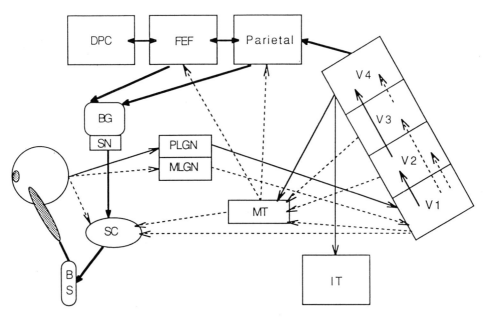

Figure 19.1 Representation of some of the main neural pathways and structures involved in visual orienting and attention in the primate brain. Solid lines indicate primarily parvocellular input, whereas the dashed arrows represent magnocellular input. Bold lines indicate mixed input. V1–V4, visual cortex; FEF, frontal eye fields; DPC, dorsolateral prefrontal cortex; BG, basal ganglia; SN, substantia nigra; MLGN and PLGN, magno and parvo portions of lateral geniculate; MT middle temporal area; IT, inferotemporal area; SC, superior colliculus; BS, brain stem.

some hypothesized roles of particular aspects of attention in structuring the young infant's interaction with the external world. It is proposed that early biases in attention contribute to the construction of the specialized cognitive architecture observed in adults.

VISUAL ORIENTING AND SPATIAL ATTENTION IN INFANTS

A number of transitions have been identified in both overt and covert visual attention during the first year of life (for recent reviews, see Johnson, 1994; Hood, 1995; Rothbart, Posner, and Rosicky, 1994), and some of those transitions have been attributed to the onset of functioning in regions of the cerebral cortex. Figure 19.1 shows a number of the neural circuits and structures that have been associated with overt and covert visual attention through neuroimaging and neuropsychological studies of human adults and through single-unit recording and lesion studies in nonhuman primates. Complementing this source of data is evidence on the postnatal development of the human cerebral cortex derived from postmortem tissue analysis and from functional and structural brain imaging. To briefly summarize this evidence, although most aspects of gross cortical structure, such as cell numbers and location, are in place at the time of birth in the human infant, more detailed aspects of cortical structure that presumably reflect functioning, such as synaptic density and glucose uptake, show prolonged postnatal development (for review, see Johnson, 1997). Furthermore, different regions of cortex show differential timing of postnatal functional development by these measures, which allows for the possibility of tracing the sequential development of neural pathways that may support particular components of visual orienting and attention. Another method for relating the functional development of brain circuits to cognitive transitions is to devise marker tasks (see Johnson and Gilmore, 1996). These are versions of tasks that have been associated with particular neural structures or circuits in cognitive neuroscience experiments and that are adapted to be suitable for infants. As discussed later, although the tasks are necessarily indirect, the use of marker tasks can provide a preliminary sketch of functional brain development and its relation to cognitive functioning.

The first systematic account of the relation between transitions in visual orienting capacities and cortical development was Bronson's (1974, 1982). He proposed that visually guided behavior in the newborn human infant is controlled primarily by means of the subcortical retinocollicular pathway, and that it is only by around two to three months of age that control shifts to cortical pathways. Thus, according to Bronson, the development of visually guided behavior can be viewed as shift from subcortical to cortical processing. The claim that the primary visual pathway is not fully functional until around three months postnatal age has been supported by a variety of electrophysiological, neuroanatomical, and behavioral studies (for more recent reviews, see Atkinson 1984; Johnson, 1990). However, as is apparent from figure 19.1, more recent evidence from cognitive neuroscience indicates that several cortical streams of information processing influence visual orienting in the primate brain. Thus, both Atkinson (1984) and Johnson (1990) have argued that the original cortical versus subcortical dichotomy for the ontogeny of visual processing inadequately captures the complexity of the likely neural developments and behavioral transitions observed.

Johnson (1990) proposed that, first, the characteristics of visually guided behavior of the infant at particular ages is determined by which of the pathways (shown in figure 19.1) is functional, and that, second, which of those pathways is functional is influenced by the developmental state of the primary visual cortex. The basis of the claim at the neuroanatomical level lies in three sets of observations: first, that the primary visual cortex is the major (though not exclusive) gateway for input to most of the cortical pathways involved in oculomotor control (Schiller, 1985); second, the primary visual cortex shows a postnatal continuation of the prenatal "inside-out" pattern of growth of the cortex, with the deeper layers (5 and 6) showing greater dendritic branching, length, and extent of myelinization than the more superficial layers (2 and 3) around the time of birth; third, there is a restricted pattern of inputs and outputs from the primary visual cortex (e.g., the efferents to area V2 depart from the upper layers) (for example, see Rockland and

Pandya, 1979; Burkhalter and Bernardo, 1989). By combining those observations with information about the developmental neuroanatomy of the primary visual cortex, Johnson (1990) hypothesized the following sequence of development of cortical pathways underlying oculomotor control: the subcortical pathway from the eye directly to the superior colliculus, followed by cortical projections from the deeper layers of area V1 to superior colliculus, followed by the pathway through MT, followed by pathways from area V1 to area V2 and on to the frontal eye fields and related structures.

To begin with the newborn infant, evidence from measures of the extent of dendritic arborization and myelinization indicate that only the deeper layers of the primary visual cortex are capable of supporting organized information-processing activity in the human newborn. Because the majority of feedforward intracortical projections depart from outside the deeper layers (5 and 6), some of the cortical pathways involved in oculomotor control may only be receiving weak or disorganized input at this stage. However, evidence from various sources, such as visual event-related potentials (ERPs), indicate that information from the eye is entering the primary visual cortex in the newborn. Thus, although some of the newborn's visual behavior can be accounted for in terms of processing in the subcortical pathway, Johnson (1990) has argued that information processing is also occurring in the deeper cortical layers at birth. Several characteristics of visually guided behavior in the newborn are consistent with predominantly, but not exclusively, subcortical control.

1. The visual tracking of a moving stimulus in the newborn has two characteristics. First, it is saccadic or steplike in manner, as opposed to the smooth manner of pursuit found in adults and in older infants. Second, the eye movements always lag behind the movement of the stimulus, rather than predicting its trajectory. Therefore, when a newborn infant visually tracks a moving stimulus, it could be described as performing a series of reorientations, behavior consistent with collicular control of orienting (for details, see Johnson, 1990).

2. Newborns more readily orient toward stimuli in the temporal, as opposed to in the nasal, visual field (e.g., Lewis, Maurer, and Milewski, 1979). Midbrain structures such as the colliculus can be driven most readily by temporal field input (Posner and Rothbart, 1980; Rafal, Smith, Kranz, Cohen, and Brennan, 1990). Recent evidence from studies of infants with complete hemispherectomy indicate that the subcortical (collicular) pathway is capable of supporting saccades toward a peripheral stimulus in the cortically blind field (Braddick et al., 1992).

3. Infants in the first few months of life do not attend to stationary pattern elements within a larger frame or pattern (e.g., Maurer, 1983) unless those elements are moving (Bushnell, 1979), the so-called externality effect. Johnson (1990) proposed that part of the explanation could be ascribed to a collicular

mechanism attempting to shift the retinal image of the largest frame or pattern elements onto the foveal field.

Around one month of age infants show obligatory attention (Stechler and Latz, 1966; Johnson, Dziurawiec, Ellis, and Morton, 1991; Hood, 1995). That is, they have great difficulty disengaging their gaze from a stimulus in order to saccade elsewhere. Although the phenomenon is still poorly understood, Johnson (1990) has suggested that it is due to the development of tonic inhibition of the colliculus via the substantia nigra (see figure 19.1). Because it projects from the deeper layers of the primary visual cortex, that pathway is hypothesized to be the first strong cortical influence on oculomotor control. One consequence of the (as yet) unregulated tonic inhibition of the colliculus is that stimuli impinging on the peripheral visual field no longer elicit an automatic exogenous saccade as readily as they do in newborns.

By about two months of age, infants begin to show periods of smooth visual tracking, although their eye movements still lag behind the movement of the stimulus. At this age they also become more sensitive to stimuli placed in the nasal visual field (Aslin, 1981) and more sensitive to coherent motion (R. Spitz, personal communication, 1992). Johnson (1990) has proposed that the onset of those behaviors coincides with the functioning of the pathway involving structure MT. The enabling of that route of eye movement control may provide the cortical magnocellular stream with the ability to regulate activity in the superior colliculus.

Due to further dendritic growth and myelinization within the upper layers of the primary visual cortex that strengthen projections to other cortical areas, around three months of age the pathways involving the frontal eye fields (FEF) may become available. That development may greatly increase the infant's ability to make anticipatory eye movements and to learn sequences of looking patterns. With regard to the visual tracking of a moving object, infants now not only show periods of smooth tracking, but their eye movements often predict the movement of the stimulus in an anticipatory manner. Experiments by Haith, Hazan, and Goodman (1988) have demonstrated that anticipatory eye movements can be readily elicited from infants by this age. They exposed 3.5-month-old infants to a series of picture slides that appeared either on the right- or left-hand side of the infant. The stimuli were either presented in an alternating sequence with fixed interstimulus interval (ISI) or with an irregular alternation pattern and irregular ISI. The regular alternation pattern produced more stimulus anticipations, and reaction times to make an eye movement were reliably faster than in the irregular series. Haith and colleagues concluded from these results that infants of this age are able to develop expectancies for noncontrollable spatiotemporal events. Canfield and Haith (1991) tested two- and three-month-old infants in a similar experiment that included more complex sequences (such as left-left-right, left-left-right). Although they failed to find significant effects with two-month-olds, three-month-olds appeared to able to acquire at least some of the more complex sequences. Additional evidence for the onset of FEF functioning in the first half year of life comes from the so-called anti-saccade task.

Frontal cortex damage in humans results in an inability to suppress involuntary automatic saccades toward targets and an apparent inability to control volitional saccades (Fischer and Breitmeyer, 1987; Guitton, Buchtel, and Douglas, 1985). For example, Guitton et al. (1985) studied normal adults and patients with frontal lobe lesions or temporal lobe lesions in an anti-saccade task. In this task participants are instructed to not look at a briefly flashed cue, but to make a saccade in the opposite direction instead (Hallett, 1978). Guitton et al. (1985) reported that, whereas normal participants and patients with temporal lobe damage could do the task with relative ease, patients with frontal damage, and especially those with damage around the FEF, were severely impaired. In particular, the frontal patients had difficulty suppressing unwanted saccades toward the cue stimulus.

Johnson (1994, 1995) developed a version of the anti-saccade task for use with infants. Clearly, one cannot give verbal instruction to a young infant to look to the side opposite from where the cue stimulus appears. Instead, infants are motivated to look at the second of two opposite peripheral stimuli more than at the first stimulus. This can be done by making the second stimulus reliably more dynamic and colorful than the first. Thus, after a number of such trials infants may learn to inhibit their tendency to make a saccade to the first stimulus (the cue) when it appears, in order to respond as rapidly as possible to the more attractive second stimulus (the target). A group of four-month-old infants showed a significant decrease in their frequency of looking to the first (cue) stimulus over a number of such trials (Johnson, 1995). A second experiment demonstrated that the decrement was not due to differential habituation to the simpler stimulus. Because six-month-olds are able to inhibit saccades to a peripheral stimulus, it is reasonable to infer that their FEF circuits are functioning by that age.

Other tasks recently conducted with infants are consistent with an increase in prefrontal cortex endogenous control over shifts of attention and saccades at around six months of age. Investigation of the neural basis of the oculomotor delayed response (ODR) task began with a study by Funahashi, Bruce, and Goldman-Rakic (1989, 1990), who demonstrated that neurons in the principal sulcus of the macaque monkey have specific patterns of activity during a delayed response task. In this task, rhesus monkeys were trained to fixate a central spot while a brief cue appeared in one of eight locations in the visual periphery. The monkeys were rewarded for maintaining fixation throughout a variable delay period of one to five seconds and for making an eye movement to the location where the cue had appeared once the central fixation stimulus had turned off. Funahashi et al. (1989, 1990) recorded neurons in the principal sulcus and in the frontal eye fields, a brain region implicated in the volitional control of eye movements. They observed that specific neurons were maintaining a representation of the cued location during the delay period. Eighty percent of the cells active during the delay

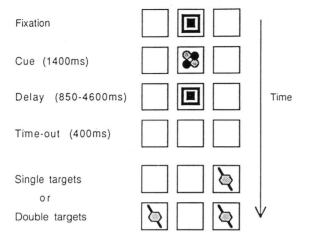

Figure 19.2 The sequence of stimuli used in Gilmore and Johnson (1995), experiment 2.

period had receptive fields that coded the direction of the cue and subsequent eye movement. Funahashi et al. (1989, 1990) argued that these results reflect the common function of the prefrontal cortex in delayed response tasks in both the visual and motor domains: specifically, the maintenance of information during short delay periods about spatial locations important for later action. This role was confirmed by reversible microlesions to the area, which resulted in selective amnesia for saccades to a localized part of the visual field. A recent positron emission tomography (PET) study on human subjects has confirmed the involvement of prefrontal cortex (and parietal cortex) in this task (Jonides et al., 1993).

Given the considerable interest in the possible functional consequences of the development of the dorsolateral prefrontal cortex (DLPC) in the human infant (see Diamond, 1991), Gilmore and Johnson (1995) devised two versions of the ODR task suitable for administering to human infants. One version is shown in figure 19.2. In terms of the sequence of stimulus presentation, this version of the task closely resembles that used by Jonides et al. (1993). Unlike the human adult version of the task, however, infants do not accept verbal instruction. Neither can a very large number of training trials be administered for food or water reward as in the monkey studies. Instead, one has to rely on the intrinsic motivation provided by attractive dynamic visual stimuli and on relatively rapid trial-by-trial learning. These differences in task motivation contribute to the caution required in interpreting the results. However, in both peripheral and central cueing versions of the task, six-month-old infants were able to tolerate delays of up to 5 seconds before making a saccade to a previously cued target location, a pattern of performance comparable to the adult monkeys studied by Funahashi and colleagues (Funahashi, Bruce and Goldman-Rakic, 1989, 1990). These results suggest that the DLPC influences oculomotor control by six months of age in the human infant.

Johnson: Developing an Attentive Brain

THE DEVELOPMENT OF COVERT ATTENTION

The discussion so far has concerned overt shifts of attention due to eye and head movements. It is evident that adults are also capable of shifting their attention covertly (without moving the receptors). One way in which evidence for covert attention in adults has been provided is by studying the effect on detection of cueing saccades to a particular spatial location. A briefly presented cue serves to draw covert attention to the location, resulting in the subsequent facilitation of detection of targets at that location (Posner and Cohen, 1980; Maylor, 1985). Although facilitation of detection and responses to a covertly attended location occurs if the target stimulus appears very shortly after the cue offset, with longer latencies between cue and target inhibition of saccades toward that location occurs (see Rafal, chapter 22, this volume).

Following lesions to the posterior parietal lobe, adults show severe neglect of the contralateral visual field. According to Posner and colleagues this neglect is due to damage to the posterior attention network—a brain circuit that includes not only the posterior parietal lobe, but also the pulvinar and superior colliculus (Posner, 1988; Posner and Petersen, 1990; see figure 19.1 for all but the pulvinar). Damage to this circuit is postulated to impair subjects' ability to shift covert attention to a cued spatial location. The involvement of those regions in shifts of visual attention has been confirmed by PET studies (see Corbetta, chapter 6, this volume). Both neuroanatomical (Conel, 1939/1967) and PET (Chugani, Phelps, and Mazziotta, 1987) evidence from the human infant indicate that the parietal lobe undergoes substantive and rapid development between three and six months after birth. The question arises, therefore, as to whether infants become capable of covert shifts of attention during this time.

Because infants do not accept verbal instruction and are poor at the motor responses that are used to study spatial attention in adults such as a key press, the only response available to demonstrate facilitation and inhibition of a cued location is eye movements. That is, overt shifts are used to study covert shifts of attention by examining the influence of a cue stimulus (which is presented so briefly that it does not normally elicit an eye movement) on infants' subsequent saccades toward conspicuous target stimuli. Using these methods, Hood and Atkinson (1991; see Hood, 1995) reported that six-month-old infants had faster reaction times to make a saccade to a target when it appeared immediately after a brief (100 ms) cue stimulus than when it appeared in an uncued location. A group of three-month-old infants did not show this effect. Johnson (1994; Johnson and Tucker, 1996) employed a similar procedure in which a brief (100 ms) cue was presented on one of two side screens before bilateral targets were presented either 100 ms or 600 ms later. It was hypothesized on the basis of the adult findings that the 200 ms stimulus onset asynchrony (SOA) would be short enough to produce facilitation, whereas the long SOA trials would result in preferential orienting toward the opposite side (inhibition of return). This result was obtained with a group of four-month-old infants, which suggests the possibility that infants are capable of covert shifts of attention at that age. Consistent with the findings discussed previously, these effects were not observed in a group of two-month-old infants.

At present it remains an open question whether the facilitation produced by the cue in these experiments is the result of direct priming of the eye movement system, or whether the eye movements are following an independent covert shift of attention. Although eye movement has also been used in some adult studies purporting to examine shifts of covert attention (e.g., Maylor, 1985; Posner, Rafal, Choate, and Vaughan, 1985), the use of this output measure raises alternative hypotheses regarding the facilitatory effects of the cue. There are at least three ways in which a spatial cue could affect saccadic latency and direction: (1) the cue stimulus itself directly initiates the saccade; (2) the cue alters the threshold for planning a saccade to a particular location (motor priming); or (3) the cue drives covert shifts of attention (independent of the mechanisms of saccade planning), which then subsequently influences eye movements. A variety of evidence has ruled out attribution of the facilitatory effects to a situation in which the cue directly drives eye movements (for discussion of this point, see Johnson, 1994; Johnson, Posner and Rothbart, 1994; Johnson and Tucker, 1996). The second possibility is that the facilitation effects observed are due to a spatially selective priming of the mechanisms that plan saccades. In this view, when the target appears, the cued location is responded to more rapidly and more frequently because the earlier presence of the cue reduces the threshold to initiate a saccade to that spatial location. Although such a mechanism may be considered an aspect of covert attention in the sense that a stimulus to which no overt response is made (the cue) influences subsequent responses to a target that occurs later, it does not require the existence of a covert attention system that is partially or wholly independent of eye movement planning and control. Currently, there is no behavioral data with infants that allows us to dissociate this possibility from an independent covert orienting system. Indeed, the relation between covert shifts of attention and saccade planning remains controversial in the adult literature (e.g., Klein, Kingstone, and Pontefract, 1992).

An alternative line of evidence relevant to covert attention in young infants comes from the research of Richards and colleagues on heart rate–defined sustained attention. Sustained attention refers to the ability of subjects to maintain the direction of their attention toward a stimulus even in the presence of distractors. Richards (1989a,b) has developed a heart rate marker for sustained attention in infants. The heart rate–defined period of sustained attention usually lasts for between 5 and 15 seconds after the onset of a complex stimulus. Figure 19.3 illustrates the heart rate–defined periods of sustained attention defined by Richards and Casey (1991).

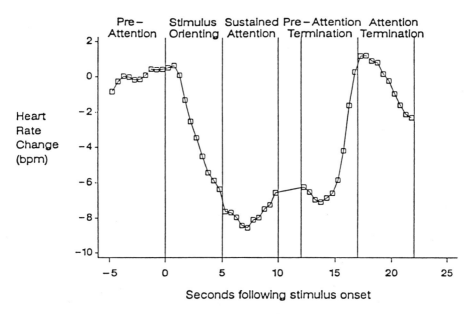

Figure 19.3 The heart rate–defined phases of sustained attention.

In order to investigate the effect of sustained attention on the response to exogenous cues, Richards (1989a,b) used an interrupted stimulus method in which a peripheral stimulus (a flashing light) was presented while the infant was gazing at a central stimulus (a complex visual pattern on a television screen). By varying the length of time between the onset of the television image and the onset of the peripheral stimulus, Richards was able to present the peripheral stimulus either within the period of sustained covert attention or outside it. Richards found that during the periods when heart rate was decreased (sustained endogenous attention) it took twice as long for the infants to shift their gaze toward the peripheral stimulus as when heart rate had returned to prestimulus levels (attention termination). Furthermore, those saccades that were made to a peripheral stimulus during sustained attention were less accurate than normal, and involved multiple hypometric saccades, which are characteristic of collicular-generated saccades (Richards, 1991). Thus, the lack of distractibility during periods of sustained attention is likely to be due to cortically mediated pathways that inhibit collicular mechanisms.

In summary, evidence for covert shifts of attention in the first six months of life is suggestive, but it is not yet conclusive. The advent of noninvasive neuroimaging methods, such as high-density ERP, offers the promise of observing measures of facilitation and inhibition other than eye movements. Studies in which heart rate measurements are correlated with ERPs during attention tasks may be particularly informative.

A number of studies have traced developments in visual attention during childhood using purely cognitive methods. Three developmental transitions that have been described are (1) the greater ability to expand or constrict a field of attention (e.g., Enns and Girgus, 1985; Chapman, 1981), (2) the greater ability to disengage attention from distracting information or invalid cueing (Akhtar and Enns, 1989; Enns and Brodeur, 1989), and (3) a faster speed of shifting attention (Pearson and Lane, 1990).

Enns and Girgus (1985) tested school-age children and adults in speeded classification tasks involving a stimulus composed of two elements that varied in distance (visual angle). Subjects had to classify stimuli on the basis of one of the two elements. Younger children (6–8 years) experienced more interference when the elements were closely spaced than did older children (9–11 years) or adults. The same stimuli were used for a second task in which both of the elements had to be taken into account. In that task the younger children had difficulty when the elements were separated by large visual angles. The authors concluded that younger children have problems in contracting and expanding the size of attentional focus. An ERP study of auditory attention also concluded that there is a development in the ability to narrow attentional focus during childhood (Berman and Freidman, 1995).

An observation that may be related is that older children and adults are often reported as being able to shift their attention more rapidly than younger children are able to. For example, Pearson and Lane (1990), using a spatial cueing paradigm, observed that younger infants took longer to covertly shift their attention to more peripheral targets, whereas they were almost as fast as adults to shift to targets very close to fixation. This indicates that it is the speed of shifting, rather than the latency to elicit a covert shift, that improves with age. The increasing speed of attentional shifts with age has also been reported during infancy (Johnson and Tucker, 1996), a report that indicates that this developmental transition may be a gradual one that begins early in life.

In several studies, younger children and infants have been argued to have greater difficulty in disengaging from distracting stimuli or invalid spatial cues. For example, Enns and Brodeur (1989) used a spatial cueing paradigm to either cue neutrally (all locations cued), unpredictably (random cueing), or predictably (cue predicted target presentation). The results from subjects aged 6, 8, and 20 years indicated that, although all age groups automatically oriented attention to the cued location, the children processed targets in noncued locations more slowly than adults, and did not take advantage of the predictability of the cues. Thus, the costs and benefits of cueing were greater in the younger subjects due to an increased cost imposed by invalid cueing. Tipper, Cameron, and Brehaut (1988) suggested that those deficits were due to the relative inability to inhibit irrelevant stimuli. Once again, similar developmental trends have been observed in infancy experiments in which younger infants were more likely to fail to disengage from competing stimuli (for reviews, see Johnson, 1995; Hood, 1995).

Very little work has been done on the neural basis of the development of covert orienting in childhood. However, some authors have attempted to study the development of visual attention in children with developmental disorders such as attention-deficit disorder (ADD) and autism and to correlate those with hypothesized neural deficits (see Swanson et al., chapter 20, this volume). For example, Courchesne and colleagues (Townsend and Courchesne, 1994; Akshoomoff and Courchesne, 1994) have tested autistic individuals on a variety of spatial cueing and attention switching tasks. They report, on the basis of autopsy and structural magnetic resonance imaging (MRI) data, that most autistic subjects have developmental damage to the cerebellum. In a number of tasks they have associated that damage with reduced ability to switch attention and with a slower shifting of covert spatial attention. Another neural deficit observed in at least some autistic subjects is bilateral parietal damage. Townsend and Courchesne (1994) have proposed that this damage gives rise to a narrowed focus of spatial attention, such that targets presented within the narrowed spotlight are detected more rapidly than normal. In contrast, targets presented at small eccentricities from fixation that would be responded to rapidly by normal subjects, are responded to much more slowly by autistic subjects because they are outside the narrow attentional focus.

THE ROLE OF ATTENTION IN DEVELOPMENT

This final section briefly outlines three of the ways in which attention is important during cognitive development (also, see Johnson, 1992). One line of evidence that visual attention is critical for normal cognitive development comes from the significant correlations that have been reported between components of visual attention in early infancy and subsequent measures of temperament and intelligence. Specifically, a number of laboratories have reported significant correlations between measures such as the extent of preferential looking to a novel stimulus (when paired with a familiar one) and subsequent IQ measures at school age (e.g., Fagan and McGrath, 1981; Fagan, 1984). Similar correlations have been reported for aspects of temperament (Rothbart and Derryberry, 1981; Johnson et al., 1991). Colombo (1993) has reviewed much of the evidence for correlations with IQ and has concluded that they are not due to methodological artefacts, and that two processes may underlie the continuity of performance: individual differences in the speed of visual information processing and the integrity of memory processes. In more recent work, Colombo (in press) has speculated on the neural basis of differences in the speed of visual information processing in infants. One hypothesis is that the magnocellular visual pathway is slower to develop than is the parvocellular. Information processing in infants whose magnocellular system development has been even further delayed would be dominated by parvocellular processing; such infants would thus be slower to process visual stimuli and would be more inclined to attend and encode detailed rather than global aspects of the stimulus. Another, nonorthogonal hypothesis is that immaturity of parietal cortex and the posterior attention system means that some individual infants continue to show the obligatory attention phenomenon, which was discussed earlier, beyond the normal age. Thus, such infants are less able to disengage their attention from the stimulus concerned and they therefore show longer looking times. These hypotheses merit further investigation.

Along with the continuity between infant attentional measures and subsequent cognitive abilities, attention in infancy and childhood is also important for the construction of normal adult neurocognitive systems. Young infants are predisposed to attend to certain types of stimuli in their world, such as novel objects, faces, and human speech. This early direction of attention may shape the specialization of cortical circuits over the first months of life. For example, Johnson and Morton (1991; Morton and Johnson, 1991) have reviewed much of the available evidence on the development of face recognition in human infants and have concluded that two mechanisms with independent neural substrates are involved: first, a preference for orienting to face-like patterns present from birth that is possibly mediated by midbrain circuitry; second, a later-emerging but more sophisticated face recognition system that is supported by cortical circuits. A key aspect of Johnson and Morton's proposal is that the first system ensures that developing cortical circuits are regularly exposed to faces, and thus plastic cortical circuits become configured to processing information about that class of stimulus. Similar general arguments have been applied to other domains, such as language acquisition (e.g., Jusczyk and Bertoncini, 1988).

A more sophisticated role for visual attention in cognitive development concerns shared attention with caregivers. This refers to the ability to detect the focus of attention of another person and to direct one's attention to the same location (Butterworth and Jarrett, 1991). Shared attention allows a child to be educated by its caregiver as to the nature of the stimulus that is the object of attention. This is a powerful mechanism for the education of the young by conspecifics, and has been argued to the basis for further developments in social as well as cognitive development (Baron-Cohen, 1991).

This chapter has briefly sketched out the importance of visual attention for cognitive development and has suggested that it can be informative about how the adult cortex develops specialization for processing certain kinds of stimuli. Conversely, taking a cognitive neuroscience approach to the development of attention has already significantly contributed to our understanding of the neural mechanisms of attention in both infants and adults.

CONCLUSIONS

1. Developments in visual orienting in infants can be related to the emergence of functioning in several cortical oculomotor pathways.

2. The development of oculomotor control in infants involves a transition to greater volitional control. This is evident from tasks in which infants are increasingly able to (1) inhibit automatic saccades, (2) produce anticipatory saccades, and (3) tolerate delays before a planned saccade.

3. By around four months of age infants may be capable of covert shifts of visual attention. However, covert attention continues to develop into childhood with regard to (1) the flexibility (changing size) of the attentional field, (2) the ability to disengage attention, and (3) the speed of attentional shifts.

4. Attention plays a critical role in cognitive development, and aspects of infant attention correlate with subsequent childhood measures of intelligence and temperament. Attention directed by endogenous biases (such as toward faces) or by caregivers (such as shared attention) plays an important role in constraining what aspects of the external environment infants and children learn about.

ACKNOWLEDGMENTS

The research was supported by the UK Medical Research Council and by the Human Frontiers Scientific Foundation. Sarah Hesketh assisted in the preparation of this chapter.

REFERENCES

Akhtar, N. and Enns, J. T. (1989) Relations between covert orienting and filtering in the development of visual attention. *J. Exp. Child Psychol.* 48: 315–334.

Akshoomoff, N. A. and Courchesne, E. (1994) ERP evidence for a shifting attention deficit in patients with damage to the cerebellum. *J. Cognitive Neurosci.* 6: 388–399.

Aslin, R. N. (1981) Development of smooth pursuit in human infants. In *Eye Movements: Cognition and Visual Perception*, edited by D. F. Fisher, R. A. Monty, and J. W. Senders, pp. 31–51. Hillsdale, NJ: Lawrence Erlbaum.

Atkinson, J. (1984) Human visual development over the first six months of life: A review and a hypothesis. *Hum. Neurobiol.* 3: 61–74.

Baron-Cohen, S. (1991) Precursors to a theory of mind: Understanding attention in others. In *Natural Theories of Mind*, edited by A. Whiten. Oxford: Blackwell. (pp. 233–251).

Berman, S., and Freidman, D. (1995) The development of selective attention as reflected by event—Related brain potentials. *J. Exp. Child Psychol.* 59: 1–31.

Braddick, O. J., Atkinson, J., Hood, B., Harkness, W., Jackson, G., and Vargha-Khadem, F. (1992) Possible blindsight in infants lacking one cerebral hemisphere. *Nature* 360: 461–463.

Bronson, G. W. (1974) The postnatal growth of visual capacity. *Child Deve.* 45: 873–890.

Bronson, G. W. (1982) The scanning patterns of human infants: Implications for visual learning. *Monographs on Infancy* 2: 136.

Burkhalter, A. and Bernardo, K. L. (1989) Organization of corticocortical connections in human visual cortex. *Proc. Natl. Acad. Sci. USA* 86: 1071–1075.

Bushnell, I. W. R. (1979) Modification of the externality effect in young infants. *J. Exp. Child Psychol.* 28: 211–229.

Butterworth, G. and Jarrett, N. (1991) What minds have in common is space: Spatial mechanisms serving joint visual attention in infancy. *Br. J. Dev. Psychol.* 9: 55–72.

Canfield, R. L. and Haith, M. M. (1991) Young infants' visual expectations for symmetric and asymmetric stimulus sequences. *Dev. Psychol.* 2: 198–208.

Chapman, M. (1981) Dimensional separability or flexibility of attention? Age trends in perceiving configural stimuli. *J. Exp. Child Psychol.* 31: 332–349.

Chugani, H. T., Phelps, M. E., and Mazziotta, J. C. (1987) Positron emission tomography study of human brain functional development. *Ann. Neurol.* 22: 487–497.

Columbo, J. (in press) On the neural mechanisms underlying developmental and individual differences in visual fixation in infanty: Two hypotheses. *Develop. Rev.*

Columbo, J. (1993). *Infant Cognition: Predicting Later Intellectual Functioning.* Individual Differences and Development Series, Vol. 5., Sage, CA.

Conel, J. L. (1967) *The Postnatal Development of the Human Cerebral Cortex.* Cambridge, MA: Harvard University Press. (Original work published 1939.)

Diamond, A. (1991) Neuropsychological insights into the meaning of object concept development. In *The Epigenesis of Mind: Essays on Biology and Cognition,* edited by S. Carey and R. Gelman. pp. 67–110. Hillsdale, NJ: Lawrence Erlbaum.

Enns, J. T. and Brodeur, D. A. (1989) A developmental study of covert orienting to peripheral visual cues. *J. Exp. Child Psychol.* 48: 171–189.

Enns, J. T. and Girgus, J. S. (1985) Developmental changes in selective and integrative visual attention. *J. Exp. Child Psychol.* 40: 315–334.

Fagan, J. F. (1984) The intelligent infant: Theoretical implications. *Intelligence* 8: 1–9.

Fagan, J. F. and McGrath, S. (1981) Infant recognition memory and later intelligence. *Intelligence* 5: 121–130.

Fischer, B. and Breitmeyer, B. (1987) Mechanisms of visual attention revealed by saccadic eye movements. *Neuropsychologia* 25: 73–83.

Funahashi, S., Bruce, C. J., and Goldman-Rakic, P. S. (1989) Mnemonic coding of visual space in the monkey's dorsolateral prefrontal cortex. *J. Neurophysiol.* 61: 331–349.

Funahashi, S., Bruce, C. J., and Goldman-Rakic, P. S. (1990) Visuospatial coding in primate prefrontal neurons revealed by oculomotor paradigms. *J. Neurophysiol.* 63: 814–831.

Gilmore, R. O. and Johnson, M. H. (1995) Working memory in six-month-old infants revealed by versions of the oculomotor delayed response task. *J. Exp. Child Psychol.* 59: 397–418.

Guitton, H. A., Buchtel, H. A., and Douglas, R. M. (1985) Frontal lobe lesions in man cause difficlties in suppressing reflexive glances and in generating goal-directed saccades. *Exp. Brain Res.* 58: 455–472.

Haith, M. M., Hazan, C., and Goodman, G. S. (1988) Expectation and anticipation of dynamic visual events by 3.5-month-old babies. *Child Dev.* 59: 467–479.

Hallett, P. E. (1978) Primary and secondary saccades to goals defined by instructions. *Vision Res.* 18: 1270–1296.

Hood, B. M. (1995) Visual selective attention in the human infant: A neuroscientific approach. In *Advances in Infancy Research 10,* edited by C. Rovee-Collier and L. Lipsitt. pp. 163–216. New York: Ablex.

Hood, B. M. and Atkinson, J. (1991) *Shifting covert attention in infants.* Paper presented at the conference of the Society for Research in Child Development, Seattle, WA.

Johnson, M. H. (1990) Cortical maturation and the development of visual attention in early infancy. *J. Cognitive Neurosci.* 2: 81–95.

Johnson, M. H. (1992) Cognitive development: Four contentions about the role of visual attention. In *Cognitive Science and Clinical Disorders*, edited by D. J. Stein and J. E. Young, pp. 43–60. San Diego: Academic Press.

Johnson, M. H. (1994) Visual attention and the control of eye movements in early infancy. In *Attention and Performance XV: Conscious and Nonconscious Processing*, edited by C. Umilta and M. Moscovitch, pp. 291–310. Cambridge, MA: MIT Press.

Johnson, M. H. (1995) The inhibition of automatic saccades in early infancy. *Dev. Psychobiol.* 28: 281–291.

Johnson, M. H. (1997) *Developmental Cognitive Neuroscience: An Introduction*. Oxford: Blackwell.

Johnson, M. H., Dziurawiec, S., Ellis, H. D., and Morton, J. (1991) Newborns' preferential tracking of face-like stimuli and its subsequent decline. *Cognition* 40: 1–19.

Johnson, M. H. and Gilmore, R. O. (1996) Developmental cognitive neuroscience: A biological perspective on cognitive change. In *Handbook of Perception and Cognition: Perceptual and Cognitive Development*, edited by R. Gelman and T. Au. pp. 333–372. Orlando, FL: Academic Press.

Johnson, M. H. and Morton, J. (1991) *Biology and Cognitive Development: The Case of Face Recognition*. Oxford: Blackwell.

Johnson, M. H., Posner, M. I., and Rothbart, M. K. (1994) Facilitation of saccades Toward a covertly attended location in early infancy. *Psychol. Sci.* 5: 90–93.

Johnson, M. H. and Tucker, L. A. (1996) The development and temporal dynamics of spatial orienting in infants. *J. Exp. Child. Psychol.* 63: 171–188.

Jonides, J., Smith, E. E., Koeppe, R. A., Awh, E., Minoshima, S., and Mintun, M. A. (1993) Spatial working memory in humans as revealed by PET. *Nature* 363: 623–625.

Jusczyk, P. W. and Bertoncini, J. (1988) Viewing the development of speech perception as an innately guided learning process. *Lang. Speech* 31: 217–238.

Klein, R. M., Kingstone, A., and Pontefract, A. (1992) Orienting of visual attention. In *Eye Movements and Visual Cognition*, edited by K. Rayner, pp. 46–65. New York: Springer.

Lewis, T. L., Maurer, D., and Milewski, A. (1979) The development of nasal detection in young infants. *Invest. Opthalmol. Vis. Sci.* Supplement 271.

Maurer, D. (1983) The scanning of compound figures by young infants. *J. Exp. Child Psychol.* 35: 437–448.

Maylor, E. A. (1985) Facilitory and inhibitory components of orienting in visual space. In *Attention and Performance XI*, edited by M. I. Posner and O. M. Marin, pp. 189–204. Hillsdale, NJ: Lawrence Erlbaum.

Morton, J. and Johnson, M. H. (1991) CONSPEC and CONLERN: A two-process theory of infant face recognition. *Psychol. Rev.* 98: 164–181.

Pearson, D. A. and Lane, D. M. (1990) Visual attention movements: A developmental study. *Child Dev.* 61: 1779–1795.

Posner, M. I. (1988) Structures and functions of selective attention. In *Clinical Neuropsychology and Brain Function: Research, Measurement, and Practice*, edited by T. Boll and B. Bryant, pp. 171–202. Washington, DC: American Psychological Association.

Posner, M. I. and Cohen, Y. (1980) Attention and the control of movements. In *Tutorials in Motor Behavior*, edited by G. E. Stelmach and J. Roguiro, pp. 243–258. Amsterdam: North Holland.

Posner, M. I. and Petersen, S. E. (1990) The attention system of the human brain. *Annu. Rev. Neurosci.* 13: 25–42.

Posner, M. I., Rafal, R. D., Choate, L. S., and Vaughan, J. (1985) Inhibition of return: neural basis and function. *Cognitive Neuropsychol.* 2: 211–228.

Posner, M. I. and Rothbart, M. K. (1980) The development of attentional mechanisms. In *Nebraska Symposium on Motivation*, edited by J. H. Flower. pp. 1–52. Lincoln, NE: University of Nebraska Press.

Rafal, R., Smith, J., Krantz, J., Cohen, A., and Brennan, C. (1990) Extrageniculate vision in hemi-anopic humans: Saccade inhibition by signals in the blind field. *Science* 250: 1507–1518.

Richards, J. E. (1989a) Development and stability of HR-defined, visual sustained attention in 14, 20, and 26 week old infants. *Psychophysiology* 26: 422–430.

Richards, J. E. (1989b) Sustained visual attention in 8-week old infants. *Infant Behav. Dev.* 12: 425–436.

Richards, J. E. (1991) Infant eye movements during peripheral visual stimulus localization as a function of central stimulus attention status. *Psychophysiology* 28, 54.

Richards, J. E. and Casey, B. J. (1991) Heart rate variability during attention phases in young infants. *Psychophysiology* 28: 43–53.

Rockland, K. S. and Pandya, D. N. (1979) Laminar origins and terminations of cortical connections of the occipital lobe in the rhesus monkey. *Brain Res.* 179: 3–20.

Rothbart, M. K., and Derryberry, D. (1981) Development of individual differences in temperament. In *Aduances in Developmental Psychology*, Vol. 1, edited by M. E. Lamb and A. L. Brown pp. 37–86. Hillsdale, NJ: Erlbaum.

Rothbart, M. K., Posner, M. I. and Rosicky, J. (1994). Orienting in normal and pathological development. *Dev. Psychopathol.* 6: 635–652.

Schiller, P. H. (1985) A model for the generation of visually guided saccadic eye movements. In *Models of the Visual Cortex*, edited by D. Rose and V. G. Dobson. pp. 62–70. Chicester, United Kingdom: Wiley.

Stechler, G. and Latz, E. (1966) Some observations on attention and arousal in the human infant. *J. Am. Acad. Child Psychiat.* 5: 517–525.

Tipper, S. P., Cameron, S., and Brehaut, J. C. (1988) Evidence for multiple internal representations of ignored objects. Unpublished manuscript.

Townsend, J. and Courchesne, E. (1994) Parietal damage and narrow "spotlight" of spatial attention. *J. Cognitive Neurosci.* 6: 220–232.

Attention-Deficit/Hyperactivity Disorder: Symptom Domains, Cognitive Processes, and Neural Networks

James Swanson, Michael I. Posner, Dennis Cantwell, Sharon Wigal, Francis Crinella, Pauline Filipek, Jane Emerson, Don Tucker, and Orhan Nalcioglu

ABSTRACT Attention-deficit/hyperactivity disorder (ADHD) is a diagnosis whose very title indicates its relation to the theme of this volume. Nonetheless, there has been a continuing dispute in the literature regarding whether clinical concepts of ADHD are related to cognitive concepts of attention, and if so, how. Modern views of attention relate cognitive concepts to neuroscience concepts. This approach is used to address the role of attention in ADHD. The goal is to relate clinical manifestation of ADHD (i.e., symptom domains) to deficits in specific neuropsychological components of attention (i.e., cognitive processes) and to make predictions about abnormalities in underlying brain anatomy and function (i.e., neural networks).

The recognition of what is now known as ADHD by physicians and its treatment with stimulant drugs (e.g., methylphenidate or amphetamine) has increased in the United States over the past half century (see Bradley, 1937), so that in 1994 approximately 6% of boys and 1.5% of girls of school age (about 2 million children) received this diagnosis and were treated with stimulants (Swanson, Lerner, and Williams, 1995). Over 9,000 articles in the literature (see Swanson, McBurnett, Wigal, et al. 1993) address general aspects of clinical diagnosis and treatment, and these well-covered topics will not be repeated here. The purpose of this chapter is to consider whether clinical concepts of attention deficit (the symptoms domains of inattention and hyperactivity/impulsivity) can be aligned with concepts of attention derived from the cognitive sciences (the neuropsychological processes of alerting, orienting, and executive control) and from the neurosciences (the neural networks with anatomical foci in right prefrontal, posterior parietal, and anterior cingulate brain regions).

Attempts to investigate this alignment are complicated by the existence of multiple clinical descriptions of the disorder and of multiple technical descriptions of cognitive processes of attention. One of the first approaches was provided by Crinella (1973), who used a clinical description (hyperactive-aggressive behavior) of a subtype of minimal brain damage from Wender (1971) and technical concepts of attention (alertness and kinetic mobility) from Luria (1966). A seminal approach, initiated by Douglas (1972), challenged the clinical descriptions that were based on informal diagnoses of hyperactivity and hyperkinesis of Clements (1966), stimulated the modern description based on the concept of attention deficit, and used descriptions of cognitive processes ("inability to sustain attention and control impulsivity") based on the classic descriptions of attention dating back to James (1890). Another important approach, initiated by Sergeant (1981), used the narrow (European) clinical description ("hyperactive and/or distractible") based on convergent and reliable ratings from multiple sources and the technical descriptions of cognitive processes (encoding, comparison, response selection, and response execution) from Sternberg (1969). A recent approach, initiated by Barkley (1993), used aspects of the broad (American) clinical description ("disinhibition or poor delay of response") of disruptive behavior disorders (DSM-III-R, 1987) and technical descriptions of cognitive processes not considered to be attentional (separation of affect, prolongation, internalization, and reconstitution) from Bronowski's theory of human language (1977). In response to his rhetorical question, "Is there an attention deficit in ADHD?" Barkley (1995) also recommended eliminating the term "attention deficit" and replacing it with the term "behavioral inhibition deficit." Before taking such a step and overturning the accumulated clinical wisdom of the past two decades, we propose to reevaluate the term "attention deficit" in terms of the refined DSM-IV (1994) clinical description of ADHD and the technical descriptions of attention from the neurosciences now being verified by brain-imaging techniques (see Posner and Raichle, 1994).

CLINICAL SYMPTOMS OF ADHD IN DSM REVISIONS

Before 1980, the core feature of ADHD was considered to be hyperactivity, and the label used to describe the disorder was hyperkinetic reaction of childhood (DSM-II, 1968). The revisions of DSM-III (1980) introduced the term attention deficit disorder (ADD) as a new label for the disorder, specified two cognitive symptom domains (inattention and impulsivity) to go along with the motor symptom domain (hyperactivity), and defined two subtypes of the disorder with (ADDH) and without (ADD) hyperactivity. The revisions of DSM-III-R (1987) changed the label only slightly to attention-deficit hyperactivity disorder (A-dHD), but the criteria were changed significantly: the polytypic concept was rejected in favor of a monotypic concept based on merging the three domains of symptoms and defining a single type of the disorder. The revisions of *DSM-IV* (1994) reestablished the use of multiple domains of symptoms and multiple subtypes of the disorder and changed the name to attention-deficit/hyperactivity disorder (A-D/HD). These perplexing changes in the DSM were intended to refine the clinical definition of what we will label ADHD. Although the specification of symptom domains and subtypes of ADHD changed often, the specific domains of symptoms have remained the same, with a gradual increase in the number of symptoms in the inattention domain, a gradual decrease in the number of symptoms in the impulsivity domain, and the addition of symptoms of verbal activity to the hyperactivity domain.

Table 20.1 DSM-IV symptoms of ADHD

Inattention	Hyperactivity/Impulsivity
Fails to give close attention to details	Fidgets with hands or feet or squirms
Has difficulty sustaining attention	Leaves seat in classroom
Does not seem to listen	Runs about or climbs when inappropriate
Does not follow through (fails to finish)	Difficulty playing quietly
Has difficulty organizing tasks	Always "on the go" or "driven by a motor"
Avoids tasks requiring sustained effort	Talks excessively
Loses things	Blurts out answers to questions
Is distracted by extraneous stimuli	Difficulty waiting turn
Is forgetful	Interrupts or intrudes on others

In DSM-IV (1994), two domains of symptoms were specified by merging the DSM-III symptom domains of impulsivity and hyperactivity into one (hyperactivity/impulsivity) and expanding the symptoms of inattention in a separate domain (inattention). In each domain, nine symptoms were listed, which are presented in an abstracted form in table 20.1. If at least six symptoms from one or both symptom domains are confirmed, a diagnosis is warranted, and so three subtypes are defined: predominately inattentive, predominately hyperactive/impulsive, and combined. The symptoms must have early onset (by age seven), must be chronic (not due to transient stressful events), must be pervasive (present in at least two settings), and must produce significant impairment.

COGNITIVE PROCESSES OF ATTENTION

Posner and Raichle (1994) offered a theory of attention based on the working hypothesis that distinct neural networks accomplish component processes of alerting, orienting, and executive control. They provided the rationale, description, and evidence for this approach, so only a summary will be presented here. *Alerting* consists of suppressing background neural noise (by inhibiting ongoing or irrelevant activity and mental effort to establish a state of vigilance) to establish readiness to react. *Orienting* consists of mobilizing specific neural resources (by facilitation of one specialized process and inhibition of others) to prepare to process an expected type of input. *Executive control* consists of coordinating multiple specialized neural processes (by detecting the presence of a target, starting and stopping mental operations, and ordering multiple responses) to direct behavior toward a goal.

NEURAL NETWORKS OF ATTENTION

Posner and Raichle (1994) proposed the neuroanatomical basis and the neural circuitry for each of the three cognitive processes of attention. Based on a review of the brain-imaging literature, they proposed that the neural network for alerting is defined by connected brain regions centered in the *right frontal* lobe (but also including the right parietal lobe and locus ceruleus), that the neural network for orienting is defined by connected brain regions centered in the *posterior parietal* lobes (but also including the superior colliculus and thalamus) that the neural network for executive control is defined by connected brain regions centered in the *anterior cingulate* gyrus (but also including the left lateral frontal lobe and basal ganglia). Posner and Raichle (1994) offered these three neural networks as examples of the anatomy and circuitry of attentional processes that operate in concert to influence how the brain processes information at brain regions specialized for sensory, motor, and other specialized functions.

RELATIONSHIP TO OTHER DESCRIPTIONS OF ATTENTION

The terms used by Posner and Raichle (1994) as technical descriptions of cognitive processes and neural networks can be related to other traditional terms used to describe attention (see Sergeant and Swanson, 1997). The alerting process and right frontal network operate to establish *sustained attention* (e.g., by maintaining a state of readiness to process nonspecific or repetitive stimuli). The orienting process and posterior parietal network operate to establish *selective attention* (e.g., by covertly disengaging, moving, and engaging an internal spotlight in response to internal or external cues signaling the type of processing required). The executive control process and anterior cingulate network operate to establish *divided attention* (e.g., by resolving conflict among multiple mental processes and responses in competition for execution in a coordinated fashion to regulate self-directed behavior).

A SELECTIVE REVIEW OF THE LITERATURE

The large literature on ADHD has been reviewed so many times (i.e., more than 350—see Swanson et al., 1993) that another review is not necessary here. Instead, we will focus on three key questions about ADHD, one for each level of analysis (clinical, cognitive, and neural): What domains of symptoms should be used to define clinical subtypes? What laboratory tests should be used to assess cognitive deficits? and What brain regions are associated with neural abnormalities?

What Domains of Symptoms Should Be Used to Define Clinical Subtypes?

The answer to this nagging question has changed in successive revisions of the DSM criteria, and unresolved issues remain about the content of the inattention domain as well as the overlap of the hyperactivity/impulsivity domain with symptom domains of non-ADHD disorders.

Content of the Inattention Domain The debate about this issue has been driven by different emphasis on symptoms of sustained attention and impulsivity. For example, the original recommendation to *include* a separate domain of inattention came from Douglas (1972), who emphasized poor sustained attention over impulsivity in her conceptualization of a basic underlying self-regulation deficit. The most recent recommendation to *exclude* a separate domain of inattention came from Barkley (1993), who emphasized the primacy of impulsivity over poor sustained attention in his conceptualization of a basic underlying behavioral inhibition deficit. Recent DSM-IV clinical descriptions of ADHD support the use of a separate inattention domain to link the clinical symptoms of ADHD to an underlying deficit in sustained attention, as well as to other aspects of attention. Only three of the nine symptoms refer to poor sustained attention (i.e., "has difficulty sustaining attention," "avoids tasks requiring sustained effort," and "does not follow through"), and these are clearly separate from symptoms of impulsivity ("blurts out answers to questions," "has difficulty waiting turn," and "interrupts or intrudes on others"), which are grouped with the symptoms of hyperactivity in the hyperactivity/impulsivity domain. Three of the remaining six symptoms in the inattention domain seem to refer to selective attention ("fails to give close attention to details," "is distracted by extraneous stimuli," and "does not seem to listen"). It is notable that the symptoms sometimes associated with ADD, as opposed to ADHD ("stares into space or reports daydreaming" and "low energy level, sluggish, or drowsy") were explicitly considered but not included in the inattention domain of DSM-IV. Thus, the DSM-IV description of inattention includes three symptoms that may be linked to the alerting network and three symptoms that may be related to the orienting network of Posner and Raichle (1994). The other three describe memory/organization deficits that may be linked to the executive cortrol network.

Overlap of Hyperactivity/Impulsivity with Other Disorders Another important issue in the clinical diagnosis of ADHD is the consideration of other disorders. DSM-IV allows for multiple diagnoses, and high rates of comorbidity have been reported with psychiatric disorders such as depression, anxiety, conduct, tic, and stress disorders (see Biederman, Newcorn, and Sprich, 1991) and with learning disorders such as reading disabilities (see Shaywitz, Fletcher, and Shaywitz, 1994). However, instead of co-occurring with ADHD, it is possible that some non-ADHD disorders masquerade as ADHD (for a discussion of how ADHD symptoms may be due to an underlying depression, see Carlson and Cantwell, 1979; for a discussion of how symptoms of ADHD may be due to an underlying reading disability, see Pennington, Grossier, and Welsh, 1993). In referred clinical samples, the most frequently recognized comorbid conditions are oppositional defiant disorder (ODD) and conduct disorder (CD), but this is controversial in Europe, where it is generally recommended that for those with both ADHD and ODD/CD, diagnostic priority should be given to ODD/CD (see Rutter, Shaffer, and Sturge, 1978) or a separate category be used for the combination (ICD-10). The symptom domains of ODD (negative, defiant, disobedient, or hostile behavior toward authority figures) and of CD (a persistent pattern of violation of the basic rights of others or of societal norms) are more highly correlated with the hyperactivity/impulsivity symptom domain than with the inattention symptom domain of ADHD (see Loney and Milich, 1982). Children with intentional problems (those who "won't pay attention) but without attentional problems (those who "can't" pay attention) are likely to manifest symptoms of disruptive behavior (restlessness and overactivity, disturbing others, low frustration tolerance, teasing and interference, and mood changes) and be misclassified by a diagnosis of ADHD. The requirement to manifest symptoms of inattention may reduce this source of misdiagnosis. It seems prudent in research studies to evaluate attentional deficits in the subgroup of ADHD cases without comorbid conditions to avoid phenocopies with false positive diagnoses of ADHD.

What Laboratory Tests Should Be Used to Assess Cognitive Deficits?

Many neuropsychological batteries have been used to assess attention deficits in ADHD, and the consistent finding across studies has been that children with ADHD do not have generalized cognitive impairment, but that they do manifest specific deficits. Pennington and Ozonoff (1996) reviewed the literature and concluded that tests of executive function (e.g., the Stroop Matching Familiar Figures, Tower of Hanoi, and Trails B tasks) were the best suited for characterization of a deficit relatively specific to ADHD. Barkley (1991) questioned the validity of laboratory tests for assessing a disorder defined on subjective behavioral ratings, but concluded that the ecological validity of tests of attention (CPT-like tests) was better than the validity of tests of impulsivity or of activity.

Instead of another review, we will present a selection of paradigms that we believe have theoretical significance for the assessment of children with ADHD: CPT paradigms, visuospatial orienting task (VOT) paradigms, and conflict resolution task (CRT) paradigms. The brain-imaging literature (see Posner and Raichle, 1994) indicates that these paradigms are effective probes of the alerting, orienting, and executive control networks.

CPT Paradigms Many CPT paradigms have been used to assess attentional deficits in ADHD, but they differ on important task variables summarized by Parasuraman (1985) (memory sequence, response rate, and event rate), which are known to affect performance on tests of sustained attention. For example, three CPT versions that have been marketed for clinical application in assessment of ADHD differ on these task variables: the GDS (Gordon Diagnostic System) (Gordon, 1983), the TOVA (Test of Variables of Attention) (Greenberg and Waldman, 1993), and the MHS (Multi-Health System)

(Conners, 1995). The GDS CPT is distinguished by the use of a memory sequence to define a target (i.e., a digit sequence, 1–9, which occurs on 10% of trials in a 9-minute task). The TOVA CPT is distinguished by variation in response rate (i.e., 22.5% of nonverbal stimuli are targets in the first 11 minutes and 77.5% are targets in the last 11 minutes of a 22-minute task). The MHS CPT is distinguished by the manipulation of event rate (i.e., 1-, 2-, and 4-second intertrial intervals within each of six blocks of trials in a 14-minute task requiring a response to any letter except X, which occurs on 90% of all trials). Thus, these versions of the CPT may probe different aspects of abnormal sustained attention. All three commercial CPTs provide norms for use in identifying abnormal performance. However, based on recommended cutoffs, these tests are limited by false positive (about .14) and false negative (about .27) probabilities, which impose limitations for use in screening of nonreferred populations (for the presence of a low base rate clinical condition) or for assessment of referred clinical populations (for differential diagnosis). For example, Baren and Swanson (1996) noted that if a CPT tests were used to screen a typical elementary school with about 500 students to identify those with ADHD (about 5% or 25 students), almost four times as many non-ADHD students (66.5) than ADHD students (18.25) would be expected to have abnormal scores. Matier-Sharma, Perachio, and Newcorn (1995) noted in an assessment of a clinical sample that CPT measures were only slightly better than chance in distinguishing ADHD from non-ADHD disorders.

Even though CPT paradigms have limited clinical value, systematic research programs have used variations of CPT paradigms to provide important information about abnormalities of sustained attention in ADHD. For example, Sergeant (1989) reviewed the results of his systematic research program using a memory scanning CPT with a fast presentation rate and concluded that the ADHD children's performance was poor at the beginning of the test, then declined at the same rate as for normal control children, suggesting a low vigilance level instead of an accelerated vigilance decrement. Placed in the framework provided by Parasuraman (1985), this suggests that low arousal instead of impaired capacity may be responsible for the performance deficit in this setting. In a continuation of this research program, event rate was varied (see Van der Meere, 1995), and when a slow presentation rate was used, a vigilance decrement (faster than normal decline in performance) was elicited in children with ADHD. Placed in the framework of Sanders (1983), this suggests that impaired state regulation may contribute to the performance deficit in this setting. These studies suggest that versions of the CPT paradigm that vary the event rate might be used to link some symptoms of inattention (those describing sustained attention) to activity in a specific neural network (the alerting network) of Posner and Raichle (1994).

VOT Paradigms Voellar and Heilman (1988) used a visuospatial cancellation test and a neurological exam to evaluate a group of children with

ADHD and found left visual field (LVF) neglect in performance and subtle left-sided neurological signs, suggesting right hemisphere dysfunction. Swanson, Posner, Potkin et al. (1991) adapted the Posner, Petersen, Fox, and Raichle (1988) visuospatial reaction time test, with 100 ms and 800 ms cue-target intervals and valid and invalid cues, and used it to test ADHD and control groups of children. The ADHD group showed a deficit consistent with right parietal lobe dysfunction (i.e., an abnormal asymmetric slowing in response time only to targets in the right visual field (RVF) after invalid cues and 800 ms cue-target intervals). Swanson, Shea, McBurnett et al. (1990) interpreted this specific abnormal lateral difference in response time as an orienting deficit in response to the target or a vigilance decrement in response to the cue. Others have tested this complex hypothesis with qualified successes: Carter, Krener, Chaderjian, Nothcutt, and Wolfe (1995) replicated this finding and extended it with an inhibition of return condition; Novak, Solanto, and Abikoff (1995) confirmed this only in baseline tests; Ottolini (1995) replicated the effect only in an ADHD group without comorbid disorders; Nigg, Swanson, and Hinshaw (1997) observed the specific effect only in biological parents of children with ADHD and not in the group of ADHD children (who showed RVF deficits in other conditions). These studies suggest that some VOT paradigms that require spatial orienting may provide a link between some clinical symptoms of inattention (those describing selective attention) and a specific neural network (the orienting network) of Posner and Raichle (1994).

CRT Paradigms Several conflict tasks that rely on inhibition of automatic responses have been identified as among the best tests to distinguish ADHD and normal groups of children. For example, Pennington and Ozonoff (1996) reviewed the literature and identified the Stroop task, which generates conflict between the reading of a word and the naming of the color in which it is printed, as one of the most sensitive tasks for documenting performance deficits in ADHD children. Tannock (1995) described a program of research using the stop task, in which a conflicting signal to inhibit a response was given at varying times after a signal to initiate a response, and reviewed the evidence that ADHD children manifested a deficit in stopping a response in progress. Sonuga-Barke (1995) described a program of research using a start task, in which a conflict was generated between two response styles (waiting for a large reward versus responding immediately for a small reward), and reviewed the evidence that ADHD children elected to not delay starting a response, even when early responding had negative economic consequences. These reviews of performance deficits on Stroop tasks, stop tasks, and start tasks suggest that some ADHD children may have executive function deficits. Posner and DiGirolamo (chapter 18, this volume) have emphasized conflict resolution as a key factor in executive control. The CRT paradigms, which depend on regulation by inhibition of the usual (or automatic) response to allow for an execution of a new response in the face of competition, may provide a link between the clinical symptoms of impulsivity and a specific neural network (the executive control network) of Posner and Raichle (1994).

What Brain Regions Are Most Likely To Show Neural Abnormalities?

Brain-imaging methods have been used to localize functional and anatomical neural abnormalities associated with ADHD. These include estimates of neural activity from electroencephalographic (EEG) source imaging (ESI), blood flow from single photon computed tomography (SPECT), glucose utilization from positron emission tomography (PET), and anatomical size and shape from magnetic resonance imaging (MRI).

ESI Satterfield, Schell, and Nicholas (1990) conducted a longitudinal study of ADHD and normal control groups of children who were tested on an extended visual and auditory selective attention task during which EEG data were collected from 19 electrode locations and used to obtain event-related potential (ERP) measures of brain function. An abnormality in an early component (N2) emerged in 6-year-old ADHD subjects but was not present at 8 years of age, when abnormalities due to smaller than normal amplitudes of P3b (maximal at parietal leads) and Nd (maximal at frontal leads) were manifested, suggesting a failure to respond to the relevant stimulus rather than an inability to block response to the irrelevant stimuli. Overall, this study was interpreted to implicate abnormalities in specific neural pathways: the frontal lobes (delayed development of Nd), parietal lobes (absence of the P3b tuning effect), the anterior cingulate (inability to attach appropriate value to stimuli), and locus ceruleus (insufficient activation of noradrenergic system to enhance P3b). Robaey, Breton, Dugas, and Renault (1992), who used a task with fewer but more salient stimuli and who collected EEG data from 16 electrode sites, reported the most diagnostic abnormality to be localized in the right parieto-occipital region (shorter P350 latency than normal, suggesting enhanced automatic processing of stimuli). Harter, Anello-Vento, Wood, and Schroeder (1988), who also used salient stimuli (color and letter matching) in a selective attention task and collected EEG data from 8 electrode locations, found ERP evidence for greater selective neural processing in right frontal regions (larger P3 and late N700), which was interpreted as a compensatory response for an early processing deficit. Novak et al. (1995), who used a visuospatial cueing task and collected EEG data from 21 electrode locations, found meager ERP data to distinguish ADHD and normal groups, but did report a significant interaction predicted from the reaction time study of Swanson et al. (1991): the group × visual field × cue interaction in the analysis of baseline P1, N1, and P3 amplitudes. That interaction suggests a lower than normal response to invalid targets in the right visual field. Overall, these ERP studies suggest abnormalities in ADHD groups in the right frontal region (implicating the alerting network) and in the right parietal region (implicating the orienting network). The ESI techniques based on dense electrode arrays of 128 (or more) EEG channels have not yet been used to test these suggestions, but we are now conducting such studies using methods developed by Tucker, Liotti, Potts, et al. (1994).

SPECT and PET Lou, Henriksen, and Bruhn (1984, 1989, 1990) used SPECT measures of blood flow to study ADHD. Despite the nonindependence of these reports (based on an overlapping series of patients), this work suggests that ADHD children have hypoperfusion (about 10% lower blood flow) to striatal and frontal brain areas and hyperperfusion of occipital brain areas. Zametkin, Nordhall, Gross, et al. (1990) and Zametkin, Liebenauer, Fitzgerald, et al. (1993) used PET measures of brain glucose metabolism in adults and adolescents with ADHD. Despite some inconsistencies (i.e., lower global glucose metabolism in ADHD adults did not hold up in a subsequent study of ADHD teenagers), there was consistency across this work when the ADHD and normal control groups were compared on the basis of normalized brain images: the prefrontal areas showed evidence of relative underactivity (i.e., about 10% lower glucose metabolism). Overall, these brain-imaging studies of individuals with ADHD suggest an abnormality in the frontal lobes (implicating the alerting and executive control networks). The new functional MRI measures of perfusion and blood flow have not yet been used to test these suggestions, but we are now conducting such studies using methods developed by Emerson, Chen, Shankle, and Nalcioglu (1995) and by Nalcioglu and Guclu (1996).

MRI Hynd, Semrud-Clikeman, and Lorys (1991) used MRI to study brain anatomy of ADHD and control groups of children and reported a trend in ADHD cases to have smaller anterior (genu) and posterior (splenium) regions of the corpus callosum, which connect the frontal and parietal brain regions of the two hemispheres. Despite some inconsistencies in the specific region, other studies have confirmed this general pattern of reduced size of the corpus callosum. Giedd, Castellanos, et al. (1994) and Baumgardner, Singer, et al. (1996) found smaller anterior regions, and Semrud-Clikeman, Filipek, et al. (1994) found smaller posterior regions. Hynd et al. (1991) and Filipek, Semrud-Clikeman, et al. (1997) also investigated the size of the frontal lobes in groups of ADHD and control children and reported smaller than average right frontal lobes, due to a lack of normal (larger right than left) asymmetry. Hynd et al. (1991), Castellanos, Giedd, Marsh, Hamburger, Vaituzis, et al. (1996), Aylward, Reiss, Reader, Singer, Brown, and Denckla (1996), and Filipek, Semrud-Clikeman, et al. (1997) investigated the size of basal ganglia structures in ADHD and control groups of children and, despite some inconsistencies in characterizing abnormalities of asymmetry, all of these studies reported smaller structures (caudate or globus pallidus) in the ADHD group. Overall, these studies of brain anatomy suggest that children with ADHD have abnormalities (smaller than normal size) in three brain structures that implicate all three neural networks specified by Posner and Raichle (1994): the corpus callosum (orienting), basal ganglia (executive control), and right frontal lobes (alerting). Full brain MRI morphometric analysis on a large sample of ADHD and control subjects has not yet been performed to link specific abnormalities to types of symptoms, but we are now conducting such a study using methods developed by Filipek et al. (1994).

ALIGNMENT OF CLINICAL, COGNITIVE, AND NEURAL LEVELS OF ANALYSIS

Based on the discussions in the previous sections, we will offer a tentative alignment of symptom domains of ADHD, cognitive processes of attention, and the neural networks of attention. We propose (1) that the three DSM-IV symptoms of inattention that describe poor sustained attention (i.e., "has difficulty sustaining attention," "does not follow through (fails to finish)," and "avoids tasks requiring sustained effort") may be related to an alerting deficit and may be linked to an abnormality in a neural network centered in the right frontal brain region; (2) that the three DSM-IV symptoms of inattention that describe poor selective attention (i.e., "fails to give close attention to details," "does not seem to listen," and "is distracted by extraneous stimuli") may be related to an orienting deficit and may be linked to an abnormality in a different neural network centered in a different brain region (bilateral parietal); (3) that the three DSM-IV symptoms of impulsivity that describe poor conflict resolution or divided attention ("blurts out answers," "difficulty awaiting turn," and "interrupts or intrudes on others") may be related to an executive function deficit and may be linked to abnormalities in a neural network centered in the anterior cingulate brain region. Our proposals are summarized in table 20.2.

Table 20.2   Alignment of symptom domains, cognitive processes, and neural networks

Symptom Domains	Cognitive Processes	Neural Networks
Inattentive-A	*Alerting*	*Right frontal*
Difficulty sustaining attention	CPT, fast (vigilance level)	Right frontal
Fails to finish	CPT, slow (vigilance decrement)	Right posterior parietal
Avoids sustained effort	CPT, high load (capacity)	Locus ceruleus
Inattentive-O	*Orienting*	*Posterior parietal*
Distracted by stimuli	VOT, cue (rapid, short response)	Bilateral parietal
Does not seem to listen	VOT, validity effect (can't engage)	Superior colliculus
Fails to give close attention	VOT, visual search (neglect)	Thalamus
Hyperactive/impulsive	*Executive control*	*Anterior cingulate*
Blurts out answers	CRT, Stroop (too automatic)	Anterior cingulate
Interrupts or intrudes	CRT, stop tasks (can't stop)	Left lateral frontal
Can't wait	CRT, start tasks (can't inhibit)	Basal ganglia

CONCLUSIONS

Our application of the Posner and Raichle (1994) theory leads to the specific prediction that ADHD is a polytypic syndrome with multiple biological bases. We have formed a multidisciplinary group to test our predictions about the biological bases of ADHD, directed by Posner and Raichle's (1994) basic science approach for defining biological bases and Cantwell's (1990) clinical science approach to defining ADHD. We plan to test specific predictions derived from the outline in table 20.2 by using the relatively new brain imaging techniques developed by members of our group: the anatomical MRI methods of Filipek et al. (1994) to investigate size and shape of brain structures, the gadolinium-enhanced MRI methods of Emerson et al. (1995) to investigate regional brain perfusion, the functional MRI methods implemented by Nalcioglu and Guclu (1996) to investigate regional blood flow, and the dense electrode EEG methods of Tucker et al. (1994) to investigate the sources and coherence of brain electrical activity.

By linking clinical symptoms of ADHD (derived from accumulated clinical wisdom) to cognitive processes and to neural networks of attention (derived from the emerging techniques of the cognitive neurosciences), we may gain a better understanding of biological bases of ADHD that will help us interpret the existing literature and evaluate apparent conflicts in speculations about brain systems involved in ADHD. For example, two recent theoretical articles about ADHD reached opposite conclusions about the hemispheric and neurotransmitter bases of ADHD: Voellar and Heilman, (1988) and Heilman, Voellar, and Nadeau (1991) proposed a right hemisphere (norepinephrine) deficit theory, whereas Malone, Kershner, and Swanson (1994) proposed a left hemisphere (dopamine) deficit theory. It is likely that these theories were developed to account for different symptom domains of ADHD: the Voellar and Heilman (1988) and Heilman et al. (1991) theory seems to emphasize the inattentive symptom domain and the Malone et al. (1994) theory seems to emphasize the hyperactive/impulsive symptom domain. Therefore, both of these theories may be correct when applied to some aspects of ADHD, with different clinical manifestations associated with multiple underlying cognitive processes and with multiple neural networks of attention.

REFERENCES

Aylward, E. H., Reiss, A. L., Reader, M. J., Singer, H. S., Brown, J. E. and Denckla, M. B. (1996) Basal ganglia volumes in children with ADHD. *J. Child Neurol.* 11: 112–115.

Baren, M. and Swanson, J. M. (1996) How not to diagnose ADHD. *Contemp. Pediat.* 13: 53–64.

Barkley, R. A. (1991) The ecological validity of laboratory and analogue assessment methods of ADHD. *J. Abnorm. Child Psychol.* 19: 149–178.

Barkley, R. A. (1993) A new theory of ADHD. *The ADHD Report* 1: 1–4.

Barkley, R. A. (1995) Is there an attention deficit in ADHD? *The ADHD Report* 3: 1–3.

Baumgardner, T. L., Singer, H. S., and Denkla, M. B., Bubin, M. A., Abrams, M. T., Colli, M. J., and Reiss, A. L. (1996) Corpus callosum morphology in children with Tourette Syndrome and Attention Deficit Hyperactivity Disorder. *Neurology* 47: 1–6.

Biederman, J., Newcorn, J., and Sprich, S. (1991) Comorbidity of ADHD with conduct, depressive, anxiety, and other disorders. *Am. J. Psychiatry* 148: 546–577.

Bradley, C. (1937) The behavior of children receiving benzedrine. *Am. J. Psychiatry* 94: 577–585.

Bronowski, J. (1977) *Human and Animal Languages.* Cambridge, MA: MIT Press.

Cantwell, D. P. (1990) Empiricism and Child Psychiatry. The 1990 C. Charles Burlingame, M. D. Award Lecture. The Institute of Living: Hartford, CT.

Cantwell, D. P. and Rutter, M. (1994) Classification: Conceptual issues and substantive findings. In *Child and Adolescent Psychiatry: Modern Approaches,* edited by M. Rutter, E. Taylor, and L. Hersov, London: Blackwell.

Carlson, G. A. and Cantwell, D. P. (1979) Unmasking masked depression in children and adolescents. *Am. J. Psychiatry* 137: 445–449.

Carter, C. S., Krener, P., Chaderjian, M., Nothcutt, C., and Wolfe, V. (1995) Asymmetrical visual-spatial atentional performance in ADHD: Evidence for a right hemisphere deficit. *Biol. Psychiatry* 37: 789–797.

Castellanos, F. X., Giedd, J. N., Marsh, W. L., Hamburger, S. D., Vaituzis, A. C., Dickstein, D. P., Sarfatti, S. E., Vauss, Y. C., Snell, J. W., Lang, N., Kaysen, D., Krain, A. L., Bitchie, B. F., Bajapakse, J. C. and Bapoport, J. L. (1996) Quantitative brain magnetic resonance imaging in attention-deficit hyperactivity disorder. *Arch. Gen. Psychiatry* 53: 607–616.

Clements, S. (1966) *Minimal Brain Dysfunction in Children* (PHS Report No. 1415). Bethesda, MD: National Institutes of Health.

Conners, C. K. (1995) *Continuous Performance Test.* Tonowanda, NY: MHS.

Crinella, F. M. (1973) Identification of brain dysfunction syndromes in children through profile analysis. *J. Abnorm. Psychol.* 82: 33–45.

Douglas, V. I. (1972) Stop, look and listen: The problem of sustained attention and impulse control in hyperactive and normal children. *Can. J. Behav. Sci.* 4: 259–282.

Diagnostic and Statistical Manual, Edition II (1968), III (1980), III-R (1987), and IV (1994). Washington DC: American Psychiatric Association.

Emerson, J. F., Chen, P. C., Shankle, W. R., and Nalcioglu, O. N. (1995) Data analysis for dynamic contrast-enhanced MRI-based cerebral perfusion measurements: Correcting for changing cortical CSF volumes. *Magma* 3: 41–48.

Filipek, P. A., Richelme, C., Kennedy, D. N., & Cauiness, V. S. Jr. et al. (1994) The young adult human brain: MRI morphometric analysis. *Cereb. Cortex* 4: 344–360.

Filipek, P. A., Semrud-Clikeman, M., Steingard, R. J., Benshaw, P. F., Kennedy, D. N., and Biederman, J. (1997) Volumetric MRI analysis comparing attention-deficit hyperactivity disorder and normal controls. *Neurology* 48: 589–601.

Giedd, J. N., Castellanos, F. X., Casey, B. J., Eckburg, P., Marsh, W. L. (1994) Quantitative morphology of the corpus callosum in attention deficit hyperactivity disorder. *Am. J. Psychiatry* 151: 665–669.

Gordon, M. (1983) *Gordon Diagnostic System.* Dewitt, NY: Gordon Systems.

Greenberg, L. M. and Waldman, I. (1993) Developmental normative data on the test of variables of attention. *J. Child Psychol. Psychiatry Allied Disciplines* 6: 1019–1030.

Harter, M. R., Anello-Vento, L., Wood, F. B., and Schroeder, M. M. (1988) Separate brain potential characteristics in children with reading disability and attention deficit disorder. *Brain Cogn.* 7: 115–140.

Heilman, K. M., Voellar, K. S., and Nadeau, S. E. (1991) A possible pathophysiological substrate of ADHD. *J. Child Neurol.* 6: S76–S81.

Hynd, G. W., Semrud-Clikeman, M., and Lorys, A. R. (1991) Corpus callosum morphology in attention-deficit hyperactivity disorder (ADHD): Morphometric analysis of MRI. *J. Learn. Disabil.* 24: 141–146.

James, W. (1890) *Principles of Psychology*. New York: Dover.

Loney, J. and Milich, R. (1982) Hyperactivity, inattention, and aggression in clinical practice. *Adv. Dev. Behav. Pediat.* 3: 113–147.

Lou, H. C., Henriksen, L., and Bruhn, P. (1984) Focal cerebral hypoperfusion in children with dysphasia and/or attention deficit disorder. *Arch. Neurol.* 41: 825–829.

Lou, H. C., Henriksen, L. and Bruhn, P. (1989) Striatal dysfunction in attention deficit and hyperkinetic disorder. *Arch. Neurol.* 46: 48–52.

Lou, H. C., Henriksen, L.,and Bruhn, P. (1990) Focal cerebral dysfunction in developmental learning disabilities. *Lancet* 335: 8–11.

Luria, A. R. (1966) *Higher Cortical Functions in Man*. New York: Basic Books.

Malone, M. A., Kershner, J. R., and Swanson, J. M. (1994) Hemispheric processing and methylphenidate effects in ADHD. *J. Child Neurol.* 9: 181–189.

Matier-Sharma, K., Perachio, N., and Newcorn, N. (1995) Differential diagnosis of ADHD. *Child Neuropsychiat.* 1: 118–127.

Nalcioglu, O. and Guclu, C. C. (1996) Hardware for real-time k-space mapping. *Book Abstr. Soc. Magn. Reson. Med.*

Nigg, J., Swanson, J. M., and Hinshaw, S. (1997) Covert visual spatial attention in boys with ADHD. *Neuropsychologia* 35: 165–176.

Novak, G. P., Solanto, M., and Abikoff, H. (1995) Spatial orienting and focused attention in ADD. *Psychophysiology* 32: 546–559.

Ottolini, Y. (1995) *Visual-Spatial Selective Attention in Children with Attention Deficits*. Unpublished doctoral dissertation, California School of Professional Psychology, San Diego, CA.

Parasuraman, R. (1985) Sustained attention: A multifactorial approach. In *Attention and Performance XI*, edited by M. I. Posner and O. S. M. Marin. Hillsdale, NJ: Lawrence Erlbaum.

Pennington, B. F., Grossier, D., and Welsh, M. C. (1993) Contrasting cognitive deficits in ADD versus RD. *Dev. Psychol.* 29: 511–523.

Pennington, B. F. and Ozonoff, S. (1996) Executive functions and developmental psychopathology. *J. Child Psychol. Psychiatry* 37: 51–87.

Posner, M. I., Petersen, S. E., Fox, P. T., and Raichle, M. E. (1988) Localization of cognitive operations in the human brain. *Science* 240: 1627–1631.

Posner, M. I. and Raichle, M. E. (1994) *Images of Mind*. Scientific American Library.

Robaey, P., Breton, F., Dugas, M., and Renault, B. (1992) An event-related potential study of controlled and automatic processes in 6- to 8- year-old boys with ADHD. *Electroencephalogr. Clin. Neurophysiol.* 82: 330–340.

Rutter, M. L., Shaffer, D., and Sturge, C. (1978, revised and corrected 1983) *A Guide to Multi-Axial Classification Scheme for Psychiatric Disorders in Childhood and Adolescence.* London: Institute of Psychiatry.

Sanders, A. F. (1983) Toward a model of stress and human performance. *Acta Psychol.* 53: 61–97.

Satterfield, J. H., Schell, A. M., and Nicholas, T. (1990) Ontogeny of selective attention effects on eventrelated potentials in attentiondeficit hyperactivity disorder and normal boys. *Biol. Psychiatry* 28: 879–903.

Semrud-Clikeman, M., Filipek, P. A., Biederman, J., Steingard, R., Kennedy, D., Renshaw, P., and Bekken, K. (1994) ADHD: Magnetic resonance imaging morphometric analysis of the corpus callosum. *J. Am. Acad. Child Adolesc. Psych.* 33: 875–881.

Sergeant, J. A. (1981) *Attentional Studies in Hyperactivity.* Groningen, The Netherlands: Veenstra.

Sergeant, J. A. (1989) In search of processing deficits of attention in ADD-H children. In *Attention Deficit Disorder Current Concepts and Emerging Trends,* edited by L. Bloomingdale and J. Swanson. Oxford: Pergamon Press.

Sergeant, J. A. and Swanson, J. M. (1997) Attention deficit in ADHD children: Localization in models of attention. Manuscript in preparation.

Shaywitz, B. A., Fletcher, J. M., and Shaywitz, S. E. (1994) Issues in the definition and classification of attention deficit disorder. *Topics Lang. Disord.* 14: 1–25.

Sonuga-Barke, E. (1995) *Impulsivity and Inhibition in Hyperactive Children.* Experimental Studies of ADHD. Amsterdam: University of Amsterdam.

Sternberg, S. (1969) Discovery of processing stages: Extensions of Donders' method. In *Attention and Performance II,* edited by A. Sanders, pp. 276–315. Amsterdam: Elsevier.

Swanson, J. M. (1995) Psychopharmacology and cognitive energetics of ADHD. In *Experimental Studies of ADHD,* edited by J. Sergeant. Amsterdam: EPOS.

Swanson, J. M., Lerner, M., and Williams, L. (1995) More frequent diagnosis of ADHD. *N. England J. Med.* 333: 944.

Swanson, J. M., McBurnett, K., Wigal, T., Pfittner, L., Lerner, M. A., Williams, L., Christian, D. L., Tarm, L., Willaitt, E., Crowley, K., Clevenger, W., Khouzom, N., Woo. C., Crinella, F. M., and Fisher, T. D. (1993) Effect of stimulant medication on children with attention deficit disorder: A review of reviews. *Excep. Child.* 60: 154–162.

Swanson, J. M., Posner, M., Potkin, S., Bonforte, S., Youpa, D., Fiore, C., Cantwell, D., and Crinella, F. M. (1991) Activating tasks for the study of visual-spatial attention in ADHD children: A cognitive anatomic approach. *J. Child Neurol.* 6: S119–S127.

Swanson, J. M., Shea, C., McBurnett, K., Potking, S. G., Fiore, T. and Crinello, F. M. (1990) Attention and hyperactivity. In *The Development of Attention: Research and Theory,* edited by J. Enns. New York: Elsevier.

Tannock, R. (1995) Cognitive and motor inhibition in hyperactives. In *Experimental Studies of ADHD,* edited by J. Sergeant. Amsterdam: EPOS.

Tucker, D. M., Liotti, M., and Potts, G. F., et al. (1994) Spatiotemporal analysis of brain electrical fields. *Human Brain. Map.* 1: 134–152.

Van der Meere, J. (1995) Energetic factors in hyperactivity. In *Experimental Studies of ADHD,* edited by J. Sergeant. Amsterdam: EPOS.

Voellar, K. K. S. and Heilman, K. M. (1988) Attention deficit disorder in children: A neglect syndrome? *Neurology* 38: 806–808.

Wender, P. H. (1971) *Minimal Brain Dysfunction in Children.* New York: Wiley.

World Health Organization. (1992) *Mental Disorders: Glossary and Guide.* Geneva: World Health Organization.

Zametkin, A. J., Liebenauer, L. L., Fitzgerald, G. A., King, A. C., Minkunas, D. V., Herscovitch, P., Yamada, E. M., and Cohen, R. M. (1993) Brain metabolism in teenagers with attention-deficit hyperactivity disorder. *Arch. of General Psychiatry* 50: 333–340.

Zametkin, A. J., Nordahl, T. T., Gross, M., King, A. C., Semple, W. E., Rumseg, J., Hamburger, S., and Cohen, R. M. (1990) Cerebral glucose metabolism in adults with hyperactivity of childhood onset. *N. England J. Med.* 323: 1361–1366.

21 Selective Attention in Aging and Dementia

Raja Parasuraman and Pamela M. Greenwood

ABSTRACT Examining the changes in selective attention associated with aging and dementia due to Alzheimer's disease (AD) can provide important information on the organization of normal cognitive systems. This chapter examines one such system—selective spatial attention—with respect to the supporting neural systems and the impact of aging and AD on those systems. Both aging and AD affect spatial attention selectively rather than globally. AD is associated with a specific deficiency in the disengagement of attention between locations and objects and in the adjustment of the spatial scale of attention. That deficit can account for much of the performance of individuals with AD on both simple discrimination and more complex visual search tasks. Comparable though smaller effects of aging on spatial attention are obtained only for "old-old" adults over 75 years of age. A distributed network linking posterior parietal and prefrontal areas with the pulvinar is proposed to support spatial attention in discrimination and search tasks. Pathological changes in AD, and to a lesser extent advanced aging, may disrupt communication between elements of the network.

The selection of events relevant to carrying out a current goal—searching for the face of a friend in a crowd, or listening for the sound of a crying child at a noisy birthday party—is a fundamental aspect of perception and action. The basic neural architecture for stimulus selection appears to mature in infancy, providing for effective exploration of the environment and social interaction (Johnson, chapter 19, this volume), although selective attention continues to develop throughout the life span (Plude, Enns, and Brodeur, 1994). Old age brings some reduction in speed of operation and in flexibility. Nevertheless, selection mechanisms continue to function quite well in healthy older adults in their 50s, 60s, and 70s (Greenwood and Parasuraman, 1997; Hartley, 1992), in "old-old" individuals more than 75–80 years old (Greenwood and Parasuraman, 1994; Greenwood, Parasuraman, and Alexander, 1997), and even in those in the early stages of dementing disorders such as Alzheimer's disease (Nebes, 1992; Parasuraman and Haxby, 1993).

Alzheimer's disease (AD) is a progressive degenerative disorder that affects many cognitive functions, with relative sparing of sensory and motor functioning (in the early stages of the disease). The study of individuals with AD therefore provides a potentially revealing probe into brain-mind relationships for a wide spectrum of cognitive processes. But AD should not be thought of as a generalized cortical disease that disrupts all aspects of cognitive functioning. A more accurate characterization would be that AD, particularly in its early stages, leads to a selective breakdown of particular cognitive functions rather than to a global loss (Nebes, 1992; Parasuraman and Nestor, 1993). Moreover, in individuals with AD there is considerable heterogeneity in the specific cognitive functions that are affected (Martin et al., 1986; Schwartz, 1990). In principle, the pattern of preservation and deterioration of cognitive functions can be linked to variations in the regional pattern of neuropathology in the AD brain.

Investigating the progression of the relatively selective impairments in cognitive functioning in persons with AD is relevant to understanding the organization of normal cognitive systems (Parasuraman and Martin, 1994). This chapter examines one such system—spatial attention—with respect to three broad issues: (1) the role of spatial attention in both simple and complex visual tasks, (2) the neural systems supporting spatial attention, and (3) the impact of aging and AD on those systems.

A RATIONALE FOR EXAMINING ATTENTIONAL FUNCTIONS

Cognitive studies in healthy and demented older adults can contribute in at least two ways to a further understanding of the neural systems of attention and memory. First, the association temporal and parietal cortices are among the neocortical areas that are affected early in the course of AD. Given the involvement of the posterior parietal cortex in attention, particularly in spatial attention (Mesulam, 1981; Posner and Petersen, 1990), studies of AD can advance knowledge of the role of the parietal cortex in different attentional tasks. Such studies can also contribute to a more general understanding of aging and dementia. Attention is affected in the very early stages of AD (for a review, see Parasuraman and Haxby, 1993). The close interrelationships between selective attention and working memory (e.g., see Awh and Jonides, chapter 16, this volume) suggest that it would not be surprising if attention deficits are coincident with or immediately follow early memory impairment, but the precise order in which cognitive impairments emerge is unknown. Neuropathological staging studies suggest that Alzheimer's-related plaques and tangles are first detectable in entorhinal cortex, and later in the hippocampal fields and then in the neocortex, particularly in association parietal and temporal cortex; primary sensory and motor areas are relatively spared until very late in the progression of the disease (Braak and Braak, 1991; Kemper, 1994). Given current knowledge of the functions associated with those brain regions, such a progression would suggest that episodic memory is the earliest cognitive function affected, followed (not necessarily in order) by attention and working memory, language, semantic memory, and visuospatial function, and finally, sensorimotor functions (Almkvist and Backman, 1993; Grady et al., 1988).

Second, the role of several subcortical neurochemical systems in attentional functioning has been examined in recent years (Robbins and Everitt,

1995). Cholinergic pathways originating in the basal forebrain have received particular scrutiny. The well-known cholinergic hypothesis of aging and dementia attributes cognitive impairments to reduction in central cholinergic function due to loss of innervation from the basal forebrain (Bartus, Dean, Beer, and Lippa, 1982). Examining attentional functions in older adults is therefore also relevant to an understanding of the role of the cholinergic system in attention. The early involvement of attention in AD suggests that treatment might profitably target attentional functions in addition to the more usual memory tests. Cholinesterase inhibitors such as tetrahydroamino-acridine (THA) that have been tested as treatments for AD may influence attentional functions in addition to memory functions (Sahakian et al., 1993). Recent studies of basal forebrain lesions in monkeys have confirmed that disruption of cholinergic input to neocortex may directly impact spatial attention (Voytko et al., 1994). For a review of the cholinergic system and its role in attentional deficits in AD, see Lawrence and Sahakian (1995).

SPATIAL ATTENTION IN DEMENTIA

Formal studies of attention in AD have only been carried out recently. A small but growing literature has examined issues within each of three domains of attention—selective, divided, and sustained attention. In reviewing those studies, Parasuraman and Haxby (1993) concluded that not all attentional operations are impaired in the early stages of AD. The pattern of preservation and impairment of different attentional functions indicates that AD neuropathology selectively affects neural networks subserving different aspects of attention. The best-understood of those aspects of attention in AD is selective attention, and spatial selective attention in particular.

Mechanisms of Selective Attention

The primate brain may have evolved selection mechanisms because of the computational limitations involved in full parallel processing of all sources of stimulation impinging on it (Broadbent, 1958; James, 1890; Niebur and Koch, chapter 9, this volume).[1] Such a processing limitation necessarily requires selectivity. Selection by location appears to be a major method of selection: information arising from a particular location is subjected to additional processing, whereas information from other locations is inhibited or attenuated (Posner, 1980). Either stimulus saliency (Theeuwes, 1994) or top-down influences from working memory (Desimone and Duncan, 1995) may lead to preferential processing of specific locations. In contrast to space-based models of selective attention, others have proposed that selectivity is implemented by perceptual groupings of stimulus attributes, otherwise known as object-based selection (Duncan, 1984). Driver and Baylis (chapter 14, this volume) suggest that there exist conditions under which both space-based and object-based selection are used.

In many studies of spatial attention, location provides important information relevant to target detection, which usually benefits as a result. Although such results are compatible with the notion of selection by location, a stronger test of the necessity of such a mechanism would be to examine whether it is used in tasks in which location information is irrelevant to target detection. In a recent study, Cave and Pashler (1995) had participants view successively presented pairs of digits displayed about 1 degree on either side of a central fixation point. Target digits were presented in one color and distractors in another color. The task was to name the highest digit of the target color. Even though location (left or right) was not relevant to a correct response, performance was better when both target digits appeared at the same location than when they appeared at different locations. Cave and Pashler (1995) concluded that selection by location is used when targets and distractors belong to the same class of objects (e.g., digits), but that other selection mechanisms are used when they belong to different classes.

Overt and Covert Shifts of Attention

These and other results point to the importance of spatial location as a selection mechanism, and perhaps even indicate that location holds a privileged position in visual selective attention. How could such a mechanism be implemented? Visual information at a particular location can be selected by eye and head movements towards the stimulus source. Because form perception is most efficient for foveated objects, saccadic eye movements, or overt shifts of attention, are necessary for complete analysis of the visual scene. However, the time taken to execute a saccade is of the order of 200–250 ms, which is too long to account for spatial selection between objects that can occur at a rate as fast as 30–40 ms per object (Briand and Klein, 1987; Koch and Ullman, 1985; Treisman and Gelade, 1980; but, see Duncan, Ward, and Shapiro, 1994). This suggests the need for another, faster spatial selection mechanism that can function even when the eyes do not move, a mechanism that has been characterized as covert attention (Posner, 1980).

Covert attention has been extensively investigated in the context of location cueing tasks, in which an advance cue directs the participant to attend to a given location while fixating another location. In a widely used task paradigm, Posner (1980) reported that a location cue speeded reaction time (RT) to detect the onset of a stimulus in the peripheral visual field. Subsequent studies have shown that precues enhance sensory processing at the attended location, as reflected in benefits for RT and for accuracy or in enhancement of early-latency event-related brain potential (ERP) components elicited by a stimulus at the attended location (Hawkins et al., 1990; Luck, Hillyard, Mouloua, Woldorff, Clark, and Hawkins, 1994). In contrast to such valid location cues, invalid cues that direct attention to another location result in costs in RT or in accuracy, presumably because of the need to shift attention away from the incorrect to the correct location.

Considerable evidence exists to suggest that the posterior parietal cortex and parts of the prefrontal cortex form a distributed network (including subcortical structures such as the pulvinar and the superior colliculus) that is involved in shifts of both covert (Corbetta, Miezin, Shulman, and Petersen, 1993; Posner, Walker, Friederich, and Rafal, 1984) and overt (Anderson et al., 1994) spatial attention (for a review, see Posner and Petersen, 1990). Positron emission tomography (PET) studies have shown that major components of that network—for example, the posterior parietal lobe—are hypometabolic in the early stages of AD (Haxby, Duara, Grady, Rapoport, and Cutler, 1985; Haxby et al., 1986). This would suggest that spatial attention shifting should be impaired in early AD.

Parasuraman, Greenwood, Haxby, and Grady (1992) examined whether this was the case by testing persons with AD and age-matched control subjects on a cued letter discrimination task. Participants were required to discriminate between different letters presented in either the left or right visual field while fixating a central point. A discrimination task was used to examine the influence of spatial attention at a level higher than simple energy detection. However, to facilitate comparisons with other neuropsychological studies that have generally only used the luminance detection task originally designed by Posner (1980), a letter detection task requiring a simple RT response was also used. The cue (an arrow) was correct (valid cue), incorrect (invalid cue), or uninformative (neutral cue) regarding the location of the target. Spatial attention shifts can occur endogenously in response to a symbolic cue, for example, an arrow presented at the central fixation point, or exogenously in response to a highly salient cue presented in the periphery near the expected stimulus location (Jonides, 1981). Both types of cueing were used in this study. Finally, in order to examine the time course of cueing effects, the stimulus onset asynchrony (SOA) or interval between cue and target was systematically varied.

For both the detection and the discrimination tasks, and for both central and peripheral cues, the AD group was faster to respond to a target in the left or right visual field with a valid cue than when the cue was neutral or invalid (see figure 21.1). This is the normal pattern of results with the covert attention task, and therefore suggests that the ability to focus attention on the target is not substantially compromised by AD. Other studies have also shown that individuals with AD, like age-matched control subjects, show an RT benefit from a warning stimulus in both simple (Sano et al., 1995) and choice RT tasks (Nebes and Brady, 1993). Those results suggest that phasic alertness and cue-driven engagement of attention are relatively well preserved in AD.

Parasuraman et al. (1992) also found that cue validity effects (invalid cue RT-valid cue RT) did not differ between the AD and control groups for the letter detection task. Similar findings were reported by Maruff, Malone, and Currie (1995) and by Faust and Balota (1997), who tested an AD and an age-matched control group on the standard Posner (1980) detection task with

A. BENEFITS

B. COSTS

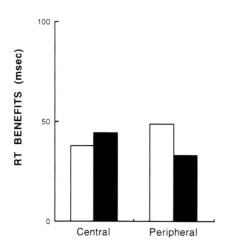

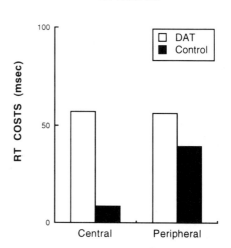

Figure 21.1   (A) Mean RT benefits of a valid spatial cue and (B) costs of an invalid cue for persons with dementia of the Alzheimer type (DAT) and for age-matched control subjects for central and peripheral cues. The DAT group had normal benefits but increased costs for both types of cues. (From Parasuraman et al., 1992.)

peripheral cues. Both studies found no overall group differences in cue validity effects, although Maruff, Malone, and Currie (1995) reported that cue validity effects in their AD group were significantly greater for right but not left visual field targets.

In contrast to the normal effects of a valid cue on RT for the discrimination task, the AD group had longer RTs to targets for invalid cues, for both central and peripheral cues (see figure 21.1) (Parasuraman et al., 1992). These results indicate that the attention shifting impairment in AD is specific to the reorienting or disengagement (Posner et al., 1984) of attention, whereas the initial shifting or engagement of attention to a location is intact. The disengagement deficit was significant only for the discrimination and not for the detection task, a result that suggests that the greater focal attention demands of discrimination exert a top-down effect on attention shifting that is particularly sensitive to dementing disease (for a similar interpretation, see Faust and Balota, 1997). Analysis of the time course of cueing effects suggested that both exogenous and endogenous attention shifting were impaired, but at different times. Exogenous shifts of attention driven by peripheral cues have been found to be most effective at short SOAs, perhaps because such cues elicit an automatic or involuntary process that is short lived and replaced by a subsequent, longer-lasting voluntary process that is elicited by central, symbolic cues (Jonides, 1981; Muller and Rabbitt, 1989). Consistent with that interpretation, the AD group showed a deficit in exogenous attention shifting only at short SOAs, whereas endogenous attention shifting was impaired only at long SOAs (figure 21.2). Although it has often been suggested that both AD (Jorm, 1986) and normal aging (Hasher and Zacks,

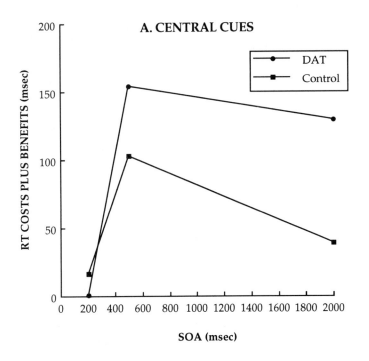

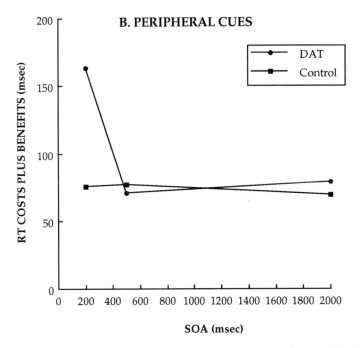

Figure 21.2 Mean RT costs plus benefits of spatial cues as a function of SOA between cue and target for (A) central and for (B) peripheral cues. Individuals with DAT had increased costs and benefits at long SOAs for central cues and at short SOAs for peripheral cues. (From Parasuraman et al., 1992.)

Parasuraman & Greenwood: Aging and Dementia

1979) primarily affect effortful processing but leave automatic processing intact, these results indicate that both forms of processing are impaired in early AD.

Using a different cued discrimination task, Oken, Kishiyama, Kaye, and Howieson (1994) confirmed a spatial disengagement deficit in early AD. Participants were required to respond to a circle presented to the left or right visual field and to withold response if a square was presented. The cue was a central arrow cue (900 ms SOA) that was either valid, invalid, or neutral. The AD group had disproportionately longer invalid RTs compared to control subjects, a result that points to a disengagement deficit in AD.

Faust and Balota (1997) tested AD, older, and young adults on a cued detection task. Single or double cues were used in order to examine inhibition of return (IOR), which occurs when a valid peripheral cue facilitates RT to a target at a short SOA but inhibits RT when the SOA is long, as if observers spontaneously shift their attention away from the cued location after some time has elapsed. The effect is also seen when a second cue appears at fixation, thus drawing attention exogeneously away from the cued location. In both cases RTs are higher at the cued (valid) than at the uncued (invalid) location (Posner, Rafal, Choate, and Vaughan, 1985). In Faust and Balota's (1997) study the single cue condition was similar to the standard Posner task except that the peripheral cue, a brightening of a peripheral box, remained brightened until the target was responded to, rather than only transiently. The authors reasoned that, if AD results in a disengagement deficit (Parasuraman et al., 1992), then it should be particularly apparent with a peripheral cue that attracts attention and remains perceptually salient. Consistent with this reasoning, whereas young adults showed a normal IOR effect at an 800 ms SOA, the AD group did not, and in fact showed facilitation. However, the AD group showed an IOR effect in the second experiment, in which double cues were used, a result that suggests that the disengagement deficit was particularly evident only when attention had to be shifted voluntarily rather than exogeneously.

The disengagement deficit in AD first reported by Parasuraman et al. (1992) is consistent with the effects of the disease on the metabolic integrity of the parietal lobe, which has also been shown to be involved in saccadic eye movements (Anderson et al., 1994). Moreover, given the many interrelationships between covert spatial attention and eye movements (Klein, Kingstone, and Pontefract, 1992), it would not be surprising if persons with AD show deficits in overt as well as covert attention shifting. Saccadic and smooth pursuit eye movements are abnormal in AD (Fletcher and Sharpe, 1988; Pirozzolo and Hansch, 1981). Because eye movements have been controlled for in the covert attention studies, the attention shifting deficit cannot be attributed to oculomotor dysfunction per se. However, as already noted, multiple covert attention shifts can occur in the time before a voluntary saccade is completed. Thus, covert attention shifts may precede and guide eye movements. Hence, if the spatial attention system is impaired in AD, then abnormal eye scan patterns should be observed in tasks requiring saccades between multiple locations. This was confirmed in a study by Scinto, Daffner, Castro, Weintraub, and Vavrik (1994). They found that individuals with AD were less accurate and were slowed in shifting their gaze between a central fixation point and a target dot presented at either two or four peripheral locations in sequence. Analysis of error patterns showed that a major contributor was perseverative fixation of the center point of one of the peripheral targets. Scinto et al. suggested that perseveration of gaze may be associated with slowed disengagement of covert attention in AD. In these studies eye movements were elicited by simple visual targets that had to be scanned in a specified manner. When they were free to attend and shift their gaze at will to a complex visual image, individuals with AD showed diminished exploration of novel or unusual parts of the display (Daffner, Scinto, Weintraub, and Mesulam, 1992). Although such lack of scanning of novel parts of a display may reflect diminished curiosity (Berlyne, 1960) it could also be a by-product of perseverative fixation of other parts of the visual image, as discussed previously.

Individuals with AD are also impaired in making anti-saccades, that is, eye movements in a direction opposite to that of a peripheral stimulus with sudden onset (Fletcher and Sharpe, 1988). This represents an inhibitory failure of overt spatial attention that is probably reflective of frontal lobe dysfunction (Guitton, Buchtel, and Douglas, 1985; Pierrot-Deseilligny, Rivaud, and Gaymard, 1991). A similar finding for covert attention was reported by Maruff and Currie (1995), who tested AD and control groups on the same Posner (1980) detection task as was used in the previously discussed study by Maruff, Malone, and Currie (1995), except that they varied the probability of the location cue. Generally, when a location cue is highly predictive (valid cue probability $\gg .5$) of the target location, normal cue validity effects are obtained. However, if the cue is not predictive (valid cue probability $\ll .5$), and in fact is more likely to indicate that the target will appear in the opposite location, then healthy participants typically adapt and have shorter RTs for invalid than for valid cues (Posner, Walker, Friderich, and Rafal 1987). Maruff and Currie (1995) found that, whereas control participants showed that pattern for a cue with a probability of .2 (i.e., they had negative cue validity scores), individuals with AD responded faster to valid cues than to invalid cues (i.e., they had positive cue validity scores) both when cues were highly predictive (.8) and when they were not (.2).

To summarize, old adults with AD can effectively use advance location information to orient covert attention to an object. However, a number of studies have pointed to an impairment in shifting covert attention in AD, or more specifically, to a disengagement deficit. The deficit is found for both automatic (exogenous) and voluntary (endogenous) shifts of attention, and is related to hypometabolism of the superior parietal lobe. The disengagement deficit also applies to overt shifts of attention associated with eye movements. The disengagement deficit may contribute to perseverative fixation and other abnormalities of visual scanning. The next section examines whether this deficit also plays a role in more complex visual tasks.

Visual Search

Shifts of attention across the visual field, whether overt or covert and whether stimulus-driven or driven top-down by a search goal, provide a selection mechanism for many visual tasks. However, the studies discussed in the previous section have mostly examined attention shifts to single objects in an otherwise empty visual field. In these studies spatial selection is involved in only a rudimentary way, given that the target is presented in isolation. Does such a mechanism also operate when there are many objects present, as in most of our visual experience, and when observers must search for a single object among distractors? Such conditions define the task of visual search, which has also been the subject of extensive investigation. In recent years a number of models of visual search have been proposed. Many of those models assume the existence of a covert spatial attention mechanism that is used to scan complex visual displays for targets (Treisman and Gelade, 1980; Wolfe, Cave, and Frankel, 1989; but, see Desimone and Duncan, 1995). The mechanism may guide or coexist with overt mechanisms for search, such as eye and head movements.

In Treisman's influential feature integration theory (Treisman and Gelade, 1980), search for targets defined by a single, unique feature is thought to occur preattentively in parallel across the visual field. For example, in a search for a colored target in a field of black items, or for a moving target among stationary objects, the targets are detected very quickly and subjectively appear to pop out from the background. For targets that are defined by the combination of two features, such as a moving object of a particular color, search is slower and increases with the number of distracting items that possess one but not both features. Since Treisman and Gelade's (1980) study, a large number of studies have been carried out to examine the conditions under which search is serial or parallel for different combinations of features and distractors. Although many of the results support the theory, certain conjunction pairs, such as motion and form, can be searched very efficiently with no effect of distractors, thus contradicting feature integration theory (Nakayama and Silverman, 1986). Those studies have led to a revision of the original theory (Treisman, 1988). At the same time, alternative search models have been put forward (Duncan and Humphreys, 1989; Wolfe et al., 1989).

Search models differ in postulating differing conditions under which search for a target is fast and independent of distractors and when it is slow and dependent on distractors. In general, search is very efficient and is associated with the subjective phenomenon of pop-out when targets are specified by a unique feature or when the overlap of target and distractor features is minimal. Search is less efficient when targets are defined by a conjunction of features or if target versus distractor discriminability is low. When search is distractor-dependent, displays with items such as letters or object forms can be searched at a rate of about 30–40 ms per item, which is consistent with the temporal characteristics of a covert attention mechanism (Koch and Ullman, 1985).

Cognitive studies suggest that the spatial attention mechanism in visual search may be the same as the one involved in covert orienting and shifting of attention in response to location cues (Parasuraman, Greenwood, and Alexander, 1995; Prinzmetal, Presti, and Posner, 1986). Furthermore, in a recent PET study, Corbetta, Shulman, Miezin, and Petersen (1995) found that in comparison to feature search, conjunction search was associated with activation of the superior parietal lobe in a region closely overlapping with the region that they had previously shown to be involved in covert shifts of attention (also, see Corbetta, chapter 6, this volume). Arguin, Joanette, and Cavanagh (1993) found that brain-damaged individuals who showed deficits in covert orienting also had slower search rates to detect targets defined by a conjunction of color and orientation, but that search was unimpaired for detection of either feature in isolation. Those results would suggest that AD individuals, who have prominent parietal lobe hypometabolism and who show an attentional disengagement deficit (Parasuraman et al., 1992), should be impaired when asked to perform a visual search task in which repeated shifts of spatial attention are required.

Nebes and Brady (1989) examined visual search performance in AD and control groups using a six-letter visual search task. On half the trials four of the letters were presented in red and two in black (the target was always black). Thus, observers could use the color cue to select the two relevant letters and effectively reduce the display size from six to two. On the remaining trials all letters were displayed in black. The advantage afforded by the color cue for search RT was the same in the AD and control groups, indicating that AD individuals could effectively select stimuli on the basis of their color. At least for simple displays, therefore, color-based selection is not markedly affected in individuals with AD, although they show prominent deficits when color selection occurs in the context of distractors that strongly activate a competing response, as in the Stroop color and word interference task (Spieler, Balota, and Faust 1996). However, this conclusion must be qualified because only simple display configurations were examined in the Nebes and Brady (1989) study. The use of a clearly defined color cue would have caused the relevant target set of letters to pop out (Treisman and Gelade, 1980), and although the target was not uniquely specified by color, only two letters had to be searched, so that the need for spatial attention was limited. Under such conditions, feature-based selection may be preserved even in moderate AD.

Although individuals suffering from AD can use spatial information to select a visual hemifield or objects of a particular color, the size of the required attentional focus is an important factor in visual selection, particularly if fine target discriminations have to be made at the attended locus and when the target set size is potentially large, unlike in the Nebes and Brady (1989) study. In visual search tasks with a target defined by a conjunction of features (e.g., color and shape), RT increases with the number of distractors, a result that suggests the use of a serial, spatial attention scanning mechanism. In Posner's (1980) conceptualization of spatial attention, the mechanism is a spotlight that illuminates a small area of the visual field. The spotlight is postulated to move across the visual field at a rate of about 30–40 ms per item in visual search tasks that are distractor-dependent. An alternative conceptualization of spatial attention, however, is that of a gradient (LaBerge and Brown, 1989) that is distributed over a relatively large area but that has a peak intensity covering only a part of that area. Studies have shown that observers can voluntarily adjust the effective area of the attentional focus from large to small or vice versa but, just like a zoom lens, resolving power must be traded off against the size of the attended area (Eriksen and Yeh, 1985).

Irrespective of which, if any, of these metaphors for spatial attention is valid, the results of cueing studies lead to the prediction that spatial cues that vary in their precision of localization should affect search efficiency. In particular, precueing should influence speed of identification of targets defined by a conjunction of features but not of targets defined by one feature. Moreover, spatial cues should affect search efficiency less in mildly demented persons than in age-matched controls. A cued visual search task that combines the orienting and search paradigms was recently developed to examine these effects (Greenwood et al., 1997; Parasuraman et al., 1995). Participants searched for feature or for conjunction targets as in the normal visual search paradigm. However, the search display was preceded by a cue that varied in size and therefore in its precision of spatial localization. This allowed for an assessment of the role of shifts of spatial attention in complex visual processing independent of factors such as display size. Cue validity was also manipulated by varying cue location, thus allowing processes of engagement and disengagement to be studied not just in a relatively empty visual field, as in the covert orienting task, but in a more complex visual scene. Individuals with AD and healthy, age-matched controls searched a display for a target characterized by a single feature (color) or by a conjunction of features (color + letter). Precues of differing sizes provided localizing information of varying precision. The more precise the cue, the greater the expected improvement in search time. Effects of display size and cue size on RT for feature search were similar in an AD group and in controls. For conjunction search, however, the AD group showed minimal effects of cue size, whereas control subjects were faster at target identification as cue size approached target size (see figure 21.3). In contrast to the previous finding of preserved engagement in a nonsearch task, these results indicated an impairment in AD in the spatial focusing (or engagement) of attention during visual search.

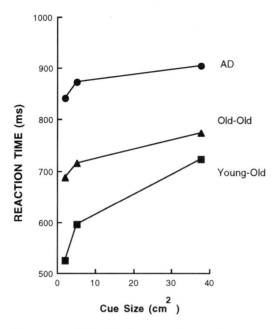

Figure 21.3 Mean RTs for conjunction search targets as a function of the size of a spatial pre-cue for AD, old-old, and young-old groups. RT decreased with increased precision (smaller size) of spatial cues for all groups, but less so for the old-old group and least for the AD group. (From Parasuraman et al., 1995.)

Spatial Scale and Object Perception

The spatial attention studies reviewed so far indicate that individuals with AD have difficulty disengaging attention from a current area of focus and shifting attention to another location. If, as suggested previously, this is a basic selection mechanism that underlies selection of objects in many different visual tasks, then this fact would suggest that the impairments that individuals with AD show on many complex visual tasks may be be due to an underlying spatial attention deficit.

AD may also impair the ability to adjust the spatial scale of attention in response to target information. But is there a deficit in shifting attention to different locations that are part of the same object? As discussed earlier, attention allocation in complex displays can be either object-based or location-based, and attentional costs can accrue if attention has to be shifted between objects or between locations within a single object (see Driver and Baylis, chapter 14, this volume). Given that previous research has shown that AD impairs divided attention (Parasuraman and Haxby 1993), individuals with AD should be particularly impaired if they have to make judgments requiring attention to multiple locations within a single object or between different objects.

Filoteo, Delis, Massman, and Buffers (1992) examined this issue by using the global/local task developed by Navon (1977). In this task, a large global

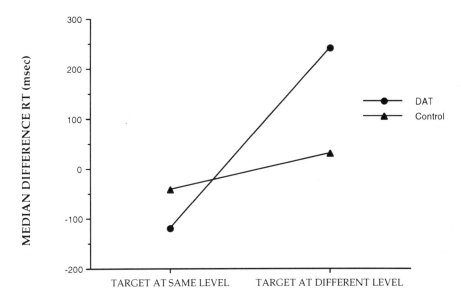

CONSECUTIVE TRIALS

Figure 21.4 Median difference in RT over consecutive trials when the target stimulus remained at the same hierarchical level (local or global) or when it switched levels on consecutive trials for persons with DAT and for age-matched control subjects. Individuals with DAT showed disproportionately increased RTs when the target switched between levels across consecutive trials. (Adapted from Filoteo et al., 1992. Reprinted with permission.)

form is made up of smaller local forms, such as a large number 1 made up of smaller 2s. Individuals were required to decide whether a target digit (e.g., 1) was present at either the local or global level (divided attention condition). The target stimulus could appear at the same level across consecutive trials (e.g., local → local) or could change level (e.g., local → global). The AD group was slowed when attention had to be switched from trial to trial from the global to the local level or vice versa (figure 21.4). When the target was at the same level across consecutive trials, RT was relatively unaffected, and if anything the AD group showed a small repetition priming effect. Both the control and AD groups responded more slowly when the target appeared at different levels on consecutive trials, but the AD group was disproportionately slowed. In a subsequent study that used the same task, Massman et al. (1993) showed that RTs of individuals with AD were disproportionately affected for detection of targets at a particular level if the opposing level contained a conflicting target (e.g., discriminating a 1 from a 2 at the local level with a 2 at the global level). These findings suggest a disengagement deficit in AD, not between spatial locations, but between different hierarchical levels of a composite object. Thus, the attention shifting deficit in AD applies not only to locations per se but also to different levels of perceptual organization at different locations within a complex stimulus.

The disengagement deficit could contribute to the difficulty individuals with AD have in performing composite object identification tasks (Filoteo et al., 1992; Thaiss and De Bleser, 1993) or cancellation tasks (Della Sala, Laicona, Spinnler, and Ubezio, 1992; Foldi, Jutagir, Davidoff, and Gould, 1992) in which attention must be successively directed to different parts of a complex visual object or to different locations. That persons with AD are less able to take advantage of spatial cues during visual search than are healthy control subjects may have implications for understanding the nature of visuospatial impairment in AD as well as in other disorders of spatial attention and visual search involving posterior parietal cortex. Thaiss and de Bleser (1994) reported a case study of a 58-year-old woman with AD who was unable to use global shape information to recognize large objects, apparently depending instead upon a feature-by-feature strategy (Farah, 1990). Thaiss and de Bleser proposed that the individual had a reduced attentional focus size because recognition improved when object size was decreased. An alternative possibility, based on the present results, is that she had difficulty in shifting attention to the appropriate scale for the required task.

Comparison to Other Dementias

The nature of the attentional deficit in AD differs from that found in other dementias such as Parkinson's disease (PD) and Huntington's disease (HD). These forms of dementia can be broadly thought of as subcortical dementias because they are associated with pathology affecting structures such as the substantia nigra (PD) and the caudate (HD), whereas AD is primarily (though not exclusively) a cortical disease. Maruff, Malone, McArthur-Jackson, et al. (1995) also found that performance of an HIV-associated dementia complex (H-ADC) group did not differ from that of HIV-negative controls in the Posner (1980) covert attention task, but the H-ADC group did show increased RTs to a nonspatial, diffuse (neutral) cue. However, the neuropathological changes associated with H-ADC are not entirely subcortical (Wiley, Masliah, and Morey, 1991), and the level of neocortical involvement is different from that in AD.

The differential effects of the dementias on selective attention are best exemplified by studies examining spatial attention in PD and AD. Whereas individuals with AD showed increased RTs to invalid location cues (Parasuraman et al., 1992), Wright, Burns, Geffen, and Geffen (1990) found that persons with PD showed *reduced* RTs. Wright et al. interpreted their results as reflecting a relative impairment in the maintenance of attention at the cued location (or abnormally fast disengagement of attention), in contrast to the delayed disengagement found in AD. Thus, although both PD and AD affect spatial attention, different components are affected. The differential pattern of a disengagement deficit in AD and a maintenance deficit in PD is also seen when attention to spatial scale is examined. As discussed previously, Filoteo et al. (1992) found that individuals with AD showed a disengagement deficit when they were required to shift attention across trials to different levels of perceptual organization in the global/local task. In a more recent study, Filoteo et al. (1995) compared the performance of three dementia groups—AD, PD, and HD—on the same global/local task. The HD group did not show a deficit in shifting attention across trials in the this task, a result that suggests that they had neither a disengagement nor a maintenance deficit. The AD group was differentially slowed in comparison to age-matched control subjects when the target level changed from global to local or vice versa across trials. In contrast, individuals with PD were *faster* than controls to respond when the target level changed across trials and *slower* when the target level remained the same. Thus, in contrast to the disengagement deficit exhibited by the AD group, and consistent with the covert attention study of Wright et al. (1990), the PD group showed a maintenance deficit. This is a striking correspondence across two quite different attentional paradigms—the covert attention task and the global/local task.

Summary of Spatial Attention Findings in AD

The ability to shift the focus of attention to a cued location or object appears to be relatively well preserved in early AD. In contrast, persons with AD display an impairment in shifting covert attention *away* from a cued location—a disengagment deficit—whether attention is shifted reflexively or voluntarily. The disengagement deficit, which also applies to overt shifts of attention associated with eye movements, is related to hypometabolism of the superior parietal lobe. Difficulties in disengaging spatial attention may also lead to slowing of visual search in AD. Although individuals with AD can engage attention at a location, they show reduced ability to adjust the spatial focus of attention around the attended location. This deficit may underly AD deficits in complex visual tasks requiring adjustment of the spatial scale of attention. Finally, the pattern of spatial attention deficits in AD is qualitatively different from attentional changes associated with some other types of dementia, notably PD and HD.

SPATIAL ATTENTION, AD, AND AGING

These studies suggest that the spatial attention deficit in AD is qualitatively distinct from that associated with other dementias, so long as they do not markedly affect the integrity of the posterior parietal lobes, which are hypometabolic in early AD. Is the spatial attention deficit in AD also qualitatively different from attentional changes associated with healthy aging? This issue is of interest, given that the cognitive and physiological changes in the early, "preclinical" stages of AD are difficult to distinguish from those associated with so-called healthy aging. Whether spatial attention changes in aging and AD differ qualitatively or quantitatively also bears on the long-standing debate of whether AD represents accelerated or exaggerated aging or a distinct disease process (Berg, 1985; Drachman, 1983). One way to examine this issue is to compare the effects of aging, especially advanced aging, and of AD on the same attentional tasks.

The study of nondemented "old-old" adults also assumes greater relevance in light of the identification of the apolipoprotein (APOE) e4 allele as a genetic risk factor for AD (Corder et al., 1993). Individuals carrying the APOE e4 allele have a greater risk of developing AD, particularly at older ages. Nondemented persons carrying the APOE e4 allele exhibit similar patterns of hemisphere-specific reduction in cerebral glucose metabolism (Small et al., 1995) that very mildly demented individuals do (Haxby et al., 1986), and they have poorer neuropsychological test scores than those without the e4 allele (Feskens, Havekes, and Kalmijn, 1994; Reed, Carmelli, and Swan, 1994). These findings are consistent with the view that, for some functions, aging and AD differ quantitatively along a continuum.

Nevertheless, the issue of a qualitative or quantitative difference in spatial attention changes between AD and aging has not been fully resolved. On the one hand, both reflexive (peripheral cues) and voluntary attention shifts (central cues) are impaired in AD, whereas only the latter is affected by aging (Greenwood and Parasuraman, 1997). However, this applies only to individuals up to about 75 years of age. Greenwood and Parasuraman (1994) reported that in a discrimination task old-old elderly (75–85 years of age) exhibited significantly greater costs of invalid cues (determined by subtraction of neutral RTs from invalid RTs) compared to young-old elderly (65–75 years of age), whether cues were central or peripheral. This is qualitatively the same pattern of results as was reported previously for AD by Parasuraman et al. (1992). Faust and Balota (1997) also found that a slightly broader age range of nondemented old-old adults (70–85 years) had increased peripheral cue validity effects.

Unfortunately, very few studies have examined attentional functions in the nondemented old-old, so that the hypothesis of a continuum between advanced age and AD must remain tentative. Examination of the neural systems of spatial attention and the effects of aging and AD on these systems may shed some light on this issue.

Neural Systems of Spatial Attention

Several proposals outlining the neural systems controlling spatial attention in the human brain have been put forward in recent years. Although the models differ in their specificity and in their focus on the importance of particular brain regions, all share in common the view that the brain systems involved are distributed across a broad network of cortical and subcortical regions (see Webster and Ungerleider, chapter 2, this volume). Mesulam (1981) proposed a network of three cortical systems for the control of both spatial and nonspatial attention. He postulated that the posterior parietal area provides a sensory representation of extrapersonal space, frontal cortex contributes a map of exploratory and orienting movements, and cingulate cortex maps motivational values to space. Goldman-Rakic (1988) proposed that visuospatial attention is mediated by a network involving frontal and parietal areas and linked to the medial pulvinar. The most specific model was put forward by Posner and Petersen (1990), who proposed that the superior parietal lobe is involved in disengaging visuospatial attention, the midbrain in shifting the focus of attention to the target area, and the pulvinar nucleus of the thalamus in obtaining data from the attended location.

The importance of posterior parietal cortex for visuospatial attention is well documented. Posner et al. (1984) observed that although individuals with superior parietal lobe lesions were unimpaired in engaging attention following a valid cue, they were selectively slowed in disengaging attention following an invalid cue, reflected in very long RTs to invalidly cued targets. Individuals in the early, mild stage of AD also showed an increase in RT costs of invalid cues, while showing no concomitant increase in benefits of valid cues (Oken, Kishiyama, Kaye, and Howieson, 1994; Parasuraman et al., 1992). Furthermore, combined RT costs and benefits were correlated with rates of resting glucose metabolism in the superior, but not in the inferior, parietal area (Parasuraman et al., 1992).

The importance of the parietal cortex to the process of disengagement has also been emphasized by single-unit recordings in monkeys. In the intra-parietal sulcus a subset of neurons discharged best after a peripheral cue directed attention away from the target (Robinson, Bowman, and Kertzman, 1991). Similarly, neurons in area 7a have been found to fire strongly to receptive field stimuli other than those that are attended (Steinmetz and Constantinidis, 1995). Behavioral manipulations of neurons in monkey intra-parietal sulcus indicate that the receptive field location is shifted before directed eye movements are (Duhamel, Colby, and Goldberg, 1992). Consistent with these findings, cerebral blood flow as measured by PET increases in the human intraparietal sulcus during a location matching task (Haxby et al., 1994), in a location-cued discrimination task (Nobre et al., 1996), and during execution of a memorized sequence of eye movements (Petit et al., 1996). These data support the view of Fischer and Breitmeyer (1987) that attention is shifted to a new location before the eyes move and suggest that the relevant mechanisms of attention shifting are dependent on the intra-parietal sulcus.

What role does the pulvinar play in selective attention? Robinson and Petersen (1992) reviewed single-unit studies in behaving monkeys and concluded that the pulvinar is involved in stimulus salience. On the basis of a PET study in a visual discrimination task, LaBerge (1990) proposed that the pulvinar acts to implement attentional filtering of targets from distractors. Studies in brain-damaged individuals also bear on the role of the pulvinar, although indirectly, because thalamic lesions are seldom confined to the pulvinar. Individuals with unilateral hemorrhagic lesions of the thalamus had abnormally slowed responses to contralateral compared to ipsilateral visual targets, regardless of whether location precues were valid or invalid (Rafal and Posner, 1987), a result that suggests reduced ability to engage attention in the visual field contralateral to the thalamic damage. A subgroup of AD individuals with particular deficits in set shifting and visual search have been reported to have decreased radiodensity in the dorsomedial thalamus (Forstl and Sahakian, 1993).

At least two other cortical regions outside the parietal lobe have been implicated in visuospatial attention: area V4 and premotor cortex. Single units in V4 responded more strongly for an attended than for an ignored stimulus within the receptive field (Luck, Chelazzi, Hillyard, and Desimone, 1997; Moran and Desimone, 1985). Motter (1994) found that this effect, seen in V4 but not in V1 or V2, could change dynamically as the selected stimulus was changed, and Motter argued that those results reflect the neuronal processes that underlie the phenomenon of pop-out (also, see Motter, chapter 4, this volume). Finally, recent work supports the proposal by Goldman-Rakic (1988) of a frontal component in the network mediating visuospatial attention. PET studies have shown that cerebral blood flow is increased by visuospatial attention in a premotor area (Haxby et al., 1994; Corbetta et al., 1993) identified as the frontal eye field in area 6 (Nobre et al., 1996). Because saccadic eye movements also activate that region (Petit et al., 1996), it cannot be determined whether the mechanisms mediating visuospatial attention and directed saccades are separable.

Effects of Aging and Dementia

These data support the view that attention is mediated by a network linking frontal and posterior parietal areas with the pulvinar (Goldman-Rakic, 1988). It is therefore of interest to examine whether pathological changes occur in these areas with aging and with AD. Neuropathological and physiological changes have been measured by cell counts, neuritic plaques and neurofibrillary tangles (NFTs), synaptic size and density, cortical volume, and cerebral metabolism and blood flow.

Greenwood and Parasuraman (1997) recently reviewed these findings in detail. They concluded that pathological changes arise in mesial temporal, orbitofrontal, superior temporal, and parietal areas in both normal aging and in AD, albeit with substantial differences in degree between the two (e.g., Arriagada, Marzloff, and Hyman, 1992). Although posterior parietal cortex and frontal cortex, which are strongly linked to visuospatial attention, are subject to pathological changes in both aging and AD, there are also alterations in brain regions not directly associated with visuospatial attention, such as mesial and superior temporal regions. AD eventually adds nearly all neocortex to the list of affected regions, although in the early, mild stages in which many cognitive studies are conducted, changes in regional metabolism occur selectively in parietal and temporal association areas. In fact, individuals in very early stage AD with only memory deficits have neocortical metabolic reductions largely confined to parietal association cortex (Grady et al., 1988; Haxby et al., 1986).

Does aging or AD affect the pulvinar? Unfortunately, this nucleus, and indeed the thalamus as a whole, is rarely studied in individuals with AD. The anterior dorsal nucleus of the thalamus and the entorhinal area may be the first sites of age-related pathological changes in the form of NFTs; those changes are magnified in AD (Braak and Braak, 1991). Thalamic NFTs have also been observed in the medial dorsal nucleus of some normally aged brains (Grossi, Lopez, and Martinez, 1989). Despite these scattered results, the thalamus has generally been characterized as a brain region that is relatively unaffected by AD neuropathology. This poses a problem for the interpretation of spatial attention deficits in AD discussed previously, because strong evidence of pulvinar involvement in spatial attention has been reported. It is therefore of considerable interest that pulvinar lesions have recently been reported in a sample of autopsy-verified cases of AD (Kuljis, 1994). Extensive clusters of NFTs in the pulvinar were found in a sample of nine AD brains. Age-matched control subjects had few lesions.

Thus, there is is evidence that all three brain regions thought to be involved in spatial attention—posterior parietal cortex, prefrontal cortex, and the pulvinar—are affected by pathological changes associated with AD, and, to a lesser extent, by aging. This indicates that pathological changes affecting components of or communication between widespread corticocortical and subcortical networks contribute to spatial attention deficits in AD. Similar though less extensive changes affect aging as well.

This conclusion contradicts a proposal by Hartley (1992, 1993), who suggested that aging affects only anterior brain regions supporting attention, and not posterior areas (e.g., parietal cortex). Hartley proposed that spatial attention is largely age invariant and that aging of frontal cortex mediates age-related decreases in other aspects of attention and cognition, such as attention to set and set shifting. Although there is some support for this view, like many generalizations, it does not fit all the data, and both assertions— that spatial attention is age invariant, and that aging does not affect the structural or functional integrity of posterior brain regions—can be disputed, as shown previously.

CONCLUSIONS

Spatial attention is not subserved by a single brain region but by distributed neural systems that support different aspects of spatial and attentional processing. The components of those systems include the posterior parietal cortex, the frontal cortex, and the pulvinar nucleus of the thalamus. Shifts of spatial attention result from the interaction of neural activity between posterior and anterior brain regions and their integration with subcortical (e.g., pulvinar) activity. Behavioral support for such an interaction is provided by the evidence, discussed previously, of top-down influences on spatial attention, which presumably reflect frontal lobe interaction with the parietal cortex.

Communication between frontal and parietal brain regions is affected by AD neuropathology, and to a lesser extent by aging, particularly by advanced aging. The pathological processes associated with AD primarily affect association cortical areas, leaving the primary sensory and motor areas relatively intact. Degeneration of particular laminae and cell types in these areas indicates selective loss of corticocortical connections, leading to the characterization of AD as a disconnection syndrome (Morrison, 1993). Correlations of glucose metabolic rates between frontal and parietal cortex (Horwitz, Grady, Schlageter, Duara, and Rapoport, 1987), as well as of EEG coherences between frontal and parietal scalp sites (Luechter, Newton, Cook, and Walter 1992), are reduced in AD, suggesting a functional dissociation that may also be indicative of corticocortical disconnection. This may produce a pattern of attentional performance in which functions such as spatial attention that depend upon communication between widely distributed brain regions are markedly disrupted.

ACKNOWLEDGMENTS

This research was supported by National Institutes of Health grants AG05769 to Raja Parasuraman and AG12387 to Pamela M. Greenwood.

NOTE

1. Although many accept this position, other views have also been postulated. Edelman (1987), for example, has argued against selective perceptual processing. He proposed instead that selectivity evolved by Darwinian principles of natural selection of one out of a set of different possible responses, i.e., as attention to action (see Allport, 1993).

REFERENCES

Allport, D. (1993) Attention and control: Have we been asking the wrong questions? A critical review of twenty-five years. In *Attention and Performance XV*, edited by D. Meyer and S. Kornblum. Cambridge, MA: MIT Press.

Almkvist, O. and Backman, L. (1993) Detection and staging of early clinical dementia. *Acta Neurol. Scand.* 88: 10–15.

Anderson, T. J., Jenkins, I. H., Brooks, D. J., Hawken, M. B., Frackowiack, R. S. J., and Kennard, C. (1994) Cortical control of saccades and fixation in a man. A PET study. *Brain* 117: 1073–1084.

Arguin, M., Joanette, Y., and Cavanagh, P. (1993) Visual search for feature and conjunction targets with an attention deficit. *J. Cognitive Neurosci.* 5: 436–452.

Arriagada, P. V., Marzloff, K., and Hyman, B. T. (1992) Distribution of Alzheimer-type pathologic changes in nondemented elderly individuals matches the pattern in Alzheimer's disease. *Neurology* 42: 1681–1688.

Bartus, R. T., Dean, R. L., Beer, B., and Lippa, A. S. (1982) The cholinergic hypothesis of geriatric memory dysfunction. *Science* 217: 408–417.

Berg, L. (1985) Does Alzheimer's disease represent an exaggeration of normal aging? *Arch. Neurol.* 42: 737–739.

Berlyne, D. (1960) *Conflict, Arousal, and Curiosity.* New York: McGraw-Hill.

Braak, H. and Braak, E. (1991) Neuropathological stageing of Alzheimer-related changes. *Acta Neuropathol.* 82: 239–259.

Briand, K. A. and Klein, R. M. (1987) Is Posner's "beam" the same as Triesman's "glue"? On the relation between visual orienting and feature integration theory. *J. Exp. Psychol. Hum. Percept. Perform.* 13: 228–241.

Broadbent, D. E. (1958) *Perception and Communication.* London: Pergamon Press.

Cave, K. R. and Pashler, H. (1995) Visual selection mediated by location: Selecting successive visual objects. *Percept. Psychophys.* 57: 421–432.

Corbetta, M., Miezin, F. M., Shulman, G. L., and Petersen, S. E. (1993) A PET study of visuospatial attention. *J. Neurosci.* 13: 1202–1226.

Corbetta, M., Shulman, G. L., Miezin, F. M., and Petersen, S. E. (1995) Superior parietal cortex activation during spatial attention shifts and visual feature conjunction. *Science* 270: 802–805.

Corder, E. H., Saunders, A. M., Strittmatter, W. J., Schmechel, D. E., Gaskell, P. C. Small, G. W., Roses, A. D., Haines, J. L., and Pericak-Vance, M. A. (1993) Gene dose of apolipoprotein E type 4 allele and the risk of Alzheimer's disease in late onset families. *Science* 261: 921–923.

Daffner, K. R., Scinto, L. F. M., Weintraub, S. J., and Mesulam, M. M. (1992) Diminished curiosity in patients with probable Alzheimer's disease as measured by exploratory eye movements. *Neurology* 42: 320–328.

De Lacoste, M. C. and White, C. L. (1993) The role of cortical connectivity in Alzheimer's disease pathogenesis: A review and model system. *Neurobiol. Aging* 14: 1–16.

Della Salla, S., Laicona, M., Spinnler, H., and Ubezio, C. (1992) A cancellation test: Its reliability in assessing attentional deficits in Alzheimer's disease. *Psychol. Med.* 22: 885–901.

Desimone, R. and Duncan, J. (1995) Neural mechanisms of selective visual attention. *Annu. Rev. Neurosci.* 18: 193–222.

Drachman, D. A. (1983) How normal aging relates to dementia: A critique and classification. In *Aging of the Brain,* edited by D. Samuel, pp. 131–148. New York: Wiley Liss.

Duhamel, J. R., Colby, C. L., and Goldberg, M. E. (1992) The updating of the representation of visual space in parietal cortex by intended eye movements. *Science* 255: 90–92.

Duncan, J. (1984) Selective attention and the organization of visual information. *J. Exp. Psychol. Gen.* 113: 501–517.

Duncan, J. and Humphreys, G. W. (1989) Visual search and stimulus similarity. *Psychol. Rev.* 96: 433–458.

Duncan, J., Ward, R., and Shapiro, K. (1994) Direct measurement of attentional dwell time in human vision. *Nature* 369: 313–315.

Edelman, G. M. (1987) *Neural Darwinism: The Theory of Neuronal Group Selection.* New York: Basic Books.

Eriksen, C. W. and Yeh, Y. (1985) Allocation of attention in the visual field. *J. Exp. Psychol. Hum. Percept. Perform.* 11: 583–597.

Farah, M. J. (1990) *Visual Agnosia.* Cambridge, MA: MIT Press.

Faust, M. E. and Balota, D. A. (1997) Inhibition of return and visuospatial attention in healthy old adults and individuals with dementia of the Alzheimer type. *Neuropsychology* 11: 13–29.

Feskens, E. J. M., Havekes, L. M., and Kalmijn, S. (1994) Apolipoprotein e4 allele and cognitive decline in elderly men. *Br. J. Med.* 309: 1202–1206.

Filoteo, J. V., Delis, D. C., Massman, P. J. and Butters, N. (1992) Directed and divided attention in Alzheimer's disease: Impairment in shifting of attention to global and local stimuli. *J. Clin. Exp. Neuropsychol.* 14: 871–883.

Filoteo, J. V., Delis, D. C., Massman, P. J., Roman, M. J., Demadura, T., Ford, E., Butters, N., Salmon, D. P., Paulsen, J., Shults, C. W., Swenson, M., and Swerdlow, N. (1995) Visual attention and perception in patients with Huntingdon's disease: Comparisons with other subcortical and cortical dementias. *J. Clin. Exp. Neuropsychol.* 17: 654–667.

Fischer, B. and Breitmeyer, B. (1987) Mechanisms of visual attention revealed by saccadic eye movements. *Neuropsychologia* 25: 73–83.

Fletcher, W. A. and Sharpe, J. A. (1988) Saccadic eye movement dysfunction in Alzheimer's disease. *Ann. Neurol.* 20: 464–471.

Foldi, N. S., Jutagir, R., Davidoff, D., and Gould, T. (1992) Selective attention skills in Alzheimer's disease: Performance on graded cancellation tests varying in density and complexity. *J. Gerontol. Psychol. Sci.* 47: P146–P153.

Forstl, H. and Sahakian, B. J. (1993) Thalamic radiodensity and cognitive performance in mild and moderate dementia of the Alzheimer type. *J. Psychiatr. Neurosci.* 18: 33–37.

Goldman-Rakic, P. (1988) Topography of cognition: Parallel distributed networks in primate association cortex. *Annu. Rev. Neurosci.* 11: 137–156.

Grady, C. L., Haxby, J. V., Horwitz, B., Sundaram, M., Berg, G., Shapiro, M., Friedland, R. P., and Rapoport, S. I. (1988) A longitudinal study of the early neuropsychological and cerebral metabolic changes in dementia of the Alzheimer type. *J. Clin. Exp. Neuropsychol.* 10: 576–596.

Greenwood, P. M. and Parasuraman, R. (1994) Attentional disengagement deficit in nondemented elderly over 75 years of age. *Aging Cog.* 1: 188–202.

Greenwood, P. M., and Parasuraman, R. (1997) Attention in aging and Alzheimer's disease: Behavior and neural systems. In *Attention, Development, and Psychopathology,* edited by J. Enns and J. Burack. New York: Guilford Press.

Greenwood, P. M., Parasuraman, R., and Alexander, G. E. (1997) Controlling the focus of spatial attention during visual search: Effects of advanced aging and Alzheimer's disease. *Neuropsychology* 11: 3–12.

Greenwood, P. M., Parasuraman, R., and Haxby, J. V. (1993) Visuospatial attention across the adult life span. *Neuropsychologia* 31: 471–485.

Grossi, D., Lopez, O. L., and Martinez, A. L. (1989) Mammillary bodies in Alzheimer's disease. *Acta Neuropathol. Scand.* 80: 41–45.

Guitton, D., Buchtel, H. A., and Douglas, R. M. (1985) Frontal lobe lesions in man cause difficulties in suppressing reflexive glances and in generating goal-directed saccades. *Exp. Brain Res.* 58: 455–472.

Hartley, A. A. (1992) Attention. In *Handbook of Aging and Cognition,* edited by F. I. M. Craik and T. A. Salthouse, pp. 3–49. Hillsdale, NJ: Lawrence Erlbaum.

Hartley, A. A. (1993) Evidence for the selective preservation of spatial selective attention in old age. *Psychol. Aging* 8: 371–379.

Hartley, A. A., Kieley, J. M., and Slabach, E. H. (1990) Age differences and similarities in the effects of cues and prompts. *J. Exp. Psychol. Hum. Percept. Perform.* 16: 523–537.

Hasher, L. and Zacks, R. T. (1979). Automatic and effortful processes in memory. *J. Exp. Psychol. Gen.* 108: 356–388.

Hawkins, H. L., Hillyard, S. A., Luck, S. J., Mouloua, M., Downing, C. J., and Woodward, D. P. (1990) Visual attention modulates signal detectability. *J. Exp. Psychol. Hum. Percept. Perform.* 16: 802–811.

Haxby, J. V., Duara, R., Grady, C. L., Rapoport, S. I., and Cutler, N. R. (1985) Relations between neuropsychological and cerebral metabolic asymmetries in early Alzheimer's disease. *J. Cereb. Blood Flow Metab.* 5: 193–200.

Haxby, J. V., Grady, C. L., Duara, R., Schlageter, N. L., Berg, G., and Rapoport, S. I. (1986) Neocortical metabolic abnormalities precede nonmemory cognitive deficits in early Alzheimer-type dementia. *Arch. Neurol.* 43: 882–885.

Haxby, J. V., Horwitz, B., Ungerleider, L., Maisog, J. M., Pietrini, P., and Grady, C. L. (1994) The functional organization of human extrastriate cortex: A PET-rCBF study of selective attention to faces and locations. *J. Neurosci.* 14: 6336–6353.

Horwitz, B., Grady, C. L., Schlageter, N. L., Duara, R., and Rapoport, S. I. (1987) Intercorrelations of regional cerebral glucose metabolic rates in Alzheimer's disease. *Brain Res.* 47: 294–306.

James, W. (1890) *The Principles of Psychology.* Cambridge, MA: Harvard University Press.

Jonides, J. (1981) Voluntary versus automatic control over the mind's eye's movement. In *Attention and Performance IX,* edited by J. B. Long and A. D. Baddeley, pp. 187–203. Hillsdale, NJ: Lawrence Erlbaum.

Jorm, A. F. (1986) Controlled and automatic information processing in senile dementia: A review. *Psychol. Med.* 16: 77–88.

Kemper, T. (1994) Neuroanatomical and neuropathological changes in normal aging and in dementia. In *Clinical Neurology of Aging* (2nd ed.), edited by M. L. Albert, pp. 3–67. New York: Oxford University Press.

Klein, R., Kingstone, A., and Pontefract, A. (1992) Orienting of visual attention. In *Eye Movements and Visual Cognition,* edited by K. Rayner. New York: Springer Verlag.

Koch, C. and Ullman, S. (1985) Shifts in selective visual attention: Towards the underlying neural circuitry. *Hum. Neurobiol.* 4: 219–227.

Kuljis, R. O. (1994) Lesions in the pulvinar in patients with Alzheimer's disease. *J. Neuropathol. Exp. Neurol.* 53: 202–211.

LaBerge, D. (1990) Thalamic and cortical mechanisms of attention suggested by recent positron emission tomographic experiments. *J. Cognitive Neurosci.* 2: 358–372.

LaBerge, D. and Brown, V. (1989) Theory of attentional operations in shape identification. *Psychol. Rev.* 96: 101–124.

Lawrence, A. D. and Sahakian, B. J. (1995) Alzheimer disease, attention, and the cholinergic system. *Alzheimer Dis. Assoc. Disord.* 9 (Suppl. 2): 43–49.

Luck, S. J., Chelazzi, L., Hillyard, S. A., and Desimone, R. (1997) Neural mechanisms of spatial selective attention in areas V1, V2, and V4 of macaque visual cortex. *J. Neurophysiol.* 77: 24–38.

Luck, S. J. and Hillyard, S. A. (1994) Spatial filtering during visual search: Evidence from human electrophysiology. *J. Exp. Psychol. Hum. Percept. Perform.* 20: 1000–1014.

Luck, S. J., Hillyard, S. A., Mouloua, M., Woldorff, M. G., Clark, V. P., and Hawkins, H. L. (1994) Effects of spatial cuing on luminance detectability: Psychophysical and electrophysiological evidence for early selection. *J. Exp. Psychol.: Hum. Percept. Perf.* 20: 887–904.

Luechter, A. F., Newton, T. F., Cook, I. A., and Walter, D. O. (1992) Changes in brain functional connectivity in Alzheimer-type and multi-infarct dementia. *Brain* 115: 1543–1561.

Martin, A., Brouwers, P., Lalonde, F., Cox, C., Teleska, P., Fedio, P., Foster, N. L., and Chase, T. N. (1986) Towards a behavioral typology of Alzheimer's disease *J. Clin. Exp. Neuropsychol.* 8: 594–610.

Maruff, P. and Currie, J. (1995) An attentional grasp reflex in patients with Alzheimer's disease. *Neuropsychologia* 33: 689–701.

Maruff, P., Malone, V., and Currie, J. (1995) Asymmetries in the covert orienting of visual spatial attention to spatial and nonspatial cues in Alzheimer's disease. *Brain* 118: 1421–1435.

Maruff, P., Malone, V., McArthur-Jackson, C., Mulhall, B., Benson, E., and Currie, J. (1995) Abnormalities of visual spatial attention in HIV infection and the HIV-associated dementia complex. *J. Neuropsychiatr. Clin. Neurosci.* 7: 325–333.

Massman, P. J., Delis, D. C., Filoteo, J. V., Butters, N., Salmon, D. P., and Demadura, T. L. (1993) Mechanisms of spatial impairment of Alzheimer's disease subgroups: Differential breakdown of directed attention to global-local stimuli. *Neuropsychology* 7: 172–181.

Mesulam, M. M. (1981) A cortical network of directed attention and unilateral neglect. *Ann. Neurol.* 19: 309–325.

Moran, J. and Desimone, R. (1985) Selective attention gates visual processing in the extrastriate cortex. *Science* 229: 782–784.

Morrison, J. H. (1993) Differential vulnerability, connectivity, and cell typology. *Neurobiol. Aging* 14: 51–54.

Morrison, J. H., Hof, P. R., Campbell, M. J., Delima, A. D., Voigt, T., Bouras, C., Cox, K., and Young, W. G. (1990) Cellular pathology in Alzheimer's disease: Implications for corticocortical disconnection and differential vulnerability. In *Imaging, Cerebral Topography and Alzheimer's disease*, edited by S. I. Rapoport, pp. 19–40. Berlin: Springer Verlag.

Motter, B. (1994) Neural correlates of feature selective memory and pop-out in extrastriate area V4. *J. Neurosci.* 14: 2190–2199.

Muller, H. J. and Rabbitt, P. M. A. (1989) Reflexive and voluntary orienting of visual attention: Time course of activation and resistance to interruption. *J. Exp. Psychol. Hum. Percept. Perform.* 15: 315–330.

Nakayama, K. and Silverman, G. H. (1986) Serial and parallel processing of visual feature conjunctions. *Nature* 320: 264–265.

Navon, D. (1977) Forest before trees: The precedence of global features in visual perception. *Cognitive Psychol.* 9: 353–383.

Nebes, R. D. (1992) Cognitive dysfunction in Alzheimer's disease. In *Handbook of Aging and Cognition*, edited by F. I. M. Craik and T. A. Salthouse, pp. 373–443. Hillsdale, NJ: Lawrence Erlbaum.

Nebes, R. and Brady, C. B. (1989) Foused and divided attention in Alzheimer's disease. *Cortex* 25: 305–315.

Nebes, R. and Brady, C. B. (1993) Phasic and tonic alertness in Alzheimer's disease. *Cortex* 29: 77–90.

Nobre, A. C., Gitelman, D. R., Sebesteyen, G. N., Meyer, J., Frith, C. D., Frackowiak, R. S. J., and Mesulam, M. M. (1996). Cortical network for visuospatial attention imaged using PET and fMRI. *Soc. Neurosci. Abstr.* 26: 1697.

Oken, B. S., Kishiyama, S. S., and Kaye, J. A. (1994) Age-related differences in visual search task performance: Relative stability of parallel but not serial search. *J. Geriatr. Psychiatry. Neurol.* 7: 163–168.

Oken, B. S., Kishiyama, S. S., Kaye, J. A., and Howieson, D. B. (1994) Attention deficit in Alzheimer's disease is not simulated by an anticholinergic/antihistaminergic drug and is distinct from deficits in healthy aging. *Neurology* 44: 657–662.

Parasuraman, R., Greenwood, P. M., and Alexander, G. E. (1995) Selective impairment of spatial attention during visual search in Alzheimer's disease. *Neuroreport* 6: 1861–1864.

Parasuraman, R., Greenwood, P. M., Haxby, J. V., and Grady, C. L. (1992) Visuospatial attention in dementia of the Alzheimer type. *Brain* 115: 711–733.

Parasuraman, R. and Haxby, J. V. (1993) Attention and brain function in Alzheimer's disease: A review. *Neuropsychology* 7: 243–273.

Parasuraman, R. and Martin, A. (1994) Cognition in Alzheimer's disease: Disorders of attention and semantic knowledge. *Curr. Opin. Neurobiol.* 4: 237–244.

Parasuraman, R. and Nestor, P. G. (1993) Preserved cognitive operations in early Alzheimer's disease. In *Adult Information Processing: Limits on Loss,* edited by J. Cerella, W. Hoyer, J. Rybash, and M. L. Commons, pp. 77–111. Orlando, FL: Academic Press.

Petit, L., Orssaud, C., Tzourio, N., Crivello, F., Berthoz, A., and Mazoyer, B. (1996) Functional anatomy of a prelearned sequence of horizontal saccades in humans. *J. Neurosci.* 16: 3714–3726.

Pierrot-Deseilligny, C., Rivaud, S., and Gaymard, B. (1991) Cortical control of reflexively guided saccades. *Brain* 114: 1473–1485.

Pirozzolo, F. and Hansch, E. C. (1981) Oculomotor reaction time in dementia reflects degree of cerebral dysfunction. *Science* 214: 349–350.

Plude, D. J., Enns, J. T., and Brodeur, D. (1994) The development of selective attention: A life-span overview. *Acta Psychol.* 86: 227–272.

Posner, M. I. (1980). Orienting of attention. *Q. J. Exp. Psychol.* 32: 3–25.

Posner, M. I. and Dehaene, S. (1994) Attentional networks. *Trends Neurosci.* 17: 75–79.

Posner, M. I. and Petersen, S. E. (1990) The attention system of the human brain. *Annu. Rev. Neurosci.* 13: 25–42.

Posner, M. I., Rafal, R. D., Choate, L., and Vaughan, J. (1985) Inhibition of return: Neural basis and function. *Cognitive Neuropsychol.* 2: 211–228.

Posner, M. I., Walker, J. A., Friederich, F. J., and Rafal, R. D. (1984) Effects of parietal injury on covert orienting of attention. *J. Neurosci.* 4: 1863–1874.

Posner, M. I., Walker, J. A., Friderich, F. J., and Rafal, R. D. (1987) How do the parietal lobes direct covert attention? *Neuropsychologia* 25: 135–146.

Prinzmetal, W., Presti, D. E., and Posner, M. I. (1986) Does attention affect visual feature integration? *J. Exp. Psychol. Hum. Percept. Perform.* 12: 361–369.

Rafal, R. D. and Posner, M. I. (1987) Deficits in human visual spatial attention following thalamic lesions. *Proc. Natl. Acad. Sci. USA* 84: 7349–7353.

Reed, T., Carmelli, D., and Swan, G. E. (1994) Lower cognitive performance in normal older adult male twins carrying the Apolipoprotein E e4 allele. *Arch. Neurol.* 52: 1189–1192.

Robbins, T. W. and Everitt, B. J. (1995) Arousal systems and attention. In *The Cognitive Neuro-sciences*, edited by M. S. Gazzaniga, pp. 703–720. Cambridge, MA: MIT Press.

Robinson, D. L., Bowman, E. M., and Kertzman, C. (1991) Covert orienting of attention in macaque. II. A signal in parietal cortex to disengage attention. *Soc. Neurosci. Abstr.* 442.

Robinson, D. L. and Petersen, S. E. (1992) The pulvinar and visual salience. *Trends Neurosci.* 15: 127–132.

Sahakian, B. J., Owen, A. M., Morant, N. J., Eagger, S. A., Boddington, S., Crayton, L., Crockford, H. A., Crooks, M., Hill, K., and Levy, R. (1993) Further analysis of the cognitive effects of tetrahydroaminoacridine (THA) in Alzheimer's disease: Assessment of attentional and mnemonic function using CANTAB. *Psychopharmacology* 110: 395–401.

Sano, M., Rosen, W., Stern, Y., Rosen, J., and Mayeux, R. (1995) Simple reaction time as a measure of global attention in Alzheimer's disease. *J. Int. Neuropsychol. Soc.* 1: 56–61.

Schwartz, M. F. (1990) *Modular Deficits in Alzheimer-Type Dementia.* Cambridge, MA: MIT Press.

Scinto, L. F. M., Daffner, K. R., Castro, L., Weintraub, S., Vavrik, M., and Mesulam, M. (1994) Impairment of spatially directed attention in patients with probable Alzheimer's disease as measured by eye movements. *Arch-Neurol.* 51: 682–688.

Small, G., Mazziota J. C., Collins, M. T., Phelphs, M. E., Mandelkern, M. A., Kaplan, A., La Rue, A., Adamson, C. F., Chang, L., Guze, B. H., Corder, E. H., Saunders, A. M., Haines, J. L., Pericak-Vance, M. A., and Rose, A. D. (1995) Apoliprotein E type 4 allele and cerebral parietal metabolism in relatives at risk for familial Alzheimer disease. *J. Am. Med. Assoc.* 273: 942–947.

Spieler, D. H., Balota, D. A., and Faust, M. E. (1996) Stroop performance in healthy younger and older adults and in individuals with dementia of the Alzheimer's type. *J. Exp. Psychol. Hum. Percept. Perform.* 22: 461–479.

Steinmzetz, M. A. and Constantinidis, C. (1995) Neurophysiological evidence for a role of posterior parietal cortex in redirecting visual attention. *Cereb. Cortex* 5: 457–469.

Thaiss, L. and De Bleser, R. (1993) Visual agnosia: A case of reduced attentional "spotlight"? *Cortex* 28: 601–621.

Theeuwes, J. (1994) Endogenous and exogenous control of visual selection. *Perception* 23: 429–440.

Treisman, A. (1988) Features and objects. *Q. J. Exp. Psychol.* 40: 201–237.

Treisman, A. and Gelade, G. (1980) A feature integration theory of attention. *Cognitive Psychol.* 12: 97–136.

Voytko, M. L., Olton, D. S., Richardson, R. T., Gorman, L. K., Tobin, J. R., and Price, D. L. (1994) Basal forebrain lesions in monkeys disrupt attention but not learning and memory. *J. Neurosci.* 14: 167–186.

Wiley, C. A., Masliah, E., and Morey, M. (1991) Neocortical damage during HIV infection. *Ann. Neurol.* 29: 651–657.

Wolfe, J. M., Cave, K. R., and Frankel, S. L. (1989) Guided search: An alternative to the feature integration model for visual search. *J. Exp. Psychol. Hum. Percept. Perform.* 15: 419–433.

Wright, M. J., Burns, R. J., Geffen, G. M., and Geffen, L. B. (1990) Covert orientation of visual attention in Parkinson's disease: An impairment in the maintenance of attention. *Neuropsychololgia* 28: 151–159.

22 Neglect

Robert D. Rafal

ABSTRACT Hemispatial neglect is a disorder of orienting that impairs awareness of signals, objects, or parts of objects on the side of space opposite a lesion in one cerebral hemisphere. The syndrome is heterogeneous, and several mechanisms may contribute to it, including disinhibited orienting to the ipsilesional field, a deranged representation of space, and deficits in disengaging attention, oculomotor corollary discharge, and representation of contralesional movement trajectories. Theories and methods for studying visual attention in normal people have contributed to our understanding of neglect, at the same time as a better understanding of neglect has elucidated some central theoretical issues in cognitive science. The study of neglect has shown that perceptual processing can proceed to the level of semantic classification in the absence of attention or conscious awareness, and that preattentive vision parses the scene to extract figure from ground, group objects and define their primary axis. Neglect appears to reflect a defect at a level of selection for action of visual objects.

The gentleman shown in figure 22.1 had recently suffered a large stroke involving the frontal and parietal lobes of the right hemisphere. His attention is directed to another person standing in front of him (not shown). He does not orient to me or to the $1 bill held just inches from his face in his left visual field (figure 22.1, left). When the same $1 is presented in his right visual field (figure 22.1, right) he orients to it promptly.

It might be thought that he is blind in his left visual field, but he is not. He suffers from the syndrome of hemispatial neglect, which most commonly results from lesions of the right cerebral hemisphere, especially from lesions involving the temporoparietal cortex. Although visual sensation is intact, he fails to detect signals in the side of space opposite the lesion or to be consciously aware of contralesional objects or parts of objects. His disability is devastating, and his behavior is a vexing puzzle to the clinician and a challenge to theories of attention and perception. Theories and methods for studying visual attention in normal people have contributed to our understanding of neglect, while at the same time, a better understanding of neglect has helped crack some of the tougher theoretical issues in cognitive science.

This chapter examines a few of those issues, including the role of attention in perceptual processing, in mediating conscious awareness, and in transducing perception into action. Investigation of these issues shows that the mutually supporting contributions of neurology and psychology have enriched both disciplines.

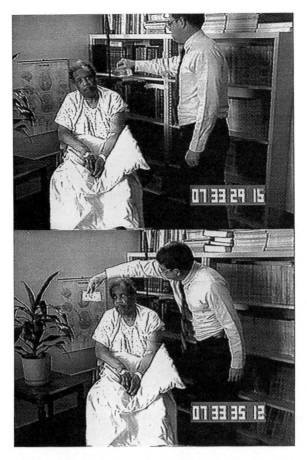

Figure 22.1 (Top) A patient with left hemispatial neglect fails to notice the examiner approaching from the left—even when a $1 bill is held inches from the left side of the patient's face. (Bottom) A moment later, however, the patient orients promptly to the $1 bill when it is held in his right field.

WHAT IS HEMISPATIAL NEGLECT?

Damage to the occipital lobe destroying the striate cortex on one side causes total and permanent blindness, called hemianopia, in the visual field contralateral to the lesion. Hemianopic individuals have no sensation of light, movement, color, or shape within the blind field (scotoma). The patient shown in figure 22.1, however, does not have any damage to primary visual pathways, and it can be shown that he is not blind in the visual field contralateral to the lesion. Figure 22.2 shows the method of confrontation testing used to assess the integrity of the visual fields at the bedside or in the clinic. The patient is told to pay attention and to expect stimuli to be presented in either the left or the right visual field, and is asked to report what he or she sees. The task may be simple detection (e.g., "tell me when you see my finger wiggle") or, as shown in figure 22.15, object identification (i.e.,

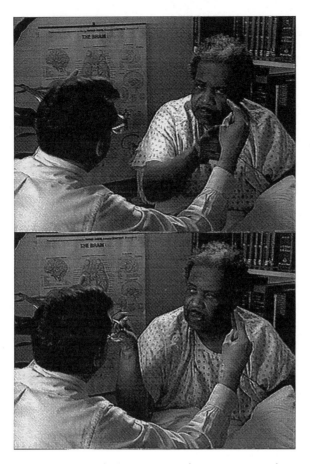

Figure 22.2 Visual extinction on confrontation testing. The patient is asked to fixate the face of the examiner and to report when a finger wiggles. (Top) When only the finger in his left field wiggles, he detects and orients to it. (Bottom) When fingers in both fields are wiggled simultaneously, he orients to the one on his right and does not see the wiggling finger in the left field.

"tell me what you see"). This patient was able to reliably report stimuli in the right (ipsilesional) field and usually reported single stimuli when presented in his left (contralesional) field (figure 22.2, top); but when he was presented two stimuli simultaneously in both fields (figure 22.2, bottom), he reported only the stimulus in the right field. He failed to detect or to orient to the other object in the left field and when asked, he denied that anything had occurred there.

This phenomenon, known as visual extinction, is quite different from what is observed in hemianopic patients. Hemianopics will never see any item presented singly in the contralesional field. The border of the scotoma is sharp and comes to the midline (or nearly to it), and is mapped in retinotopic coordinates; that is, the scotoma moves with the eye. If a patient with a left hemianopia tilts his head 90 degrees to the right, the upper part of the world is no longer visible. In contrast, the patient with visual extinction often will

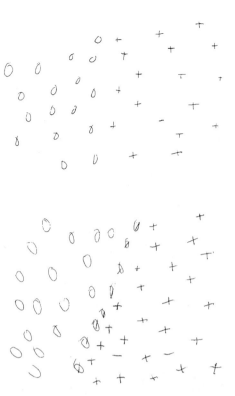

Figure 22.3 Neglect in a cancellation task. A patient with left hemispatial neglect fails to cancel out items on the left side of the page. (Top) Cancellation stops at the boundary between two areas of different texture. (Bottom) Cancellation stops when she finishes crossing out the first item on the other side of the boundary.

see a single item presented in the contralesional field. Unlike the sharp retinotopic border of hemianopia, the likelihood of a patient with visual neglect detecting a visual event declines as a gradient from ipsilesional to contralesional locations. When two targets are presented, visual extinction of the more contralesional object may occur even if both items are presented in the right visual field. As will be discussed later, the deficit in neglect is not defined retinotopically; the neglected object or part of an object can move or rotate as the reference frame of the object(s) relative to the viewer changes.

Also unlike the patient with neglect, a hemianopic individual learns that he or she has a sensory impairment and will make compensatory efforts to explore the side of space affected by the deficit. Visual extinction, by contrast, is often accompanied by a pronounced deficit in exploratory behavior. In conventional practice, the deficit in exploratory behavior is tested using a cancellation task like that shown in figure 22.3, by asking the patient to draw a familiar object like a clock or a tree or, as shown in figure 22.4, to copy a simple drawing. Another common test of neglect is a line bisection task. The patient is shown lines on a piece of paper (usually arrayed horizontally) and asked to bisect the line in the middle. The patient bisects the line closer to the

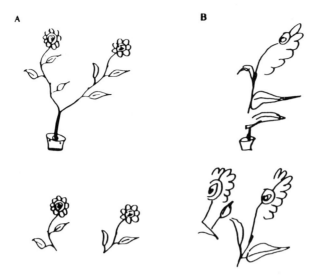

Figure 22.4 Neglect in a copying task. Whether one or both flowers is neglected depends upon whether they are part of the same plant. Even when both flowers are copied, the left side of each was neglected. (From Marshall and Halligan, 1993.)

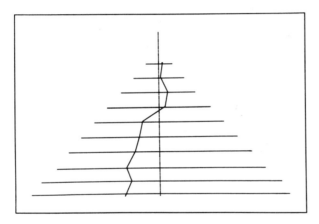

Figure 22.5 Bisection error in patients with hemispatial neglect is proportional to the length of the line being bisected. (From Marshall and Halligan, 1990.)

ipsilesional end and, interestingly, the degree of bisection error is typically proportional to the length of the line to be bisected (figure 22.5) (Marshall and Halligan, 1990).

Such deficits in exploratory behavior are not seen in hemianopic patients. It is paradoxically true that, whereas the hemianopic patient is in some sense more blind (after all, the patient with neglect often can see some things in the contralesional field), the patient with neglect is far more disabled. When neglect manifests in its most severe form, the patient acts as if the contralesional side of the world does not exist, and the head and eyes deviate to the ipsilesional side. When approached from the contralesional side and addressed, the patient does not turn, but instead responds to anyone else located ipsilesionally. He doesn't dress, shave, or comb the contralesional side of the body, and fails to eat food on one side of the plate. He begins reading or writing in the middle of the page. When copying or drawing (see figures 22.3 and 22.4), the contralesional sides of objects are omitted and the patient is quite satisfied with the production. The afflicted individual may be unaware that half of his world, or even half of his body, is gone. He may deny that the contralesional arm and leg are paralyzed, proclaim himself fit, and act puzzled as to why he might be in the hospital.

FRACTIONATION OF THE SYNDROME OF HEMISPATIAL NEGLECT: PERCEPTUAL AND MOTOR CONTRIBUTIONS TO NEGLECT

The clinical manifestations of hemispatial neglect constitute a symptom complex that is a heterogeneous constellation. The occurrence of its various component symptoms—impaired social orienting, extinction, impaired motor exploration—can vary from patient to patient, and the component symptoms may be dissociated from one another in any given patient. Some patients without extinction on confrontation testing may exhibit neglect in cancellation or line bisection tasks. Others may exhibit consistent extinction but no impairment on the conventional pencil and paper tasks. Other patients may demonstrate the florid neglect syndrome with all those signs in the acute phase of the illness but seem to recover, and may then show none of the signs of the neglect syndrome on clinical examination using those bedside tests. These individuals might not, then, be diagnosed as having neglect, and would not be included in studies of neglect. Nevertheless, families of such individuals often report neglect as a continuing disability, the patient often failing to find things that happen to be in the contralesional field, or the embarrassing experience of a man walking into the ladies room because he misses the first two letters in the sign "WOMEN."

Many Circuits and Many Forms of Neglect

Which components of the neglect symptom complex are manifest in a given individual may depend upon the extent and chronicity of the lesion, which brain structures are involved, and perhaps the patient's individual brain architecture and personal history. The neural circuitry controlling spatial attention is a distributed network involving cortical and subcortical structures (Mesulam, 1981). Within that network there appear to be several specialized and interconnected circuits for regulation of different kinds of behavior. Consider the different kinds of representations of space that are necessary for performance of some common, simple tasks. A representation of space for generating an eye movement to a visual signal requires retinotopic coordinates. One for controlling reaching requires an egocentric representation of space—a scene-based representation in which location in the environment is coded and remains constant even if the eyes move. In monkeys, areas of parietal lobe have been identified, in which retinotopically mapped information is gated by eye positiont (Zisper and Anderson, 1988). For reaching, moreover, the representation must be integrated with a reference frame mapped relative to hand position (Graziano, Yap, and Gross, 1994). That kind of representation of near peripersonal space may not be, however, adequate for throwing. Throwing may require a separate representation of distant space (Rizzolatti and Camarda, 1987). The representations of space that may be adequate for reaching to a stationary object may not suffice for reaching for a moving object. For this, one wants an object-based representation that updates the changing location of parts of the object relative to an egocentric reference frame. Finally, consider the problem of remembering the location of a cache of food relative to some geographical landmark, or the problem of remembering the locations of cities on a map. For those tasks one wants an allocentric reference frame in which the relative locations of objects are represented in a frame of reference totally independent of the viewpoint of the individual. For navigating while moving in the environment, the allocentric map must be continually updated and integrated with some enduring record of changes in body position with regard to the allocentric reference frame; for example, the "place" cells that have been identified in rat hippocampus (O'Keefe, 1993).

Given that there may be many such independent circuits that might be affected by some lesions and spared in others, it is not surprising that the manifestations of visual neglect may vary from patient to patient. Performance on many of the tests used clinically to diagnose neglect and to measure its severity can be influenced by both motor and perceptual factors. Errors in line bisection or missed items in a cancellation task may be caused by perceptual neglect, motor neglect, or a combination of both. Failure to cross out the left-most items on a cancellation task, for example, could be due to failure to see the left-most items or to a motor bias against moving the hand toward the left. In some patients neglect may be more perceptual and in others more motor. Although this distinction may be better appreciated as a continuum rather than as a dichotomy, the distinction between disorders of attention and of intention has been a useful one (Heilman, Valenstein, and Watson, 1985). Some patients with a more pure attentional disorder (typically those with more posterior lesions that spare frontal lobes) may have visual extinction and other perceptual deficits, but no motor bias against turning contralesionally, moving the limbs contralateral to the lesion, or reaching into the contralesional field (directional hypokinesia) (Coslett, Bowers, Fitzpatrick, Haws, and Heilman, 1990; Heilman, Bowers, Coslett, Whelan, and Watson, 1985). Other patients who do not show extinction or other signs of perceptual neglect may, nevertheless, have a motor bias that causes neglect behavior in cancellation and construction tasks. Many patients with neglect have both perceptual and motor components affecting performance in these types of tasks. The relative contributions of the components may vary from patient to patient depending on the size and location of the lesion and on the task used to assess neglect.

Separating Perceptual and Motor Components of Neglect

Several ingenious studies have recently dissociated perceptual and motor components of neglect to measure their effects independently. Bisiach, Geminiani, Berti, and Rusconi (1990) first demonstrated that dissociation by using a pulley device in a bisection task. Patients with neglect bisected lines under two conditions. Under one, movement of the pencil toward the left (contralesional) direction required movement of the hand to the left. In this standard version of the task, a deficit in bisection could be due to perceptual neglect, motor neglect, or a combination of both. In the other version of the task, the pulley device required rightward movement of the hand to move the pencil to the left. Patients in whom neglect was exclusively due to a motor bias against moving the hand toward the left could be expected to improve their bisection performance in the second version of the task. Some patients, those in whom neglect was dominantly perceptual, showed an equal amount of neglect in both versions of the task. Some patients showed some improvement in bisection with the pulley; and some, those in whom neglect was dominantly a motor bias, had no neglect under the pulley condition. The patients with more pure motor neglect tended to have more frontal lesions. Similar dissociations between perceptual and motor neglect have been also demonstrated using other devices to separate out motor bias contributions to neglect by using television cameras (Coslett et al., 1990) and mirrors (Tegner and Levander, 1991). While there are clear tendencies for motor neglect to be more associated with more frontal lesions, the anatomical substrates relating to perceptual and motor neglect remain to be more precisely specified (Mattingley, Bradshaw, and Phillips, 1992).

An elegant companion test to line bisection has been introduced (Milner, Harvey, Roberts, and Forster, 1993) to determine whether motor neglect contributes to bisection errors in an individual patient. Patients who manifest bisection errors were shown prebisected lines that were bisected in the middle or to the left or right of midline. The patients were asked to point to the end of the line that was closest to the bisection mark. The critical condition is that in which the line is bisected in the middle. Patients in whom bisection error is due exclusively to a motor bias to the right would be expected to point to the right end of the line. Milner et al. have reported several patients with left hemispatial neglect who pointed to the left end of the line. That result suggests that, in those patients, bisection errors were not due to a motor bias toward the right but rather to perceptual distortion causing them to perceive the left side of the line as being shorter than the right.

A more recent study has confirmed that neglect reduces perceived length. Milner and Harvey (1995) showed patients with neglect two horizontal rectangles on a sheet of paper, one in each visual field, and asked them to judge which rectangle was shorter. On the critical trial in which the shapes were equal in length, the patients indicated those in the left field to be shorter. In a control test in which vertical lines were shown, no such asymmetry in length judgment was evident. Those findings indicate that patients with perceptual neglect experience the left side of space as horizontally compressed.

METHODOLOGICAL CONSIDERATIONS: HOW WE STUDY VISUAL NEGLECT AND WHAT WE CAN LEARN FROM IT

Given the heterogeneity of the population of individuals who manifest symptoms of neglect, and the fact that different patients may show similar symptoms for different reasons, how are we to go about studying these phenomena in order to gain a better understanding of the psychobiology of normal perception and behavior and the neural substrates that mediate them? The best approach depends on the specific problem being addressed.

For example, patients with hemispatial neglect afford a unique opportunity to investigate one critical issue in cognitive science: how much perceptual processing proceeds in the absence of attention and awareness? To address that question, we can use implicit measures to infer the degree to which neglected stimuli in the contralesional field are processed, and then compare those effects to those produced by the same stimuli presented in the "good," ipsilesional field that the patient does see. If the patient has no explicit awareness of the stimuli in the neglected field, yet produces behavioral effects on indirect measures of processing that are equivalent to those produced by stimuli in the ipsilesional field, this result is strong evidence for processing without awareness. This kind of within-subject comparison can help us determine whether the processing required to produce the effect being implicitly measured requires attention and conscious awareness. If comparable effects are observed for contralesional neglected and for ipsilesionally perceived stimuli, then the inference is that the perceptual process being measured can proceed without attention and in the absence of conscious awareness.

Note that patients for this kind of investigation must be selected based upon behavioral criteria; namely, extinction of contralesional stimuli. The anatomy of the responsible lesion is not directly relevant to the question being addressed, nor is the presence or absence of other signs of neglect. Because the critical manipulation is done within subjects, the performance of selected patients need not be compared to normal performance or to the performance of any group of individuals. On the other hand, the selection criteria for this kind of study must be quite stringent. Not every patient who might be classified as showing neglect or extinction would be suitable for testing the hypothesis under consideration. For example, the patient must not also have an occipital lesion that impairs sensory processing. Further, the degree of extinction required to permit a reasonable test of the hypothesis must be quite dense. If the patient only exhibits extinction inconsistently, then the demonstration of processing of contralesional stimuli might only reflect those trials on which the patient does perceive the stimulus, not those in which the stimulus is extinguished. The ideal test of this kind of hypothesis requires (1) that there be no explicit awareness of contralesional stimuli being used in the test, and (2) that the effects being measured be equal for contralesional and ipsilesional stimuli. It is not common for such severe extinction to persist for long; when it is present, the patient is often quite ill and the investigator is unlikely to have the opportunity for prolonged testing that extends over several sessions.

For that kind of problem then, single case designs are not only adequate, but necessary. The prospects for testing a large group of patients meeting these criteria are not good. Obviously, replication of the result in additional patients is desirable to confirm the generality of the conclusions; if the neuropsychological observations converge with studies in normal subjects (for example, using masked primes to measure implicitly the processing of stimuli that are not perceived), so much the better.

On the other hand, if the goal is to specify the neural substrate for a cognitive operation, single case studies may not be helpful. If one finds that a patient who has a lesion that includes a certain brain region exhibits a certain performance, we cannot know whether the performance results from the lesion in that area, from some other area also involved by the lesion, or from some other characteristic of that individual. Even if we could be confident that the lesion of the specified region was responsible for the performance in that individual, we could not know whether the neural substrate for the behavior in that person was typical or anomalous with regard to the general population.

Therefore, although single case studies can reveal much about the architecture of normal cognition, a very different approach is necessary to answer questions about the neuroanatomical basis of a cognitive process. If the goal is to investigate the specific contributions to perception and attention of the parietal lobe, midbrain, pulvinar, or prefrontal cortex—or their dynamical interaction—it is necessary to study groups of patients with well-circumscribed lesions affecting one of the structures in the network but sparing others. This approach generally requires the selection of patients with relatively small lesions who may not manifest, in the chronic stage of illness when the remote (diaschesis) effects on other parts of the network have resolved, any clinically obvious attentional disorder.

This kind of analysis has only become possible in the past decade or so with the development of neuroimaging techniques with high resolution, such as computerized axial tomography (CT) and magnetic resonance imaging (MRI). During the same period that the lesion method has matured in the study of human cognition, other methods of dynamic brain imaging, such as event-related potential (ERP) recordings (from scalp or implanted electrodes), positron emission tomography (PET), magneto-encephalography and functional MRI, have provided converging findings both in brain-injured and normal human subjects.

The remainder of this chapter reviews investigations that have used both single case studies and group studies to address some of the dominant issues in the psychobiology of attention: (1) What is the neural substrate for orienting attention? (2) In what reference frames does attention operate? (3) To what degree is unattended visual information processed in the absence of attention and awareness, and to what degree does that information influence behavior?

DISENGAGING ATTENTION AND THE MECHANISM OF EXTINCTION

Does the phenomenon of extinction indicate that the parietal lobe is involved in controlling the orienting of attention? It had been argued (Bay, 1953; Bender and Feldman, 1972) that an attentional explanation may not be necessary to explain extinction. Instead, extinction could simply result from sensory competition. That is, although parietal lobe lesions do not produce hemianopia, they might nevertheless cause visual perceptions to be more weakly represented in the contralesional than in the ipsilesional field. Under conditions of sensory competition (especially if the general effects of brain damage also cause attentional resources to be limited), the weakest sensory signal might not be perceived.

The most direct evidence for an attentional explanation of extinction was provided in an experiment in which it was shown that attending to the ipsilesional visual field could cause extinction even under conditions in which there was no competing visual target to be reported in the ipsilesional field (Posner, Walker, Friedrich, and Rafal, 1984). The subject was asked respond, by pressing a key, to the appearance of a target at a peripheral location. The target was preceded by a precue that summoned attention either to the location of the forthcoming target (valid cue) or to the wrong location (invalid cue). The cue could be, for example, a flash of light at one of the possible target locations. This experimental paradigm has the virtue of revealing several putative components of visual orienting. When an individual is attending to an object of interest, attention is assumed to be *engaged* at the location of that object. If attention is to be deployed elsewhere, it must first be *disengaged* from its current focus, and then *moved* to the new location. In this paradigm, normal detection when the cue is valid implies that the individual is able to move attention in response to the cue. If a valid cue affords no benefit in performance and if no difference in detection is observed between valid and invalid cue conditions, it could be inferred that the individual is unable to move attention. If, on the other hand, the individual is able to move attention in response to a valid cue, but is selectively impaired in detection when the cue is invalid, then there will be a large difference in detection performance in valid and invalid cue conditions and a deficit in disengaging attention can be inferred.

As described earlier, a patient with a parietal lobe lesion causing extinction is relatively unimpaired in detecting a signal presented alone in the contralesional field, and therefore is evidently competent to move attention toward that field. When a competing stimulus is presented simultaneously in the ipsilesional field, however, attention becomes stuck there and the patient is unable to disengage attention to detect the contralesional stimulus.

The investigations of Posner et al. showed that patients with lesions of the posterior association cortex, even those who did not have neglect or show clinical extinction on conventional examination, demonstrated an extinctionlike response time (RT) pattern (Posner et al., 1984; Posner, Inhoff, Friedrich, and Cohen, 1987; Posner, Walker, Friedrich, and Rofal, 1987). Detection RT in the field opposite to the lesion (contralesional field) was not much slowed (and in some patients was not slowed at all compared to the ipsilesional field) if a valid cue was given. So, the patients were able to use the precue to move their attention to the contralesional field, and when they did so their performance for contralesional targets was relatively unimpaired. When, however, a cue summoned attention toward the ipsilesional field and the target subsequently occurred in the opposite, contralesional field (invalid cue), detection RT slowed dramatically. This extinctionlike RT pattern occurred not only when the cue was a flashing box in the ipsilesional field, but also for several hundred milliseconds after the cue disappeared—or even when the cue was an arrow in the center of the screen pointing to the ipsilesional field. That is, the extinction effect occurred when attention was directed ipsilesionally, even though there was no competing target signal to detect in that field.

The Neural Substrate for Disengaging Attention

In our initial study of covert orienting in patients with parietal lesions (Posner et al., 1984), patients were selected solely on the basis of having a lesion involving the parietal lobe. Some had acute lesions and clinical signs of neglect or visual extinction. Some patients had chronic lesions and no clinical signs of visual inattention. The etiologies and anatomical extent of the lesions were also heterogeneous. Some lesions were strokes, some tumors or other etiologies, and in many patients the lesion also extended beyond the parietal lobe to involve the frontal lobe as well. That study was not designed to specify the area of posterior association cortex (PAC) that was responsible for the disengagement of attention. A post hoc correlational analysis suggested that the superior parietal lobe might be most responsible for disengaging attention. However, because the patients with lesions in the superior parietal lobe were not matched with other patients on several other critical variables (right or left hemisphere lesion, vintage of the lesion, etiology—stroke versus tumor with swelling), the conclusions derived from the post hoc correlation were tentative.

A more recent study (Friedrich, Egly, Rafal and Beck, in press) was designed to extend the findings of Posner et al. (1984). One major goal was to specify the anatomical basis of the disengage deficit. In order to permit a more valid functional-anatomical analysis uncontaminated by the effects of diaschesis on regions remote from those that could be defined with MRI or CT, only patients who had chronic lesions (at least six months after the stroke) restricted to the posterior association cortex in one hemisphere and sparing the frontal lobes were selected. None of these patients had any residual clinical neglect or extinction. The effects of valid and invalid cues on detection were compared for targets appearing in the contralesional and the ipsilesional fields.

Subgroups of patients with posterior association cortex lesions were compared with one another. Because the initial study of Posner et al. (1984) gave some suggestion that involvement by the lesion of the superior parietal lobe (SPL) most correlated with the extinctionlike RT pattern, one analysis compared a subgroup in whom the lesion involved the SPL with another subgroup in whom the lesions spared the SPL. Because clinico-anatomical studies have consistently correlated the neglect syndrome with lesion of the temporo-parietal junction (TPJ), another analysis compared a subgroup of patients with TPJ involvement (including the superior temporal gyrus) with a subgroup of patient in whom the lesion spared the TPJ. Figure 22.6 shows the MRI scan of one of the patients with a discrete lesion of the TPJ. The results showed that the extinctionlike RT pattern deficit was greatest in the

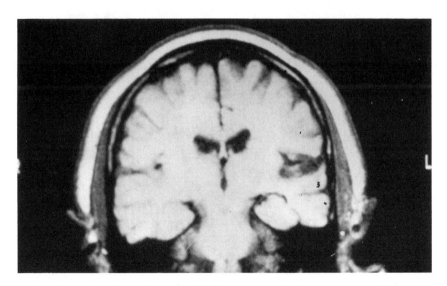

Figure 22.6 Coronal MRI of patient with a lesion restricted to the posterior part of the superior temporal gyrus and the adjacent temporo-parietal cortex.

TPJ lesion patient subgroup. There was no evidence that a lesion of the SPL contributed at all to the extinctionlike RT pattern.

Is There a "Disengager" in the Temporo-Parietal Junction?

The finding of an extinctionlike RT pattern observed in patients with posterior association cortex lesions led Posner et al. (1984) to suggest that clinical extinction could be characterized as a difficulty in disengaging attention. Although that is certainly a reasonable description of the behavior, a framework proposed by Posner and Petersen (1990) makes a somewhat stronger theoretical claim; namely, that the difficulty in disengaging attention identifies a cortical region that is the neural substrate for a specific elementary operation of disengaging attention. Cohen, Romero, Servan-Schreiber, and Farah (1994) questioned that interpretation by demonstrating a connectionist model that, when "lesioned," produces an extinctionlike RT pattern, even though it does not incorporate a specific "disengager." In their model, attention "units" mutually inhibit one another. Damage to one such unit disinhibits its partner. The disinhibited engagement of the units results in a deficit in disengaging attention from an engaged signal as an emergent property of the system—without the need to invoke a specific disengager. Thus, the demonstration of a pattern of behavior that can be characterized as a disengagement deficit need not necessarily imply the existence of a specific disengager.

On the other hand, the fact that one need not postulate a disengager to account for the observed pattern of performance does not provide direct evidence against the existence of a disengager either. Nor does the model of Cohen and Farah (1991) fully account for all the experimental data upon which Posner and Petersen based their account. The Posner and Petersen hypothesis was not predicated solely on the data from patients with lesions of posterior association cortex in the covert orienting task, but on a dissociation between two patient groups: one with posterior association cortex lesions that evidenced a pattern of performance on the covert orienting task consistent with a deficit in disengaging attention; and another patient group with midbrain lesions that evidenced a pattern of performance on the covert orienting task consistent with a deficit in moving attention.

Figure 22.7 illustrates the dissociation by comparing the results in patients with TPJ lesions with the same experiment that we conducted in patients with midbrain lesions due to a degenerative disease called progressive supranuclear palsy (PSP) (Rafal, Posner, Friedman, Inhoff, and Bernstein, 1988). Figure 22.7 compares the effects of valid and invalid cues on detection as the difference in RT between the affected visual field and the more normal field. For TPJ lesion patients the difference is between contralesional and ipsilesional field; for PSP patients the comparison is between vertical and horizontal attention shifts (because in PSP patients' eye movements are more affected

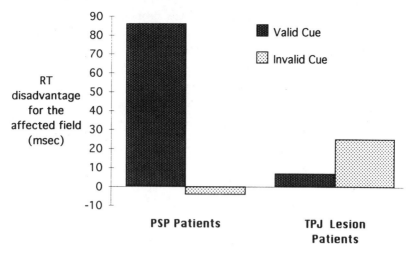

Figure 22.7 Covert orienting in patients with progressive supranuclear palsy (PSP) and temporo-parietal junction (TPJ) lesions. Targets appeared 50, 150, 300, or 500 ms following an uninformative peripheral precue. The results are depicted as the difference in detection RT between the more affected and the more normal visual fields in the valid and invalid cue conditions. For the PSP patients (left) attention shifts were compared in the vertical (more affected) and horizontal (less affected) planes, whereas in the TPJ lesion patients (right) the effects of orienting were compared for contralesional and ipsilesional targets. In the PSP patients a significant asymmetry between the more affected and less affected fields occurred only in the valid cue condition (Rafal et al., 1988), whereas in the TPJ lesion patients, detection was significantly impaired for contralesional targets only in the invalid cue condition (Senechal, unpublished observations.)

in the vertical than in the horizontal plane). The figure shows that, for the patients with midbrain lesions, the deficit in orienting is present only for valid cues, suggesting that these patients are slow to move attention toward a valid cue but are not impaired in disengaging attention when the cue is invalid (Rafal et al., 1988). In contrast, the TPJ lesion patients show no impairment when the cue is valid, indicating that they are able to move their attention normally to the contralesional field if it is not already engaged in the ipsilesional field. However, when attention is engaged in the ipsilesional field by an invalid cue presented there, the extinctionlike RT pattern is manifest.

The dissociation between patient groups in this experiment is consistent with the framework advanced by Posner and Petersen (1990) that there are separate elementary operations involved in the orienting of spatial attention. They suggest that the midbrain is involved in moving attention, whereas the TPJ functions in disengaging attention. According to that framework clinical extinction might be thought of as a deficit in the disengagement operation.

Orienting Bias and Hemispherical Rivalry

One model of the neurobiology of spatial attention that postulates the kind of reciprocal inhibition modeled by Cohen et al. (1994) is Kinsbourne's hemispheric rivalry account. He proposed that each hemisphere, when activated, mediates an orienting response in the contralateral direction (Kinsbourne, 1977, 1993, 1994). According to that account, neglect results from a unilateral lesion because of a breakdown in the balance of hemispheric rivalry such that the nonlesioned hemisphere generates an unopposed orienting response toward the side of the lesion. Experimental observations in patients with hemi-neglect provide some support for this view. Ladavas, Del Pesce, and Provinciali (1989) showed in patients with neglect that detection performance followed a gradient, with detection improving systematically for more ipsilesional targets. Of particular interest was the observation that detection of the most ipsilesional targets was even better than for normal control subjects. Those results suggest that patients with neglect hyperorient toward the ipsilesional field.

However, a hyperorienting deficit and a disengagement deficit need not be mutually exclusive explanations for neglect. A patient with neglect could have both ipsilesional hyperorienting, causing the patient to become more engaged on ipsilesional objects, and an additional deficit in disengaging attention. Both the hyperorienting and the disengagement difficulty could act synergistically with one another to aggravate neglect. One interesting prediction of the hemispheric rivalry account of neglect that does not also involve a disengagement deficit is that neglect produced by a lesion in one hemisphere may be reversed by a second lesion in the other. The model of Cohen et al. (1994) does simulate that effect, and a recent case report has demonstrated the same result in a patient with whose neglect recovered after a second lesion in the opposite hemisphere (Vuileumier, Hester, Assal, and Regli, 1996).

What might be the neural basis for reciprocal hemispherical inhibition? One account emphasizes mutually inhibitory callosal connections between the hemispheres. According to that account, when one hemisphere is lesioned, homologous regions of the opposite hemisphere, which normally receive inhibitory projections from the damaged region through the corpus callosum, become disinhibited and the disinhibited regions produce hyperorienting of attention to the ipsilesional side. We have recently (Seyal, Ro, and Rafal, 1995) obtained some support for that hypothesis by examining the effects of transcranial magnetic stimulation (TMS) on sensory thresholds for tactile detection in normal subjects. A suprathreshold (i.e., sufficiently strong to activate a twitch in the contralateral thumb when applied over motor cortex) TMS stimulus transiently inactivates subjacent cortex. This study examined whether the hemisphere opposite the TMS stimulus would show signs of disinhibition, manifested as a reduced threshold to detect a tactile stimulus in the thumb *ipsilateral* to the TMS lesion. Results supported the attentional disinhibition account by showing a reduced ipsilateral tactile threshold after parietal (3 or 5 cm posterior to motor cortex) TMS, but not when TMS was applied at control locations over the motor cortex or 5 cm anterior to it.

Another mechanism that has been suggested for ipsilesional hyperorienting postulates an interaction between cortex and subcortex. According to this account, the unlesioned parietal lobe becomes disinhibited and tonically increases activity in the superior colliculus ipsilateral to it, whereas the colliculus on the side of the lesion loses some normally present tonic activation. As a result, parietal lesions also produce an imbalance in the activity of subcortical structures involved in orienting, such as the superior colliculus. The contralesional superior colliculus becomes disinhibited, and this results in exaggerated reflexive orienting to signals in the ipsilesional field. Sprague's experiments in the cat confirmed that this kind of cortical-subcortical interaction is important in regulating visually guided orienting behavior (Sprague, 1966). Cats were first rendered blind in one visual field by removal of occipital and parietal cortex. It was then shown that vision in this field improved if the opposite superior colliculus were removed. A similar result was obtained when the inhibitory connections were severed between the contralesional substantia nigra pars reticulata and the ipsilesional colliculus (Wallace, Rosenquist, and Sprague, 1989, 1990).

The Sprague effect is thought to work in the following way. Parieto-occipital projections to the ipsilateral superior colliculus normally exert a tonic facilitation on it. After parietal lesions the colliculus loses tonic activation, and at the same time the opposite (contralesional) colliculus becomes hyperactive due to increased activation from its parietal lobe that, as noted earlier, is disinhibited. This imbalance is sustained and aggravated by the mutually inhibitory connections between the two colliculi themselves. The more active contralesional superior colliculus is released from inhibition and produces disinhibited reflexive orienting to ipsilesional signals. Once attention is reflexively drawn to the ipsilesional field, the disengagement deficit causes attention to get stuck there—resulting in neglect. If the contralesional superior colliculus (or the fibers of passage from the substantia nigra pars reticulata to the opposite colliculus) is then removed, hyperorienting, and hence neglect, is ameliorated.

The Sprague effect demonstrates (at least in cats) that neglect is aggravated by disinhibition of subcortical visual pathways on the side opposite the cortical lesions; and that prevention of visual input to that colliculus can alleviate neglect. Are there any practical applications of this phenomenon in rehabilitation? Now it is obviously not an option to surgically remove the contralesional superior colliculus in humans who have suffered parietal lobe strokes. It is possible, however, to decrease contralesional collicular activation, and reflexive orienting, by occluding the ipsilesional eye with a patch (Posner and Rafal, 1987), and that procedure helps reduce symptoms of neglect (Butter, Kirsch, and Reeves, 1990).

It seems likely that both cortical and subcortical imbalances contribute to the rightward bias of attention in patients with neglect. The subcortical imbalance is presumably more pronounced during the period of extensive diaschesis in the acute stage following the ictus. The imbalance is thought to produce not just a turning bias, but also a shift in the spatial frame of reference such that the contralesional space is more weakly represented (Karnath, 1994; Kinsbourne, 1994). The effect of the rightward bias on spatial representation can be reduced transiently by production of a countervailing orienting bias through vestibular activation. One way to activate the vestibular apparatus is with caloric stimulation. The ear canal is irrigated with cold (or warm) water to deactivate the inner ear or to induce conduction currents of the endolymph in the inner ear. This produces vertigo—a spinning sensation similar to what one gets after getting off a spinning bar stool or rolling down a hill. The world is perceived to spin in the opposite direction—a displacement of the spatial frame of reference. Caloric stimulation has been shown to transiently alleviate not only visual (Cappa, Sterzi, Vallar, and Bisiach, 1987; Rubens, 1985) and somatosensory (Vallar, Bottini, Rusconi, and Sterzi, 1993) neglect, but also the lack of awareness of the deficit (anosognosia) (Bisiach, Rusconi, and Vallar, 1991). A shift in spatial representation by vibration of neck muscles (Karnath, Christ, and Hartje, 1993) or by optokinetic stimulation (a striped drum rotated in front of the eyes) (Pizzamiglio, Frasca, Guariglia, Inaccia, and Antonucci, 1990) can also decrease neglect.

Extinction and Neglect: Disengaging Attention During Visual Search and Exploration

The covert orienting studies that showed a difficulty in disengaging attention examined the effect of lesions on detection of a luminance change in a relatively uncluttered field. To understand how the deficit in disengaging attention can contribute to deficient exploration in situations like drawing and cancellation tasks, it is necessary to examine attentional search in a cluttered field in which many objects compete for attention.

Eglin, Robertson, and Knight (1989) studied visual search in patients with neglect using a task developed by Treisman and Gelade (1980). They varied the side of a predesignated conjunction target (one defined by a specific color and shape, requiring the conjunction of more than one feature to identify) among a variable number of distractors, and measured the time to find the target. When distractors were present, they could occur in either the ipsilesional field or the contralesional field. As long as no distractors appeared on the ipsilesional side of the display, no differences were found in locating a target on the neglected and intact sides. In other words, in displays that were limited to the contralesional side of a page, there were no objects to attract attention to the intact side and so nothing from which to disengage attention. Under those circumstances, the patients searched the display on the left as readily as they searched displays on the right. In contrast, for bilateral displays, in which distractors were present in both fields, search times increased as a function of the number of distractors or objects in the ipsilesional field. Each distractor on the intact side tripled the search time to locate the contralesional target. That is, the difficulty in disengaging attention from the ipsilesional field of distractors to move attention to the contralesional field depended on the number of items in the display.

Using a modified cancellation task, Mark, Kooistra, and Heilman (1988) provided an elegantly simple demonstration that the deficit in disengaging attention contributes to neglect during searches of a cluttered field. They compared a conventional cancellation task, in which the patient was shown a page filled with lines and asked to cross them all out, with another condition in which they asked the patient to erase all the lines. As each line was erased, and thus no longer present, the patient no longer had to disengage from it before moving on. Performance was strikingly better in this erasure task than in the conventional line cancellation task.

Local Perceptual Biases After Right Temporo-Parietal Junction Lesions Exacerbate Visual Neglect

Some patients with parietal lobe lesions may have extinction but may not exhibit any of the exploratory deficits of neglect as assessed by drawing, copying, cancellation, or bisection tasks. In fact, extinction appears to be just as frequent after left as after right hemisphere lesions; but other components of the syndrome, including deficits in exploration of contralesional space, are much more frequent after right hemisphere lesions, especially after lesions involving the right TPJ (Vallar, 1993). So, although a deficit in disengaging attention may be a satisfactory explanation for extinction, it seems that other factors, perhaps specific to right hemisphere lesions, are at work in patients with the full-blown syndrome of neglect.

As discussed earlier, factors that cause attention to become more actively engaged in the ipsilesional field, such as hyperorienting to it or the presence of more distractors in it, will exacerbate the problem of disengaging attention and, hence, will exacerbate visual neglect. Another effect specific to a lesion of the right TPJ but not to the left TPJ is that it causes attention to become locked onto local perceptual details (Robertson, Lamb, and Knight, 1988). Figure 22.8 (Delis, Robertson, and Efron, 1986) shows the copying of a patient with a large stroke of the right hemisphere, and that of a patient with a large stroke involving the left hemisphere. The right hemisphere lesion caused almost the complete exclusion of the global organization of the figure, whereas the left hemisphere lesion caused the exclusion of local detail.

The conjoint effects of the local bias with a difficulty in disengaging attention combine in producing some classic constructional signs of neglect in paper and pencil tasks. Consider, for example, a patient writing a number onto a clock face. She will be more successful if, as she is writing in each number, she remains oriented to her task with reference to the whole clock. If her attention becomes excessively focused on the number she is writing and she loses sight of the whole clock, she will have more difficulty disengaging from that number to fill in the rest of the numbers in the correct

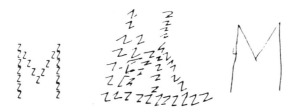

Figure 22.8 Drawing of hierarchical stimuli by two patients. (Left) The figure that the patients were asked to copy is a hierarchical pattern in which the large letter at the global level is an *M* constructed from small *Z*s at the local level. (Middle) Global organization was lost in this drawing by a patient with a right hemisphere lesion. (Right) Only the global organization of the figure is preserved, whereas the local details are lost in this copy by a patient with a left hemisphere lesion. (From Delis et al., 1986.)

locations on the clock face. As she writes a number in the clock face, her attention gets stuck there, and the difficulty in disengaging attention causes the numbers drawn subsequently to be bunched up together next to it. On the other hand, if the clock face remains uncluttered with other numbers, patients with neglect are better able to remain oriented to the whole clock face. Di Pellegrino (1995) showed that neglect patients could put a single number in the appropriate location on a clock face as long as they were given a separate sheet for each number.

Halligan and Marshall (1994) have shown the importance of the local bias as a contributor to neglect and how the local bias and the deficit in disengaging attention interact to determine neglect behavior. They asked their patient with left hemispatial neglect to bisect a horizontal line. In one condition they also presented a vertical line at the right end of the line that was to be bisected. Before asking the patient to bisect the horizontal line, they gave their patient a task that required attending to the full extent of the vertical line. This obliged the patient to expand the attentional spotlight from the point at the end of the horizontal line—and improved subsequent bisection performance on the horizontal line. The condition helped the patient to overcome the tendency to become hyperengaged in a small focus of attention at the end of the line to be bisected, and neglect was improved. Perhaps the expansion of attention to a more global level explains why patients with neglect make less bisection error when bisecting a rectangle than when bisecting a line—and why the higher the vertical extent of the rectangle, the less the bisection error (Vallar, 1994).

REFERENCE FRAMES FOR VISUAL ATTENTION: WHAT IS NEGLECTED IN NEGLECT?

Extrapersonal space exists independent of the viewpoint of the observer. Even when we are lying down (or standing on our heads), "up" and "down" remain the same, determined by the gravitational field. Ladavas (1987) first

Development and Pathologies of Attention

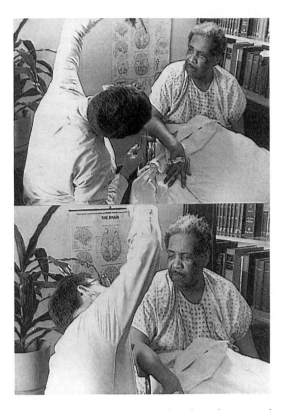

Figure 22.9 Reference frames and neglect. This patient detected a single finger wiggling in his contralesional field, but did not see it if a finger was also wiggled simultaneously in the ipsilesional (right) field (extinction). The test illustrated here demonstrates the dependence of extinction on the reference frame of the patient. When the examiner rotates clockwise (top), there is extinction of the lower stimulus, which is still the left side of the object, and the patient looks up. When the examiner rotates counter-clockwise (bottom), there is extinction of the upper stimulus, which is still the left side of the object, and the patient looks down. (From Rafal, 1994.)

showed that when patients with neglect tilted their heads, neglect was manifest not in terms of visual field, but in terms of gravitational coordinates.

However, figure 22.9 strikingly demonstrates, using a test devised by Lynn Robertson, that neglect is not always manifest in simple environmental (gravitational) coordinates. Here I was testing for extinction by wiggling fingers on both of my hands. In one condition my body and face were rotated to the left (i.e., the reference frame was rotated counterclockwise). In that condition the patient detected the upper finger wiggle and extinguished the lower; that is, there was extinction of the left side of the reference frame (the reference frame being me). In contrast, when my body and face were rotated to the right (i.e., the reference frame was rotated clockwise), the patient detected the lower finger wiggle and extinguished the upper; that is, there was extinction of the opposite spatial location, but again it was on the left side of the reference frame. In that case, then, neglect was not manifest with reference to gravitational coordinates, but with reference to the principal axis of the attended object.

It seems that visual neglect does not simply affect a visual field mapped in retinotopic coordinates, nor even simply one side of egocentric space. It can be manifest in object-based coordinates. The phenomenon of object-based neglect, however, highlights a paradox in which the reference frame in which neglect is manifest can be defined by objects or by parts of objects that are neglected. To understand how neglect can operate in object-based coordinates for objects that are neglected, we first need to consider to what degree visual objects can be represented in the neglected field outside of the focus of attention.

Figure-Ground Segregation and Grouping in Visual Neglect

When the two drawings on the left (a) and right (b) of figure 23.10 are viewed, bright green objects on a dim red background are normally seen (both because the green is brighter and because its area is smaller than the dim red). Driver, Baylis, and Rafal (1993) showed a patient with left hemineglect figures like these and asked him to remember the shape of the dividing line between red and green, and to then match that line with the probe shapes (shown under the study shapes in figure 22.10). Notice that the

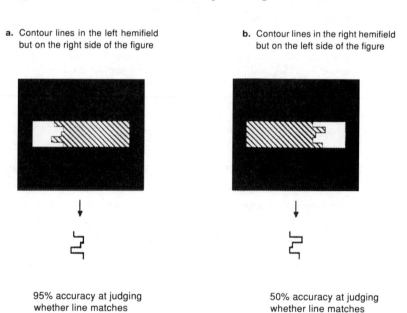

a. Contour lines in the left hemifield but on the right side of the figure

b. Contour lines in the right hemifield but on the left side of the figure

95% accuracy at judging whether line matches

50% accuracy at judging whether line matches

Figure 22.10 A patient with left hemispatial neglect was shown figures like those shown here and was asked to report verbally whether the contour dividing red areas (shown as hatched) and bright green areas (shown as white) of a rectangle matched the probe line presented immediately below the rectangle following its offset. Normally the small bright green region is seen as figure against the dim, red background. Although not required to identify figure or ground, the patient showed more neglect for the left side of the figure (b), even though this figure was in the right visual field. (From Driver et al., 1993.)

Development and Pathologies of Attention

boundary to be remembered is on the left side of the page in (a) and on the right in (b); yet for (a) the boundary to be remembered lies on the right side of the green object, whereas in (b) it lies on the left side of the green object. The patient's task did not require any judgment about either the perceived object (green) or its ground (red). His task was only to attend to the shape of the line bordering the two colored areas. Were neglect manifest strictly with respect to egocentric space, more errors would have been expected for (a) than for (b). The results showed the exact opposite pattern. The patient was much more accurate in condition (a), in which the to-be-remembered contour was on the right side of the object but on the left side of the page, than in condition (b), in which the to-be-remembered contour was on the left side of the object but on the right side of the page. Although the green shape on the left side in (a) was in the neglected field and judgments about the object were not relevant to the task at hand, the patient's attention was nevertheless summoned to it.

In that example, neglect operated with regard to the reference frame of the object. These observations tell us two important things: (1) the processes for segregating figure from ground can operate preattentively in the neglected field, and (2) attention operates at a later stage on candidate objects generated by those preattentive processes. The object-based neglect of objects segregated from ground is nicely shown by the drawings of similar shapes shown in figure 22.11 (Marshall and Halligan, 1994). Notice also in figure 22.3 (top) that the patient stopped canceling items right at the boundary of the two textures at the edge of the group defined on the right.

Another preattentive process that is preserved in patients with unilateral neglect is the segregation of figure from ground based on symmetry. The effect of symmetry in preattentive generation of candidate objects was first demonstrated by showing a patient with visual neglect pictures like those shown in figure 22.12 (Driver et al., 1993). When the patient was asked to report which color was "in front" of the background, he, like normal individuals, identified the symmetrical objects as the figure; but when asked to judge whether the shapes were symmetrical or not, he performed at chance. That is, even though his neglect prevented him from reporting whether or not shapes were symmetrical, he nevertheless perceived symmetrical shapes as the objects in the visual scene.

Once candidate objects are preattentively segregated from background, they may then be grouped with other objects based on Gestalt principles. Figure 22.13 shows a task used to test whether grouping is preserved in visual neglect (Driver, Baylis, Goodrich, and Rafal, 1994). The patients' task was simply to determine whether or not there was a gap in the top of the central triangle. The principal axis of the triangle (i.e., which way it appeared to point) was manipulated by the way in which the central triangle was grouped with the others. In the figure on the right, the alignment of the triangles (from southwest to northeast) causes them to appear to be pointing toward the northwest, and the gap in the top of the central triangle is per-

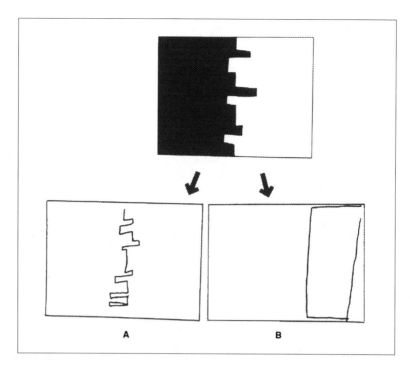

Figure 22.11 Object-based neglect is demonstrated by the copying performance of a patient with left hemispatial neglect. When asked to copy the black object, the patient does well, because the jagged contour is on the right side of the black object. When asked to copy the white object, the patient is unable to copy the jagged contour, because it is on the left side of the object being attended. (From Marshall and Halligan, 1994.)

ceived to appear on the right side of its perceived principal axis. In the figure on the left, the alignment of the triangles (from southeast to northwest) causes them to appear to be pointing toward the northeast, and the gap in the top of the central triangle is perceived to appear on the left side of its perceived principal axis. Results in three patients with left hemineglect showed that all missed more of the gaps in the condition in which the gap was on the perceived left of the triangle. Those results demonstrate that grouping is preserved in visual neglect and that attention operates in the reference frame of the group such that visual neglect is determined based on the principal axis of the group.

Ro and Rafal (1996) have shown recently that neglected visual features contribute to the perception of geometric illusions that influence the perception of line length. Recall that bisection errors in patients with hemispatial neglect are proportionate to line length (Marshall and Halligan, 1990). After determining that our patient had no explicit awareness of the left side of the figures shown in figure 22.14, we asked her to bisect the shaft lines of the drawings. Normal subjects judge the shaft on the bottom left to be longer than the shaft on the bottom right—the Müller-Lyer illusion. The patient made greater bisection errors for the bottom left figure than for the bottom

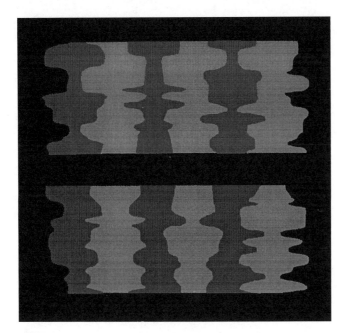

Figure 22.12 Normally, symmetrical regions of figures like these are perceived as objects in front of the background. The patient reported by Driver et al. (1993) also reported the symmetrical regions as being in front of the background, even though his neglect prevented him from explicitly determining whether or not the shapes where symmetrical.

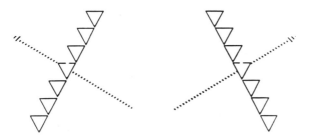

Figure 22.13 The figures used by Driver et al. (1994) to study axis-based visual neglect. Three patients with left hemispatial neglect were asked to report whether or not the triangle in the center had a gap in it. Because of grouping of the triangles, triangles on the left are seen as pointing toward the northwest, so that the gap in the top of the central triangle is on the right side of its principal axis; whereas the triangles on the right are seen as pointing toward the northeast, so that the gap in the top of the central triangle is on the left side of its principal axis. All three patients had more neglect (missed seeing the gap) in the condition shown on the right than in the condition shown on the left.

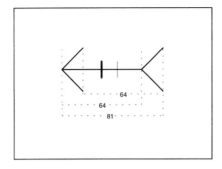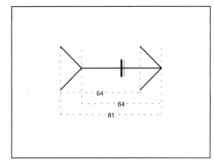
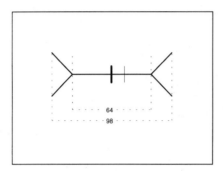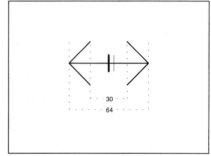

Figure 22.14 The four fin configurations producing the Judd illusion (top row) and the Müller-Lyer illusion (bottom row). The solid black line shows the true midpoint of the shaft. The reader can experience the Judd illusion in the top figures, which do not appear to be bisected in the middle. The reader can also experience the Müller-Lyer illusion, in which the left shaft appears to be longer than the right. The fine lines indicate the median bisection point produced by the patient.

right figure, showing both that she was subject to the Müller-Lyer illusion and that her bisection performance was affected by the *perceived* length of the line. Furthermore, comparison of bisection errors for the two top figures (the Judd illusion) revealed that features on the left side of the shaft affected bisection performance as much as did features on the right side of the shaft. These observations indicate that geometric illusions are generated preattentively to determine perceived size, and that bisection errors in hemispatial neglect are amplified by perceived line length induced by those illusions.

Object-Centered Neglect

Behrmann and Tipper (1994) have shown object-based neglect that actually moved to the ipsilesional side of the object after it rotated. RT was measured to targets appearing in either the left (contralesional) or right (ipsilesional) side of a dumbbell. Patients were slower to respond to targets on the left. If the dumbbell rotated, however, such that the two sides of the dumbbell reversed fields, RTs were prolonged for targets on the right.

An elegant demonstration of object based neglect is demonstrated by the copying performance of the patient reported by Marshall and Halligan (1993) and shown in figure 22.4. When copying the flower shown on the top left, in which the two flowers are part of the same plant, the patient copied only the right side of the right flower and neglected the left flower entirely (top right). When the patient was to copy the figure on the bottom left, which contained the same two flowers but not depicted as part of the same plant, the two flowers were treated as separate objects and the patient copied the right side of each and neglected the left side of each (bottom right).

Object-based neglect has also been inferred from the reading errors of neglect patients. In a striking demonstration of neglect dyslexia reported by Hillis and Caramazza (1991), a patient with right hemineglect made more errors at the end of the word regardless of the orientation of the word on the page; that is, even when the word was upside-down such that the right end of the word was in the left visual field. Patients with neglect also have been shown to make more reading errors when they read pronounceable non-words than when they read words (Brunn and Farah, 1991; Friedrich, Walker, and Posner, 1985; Sieroff, Pollatsek, and Posner, 1988) This shows that word forms are preattentively processed and integrate the constituent letters into a single object. The study by Brunn and Farah (1991) incorporated cancellation or line bisection tasks along with the reading task. Less neglect was found on the secondary task when the primary task required reading a word than a nonword. This finding suggests that word processing causes an automatic deployment of attention to encompass the entire word.

Not all attempts to identify object-based neglect have been successful; and a contrast of those studies that have demonstrated object-based neglect and those that have not is instructive. Farah, Brunn, Wong, Wallace, and Carpenter (1990) asked patients to name colors surrounding pictures of common objects. When the pictures were rotated, the colors neglected did not rotate with the object; that is, neglect remained location-based rather than object-based. Behrmann and Moscovitch (1994) used the same paradigm and confirmed the lack of object-based neglect with object drawings. However, object-based neglect was manifest in the special case in which the objects were asymmetrical letters. That is, object-based neglect was manifest when the object's identity was uniquely defined by its principal axis.

PREATTENTIVE PERCEPTUAL PROCESSING WITHOUT CONSCIOUS AWARENESS: EVIDENCE FROM THE NEGLECT SYNDROME

Demonstrations like those depicted in figures 22.10–22.14 show that candidate objects in the visual field can segregate from the background in the absence of attentive awareness, that those candidate objects are also grouped by preattentive mechanisms, and that attention then operates on object-based representations. The autonomy of early vision from attentional mechanisms, demonstrated in patients with neglect, indicates that much visual information is processed outside of conscious awareness. The study of neglect can teach us how much information processing goes on in the absence of conscious awareness. Recent studies have shown that neglected visual information is in fact processed to a high level in which the identity of objects and words is registered outside of the patient's awareness

In a seminal study Volpe, Ledoux, and Gazzaniga (1979) showed that some patients with neglect were able to tell whether an object in the contralesional field was same or different from one in the ipsilesional field—even though they could not tell what the object was. So some information is available from the extinguished object. However, it has been shown that perceptual degradation of stimuli in normal subjects also causes a loss of the ability to identify objects before the ability to make same-different judgments is lost (Farah, Wong, Monheit, and Morrow, 1989). The findings of Volpe et al. thus do not necessarily, in themselves, indicate that perceptual processing is fully preserved in extinguished stimuli.

A modification of the simple clinical test for extinction provides evidence for processing of information in the neglected field (figure 22.15). I have found that when some patients with relatively mild neglect are simultaneously presented with two different objects, they can be much less likely to show extinction than when two identical objects are shown. Information in the unattended field is clearly processed sufficiently for it to be distinguished as different than its counterpart in the ipsilesional field. This difference signal triggers an orienting response leading to detection and ultimately discrimination. Figure 22.3 (bottom) shows a second example of cancellation performance being affected by texture segregation. Unlike the example in the top of the figure, however, the patient, on one occasion, did notice an item to the left of the boundary and then crossed it out along with all the other similar items along the boundary. Perhaps in that instance she crossed the boundary because the item on the other side of the boundary was different from those she had been crossing out and attracted her attention. Thereafter, however, all the items to the left of it were similar, so she extinguished them and stopped canceling.

But do the objects need to be identical or just similar for extinction to occur? If they do not have to be identical, in what way must they be similar for extinction to occur? I became intrigued by that question one day when I showed a patient two different types of fork (a white, plastic picnic fork in one field, and a silver, metal dinner fork in the other). He reported only seeing one fork in his right field (figure 22.15). Even though the objects differ visually, the fact that they are classified the same seemed to determine whether the patient oriented to one or to both.

Baylis, Driver, and Rafal (1993) extended that clinical observation with an experiment conducted with the patient shown in figure 22.15 and with four other patients. All had recently shown clinical signs of extinction and neglect. Some had recovered to the point that clinical extinction was no longer evident on bedside confrontation testing and they no longer had neglect on

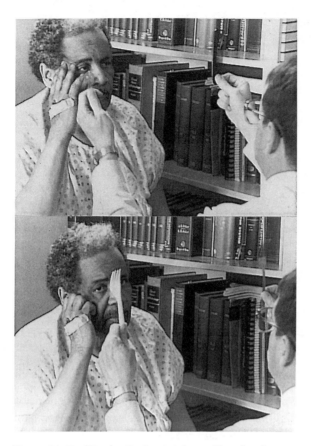

Figure 22.15 Visual extinction is influenced by what the competing objects are. When shown two different objects the patient first named the key in the ipsilesional field, and then (top) also reported the comb in his contralesional (left) field. When shown two forks (bottom) he reported only the one in his ipsilesional (right) field, and failed to notice the other fork in the contralesional (left) field (even though it was a different color). (From Rafal, 1994.)

standard pencil and paper tasks. Nevertheless, in all of them the exposure duration of briefly presented colored letters could be titrated to a point at which they reliably identified single letters in either field, but showed extinction on many trials with bilateral stimuli. Once that exposure duration was determined for each patient, colored letters were randomly presented either unilaterally or bilaterally and the patients were asked to report what they saw on each side. The critical trials were those with bilateral targets in which the patient showed extinction; that is, when the partient correctly reported the ipsilesional target but reported seeing nothing in the contralesional field. In one condition they were asked to name only the letter(s) (X or E), and in another to report only the color(s) (red or green). The results showed that extinction occurred much more frequently when the bilateral stimuli were identical *in the attribute to be reported*. On blocks in which the task was to report the name of the letter, extinction was not ameliorated if the stimuli were of different colors, and vice versa for the color report blocks. Those results confirm that information about shape and color of neglected objects are processed. More importantly, they demonstrate that access of this information to conscious awareness is contingent upon the goals dictated by the task at hand.

Berti and Rizzolatti (1992) provided evidence from neglect patients that extinguished objects are processed to a categorical level of representation. Their subjects categorized line drawings of pictures presented in the ipsilesional field. Their performance was better not only when the same picture was presented simultaneously in the contralesional, extinguished visual field, but also when the picture in the contralesional field was a different object in the same category as the target object in the ipsilesional field. Ladavas, Paladini, and Cubelli (1993) have more recently confirmed those findings, and have also provided data showing that the patients performed at levels predicted by chance on explicit report of the stimuli in the neglected field. McGlinchey-Berroth, Milberg, Verfaellie, Alexander, and Kilduff (1993) gave a lexical decision task to four patients with left hemineglect. A letter string was presented in the center of the display and the patients' reaction time was measured to respond whether or not the letter string constituted an English word. Each trial began with a picture presented briefly in either the ipsilesional or contralesional field, and that prime could either be semantically related to the target word or unrelated. That kind of priming generally facilitates RT responses in the lexical decision task when the target word is semantically related to the prime stimulus. In the patients, primes presented in the contralesional field produced just as much priming as did those in the ipsilesional field, even though the patients were not able to identify the contralesional primes in an explicit report task.

The emerging evidence suggests that extinguished objects undergo extensive perceptual and categorical processing outside of the focus of attention, and that access to awareness of that information is inhibited quite late in selection. A dramatic example was reported by Marshall and Halligan (1988). Their patient with left neglect was shown a picture of two houses, one on the right and the other on the left. The picture depicted the house on the left as being on fire. The patient did not notice that detail and reported that the two houses looked just alike. Nevertheless, when asked to choose which house she would prefer to live in, she chose the house on the right— although she couldn't offer any explanation for her preference. Although such a dramatic example may not be typical of most patients with neglect, that kind of observation is consistent with experimental findings that information that is extinguished can influence feelings and behavior even though the patient is not consciously aware of it.

These examples show that neglected information is processed to an advanced stage in which the meaning of the neglected objects are, in fact, encoded. Yet the information is somehow prevented from making contact with neural systems that permit access to awareness. Does the neglected information have direct contact with systems controlling motor activity? In a situation in which a given stimulus is tightly associated with a specific motor act (moving the foot to the break pedal when the light turns red), does neglected information activate response channels with which it has become associated?

To examine whether extinguished information is effective in activating associated motor response channels, Cohen, Ivry, Rafal, and Kohn (1995) used a flanker interference paradigm in patients with visual neglect. The patients were asked to respond to color patches (red or green) presented in the center of a display screen. On each trial a flanking color patch was presented simultaneously with the visual target either in the neglected visual field contralateral to the lesion or in the ipsilesional field. The flanker, which the patients were instructed to ignore, could either be the same as the target and therefore congruent with the required response, or it could code the opposite, incongruent response, or it could be blue (a neutral color). The results indicated comparable flanker interference effects from the neglected flankers as from the flankers in the intact visual field. Those findings, and others using flanker effects in patients with neglect (Audet, Bub, and Lecours 1991), indicate not only that perceptual processing of the flankers is preserved in the neglected visual field, but that they are also effective in activating response channels with which they have been associated. Moreover, these findings indicate that the anatomical pathways involved in transducing stimulus to response code activation do not require intact parietal lobe function or conscious awareness of the stimulus.

Spatial Representations and Neglect

Neglect can result not only in the failure to perceive or to respond to contralesional signals or objects, but also to a lack of conscious access to the contralesional side of visual images stored in memory (Bisiach, 1993). Bisiach and Luzzatti (1978) asked patients with left hemineglect to imagine themselves in the Piazza del Duomo in Milan. In one condition they asked the patients to imagine themselves at one end of the square, looking toward the cathedral dominating the other end of the square, and asked them to describe what they would be able to see. In another condition the patients were asked to imagine themselves standing on the cathedral steps facing the opposite way. In both circumstances the patients reported fewer landmarks on the contralesional side of the mental image.

These kinds of observations have engendered an account of neglect in which the parietal lobes are assumed to maintain a representation of space in viewer-centered coordinates, and in which parietal lesions are assumed to produce a degradation of the contralesional representation. In an elegant experimental test of this account, Bisiach, Luzzatti, and Perani (1979) had patients view cloudlike shapes that were passed slowly behind a slit (so that only part of the shape could be seen at any moment). The task required that a mental image be generated and maintained as the slit moved over the shape that the patients were attempting to remember. The patients were shown two shapes that could be either the same or different, and they were asked to respond whether the shapes were the same or not. On the trials in which the shapes were different, they could be different on their left or right sides. The patients made more errors on this task when shapes were different from each other on the contralesional end than on the ipsilesional end.

We need to know more about the neuroanatomical and pathophysiological basis for the deficit of spatial representation in neglect (Kinsella, Oliver, Ng, Packer, and Stark, 1993). Some authors have considered spatial representation in terms of oculomotor coding (Duhamel, Colby, and Goldberg, 1992; Gianotti, 1993), whereas others have emphasized spatial working memory (Funahashi, Bruce, and Goldman, 1993). Recent reports show that perceptual neglect and neglect of internal imagery may be dissociated. Two patients with perceptual neglect and mainly parietal lesions did not evidence neglect in visual imagery (Anderson, 1993), whereas a patient with a frontal lesion causing neglect of imagined scenes did not have perceptual neglect (Guariglia, Padovani, Pantano, and Pizzamiglio, 1993).

CONCLUSIONS

In neglect, a constellation of symptoms is seen that affect both perception and exploratory behavior. Which symptoms (and with what severity) occur in any given patient depend upon the extent and location of the lesion, its chronicity, as well as the premorbid cognitive architecture of the individual. Across the rather heterogeneous population of patients with elements of the neglect syndrome, the pathophysiological mechanisms underlying each of the component symptoms are diverse. We are just beginning to understand some of these: hyperreflexive orienting toward the ipsilesional side or to local elements in the visual scene; impaired ability to disengage attention; a deranged internal representation of space that is not only shifted but contracts contralesionally; impaired voluntary orienting toward the contralesional field; a motor bias toward the ipsilesional side that causes defective contralesional exploratory behavior; deficient ability to generate contralesional voluntary saccades; failure of contralesional stimuli to produce arousal. The manifestations of neglect in an individual patient may not simply represent the additive contributions of each of those mechanisms, but rather an interaction between them (Humphreys and Riddoch, 1993).

The study of neglect has advanced our understanding of preattentive vision and of the functions of attention in object recognition and in the control of goal-directed behavior. We have learned that the visual scene is parsed preattentively into candidate objects, and that attention then operates on those objects to afford awareness and recognition of them, and to guide subsequent action. Information about neglected objects is processed to an advanced level, and neglect appears to occur quite late at a stage of selection for action. Nevertheless, unattended information does influence behavior and may guide subsequent orienting, leading, ultimately, to awareness of the previously neglected object. Thus, the study of neglect also aids our understanding of the interactions of conscious and unconscious processing (Humphreys and Riddoch, 1993; Young, Hellawell, and Welch, 1992). We are developing a better understanding of the plight of these patients and of their perplexing behavior. These insights can be applied to fashioning more rational approaches to their rehabilitation (Diller and Riley, 1993; Robertson, Halligan, and Marshall, 1993).

REFERENCES

Anderson, B. (1993) Spared awareness for the left side of internal visual images in patients with left-sided extrapersonal neglect. *Neurology* 43: 213–216.

Audet, T., Bub, D., and Lecours, A. R. (1991) Visual neglect and left-sided context effects. *Brain Cogn.* 16: 11–28.

Bay, E. (1953) Disturbances of visual perception and their examination. *Brain* 76: 515–530.

Baylis, G., Driver, J., and Rafal, R. (1993) Extinction and stimulus repetition. *J. Cognitive Neurosci.* 5: 453–466.

Behrmann, M. and Moscovitch, M. (1994) Object-centered neglect in patients with unilateral neglect: Effects of left-right coordinates of objects. *J. Cognitive Neurosci.* 6: 1–16.

Behrmann, M. and Tipper, S. P. (1994) Object-based visual attention: Evidence from unilateral neglect. In *Attention and Performance XIV: Conscious and Nonconscious Processing and Cognitive Functioning*, edited by C. Umilta and M. Moscovitch, pp. 351–376. Hillsdale, NJ: Lawrence Erlbaum.

Bender, M. B. and Feldman, M. (1972) The so-called "visual agnosias." *Brain* 95: 173–186.

Berti, A. and Rizzolatti, G. (1992) Visual processing without awareness: Evidence from unilateral neglect. *J. Cognitive Neurosci.* 4: 345–351.

Bisiach, E. (1993) Mental representation in unilateral neglect and related disorders: The twentieth Bartlett memorial lecture. *Q. J. Exp. Psychol.* 46A: 435–462.

Bisiach, E., Geminiani, G., Berti, A., and Rusconi, M. L. (1990) Perceptual and premotor factors of unilateral neglect. *Neurology* 40: 1278–1281.

Bisiach, E. and Luzzatti, C. (1978) Unilateral neglect of representational space. *Cortex* 14: 129–133.

Bisiach, E., Luzzatti, C., and Perani, D. (l979) Unilateral neglect, representational schema and consciousness. *Brain* 102: 609–618.

Bisiach, E., Rusconi, M. L., and Vallar, G. (1991) Remission of somatoparaphrenic delusion through vestibular stimulation. *Neuropsychologia* 29: 1029–1031.

Brunn, J. L. and Farah, M. J. (1991) The relationship between spatial attention and reading: Evidence from the neglect syndrome. *Cognitive Neuropsychol.* 8: 59–75.

Butter, C. M., Kirsch, N. L., and Reeves, G. (1990) The effects of lateralized dynamic stimuli on unilateral spatial neglect following right hemisphere lesions. *Restor. Neurol. Neurosci.* 2: 39–46.

Cappa, S. F., Sterzi, R., Vallar, G., and Bisiach, E. (1987) Remission of hemineglect and anosognosia after vestibular stimulation. *Neuropsychologia* 25: 775–782.

Cohen, A., Ivry, R., Rafal, R., and Kohn, C. (1995) Response code activation by stimuli in the neglected visual field. *Neuropsychology* 9: 165–173.

Cohen, J. and Farah, M. (1991) *Disengaging from the disengage operation*. Paper presented at the annual meeting of the Psychonomic Society, San Francisco.

Cohen, J. D., Romero, R. D., Servan-Schreiber, D., and Farah, M. J. (1994) Mechanisms of spatial attention: The relation of macrostructure to microstructure in parietal neglect. *J. Cognitive Neurosci.* 6: 377–387.

Coslett, H. B., Bowers, D., Fitzpatrick, E., Haws, B., and Heilman, K. M. (1990) Directional hypokinesia and hemispatial inattention in neglect. *Brain* 113: 475–486.

Delis, D. C., Robertson, L. C., and Efron, R. (1986) Hemispheric specialization of memory for visual hierarchical stimuli. *Neuropsychologia* 24: 205–214.

Diller, L. and Riley, E. (1993) The behavioral management of neglect. In *Unilateral Neglect: Clinical and Experimental Studies*, edited by I. H. Robertson and J. C. Marshall, pp. 293–310. Hillsdale, NJ: Lawrence Erlbaum.

Di Pellegrino, G. (1995) Clock-drawing in a case of left visuospatial neglect: A deficit of disengagement. *Neuropsychologia* 33: 353–358.

Driver, J., Baylis, G., and Rafal, R. (1993) Preserved figure-ground segmentation and symmetry perception in a patient with neglect. *Nature* 360: 73–75.

Driver, J., Baylis, G. C., Goodrich, S. J., and Rafal, R. D. (1994) Axis-based neglect of visual shapes. *Neuropsychologia* 32: 1353–1365.

Duhamel, J. R., Colby, C. L., and Goldberg, M. E. (1992) The updating of the representation of visual space in parietal cortex by intended eye movements. *Science* 255: 90–92.

Eglin, M., Robertson, L. C., and Knight, R. T. (1989) Visual search performance in the neglect syndrome. *J. Cognitive Neurosci.* 1: 372–385.

Farah, M. J., Brunn, J. L., Wong, A. B., Wallace, M. A., and Carpenter, P. A. (1990) Frames of reference for allocating attention to space: Evidence from the neglect syndrome. *Neuropsychologia* 28: 335–347.

Farah, M. J., Wong, A. B., Monheit, M. A., and Morrow, L. A. (1989) Parietal lobe mechanisms of spatial attention: Modality-specific or supramodal? *Neuropsychologia* 27: 461–470.

Friedrich, F. J., Walker, J. A., and Posner, M. I. (1985) Effects of parietal lesions on visual matching: Implications for reading errors. *Cognitive Neuropsychol.* 2: 253–264.

Friedrich, F. J., Egly, R. D., and Beck, D. (in press). Spatial attention deficits in humans: a comparison of superior parietal and temporal-parietal junction lesions. *Neuropsychology.*

Funahashi, S., Bruce, C. J., and Goldman, R. P. (1993) Dorsolateral prefrontal lesions and oculomotor delayed-response performance: Evidence for mnemonic "scotomas." *J. Neurosci.* 13: 1479–1497.

Gianotti, G. (1993) The role of spontaneous eye movements in orienting attention and in unilateral neglect. In *Unilateral Neglect: Clinical and Experimental Studies*, edited by I. H. Robertson and J. C. Marshall, pp. 107–122. Hillsdale, NJ: Lawrence Erlbaum.

Graziano, M. S. A., Yap, G. S., and Gross, C. G. (1994) Coding of visual space by premotor neurons. *Science* 266: 1054–1057.

Guariglia, C., Padovani, A., Pantano, P., and Pizzamiglio, L. (1993) Unilateral neglect restricted to visual imagery. *Nature* 364: 235–237.

Halligan, P. W. and Marshall, J. C. (1994) Right-sided cueing can ameliorate left neglect. *Neuropsychol. Rehab.* 4: 63–73.

Heilman, K. M., Bowers, D., Coslett, H. B., Whelan, H., and Watson, R. T. (1985) Directional hypokinesia: Prolonged reaction times for leftward movements in patients with right hemisphere lesions and neglect. *Neurology* 35: 855–859.

Heilman, K. M., Valenstein, E., and Watson, R. T. (1985) The neglect syndrome. In *Clinical Neuropsychology*, edited by J. A. M. Fredricks, pp. 153–183. New York: Elsevier Science.

Hillis, A. E. and Caramazza, A. (1991) Deficit to stimulus-centered, letter shape representations in a case of "unilateral neglect." *Neuropsychologia* 29: 1223–1240.

Humphreys, G. W. and Riddoch, M. J. (1993) Interactive attentional systems in unilateral visual neglect. In *Unilateral Neglect: Clinical and Experimental Studies*, edited by I. H. Robertson and J. C. Marshall, pp. 139–168. Hillsdale, NJ: Lawrence Erlbaum.

Karnath, H. O. (1994) Disturbed coordinate transformation in the neural representation of space as the crucial mechanism leading to neglect. *Neuropsychol. Rehab.* 4: 147–150.

Karnath, H. O., Christ, K., and Hartje, W. (1993) Decrease of contralateral neglect by neck muscle vibration and spatial orientation of trunk midline. *Brain* 116: 383–396.

Kinsbourne, M. (1977) Hemi-neglect and hemisphere rivalry. In *Advances in Neurology*, edited by E. A. Weinstein and R. P. Friedland, pp. 41–49. New York: Raven Press.

Kinsbourne, M. (1993) Orientational bias model of unilateral neglect: Evidence from attentional gradients within hemispace. In *Unilateral Neglect: Clinical and Experimental Studies*, edited by I. H. Robertson and J. C. Marshall, pp. 63–86. Hillsdale, NJ: Lawrence Erlbaum.

Kinsbourne, M. (1994) Mechanisms of neglect: Implications for rehabilitation. *Neuropsychol. Rehab.* 4: 151–153.

Kinsella, G., Oliver, J., Ng, K., Packer, S., and Stark, R. (1993) Analysis of the syndrome of unilateral neglect. *Cortex* 29: 135–140.

Ladavas, E. (1987) Is the hemispatial deficit produced by right parietal damage associated with retinal or gravitational coordinates? *Brain* 110: 167–180.

Ladavas, E., Del Pesce, M., and Provinciali, L. (1989) Unilateral attention deficits and hemispheric asymmetries in the control of visual attention. *Neuropsychologia* 27: 353–366.

Ladavas, E., Paladini, R., and Cubelli, R. (1993) Implicit associative priming in a patient with left visual neglect. *Neuropsychologia* 31: 1307–1320.

Mark, V. W., Kooistra, C. A., and Heilman, K. M. (1988) Hemispatial neglect affected by non-neglected stimuli. *Neurology* 38: 1207–1211.

Marshall, J. C. and Halligan, P. W. (1988) Blindsight and insight in visuo-spatial neglect. *Nature* 336: 766–767.

Marshall, J. C. and Halligan, P. W. (1990) Line bisection in a case of visual neglect: Psychophysical studies with implications for theory. *Cognitive Neuropsychol.* 7: 107–130.

Marshall, J. C. and Halligan, P. W. (1993) Visuo-spatial neglect: A new copying test to assess perceptual parsing. *J. Neurol.* 240: 37–40.

Marshall, J. C. and Halligan, P. W. (1994) Left in the dark: The neglect of theory. *Neuropsychol. Rehab.* 4: 161–167.

Mattingley, J. B., Bradshaw, J. G., and Phillips, J. G. (1992) Impairments of movement initiation and execution in unilateral neglect: Directional hypokinesia and bradykinesia. *Brain* 115: 1849–1874.

McGlinchey-Berroth, R., Milberg, W. P., Verfaellie, M., Alexander, M., and Kilduff, P. T. (1993) Semantic processing in the neglected visual field: Evidence from a lexical decision task. *Cognitive Neuropsychol.* 10: 79–108.

Mesulam, M. M. (1981) A cortical network for directed attention and unilateral neglect. *Ann. Neurol.* 4: 309–325.

Milner, A. D. and Harvey, M. (1995) Distortion of size perception in visuospatial neglect. *Curr. Biol.* 5: 85–89.

Milner, A. D., Harvey, M., Roberts, R. C., and Forster, S. V. (1993) Line bisection errors in visual neglect: Misguided action or size distortion? *Neuropsychologia* 31: 39–49.

O'Keefe, J. (1993) Hippocampus, theta, and spatial memory. *Curr. Opin. Neurobiol.* 3: 917–924.

Pizzamiglio, L., Frasca, R., Guariglia, C., Inaccia, R., and Antonucci, G. (1990) Effect of optokinetic stimulation in patients with visual neglect. *Cortex* 26: 535–540.

Posner, M. I., Inhoff, A. W., Friedrich, F. J., and Cohen, A. (l987) Isolating attentional systems: A cognitive-anatomical analysis. *Psychobiology* 15: 107–121.

Posner, M. I. and Petersen, S. (1990) The attention system of the human brain. *Annu. Rev. Neurosci.* 13: 25–42.

Posner, M. I. and Rafal, R. D. (1987) Cognitive theories of attention and the rehabilitation of attentional deficits. In *Neuropsychological Rehabilitation*, edited by R. J. Meir, L. Diller, and A. L. Benton, pp. 182–201. London: Churchill and Livingston.

Posner, M. I., Walker, J. A., Friedrich, F. J., and Rafal, R. (1984) Effects of parietal injury on covert orienting of visual attention. *J. Neurosci.* 4: 1863–1874.

Posner, M. I., Walker, J. A., Friedrich, F. J., and Rafal, R. D. (1987) How do the parietal lobes direct covert attention? *Neuropsychologia* 25: 135–146.

Rafal, R. D. (1994) Neglect. *Curr. Opin. Neurobiol.* 4: 2312–2316.

Rafal, R. D., Posner, M. I., Friedman, J. H., Inhoff, A. W., and Bernstein, E. (1988) Orienting of visual attention in progressive supranuclear palsy. *Brain* 111: 267–280.

Rizzolatti, G. and Camarda, R. (1987) Neural circuits for spatial attention and unilateral neglect. In *Neurophysiological and Neuropsychological Aspects of Spatial Neglect*, edited by M. Jeannerod, pp. 289–314. Amsterdam: North Holland.

Ro, T. and Rafal, R. D. (1996) Perception of geometric illusion in visual neglect. *Neuropsychologia* 34: 1197–1202.

Robertson, I. H., Halligan, P. W., and Marshall, J. C. (1993) Prospects for the rehabilitation of unilateral neglect. In *Unilateral Neglect: Clinical and Experimental Studies*, edited by I. H. Robertson and J. C. Marshall, pp. 279–292. Hillsdale, NJ: Lawrence Erlbaum.

Robertson, L. C., Lamb, M. R., and Knight, R. T. (1988) Effects of lesions of the temporal-parietal junction on perceptual and attentional processing in humans. *J. Neurosci.* 8: 3757–3769.

Rubens, A. B. (1985) Caloric stimulation and unilateral visual neglect. *Neurology* 35: 1019–1024.

Seyal, M., Ro, T., and Rafal, R. (1995) Increased sensitivity to ipsilateral cutaneous stimuli following transcranial magnetic stimulation of the parietal lobe. *Ann. Neurol.* 38: 264–267.

Sieroff, E., Pollatsek, A., and Posner, M. I. (1988) Recognition of visual letter strings following injury to the posterior visual spatial attention system. *Cognitive Neuropsychol.* 5: 427–449.

Sprague, J. M. (1966) Interaction of cortex and superior colliculus in mediation of peripherally summoned behavior in the cat. *Science* 153: 1544–1547.

Tegner, R. and Levander, M. (1991) Through a looking glass: A new technique to demonstrate directional hypokinesia in unilateral neglect. *Brain* 113: 1943–1951.

Treisman, A. and Gelade, G. (1980) A feature integration theory of attention. *Cognitive Psychol.* 12: 97–136.

Vallar, G. (1993) The anatomical basis of spatial neglect in humans. In *Unilateral Neglect: Clinical and Experimental Studies,* edited by I. H. Robertson and J. C. Marshall, pp. 27–62. Hillsdale, NJ: Lawrence Erlbaum.

Vallar, G. (1994) Left spatial hemineglect: An unmanageable explosion of dissociations? No. *Neuropsychol. Rehab.* 4: 209–212.

Vallar, G., Bottini, G., Rusconi, M. L., and Sterzi, R. (1993) Exploring somatosensory hemineglect by vestibular stimulation. *Brain* 116: 71–86.

Volpe, B. T., Ledoux, J. E., and Gazzaniga, M. S. (1979) Information processing in an "extinguished" visual field. *Nature* 282: 722–724.

Vuileumier, P., Hester, D., Assal, G., and Regli, F. (1996) Unilateral spatial neglect recovery after sequential strokes. *Neurology* 19: 184–189.

Wallace, S. F., Rosenquist, A. C., and Sprague, J. M. (1989) Recovery from cortical blindness mediated by destruction of nontectotectal fibers in the commisure of the superior colliculus in the cat. *J. Comp. Neurol.* 284: 429–450.

Wallace, S. F., Rosenquist, A. C., and Sprague, J. M. (1990) Ibotenic acid lesions of the lateral substantia nigra restore visual orientation behavior in the hemianopic cat. *J. Comp. Neurol.* 296: 222–252.

Young, A. W., Hellawell, D. J., and Welch, J. (1992) Neglect and visual recognition. *Brain* 115: 51–71.

Zisper, D. and Anderson, R. (1988) A back-propagation programmed network that simulates response properties of a subset of posterior parietal neurons. *Nature* 331: 679–684.

23 The Mind Adrift: Attentional Dysregulation in Schizophrenia

Paul G. Nestor and Brian F. O'Donnell

ABSTRACT Schizophrenia is characterized by disturbances in both sustained and selective attention. These disturbances have long been thought to reflect a breakdown in higher-order, top-down processes, with early preattentive processes relatively spared. Evidence is presented to show, however, that schizophrenic attentional deficits are not necessarily limited to voluntary, conscious operations, such as those involved in working memory, but also include fast-acting, involuntary inhibitory mechanisms. These inhibitory mechanisms may reflect intrinsic properties of neuronal circuits that underlie higher-order complex systems. In schizophrenia, faulty inhibition at the cellular level may produce gain dysregulation of a complex system. A biophysical model is presented to show how gain or neuromodulation dysfunction in schizophrenia may be understood in reference to intrinsic properties of specific neuronal circuits.

Schizophrenia is a severe psychiatric disorder that profoundly alters emotional, cognitive, and social function. Although the course and the symptomatology of the disease vary greatly, attentional and cognitive deficits usually accompany the disorder, and may precede the onset of psychiatric symptoms. A neuropathological basis has yet to be established, although gross neuroanatomical abnormalities observed on quantitative brain imaging in schizophrenia include increased ventricular size, decreased brain volume or weight, and decreased grey matter. Recent quantitative magnetic resonance imaging (MRI) studies have shown volumetric abnormalities in thalamic structures (Andreasen et al., 1994) as well as reductions in the medial temporal lobe and the superior temporal gyrus, often more severe on the left side (e.g., Barta et al., 1990; Shenton et al., 1992). Subtle abnormalities of limbic system structures, including the hippocampus (Kovelman and Scheibel, 1984), entorhinal cortex (Arnold, Hyman, Van Hoesen, and Damasio, 1991), and cingulate gyrus (Benes and Bird, 1987), have been reported.

The neuropharmacology of schizophenic cognitive abnormalities and the psychiatric symptomatology have focused primarily on dopaminergic transmission in basal ganglia and mesolimbic structures, although other neuromodulatory systems, such as serotonergic systems, have also been implicated. Schizophrenic symptoms are induced or worsened by dopamine agonists and are reduced by dopamine antagonists, implicating hyperdopamingeric transmission in the expression of the disease. Others have suggested that the disease may be viewed more precisely in terms of dopamine dysregulation (e.g.,

Davis et al., 1986), with positive acute symptoms, such as paranoia or delusions, linked to hyperdopaminergic activity (e.g., Frecska, Perenyl, Bagdy, and Reval, 1985), and negative symptoms, such as blunted affect or poverty of speech, linked to hypodopaminergic activity (Tandon and Greden, 1989). There is, however, little direct support for increased dopamine receptors in schizophrenia (Farde et al., 1990; Martinot et al., 1990), and dopaminergic transimission may be intimately related to other neuromodulators, particularly glutamate (Sarter, 1991).

ATTENTION AND SCHIZOPHRENIA

Severe attentional disturbances have been noted in schizophrenia since the advent of modern descriptions of the illness by Bleuler (1911/1950) and Kraepelin (1919/1971) at the turn of the century. Patients suffer from difficulties in both sustaining and shifting attention in response to situational or conversational demands. At other times, they orient to and fixate on trivial aspects of the environment. Spoken and written language in patients is often affected by "thought disorder," which includes loose associations, tangentiality, and disrupted syntax.

This chapter examines attention at various levels of brain organization from basic cellular functioning to distributed neural systems. Such a framework is useful for the study of attention deficits in diseases in which localized brain circuits with corresponding neurotransmitter and cellular abnormalities have been identified (see Shepherd, 1995). In schizophrenia, the framework is also helpful, but is obviously limited by the absence of a firmly established neuropathological basis for the disease. Therefore, this review is limited to studies that have used direct, specific, and precisely controlled experimental measures that permit an analysis of the role of attention in various operations and mechanisms that may eventually be related to discrete neural systems. Both sustained and selective attention are examined.

Sustained Attention

Among the most frequently used measures of sustained attention with schizophrenic patients is the continuous performance test (CPT), first developed by Rosvold, Mirsky, Sarason, Bransome, and Beck (1956) and subsequently modified by others (e.g., Kornetsky and Mirsky, 1966; Wohlberg and Kornetsky, 1973). The conventional CPT, which often requires only the detection of an infrequent and unpredictable target, is highly sensitive to schizophrenia and may distinguish patients with schizophrenia from other clinical groups, including alcoholics (e.g., Orzack and Kornetsky, 1966). Schizophrenic patients often perform more poorly on the CPT than on other neuropsychological tests, a result that leads some to suggest that the CPT reflects a selective impairment in attention, as opposed to a generalized cognitive deficit (e.g., Kornetsky and Mirsky, 1966; Orzack and Kornetsky, 1966). Neuroleptic medication may improve but does not normalize CPT performance in schizophrenic patients (Orzack, Kornetsky, and Freeman, 1967).

Cognitive Vigilance Although highly sensitive to schizophrenic performance deficit, the conventional CPT is generally insensitive to behavioral changes in normal controls, who tend to perform at ceiling levels. Cornblatt and Keilp (1994) recently developed the CPT identical pairs paradigm (CPT-IP), which is not confounded by ceiling effects. The CPT-IP includes two versions: a number version, in which a target is defined as two consecutive, identical number strings; and a spatial version, in which a target is defined as two consecutive, identical nonsense shapes. Target detection requires successive discrimination, placing considerable demands on working memory, and in that sense, the CPT-IP may be classified as a cognitive vigilance test (Parasuraman and Davies, 1977; See, Howe, Warm, and Dember, 1995).

In their comprehensive literature review, Cornblatt and Keilp (1994) presented fairly strong evidence that the CPT-IP may be a particularly sensitive and specific measure of both schizophrenia and of genetic risk for schizophrenia. They noted that the CPT-IP discriminated schizophrenic patients from affective psychiatric patients, as well as from unaffected offspring of parents with schizophrenia, from unaffected adult siblings of schizophrenic patients, and from persons diagnosed with schizotypal personality disorder, a suspected schizophrenic genotype without an overt schizophrenic phenotype.

Sensory Vigilance On the perceptually degraded CPT, blurred stimuli, such as numbers, are presented rapidly and singly, and subjects must respond to a predesignated target (e.g., 0) that occurs infrequently. Although cognitive in nature, the stimuli (numbers) are perceptually degraded so as to burden early sensory processing (Nuechterlein, Parasuraman, and Qiyuan, 1983). The degraded CPT may thus be viewed more as a test of sensory vigilance than of cognitive vigilance (see See et al., 1995). Nuechterlein (1983) compared various versions of the conventional CPT with the perceptually degraded CPT, and found that only the degraded CPT distinguished children at risk for schizophrenia from other contrast groups, including hyperactive children with attentional deficits. In a longitudinal study, Nuechterlein (1991) found that patients in the early stages of schizophrenia had lower hit rates and reduced sensitivity than did control subjects, and those patients showed a similar performance deficit upon follow-up, independent of clinical status at the time of testing. Schizophrenic deficits on the degraded CPT may therefore reflect an enduring trait that is evident during periods of both acute decompensation and relative remission.

Although patients with schizophrenia show an overall performance decrement, it is not clear that they show a more rapid vigilance decrement on the

CPT. Nestor, Faux, McCarley, Shenton, and Sands (1990) used the perceptually degraded CPT to investigate the nature of vigilance decrement in patients with schizophrenia. Schizophrenic patients were first given training with undegraded stimuli, and then with degraded stimuli. Both groups showed a vigilance (hit rate) decrement over time on task in the degraded condition, with control subjects showing a 5.6% decline and schizophrenic patients showing a 13.6% decline. Signal detection analysis indicated that patients had a more rapid decline in A' (perceptual sensitivity) over time on task than did control subjects. In contrast, both groups showed similar changes in B'' (response bias) over time on task. These results indicate that under experimental conditions that provide training to insure a reasonable level of performance stability (see Parasuraman and Giambra, 1991), patients with schizophrenia may show an impairment in sustained attention, as defined by a more rapid decline in A', independent of B''. This impairment in sustained attention may be evident for only sensory vigilance tasks under conditions designed to tax processing resources. It may also be further exacerbated by neuroleptic withdrawal (Nestor et al., 1991). How that schizophrenic impairment in sustained attention relates to the findings of other CPT studies reviewed previously is unknown.

Summary Schizophrenic patients perform poorly on virtually all tests of sensory and cognitive vigilance, although the precise nature of the impairment is not entirely clear. For example, performance over time on task is generally thought to be a critical dimension of vigilance (e.g., Parasuraman and Davies, 1977). In normal controls, performance generally declines over time for sensory vigilance tasks but remains stable, if not improved over time, for cognitive vigilance tasks (See et al., 1995). For sensory vigilance tasks, sustained attention is most rigorously defined by a decline in perceptual sensitivity independent of response bias (Parasuraman, 1984). With the exception of the studies by Nestor and colleagues, evidence of a more rapid decline in perceptual sensitivity on tests of sensory vigilance has not been reported in patients with schizophrenia.

Selective Attention

Selective attention refers to mechanisms that serve to facilitate processing of task-relevant stimuli or features and to inhibit processing of irrelevant information. These mechanisms may operate on sets of stimuli presented simultaneously, as in a visual search task, or between stimuli across a temporal interval. Abnormalities of selective attention in schizophrenia have been observed for both simultaneously presented and for temporally asynchronous stimuli, within both the nonverbal and semantic domains. Historically, abnormal reaction time to imperative stimuli after a warning period and disruption of semantic processing are robust schizophrenic deficits that have been attributed to a disease-related selective attention deficit (Neale and Oltmanns,

1980). More recent investigations with schizophrenic patients have used information-processing techniques to examine the more basic operations of selective attention, such as search, facilitation, and inhibition. Those studies have provided evidence of problems of attentional selectivity at virtually all levels of information processing—sensory, perceptual, cognitive, and response selection.

Sensory Processing Deficits in selective attention may arise from disturbances of habituation or from reflexive inhibition at a sensory level of processing. In normal individuals, for example, presentation of a tone inhibits the startle response to a loud white noise burst, as measured by reduced latency and amplitude of eye blinks to the white noise burst. This effect, referred to as prepulse inhibition, is apparent as early as 30 ms after prepulse presentation. Using this paradigm, Braff, Sacuzzo, and Geyer (1991) demonstrated that patients with schizophrenia show less startle inhibition after a tone prepulse. Likewise, for sensory gating in which the auditory P50 is attenuated by a prestimulus click, schizophrenic patients show a similar pattern of results. Indeed, schizophrenic patients, and about half their first-degree relatives, show less P50 inhibition to the second click than do control subjects (Adler and Waldo, 1991; Freedman, Adler, Waldo, Pachtman, and Franks, 1983).

Perceptual Selection Span of apprehension studies provide additional evidence of an early-stage problem in selective attention. In the span of apprehension task, subjects view a visual display of elements, usually letters, presented in an imaginary rectangular matrix for about 70 ms. Display size, as measured by the number of letters, is varied, and subjects are instructed either to report as many letters as possible (full report version) or to indicate which one of two target letters, such as a T or an F, is present in each display (forced choice version). Several studies have demonstrated schizophrenic deficits on forced choice tasks (e.g., Asarnow and MacCrimmon 1978; Davidson and Neale, 1974). In contrast, for the full report version, results have suggested no deficit for either adult (Cash, Neale, and Cromwell, 1972) or child (Asarnow and Sherman, 1984) schizophrenic patients. Although not always replicated (Miller, Chapman, Chapman, and Barnett, 1990), this apparent dissociation between forced choice and full report versions suggests that schizophrenic patients may not have difficulties searching a visual display (full report) but have problems identifying targets from a cluttered display in which nontarget letters must be suppressed or inhibited (forced choice).

For backward masking studies, subjects identify a briefly presented visual target, such as the letter O, presented at or just above threshold, followed by (and thus referred to as backward) a noninformational patterned mask of Xs. The time between target and mask, computed as either the interstimulus interval (ISI) or as the stimulus onset asynchrony (SOA), the energy of the mask (luminance), and the spatial location of the mask in reference to the target are all important factors that influence target identification. For a low-energy mask presented in close spatial proximity to but not overlapping with the target, masking effects are greatest for midrange ISIs of 20 to 70 ms, and are negligible for very short ISIs below 20 ms and for longer ISIs above 70 ms (e.g., Braff and Sacuzzo, 1985; Green, Nuechterlein, and Mintz, 1994). Patients with schizophrenia, remitted schizophrenic patients, and schizotypal patients all show backward masking deficits, particularly for midrange ISIs of 20 to 70 ms (e.g., Sacuzzo and Schubert, 1981; Steronko and Woods, 1978). Schizophrenic deficits are limited to backward but not forward masking procedures, which is important because the former is thought to be mediated by central processes and the latter by peripheral processes (e.g., Slaghuis and Bakker, 1995). And finally, schizophrenic masking deficits are not attributable to a disease-related generalized deficit (Brody, Sacuzzo, and Braff, 1980).

Originally thought to reflect either slow transfer of information from iconic memory to short-term memory (e.g., Sacuzzo and Braff, 1981) or a failure to reject or inhibit irrelevant stimuli (Green and Walker, 1984; Knight, 1984), masking deficits in schizophrenia may reflect the integrity of two highly related but anatomically and functionally distinct visual channels, known as transient and sustained neural pathways (Breitmeyer and Ganz, 1976; Hubel and Livingstone, 1987). The transient channel, which is sub-served by retinal A cells and by the magnocellular pathway postretinally, responds to low spatial frequencies, has short neuronal response latencies, and is sensitive to contrast and movement. In contrast, the sustained channel, which is subserved by retinal B cells and the parvocellular pathway, re-sponds to high spatial frequencies, has long neuronal response latencies, and may be involved in form identification. Masking deficits in schizophrenia may reflect a failure of sustained channel activity to inhibit transient channel activity (Elkins, Cromwell, and Asarnow, 1992).

Schizophrenic patients may also show abnormal latent inhibition, a type of inhibitory conditioning that has been demonstrated across species (Lubow and Gewirtz, 1995). In a latent inhibition paradigm, a stimulus of no con-sequence and requiring no response is presented repeatedly, presumably re-sulting in a passive buildup of inhibition. If that stimulus subsequently becomes a conditional stimulus, conditioning is slower in healthy subjects in relation to schizophenic patients.

Faulty inhibition in patients with schizophrenia may impact on a wide range of attentional behaviors. Nestor et al. (1992), for example, used a covert orienting paradigm (Posner, 1980) to examine specific operations of visual selective attention in patients with schizophrenia. In relation to normal controls, schizophrenic patients showed slightly, but not statistically signif-icant, faster RT for validly cued targets—an unexpected finding that may be indicative of hyperattentional facilitation. Even more important, however, schizophrenic patients showed a significant reduction in cost for invalidly cued targets, suggesting that invalid cues did not inhibit RT as they did in normal controls. This latter finding was similar to that reported for both Parkinsonian patients (Clark, Geffen, and Geffen, 1989) and for healthy control subjects who were administered dopaminergic antagonists (Wright, Burns, Geffen, and Geffen, 1990). Nestor et al. (1992) interpreted these data as evidence of a disease-related impairment in inhibitory processes, perhaps modulated by dopaminergic systems, that help maintain a selected focus of attention.

In a similar vein, Beech, Powell, McWilliam, and Claridge (1989) demonstrated reduced negative priming (as measured by RT to targets that were previously distractors) in schizophrenic patients. Elkins and Cromwell (1994) adapted a flanking priming paradigm to examine facilitation and inhibition in patients with schizophrenia and found that flankers incompatible with targets produced significantly less interference for schizophrenic patients than for normal controls and depressed patients. Elkins and Cromwell noted that reduced interference occurred for SOAs of no more than 200 ms. They interpreted such reduced interference as evidence of a disease-related disturbance in fast, automatic attentional inhibition, which they distinguished from the more strategic, controlled inhibition that is thought to underlie reduced negative priming and reduced attentional cost in patients with schizophrenia.

Semantic Processing   Several studies have now demonstrated that patients with schizophrenia show enhanced semantic priming as measured by either RT (Spitzer et al., 1994) or performance accuracy (Kwapil, Hegley, Chapman, and Chapman, 1990). For example, Kwapil et al. developed a methodologically elegant word pair priming task to compare semantic facilitation in schizophrenic patients with bipolar patients and normal controls. Kwapil et al. controlled for overall performance accuracy by perceptually degrading target words and by titrating the level of perceptual degradation of the targets for each subject. In comparison to both bipolar patients and control subjects, schizophrenic patients showed a significant increase in performance accuracy to target words preceded by semantically related primes. These findings indicated enhanced semantic facilitation in patients with schizophrenia, which was not an artifact of poor performance, and which again may reflect faulty inhibition (see Maher, 1983).

Semantic activation may be indexed by an event-related potential (ERP) measure, the N400 component, which is thought to reflect semantic expectancy, as operationalized in terms of cloze probability (Kutas and Hillyard, 1984). In healthy subjects, N400 is influenced by sentence context (e.g., Kutas, Van Petten, and Besson, 1988) and by the degree of association among words (e.g., Bentin, McCarthy, and Wood, 1985) or their conceptual representations (Nigam, Hoffman, and Simmons, 1992). Relatively large negative potentials are elicited for semantically unrelated word pairs (e.g., "doctor" and "table"), semantically incongruent sentences (e.g., "Every Sunday people pray in their

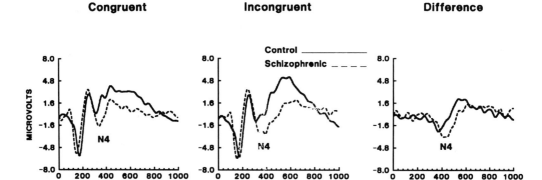

Figure 23.1 Grand averaged ERPs to congruent and incongruent words from a group of patients with schizophrenia (dotted line) and a group of control subjects (solid line). Note the increased negative potential (N400) in the schizophrenic group in both congruent and incongruent conditions.

local nest"), and for words at the beginning of a sentence in comparison to words at the end of a sentence. Word pair priming studies have indicated that in relation to normal control subjects, schizophrenic patients show longer N400 latency but do not differ in N400 amplitude (Grillon, Ameli, and Glazer, 1991; Koyama et al., 1991). However, for studies using sentences instead of word pairs, recent evidence (Nestor et al., 1997; Niznikiewicz et al., 1997) has demonstrated that schizophrenic patients show both prolonged latency and increased negativity regardless of sentence type (sensible versus nonsensible) or modality (auditory versus visual). Nestor et al. (1997) suggested that in patients with schizophrenia, semantic activation may be more diffuse and less constrained, as reflected by enhanced N400 negativity, which in turn results in reduced speed of activation, as reflected by prolonged N400 latency (figure 23.1).

ERP Measures of Selective Attention In addition to studies of the N400 component associated with semantic processing, ERPs elicited during tonal discrimination tasks have been used to study both early and last stages of selectivity. For these tasks, subjects typically count or respond to low-probability target tones appearing in a sequence of frequent distractor tones. ERP measures provide a tool to investigate the time course of selective attention operations that occur prior to, or in the absence of, a behavioral response. These measures are frequently abnormal in patients with schizophrenia, are usually evident as amplitude reduction in attentionally modulated ERP components, and affect both early (100–200 ms) and late (200–600 ms) components to target and nontarget tones (O'Donnell et al., 1994) (figure 23.2). Most consistently, there are amplitude reductions in the N200 and P300 components elicited by low-probability target tones, which persist across changes in medication and clinical state (Ford et al., 1994).

FREQUENT   TARGET

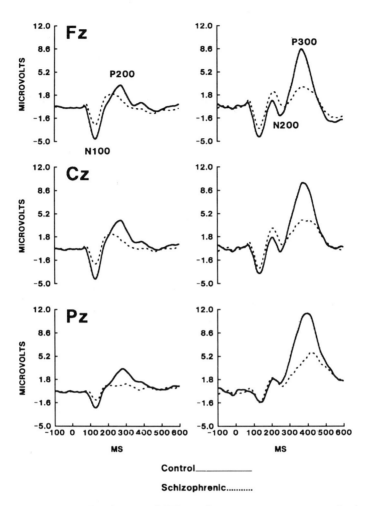

Figure 23.2 Grand averaged ERPs to frequent, nontarget tones and infrequent, nontarget tones recorded from a group of patients with schizophrenia (dotted line) and a group of control subjects (solid line). Note the marked reduction in amplitude of the positive P300 component and the immediately preceding negative deflection, N200.

Because P300 and the immediately preceding N200 component are thought to index detection and categorization of task-relevant stimuli and associated working memory operations, these findings suggest a severe disturbance of the physiological substrates of selective attention in schizophrenia. These physiological substrates may include the left posterior superior temporal gyrus for the P300 component, and both superior temporal gyrus and medial temporal structures for N200 (O'Donnell et al., 1993).

These findings from nonlinguistic paradigms differ from N400 abnormalities in semantic paradigms, in that they suggest reduced activation to stimuli

Nestor & O'Donnell: Schizophrenia

but normal processing speed, whereas N400 amplitude may be enhanced in schizophrenia and processing speed may be slowed. This dissociation suggests that the processing of linguistic stimuli may be associated with failure of inhibitory processes driven by semantic context or associations, whereas processing of nonlinguistic, auditory stimuli is associated with a lack of facilitation associated with probability-based expectancies. Despite these differences, both P300 and N400 abnormalities appear to index failure to utilize preceding context, either semantic or probabilistic, to modulate stimulus processing.

Summary   Schizophrenia may very well be associated with a fundamental problem with selectivity that operates at virtually all levels of information processing, from basic sensory to higher-order semantic processing. The foregoing studies have provided fairly strong evidence that the selective deficit may reflect faulty inhibition and, to a lesser extent, abnormal facilitation. Indeed, span of apprehension studies have suggested relatively intact visual search but clearly impaired inhibitory processes. Similarly, schizophrenic deficits of prepulse inhibition may reflect an early-stage, automatic failure of inhibitory processes. Reduced negative priming and reduced attentional cost in schizophrenic patients may also reflect faulty inhibition. Finally, prolonged latency and enhanced negativity of N400 point to semantic overactivation in schizophrenia, which may reflect a failure to use contextual constraints.

DISCUSSION: GAIN DYSREGULATION IN SCHIZOPHRENIA

The foregoing studies have provided consistent evidence of a schizophrenic disturbance in operations involved in sustained and selective attention. Although the relationship between sustained and selective abnormalities has yet to be established in schizophrenia, it seems likely that both are intimately related to the neural disturbance that is central to the disease. Both sustained and selective attention involve the suppression of irrelevant stimuli. In schizophrenia, these deficits may reflect a specific weakening of attentional inhibitory processes that operate at virtually all levels of the central nervous system from sensory to higher-order attentional processing. For example, within approximately 30 ms, a masking stimulus significantly interferes with perceptual processing in patients with schizophrenia. Such effects probably operate at a preconscious, automatic level before higher-order, controlled, strategic, and voluntary processes are engaged, and well before other extraneous variables, such as motivation or cooperation, are likely to influence performance. Moreover, the pervasiveness of these effects suggests that the disturbance probably affects many regions of the brain, although in particular patients specific systems may be more disrupted than others. For example, auditory hallucinations and the semantic aspects of thought disorder may be specifically related to disturbance of medial temporal and superior temporal gyrus circuits (Shenton et al., 1992; Nestor et al., 1993). We think it is unlikely, however, that the spectrum of attentional deficits in schizophrenia can be attributed to a local disruption of one particular region or lobe of the brain.

How, then, might these abnormalities be formally described? Attention is often described in terms of a modulatory or gain function that increases the strength of selected sensory input and decreases the strength of unselected sensory input. Gain may be modulated by various neurotransmitters, such as dopamine, serotonin, or glutamate. Low gain produces excessive shifts of attention, reduced sustained attention, and diffuse spread of activation within various modules, such as semantic or associative memory. By contrast, high gain biases responses to the most dominant, prepotent stimuli, with attention rigidly focused and difficult to shift. Consider, for example, the idea that schizophrenia is associated with gain dysregulation. There is now fairly strong evidence that auditory and visual selective attention involves an early gain mechanism that modulates processing within approximately 100 ms poststimulus (e.g., Hillyard, Mangun, Woldorff, and Luck, 1995). For visual stimuli, these modulatory effects are seen in extrastriate but not in primary cortical areas (Colby, 1991; Corbetta, Miezin, Dobmeyer, Shulman, and Petersen, 1991; Haxby et al., 1991); for auditory stimuli, these effects are located in temporal but not in brainstem areas (e.g., Hillyard et al., 1995). In schizophrenia, information-processing disturbances occur early, as demonstrated by masking and span of apprehension studies. Electrical recordings of brain activity in patients with schizophrenia also reveal reduced amplitude in early sensory components, such as the auditory P50 and N100. Thus, within that framework, these behavioral and neurophysiological abnormalities may be understood in terms of a faulty gain mechanism such that early stimulus representations are degraded in schizophrenia.

A gain abnormality also accounts for some anomalous findings, such as those related to latent inhibition or negative priming, in which patients arguably outperform normals subjects. A low gain may reduce the inhibitory effects of recently ignored stimuli. Under those conditions, a recently ignored stimulus will be processed as efficiently as a novel stimulus, as is the case in both negative priming and latent inhibition paradigms. By contrast, in healthy subjects, an early gain mechanism suppresses responses to an ignored stimulus, and the inhibitory effects are more powerful and long-lasting so that responses will be slower when the previously ignored stimulus becomes salient. One advantage of this account is that it does not require the often troubling assumption of a so-called homunculus, or a central executive, typically located in the frontal lobe, which is thought to control attention. Rather, gain influences are a by-product of computations performed by populations of selected neurons, particularly by those of the associative cortices that have been shown to have specific attentional effects across a variety of activation paradigms (e.g., Corbetta et al., 1990; Spitzer, Desimone, and Moran, 1988; Moran and Desimone, 1985). In schizophrenia, one consequence of gain dysregulation may be reduced intensity of neuronal response to attended stimuli.

Grunze, Rainne, Hasselmo, Barkai, and Hearn, (1996) have recently proposed a biophysical model of how a gain or neuromodulation dysfunction in schizophrenia may be understood in reference to intrinsic properties of specific neuronal circuits. Based on their studies of local hippocampal circuits in region CA1 of a rat, Grunze and colleagues have suggested that schizophrenia may be associated with a disturbance in local inhibitory circuits and the inhibitory neurotransmitter, GABA. In their model, activation of projection neurons results in excitation of GABAergic inhibitory interneurons, which in turn inhibit other projection neurons within the circuit. Activation of those inhibitory circuits appears to modulate NMDA receptors, and produces long term potentiation, suggesting that this feedback inhibitory system may be involved in associative learning. Biophysical simulations using this circuit have suggested that partial blockade of the recurrent inhibitory circuit with NMDA antagonists disrupts the ability of the circuit to recognize patterns with overlapping elements. This was due to a failure of recurrent inhibition to prevent aberrant spread of activation during associative learning. Grunze et al. suggested that some of the hallmark clinical symptoms of schizophrenia, most notably loose associations, may originate from a breakdown in neuronal inhibition (see figure 23.3).

Cohen and Servan-Schreiber (1992) proposed a similar formal computational model of schizophrenic cognitive dysfunction, but their model does not attempt to simulate actual neural circuits. In this model, a dopaminergic-mediated gain dysregulation is thought to account for at least a subset of the neuropsychological abnormalities of schizophrenia. These investigators have suggested that schizophrenic disturbances on CPT, Stroop, and lexical disambiguation tasks may be related to a single disturbance in the use and maintenance of contextual information. This context module is dependent upon a mesocortical and prefrontal system, modulated by dopamine. They propose that dopaminergic abnormality of schizophrenia reduces the gain function of processing units within the module, which causes increased noise in the internal representation of context. Because higher levels of noise cause rapid degradation of contextual representation, the model suggests that the failures of contextual modulation of performance observed on both behavioral and physiological measures will become more severe at greater temporal intervals (Braver, Cohen, and Servan-Schreiber, in press).

Although the specific neural structures differ in these models and may very well prove to be incorrect, the models of both Cohen and Servan-Schreiber and Grunze et al. provide testable behavioral predictions regarding normal and schizophrenic performance. In many ways, both models may be viewed as complementary, representing distinct levels of analysis from cellular to complex neural systems. Yet at the same time, the models differ on many dimensions, particularly with regard to the neuropharmacological basis of gain dysregulation in schizophrenia. Behavioral predictions may also differ. For example, on tasks involving detection of targets preceded by cues, the Cohen and Servan-Schreiber model predicts a decline in schizophrenic performance with increasing interstimulus intervals. By contrast, the model by Grunze and colleagues provides a cellular basis for fast-acting, inhibitory mechanisms that are not dependent upon voluntary, conscious attention. In schizophrenia, faulty inhibitory mechanisms may produce disturbances in the very early stages of processing, and those effects do not necessarily worsen with increasing time intervals. Moreover, patients may have no awareness of the extent to which the product of the faulty operations is degraded or compromised. In that sense, some of their deficits may be described as unconscious (see Kihlstrom, 1987). This may contribute to the failure of many patients to recognize that their perceptions and experiences are psychotic.

Attentional abnormalities of schizophrenia may be due to a disturbance in an early gain mechanism arising from a circuitry disturbance related to GABAergic inhibitory interneurons. Those neural circuits are widely distributed but are highly represented in limbic regions, an area long thought to play an important role in the pathogenesis of schizophrenia. In this model, schizophrenic attentional abnormalities may not necessarily be dependent on a complex system, but may be related to intrinsic properties of neuronal circuits. In addition, the behavioral manifestations of such a disturbance would vary with the functional properties of different complex systems and would therefore be consistent with the heterogeneity of behavioral disturbances observed in the disease. Finally, the dependence of recurrent inhibition of NMDA receptors is particularly interesting in the context of schizophrenia, given that phencyclidine, an NMDA antagonist, can induce psychotic symptoms in humans.

CONCLUSIONS

Gain dysregulation due to faulty inhibition would clearly have profound effects on information processing in patients with schizophrenia, as suggested by the consequences of dampening of recurrent inhibition during associative learning of overlapping (or related) patterns in the Grunze et al. (1996) cellular model, and by the failure of contextual inhibition on dominant responses in the more abstract model of Cohen and Servan-Schreiber (1992). Although these effects may be diffuse and widespread, there may be some distinctive characteristics of schizophrenic gain dysregulation that would be open to empirical falsification. One fundamental consequence of such dysregulation may be evident in how predictive rules are developed and how expectancies are generated. Predictability and expectancies may emerge from either top-down or bottom-up processes. The bottom-up processes may be of particular interest in that they may be directly related to regularities in the firing of selected neuronal populations. In this framework, statistical properties governing the activation functions of these neuronal populations are altered in

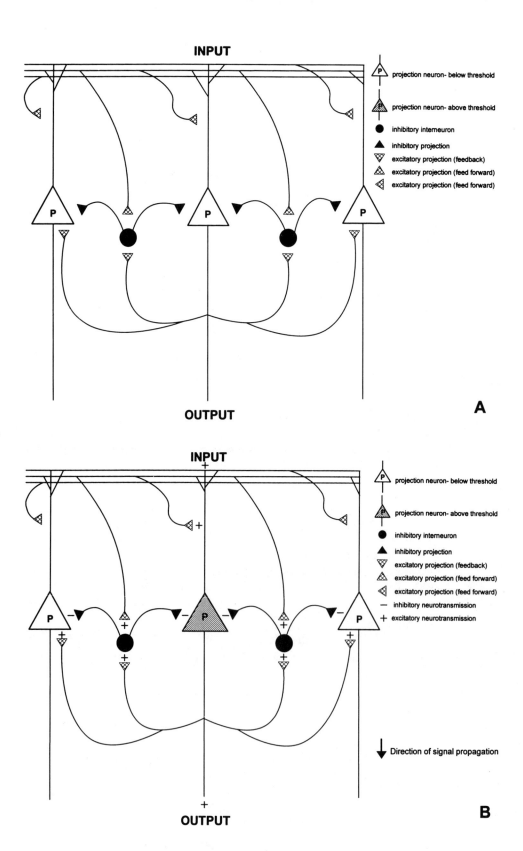

Development and Pathologies of Attention

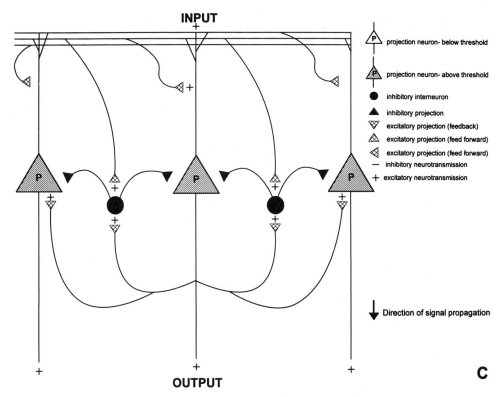

Figure 23.3 (A) A local circuit within the CA1 region of the rat hippocampus, comprising three projection neurons (large triangles) and two inhibitory interneurons. In this figure, all neurons are in resting state, and there is no input from the feedforward excitatory inputs. In addition to efferent projections beyond the local circuit, the projection neurons have excitatory projections to each other, and to the inhibitory interneurons. (B) The effect of excitatory neurotransmission on the central projection neuron in the presence of long term inhibition via the inhibitory interneurons. Plus signs indicate excitatory synapses, and minus signs indicate inhibitory synapses. The central projection neuron depolarizes, which results in feedback excitation of adjacent projection neurons, as well as excitation of both inhibitory interneurons. The interneurons, in turn, inhibit further depolarization of the adjacent projection neurons, and quickly restore the depolarized central neuron to resting state. Consequently, the output of the local circuit preserves the pattern of stimulation applied through the input projections. (C) The effect of excitatory neurotransmission on the central projection neuron in the absence of effective recurrent inhibition. When the central projection neuron fires, it also excites the adjacent projection neurons in the local circuit. Because the interneurons do not inhibit these adjacent neurons, the excitation results in depolarization of these projection neurons. This spread of activation causes input to a single projection neuron to spread across the circuit, resulting in output from multiple neurons and loss of the original input pattern.

schizophrenia. The hypothesized gain dysregulation via faulty inhibition would have a dramatic effect on those tasks, however elemental, that involve an implicit or explicit rule of contingency whereby the occurrence of one stimulus predicts the occurrence of another stimulus, as in classical conditioning (e.g., Abrams and Kandel, 1988), or that involve the modulation of a response based on preceding context, as in prepulse inhibition or negative priming.

REFERENCES

Abrams, T. W. and Kandel, E. R. (1988) Is contiguity detection in classical conditioning a system or a cellular property? Learning in *Aplysia* suggests a possible molecular site. *Trends Neurosci.* 4: 128–135.

Adler, L. E. and Waldo, M. C. (1991) Counterpoint: Sensory gating-hippocampal model of schizophrenia. *Schizophr. Bull.* 17: 19–24.

Andreasen, N. C., Arndt, S., Swayze, V., Cizadlo, T., Flaum, M., O'Leary, D., Ehrhardt, J. C., and Yuh, W. T. C. (1994) Thalamic abnormalities in schizophrenia visualized through magnetic resonance image averaging. *Science* 266: 294–298.

Arnold, S. E., Hyman, B. T., Van Hoesen, G. W., and Damasio, A. R. (1991) Some cytoarchitectural abnormalities of the entorhinal cortex in schizophrenia. *Arch. Gen. Psychiatry* 48: 625–632.

Asarnow, R. F. and MacCrimmon, D. J. (1978) Residual performance deficit in clinically remitted schizophrenics: A marker of schizophrenia? *J. Abnorm. Psychol.* 87: 597–608.

Asarnow, R. F. and Sherman, T. (1984) Studies of visual information processing in schizophrenic children. *Child Dev.* 55: 249–261.

Barta, P. E., Pearlson, G. D., Powers, R. E., Menon, R., Richards, S., and Tune, L. E. (1990) Auditory hallucinations and smaller superior temporal gyral volume in schizophrenia. *Am. J. Psychiatry* 147: 1457–1462.

Beech, A., Powell, T., McWilliam, J., and Claridge, G. (1989) Evidence of reduced "cognitive inhibition" in schizophrenia. *Br. J. Clin. Psychol.* 28: 109–117.

Benes, F. M. and Bird, E. D. (1987) An analysis of the arrangement of neurons in the cingulate cortex of schizophrenic patients. *Arch. Gen. Psychiatry* 44: 608–616.

Bentin, S., McCarthy, G., and Wood, C. C. (1985) Event-related potentials associated with semantic priming. *Electroencephalogr. Clin. Neurophysiol.* 60: 343–355.

Bleuler, T. (1950) *Dementia Praecox of the Group of Schizophrenias* (trans.). New York: International Universities Press. (Original work published in 1911.)

Braff, D. L. and Sacuzzo, D. P. (1985) The time course of information processing deficits in schizophrenia. *Am. J. Psychiatry* 142: 170.

Braff, D. L., Sacuzzo, D. P., and Geyer, M. A. (1991) Information processing dysfunctions in schizophrenia: Studies of visual backward masking, sensorimotor gating, and habituation. In *Handbook of Schizophrenia: Neuropsychology, Psychophysiology, and Information Processing*, edited by R. H. Steinhauer, J. H. Grunzelier, and J. Zubin, pp. 303–334. New York: Plenum Press.

Braver, T. S., Cohen J. D., and Servan-Schreiber, D. (in press) A computational model of prefrontal cortex function. In *Advances in Neural Information Processing Systems* (Vol. 7) edited by D. S. Touretzky, G. Tesauro, and T. U. Leen. Cambridge, MA: MIT Press.

Breitmeyer, B. and Ganz, L. (1976) Implications of sustained and transient channels for theories of visual pattern masking, saccadic suppression, and information processing. *Psychol. Rev.* 83: 1–27.

Brody, D., Sacuzzo, D. P., and Braff, D. L. (1980) Information processing for masked and unmasked stimuli in schizophrenia and old age. *J. Abnorm. Psychol.* 89: 617.

Cash, T. F., Neale, J. M., and Cromwell. R. L. (1972) Span of apprehension in acute schizophrenics: A full report technique. *J. Abnorm. Psychol.* 79: 322–326.

Clark, C. R., Geffen. G. M., and Geffen, L. B. (1989) Catecholamines and covert orientation of attention in humans. *Neuropsychologia* 27: 131–139.

Cohen, J. D. and Servan-Schreiber, D. (1992) Context, cortex, and dopamine: A connectionist approach to behavior and biology in schizophrenia. *Psychol. Rev.* 99: 45–77.

Colby, C. L. (1991) The neuroanatomy and neurophysiology of attention. *J. Child Neurol.* 6: S90–S118.

Corbetta, M., Miezin, F. M., Dobmeyer, S., Shulman, G. L., and Petersen, S. E. (1990) Attentional modulation of neural processing of shape, color, and velocity in humans. *Science* 248: 1556–1559.

Corbetta, M., Miezin, F. M., Dobmeyer, S., Shulman G. L., and Petersen, S. E. (1991) Selective and divided attention during visual discrimination of shape, color, and speed: functional anatomy by positron emission tomography. *J. Neurosci.* 11: 2383–2402.

Cornblatt, B. A. and Keilp, J. G. (1994) Impaired attention, genetics, and the pathophysiology of schizophrenia. *Schizophr. Bull.* 20: 31–46.

Davidson, G. S. and Neale, J. M. (1974) Effects of signal-noise similarity on information processing of schizophrenics. *J. Abnorm. Psychol.* 83: 683–686.

Davis, K. L., Fiori, M., Davis, B. M., Mohs, R. C., Horvath, T. B., and Davidson, M. (1986) Dopaminergic disregulation in schizophrenia: A target for new drugs. *Drug Dev. Res.* 9: 71–83.

Elkins, I. J. and Cromwell, R. L. (1994) Priming effects in schizophrenia: Associative interference and facilitation as a function of visual context. *J. Abnorm. Psychol.* 103: 791–800.

Elkins, I. J., Cromwell, R. L., and Asarnow, R. F. (1992) Span of apprehension in schizophrenic patients as a function of distractor masking and laterality. *J. Abnorm. Psychol.* 101: 53–60.

Farde, L., Wiesel, F. A., Stone-Elander, S. S., Halldin, C., Nordstrom, A. L., Hall, H., and Sedvall, G. (1990) D2 dopamine receptors in neuroleptic naive schizophrenic patients. *Arch. Gen. Psychiatry* 47: 213–219.

Ford, J. M., White, P. M., Csernansky, J. G., Faustman, W. O., Roth, W. T., and Pfefferbaum, A. (1994) ERPs in schizophrenia: Effects of antipsychotic medication. *Biol. Psychiatry* 36: 153–170.

Frecska, E., Perenyl, A., Bagdy, G., and Reval, K. (1985) CSF dopamine turnover and positive schizophrenic symptoms after withdrawl of long-term neuroleptic treatment. *Psychiatr. Res.* 16: 221–226.

Freedman, R., Adler, L. E., Waldo, M. C., Pachtman, E., and Franks, R. D. (1983) Neurophysiological evidence for a deficit in inhibitory pathways in schizophrenia: Comparison of medicated and drug-free patients. *Biol. Psychiatry* 18: 537.

Green M. F., Nuechterlein, K. H., and Mintz, J. (1994) Backward masking in schizophrenia and mania: I. Specifying a mechanism. *Arch. Gen. Psychiatry* 51: 939–944.

Green, M. and Walker, E. (1984) Susceptibility to backward masking in schizophrenic patients with positive versus negative symptoms. *Am. J. Psychiatry* 141: 1273.

Grillon, C., Ameli, R., and Glazer, W. (1991) N400 and semantic categorization in schizophrenia. *Biol. Psychiatry* 29: 467–480.

Grunze, H. C. R., Rainnie, D. G., Hasselmo, M. E., Barkai, E., Hearn, E. F., McCarley, R. W., and Greene, R. W. (1996) NMDA-dependent modulation of CA1 local circuit inhibition. *J. Neurosci.* 16: 2034–2043.

Haxby, J. V., Grady, C. L., Horwitz, B., Ungerleider, L. G., Mishkin, M., Carson, R. E., Herscovitch, P., Schapiro, M. B., and Rappoport, S. I. (1991) Dissociation of object and spatial visual processing pathways in human extrastriate cortex. *Proc. Natl. Acad. Sci. USA* 88: 1621–1625.

Hillyard, S. A., Mangun, G. R., Woldorff, M. G., and Luck, S. J. (1995) Neural systems mediating selective attention. In *The Cognitive Neurosciences*, edited by M. S. Gazzaniga, pp. 665–681. Cambridge, MA: MIT Press.

Hubel, D. H. and Livingstone, M. S. (1987) Segregation of form, color, and stereopsis in primate area 18. *J. Neurosci.* 7: 3378–3415.

Kihlstrom, J. F. (1987) The cognitive unconscious. *Science* 237: 1445–1452.

Knight, R. A. (1984) Converging models of cognitive deficit in schizophrenia. In *Theories of Schizophrenia and Psychosis*, edited by W. Spaulding, and J. K. Cole. pp. 93–156. Lincoln, Nebraska: University of Nebraska Press.

Kornetsky, C. and Mirsky, A. F. (1966) On certain psychopharmacological and physiological differences between schizophrenics and normal persons. *Psychopharmacologia* 8: 309–318.

Kovelman, J. A. and Scheibel, A. B. (1984) A neurohistological correlate of schizophrenia. *Biol. Psychiatry* 19: 1601–1621.

Koyama, S., Nageishi, Y., Shimokochi, M., Hokama, H., Miyazato, Y., Miyatani, M., and Ogura, C. (1991) The N400 component of event-related potentials in schizophrenic patients: A preliminary study. *Electroencephalogr. Clin. Neurophysiol.* 78: 124–132.

Kraepelin, E. (1971) *Dementia Praecox* (translated by E. Barclay and S. Barclay) New York: Churchill Livingstone. (Original work published in 1919.)

Kutas, M. and Hillyard, S. A. (1984) Brain potentials during reading reflect word expectancy and semantic association. *Nature* 307: 161–163.

Kutas, M., Van Petten, C., and Besson, M. (1988) Event-related potential asymmetries during the reading of sentences. *Electroencephalogr. Clin. Neurophysiol.* 69: 218–233.

Kwapil, T. R., Hegley, D. G., Chapman, L. J., and Chapman, J. P. (1990) Facilitation of word recognition by semantic priming in schizophrenia. *J. Abnorm. Psychol.* 99: 215–221.

Lubow, R. E. and Gewirtz, J. C. (1995) Latent inhibition in humans: Data, theory, and implications for schizophrenia. *Psychol. Bull.* 117: 87–103.

Maher, B. A. (1983) A tentative theory of schizophrenic utterance. In *Progress in Experimental Personality Research: Vol 12. Psychopathology*, edited by B. A. Mather and W. B. Maher, pp. 1–52. New York: Academic Press.

Martinot, J. L., Péron-Magnan, P., Huret, J. D., Mazoyer, B., Baron, J. C., Boulenger, J. P., Loc'h, C., Mazière, B., Caillard, V., and Loo, H. (1990) Striatal D*2 dopaminergic receptors assessed with positron emission tomography and [76Br] bromospiperone in untreated schizophrenic patients. *Am. J. Psychiatry* 147: 44–50.

Miller, M. B., Chapman, L. J., Chapman, J. P., and Barnett, E. M. (1990) Schizophrenic deficit span of apprehension. *J. Abnorm. Psychol.* 99: 313–316.

Moran, J. and Desimone, R. (1985) Selective attention gates visual processing in the extrastriate cortex. *Science* 229: 782–784.

Neale, J. M. and Oltmanns, T. F. (1980) *Schizophrenia*. New York: Wiley.

Nestor, P. G., Faux, S. F., McCarley, R. W., Penhune, V., Shenton, M. E., and Pollak, S. (1992) Attentional cues in chronic schizophrenia: Abnormal disengagement of attention. *J. Abnorm. Psychol.* 101: 682–689.

Nestor, P. G., Faux, S. F., McCarley, R. W., Sands, S. F., Horvath, T. B., and Peterson, A. (1991) Neuroleptics improve sustained attention in schizophrenia: A study using signal detection theory. *Neuropsychopharmacology* 4: 145–149.

Nestor, P. G., Faux, S. F., McCarley, R. W., Shenton, M. E., and Sands, S. F. (1990) Measurement of visual sustained attention in schizophrenia using signal detection analysis and a newly developed computerized CPT task. *Schizophr. Res.* 3: 329–332.

Nestor, P. G., Kimble, M. O., O'Donnell, B. F., Smith, L., Niznikiewicz, M., Shenton, M. E., and McCarley, R. W. (1997) A neurophysiological study of semantic processing in schizophrenia. *Am. J. Psychiatry* 154: 640–646.

Nestor, P. G., Shenton, M. E., McCarley, R. W., Haimson, J., Smith, R. S., O'Donnell, B. F., Kimble, M., Kikinis, R., and Jolesz, F. A. (1993) Neuropsychological correlates of MRI temporal lobe abnormalities in schizophrenia. *Am. J. Psychiatry* 150: 1849–1855.

Nigam, A., Hoffman, J. E., and Simmons, R. F. (1992) N400 to semantically anomalous pictures and words. *J. Cognitive Neurosci.* 4: 15–22.

Niznikiewicz, M. A., O'Donnell, B. F., Nestor, P. G., Smith, L., Law, S., Karapelou, M., Shenton, M. E., and McCarley, R. W. (1997) ERP assessment of visual and auditory language processing in schizophrenia. *J. Abnorm. Psychol.* 106: 85–94.

Nuechterlein, K. H. (1983) Signal detection in vigilance tasks and behavioral attributes among offspring of schizophrenic mothers and among hyperactive children. *J. Abnorm. Psychol.* 92: 4–28.

Nuechterlein, K. H. (1991) Vigilance in schizophrenia and related disorders. In *Handbook of Schizophrenia: Vol. 5. Neuropsychology, Psychophysiology, and Information Processing*, edited by S. R., Steinhauer, J. H. Gruzelier, and J. Zubin. Amsterdam: Elsevier.

Nuechterlein, K. H., Parasuraman, R., and Qiyuan, J. (1983) Visual sustained attention: Image degradation produces rapid sensitivity decrements over time. *Science* 220: 327–329.

O'Donnell, B. F., Hokama, H., McCarley, R. W., Smith, R. S., Salisbury, D. F., Mondrow, E., Nestor, P. G., and Shenton, M. E. (1994) Auditory ERPs to nontarget stimuli in schizophrenia: Relationship to probability, task-demands, and target ERPs. *Int. J. Psychophysiol.* 17: 219–231.

O'Donnell, B. F., Shenton, M. E., McCarley, R. W., Faux, S. F., Smith, R. S., Salisbury, D. F., Nestor, P. G., Pollak, S. D., Kikinis, R., and Jolesz, F. A. (1993) The auditory N2 component in schizophrenia: Relationship to MRI temporal lobe grey matter and to other ERP abnormalities. *Biol. Psychiatry* 34: 26–40.

Orzack, M. H. and Kornetsky, C. (1966) Attention dysfunction in chronic schizophrenia. *Arch. Gen. Psychiatry* 14: 323–3

Orzack, M. H., Kornetsky, C., and Freeman, H. (1967) The effects of daily carphenazine on attention in the schizophrenic patient. *Psychopharmacologia* 11: 31–38.

Parasuraman, R. (1984) Sustained attention in detection and discrimination. In *Varieties of Attention*, edited by R. Parasuraman and D. R. Davies, pp. 243–267. Orlando, FL: Academic Press.

Parasuraman, R. and Davies, D. R. (1977) A taxonomic analysis of vigilance. In *Vigilance: Theory, Operational Performance, and Physiological Correlates*, edited by R. R. Mackie, pp. 559–574. New York: Plenum Press.

Parasuraman, R. and Giambra, L. (1991) Skill development in vigilance: Effects of event rate and age. *Psychol. Aging* 6: 155–169.

Posner, M. I. (1980) Orienting of attention. *Q. J. Exp. Psychol.* 32: 3–25.

Rosvold, H. E., Mirsky, A., Sarason, I., Bransome, E. D., Jr., and Beck, L. H. (1956) A continuous performance test of brain damage. *J. Consult. Psychol.* 20: 343–350.

Sacuzzo, D. P. and Braff, D. L. (1981) Early information processing deficits in schizophrenia: New findings using schizophrenic subgroups and manic controls. *Arch. Gen. Psychiatry* 38: 175.

Sacuzzo, D. P. and Schubert, D. L. (1981) Backward masking as a measure of slow processing in schizophrenic spectrum disorders. *J. Abnorm. Psychol.* 90: 305.

Sarter, M. (1991) Dopamine-GABA-cholinergic interactions and negative schizophrenic symptomatology. *Behav. Brain Sci.* 14: 46–47.

See, J. E., Howe, S. R., Warm, J. S., and Dember, W. N. (1995) Meta-analysis of the sensitivity decrement in vigilance. *Psychol. Bull.* 117: 230–249.

Shenton, M. E., Kikinis, R., Jolesz, F. A., Pollack, S. D,. LeMay, M., Wible, C. G., Hokama, H., Martin, J., Metcalf, D., Coleman, M., and McCarley, R. W. (1992) Abnormalities of the left temporal lobe and thought disorder in schizophrenia: A quantitative magnetic resonance imaging study. *N. England J. Med.* 327: 604–612.

Shepherd, G. M. (1995) Toward a molecular basis for sensory perception. In *The Cognitive Neurosciences*, edited by M. S. Gazzaniga. Cambridge, MA: MIT Press.

Slaghuis, W. L. and Bakker, V. J. (1995) Forward and backward visual masking of contour by light in positive- and negative-symptom schizophrenia. *J. Abnorm. Psychol.* 104: 41–54.

Spitzer, H., Desimone, R., and Moran, J. (1988) Increased attention enhances both behavioral and neuronal performance. *Science* 240: 338–340.

Spitzer, M., Weisker, I., Winter, M., Maier, S., Hermle. L., and Maher, B. (1994) Semantic and phonological priming in schizophrenia. *J. Abnorm. Psychol.* 103: 485–493.

Steronko, R. J. and Woods, D. J. (1978) Impairment in early stages of visual information processing in nonpsychotic schizotypic individuals. *J. Abnorm. Psychol.* 87: 481.

Tandon, R. and Greden, J. F. (1989) Cholinergic overactivity and negative schizophrenic symptoms. A model of cholinergic/dopaminergic interactions in schizophrenia. *Arch. Gen. Psychiatry* 46: 745–753.

Wohlberg, G. W. and Kornetsky, C. (1973) Sustained attention in remitted schizophrenics. *Arch. Gen. Psychiatry* 28: 533–537.

Wright, M. J., Burns, R. J., Geffen, G. M., and Geffen, L. B. (1990) Covert orientation of visual orientation in Parkinson's disease: An impairment in the maintenance of attention. *Neuropsychologia* 28: 151–159.

Contributors

Edward Awh
Department of Psychology
University of Michigan
Ann Arbor, Michigan

Gordon C. Baylis
Department of Psychology
University of South Carolina
Columbia, South Carolina

Jochen Braun
Division of Biology
California Institute of Technology
Pasadena, California

Dennis Cantwell
Center for the Biological Study of
ADHD
University of California
Irvine, California

Vincent P. Clark
Laboratory of Brain and Cognition
National Institute of Mental Health
Bethesda, Maryland

Susan M. Courtney
Laboratory of Brain and Cognition
National Institute of Mental Health
Bethesda, Maryland

Francis Crinella
Center for the Biological Study of
ADHD
University of California
Irvine, California

Maurizio Corbetta
Department of Neurology
Washington University School of
Medicine
St. Louis, Missouri

Matthew C. Davidson
Department of Psychology
University of Oregon
Eugene, Oregon

Jon Driver
Department of Psychology
University College London
London, United Kingdom

Jane Emerson
Center for the Biological Study of
ADHD
University of California
Irvine, California

Pauline Filipek
Center for the Biological Study of
ADHD
University of California
Irvine, California

Ira Fischler
Department of Psychology
University of Florida
Gainesville, Florida

Gregory J. DiGirolamo
Department of Psychology
University of Oregon
Eugene, Oregon

Massimo Girelli
Department of Psychology
University of Verona
Verona, Italy

Pamela M. Greenwood
Cognitive Science Laboratory
The Catholic University of America
Washington, DC

James V. Haxby
Laboratory of Brain and Cognition
National Institute of Mental Health
Bethesda, Maryland

Mark H. Johnson
MRC Cognitive Development Unit
London, United Kingdom

John Jonides
Department of Psychology
University of Michigan
Ann Arbor, Michigan

Julian S. Joseph
Department of Psychology
University of Nevada
Reno, Nevada

Robert T. Knight
Neurology Service
VA Medical Center
Martinez, California

Christof Koch
Division of Biology
California Institute of Technology
Pasadena, California

Steven J. Luck
Department of Psychology
University of Iowa
Iowa City, Iowa

Richard T. Marrocco
Department of Psychology
University of Oregon
Eugene, Oregon

Brad C. Motter
Research Service
Medical Center
Syracuse, New York

Ken Nakayama
Department of Psychology
Harvard University
Cambridge, Massachusetts

Orhan Nalcioglu
Center for the Biological Study of
ADHD
University of California
Irvine, California

Paul G. Nestor
Department of Psychology
University of Massachusetts
Boston, Massachusetts

Ernst Niebur
Department of Neuroscience
The Johns Hopkins University
Baltimore, Maryland

Brian F. O'Donnell
Department of Psychology
Harvard Medical School
Boston, Massachusetts

Raja Parasuraman
Department of Psychology
The Catholic University of America
Washington, DC

Michael I. Posner
Department of Psychology
University of Oregon
Eugene, Oregon

Robert D. Rafal
Neurology Service
VA Medical Center
Martinez, California

Trevor W. Robbins
Department of Experimental
Psychology
University of Cambridge
Cambridge, United Kingdom

Lynn C. Robertson
Neurology Service
VA Medical Center
Martinez, California

Judi E. See
Logicon Technical Services
Dayton, Ohio

James Swanson
Center for the Biological Study of
ADHD
University of California
Irvine, California

Diane Swick
Neurology Service
VA Medical Center
Martinez, California

Don Tucker
Department of Psychology
University of Oregon
Eugene, Oregon

Leslie G. Ungerleider
Laboratory of Brain and Cognition
National Institute of Mental Health
Bethesda, Maryland

Joel S. Warm
Department of Psychology
University of Cincinnati
Cincinnati, Ohio

Maree I. Webster
Stanley Foundation Research
Institute
NIMH Neuroscience Center at
St. Elizabeths Hospital
Washington, DC

Sharon Wigal
Center for the Biological Study of
ADHD
University of California
Irvine, California

Author Index

Abdullaev, Y. G., 101, 121, 391, 399, 410–411, 418, 423
Abikoff, H., 453, 453, 458
Abney, O. L., 42, 49
Abrams, R. A., 334, 350
Abrams, T. W., 541, 542
Ackles, P., 240, 256
Acuna, C., 57, 68
Adams, J. A., 246, 249
Adams, M. M., 134, 141
Adamson, C. F., 477, 487
Adelson, E., 175, 182
Adler, L. E., 531, 542–543
Agis, I. F., 385, 397
Agresti, A., 386, 398
Akhtar, N., 437, 440
Akshoomoff, N. A., 438, 440
Alavi, A., 96, 121
Alexander, G. E., 28, 30, 461, 471–472, 474, 483, 486
Alexander, M. P., 154, 161, 518, 523
Alexinsky, T., 44, 48, 199, 213, 228, 234, 249
Aliminosa, D., 144, 161
Alivisatos, B., 362, 378
Allen, M., 242–243, 249
Allison, T., 75, 91
Allman, J. M., 329–330, 347
Allport, D. A., 4, 7, 13, 105, 117, 335, 347, 402–404, 419, 481
Alluisi, E. A., 233, 252
Almkvist, O., 462, 481
Aloimonos, J., 171, 181
Alpert, N. M., 144, 159, 366, 377, 379
Amaral, D. G., 153, 157
Ameli, R., 534, 543
Ames, C. T., 80, 93
Andersen, C., 59, 68, 177, 181
Andersen, R. A., 57, 68, 166, 175, 184, 257, 261, 275

Anderson, B., 520–521
Anderson, C. H., 101, 120
Anderson, E., 285, 292, 297
Anderson, J. R., 387, 395
Anderson, R. A., 495, 525
Anderson, T. J., 111–112, 117, 465, 468, 481
Andreasen, N. C., 154, 157, 527, 542
Andrewes, D. G., 151, 160
Anello-Vento, L., 453, 458
Annett, L. E., 207, 213
Antonucci, G., 506, 524
Appel, J. B., 200, 213
Appenzeller, T., 5, 14
Apple, C., 201, 213
Arezzo, J. C., 75, 93
Arguin, M., 271, 275, 471, 481
Arndt, S., 154, 157, 527, 542
Arnell, K. M., 404, 422–423
Arnold, S. E., 527, 542
Arnsten, A. F. T., 42, 45, 47–48, 196, 213
Arriagada, P. V., 479, 481
Arruda, J. E., 229, 255
Arthur, D. L., 150, 157
Asan, E., 38, 48
Asarnow, R. F., 240, 250, 531–532, 542–543
Ashbridge, 112
Ashby, F. G., 260, 275
Aslin, R. N., 431, 440
Assal, G., 504, 525
Aston-Jones, G., 44, 48–49, 199, 212–213, 228, 236, 249
Atkinson, J., 429–430, 440–441, 434
Attneave, F., 287, 296, 418, 419
Auburtin, 143
Audet, T., 519, 521
Awh, E. S., 112–114, 121, 353, 369–372, 374–375, 378–379, 418, 421, 433, 442
Axford, J. G., 77, 92
Aylward, E. H., 454, 456

Bacharach, V. R., 332, 339, 347
Backman, L., 462, 481
Bacon, W. F., 170, 182
Baddeley, A. D., 7, 13, 415, 418–419
Bagdy, G., 528, 543
Bahri, T., 7, 13
Baizer, J. S., 28, 30, 60, 66
Baker, D., 233, 255
Bakker, V. J., 532, 546
Baleydier, C., 27–28, 30–31
Balint, R., 269, 275
Ballantine, H. T., 413, 419
Ballard, D., 171–172, 182
Balota, D. A., 465–466, 468, 471, 477, 483,
    487
Bandettini, P. A., 128, 130, 140
Banks, W. P., 309, 324
Barbas, H., 27, 31
Baren, M., 150, 161, 451, 456
Barett, A., 319, 323
Barkai, E., 538–539, 543
Barkley, R. A., 446, 449, 450, 456–457
Barnes, J. C., 195, 215
Barnett, E. M., 531, 544
Baron, J. C., 528, 544
Baron-Cohen, S., 439–440
Barta, P. E., 527, 542
Bartus, R. T., 45, 48, 148, 157, 463, 481
Bashinski, H. S., 332, 339, 347
Baudena, P., 145, 151, 158
Bauer, R. H., 149, 158
Bauer, R. M., 385, 386, 398
Baumgardner, T. L., 454, 457
Bay, E., 499, 521
Baylis, G. C., 299, 301–303, 306–311, 316,
    318–319, 321–322, 463, 510–511, 513,
    516, 521–522
Baylis, L., 319, 322
Beatty, J., 229, 253
Beaumont, J. G., 242, 251
Beck, L. H., 191, 218, 528, 545
Beck, L. N., 237, 256
Becker, D. P., 239, 256
Beech, A., 533, 542
Beer, B., 463, 481
Behrmann, M., 164, 184, 261, 276, 317–318,
    322, 514–515, 521
Belliveau, J. W., 107, 121, 124, 131, 142
Belyavin, A., 229, 249
Bench, C. J., 406–407, 419
Bender, M. B., 499, 521
Benes, F. M., 415–416, 419, 527, 542
Benson, D. F., 145, 161, 384, 387, 395

Benson, E., 475, 485
Bentin, S., 382, 395, 392, 394, 533, 542
Bentivoglio, M., 21, 31
Berch, D. B., 221, 250
Berg, G., 462, 465, 477, 480, 483–484
Berg, L., 477, 482
Berg, P., 79, 91
Berkovic, S. F., 151, 160
Berlyne, D., 469, 482
Berman, K. F., 240, 250
Berman, S., 437, 440
Bernardo, K. L., 430, 440
Bernstein, E., 270, 276, 502–503, 524
Berthoz, A., 111–112, 120, 478–479, 486
Berti, A., 496, 518, 521
Bertoncini, J., 439, 442
Bertucci, P., 339, 347
Besner, D., 389, 395
Besson, M., 386, 392, 395–396, 533, 544
Biederman, I., 404, 423
Biederman, J., 449, 454, 457, 459
Biraben, A., 145, 151, 158
Bird, E. D., 527, 542
Bisiach, E., 19, 26, 31, 496, 506, 519, 521
Biswal, B., 134, 139–140
Black, S. E., 318, 322
Blackstad, T. W., 20, 31
Bladin, P. F., 151, 160
Blamire, A. M., 373–375, 379, 381, 391, 397
Blaser, E., 285, 292, 297
Bloch, G., 373–375, 379
Bloom, F. E., 44, 48, 81, 93
Blueler, T., 528, 542
Blume, H. W., 367, 380
Blumstein, S. E., 388, 397
Boaz, T., 392, 395
Bobrow, D. G., 233, 253, 283, 286, 298
Boch, R., 60, 66, 67, 358, 378
Boddington, S., 463, 487
Boies, S. J., 6, 15, 199, 217
Boller, F., 240, 256
Bonforte, S., 453, 459
Bonnel, A. M., 336, 337, 339, 347, 349
Boone, J. R., 390, 397
Bormans, G., 105, 107, 109, 111–112, 118,
    122, 364–365, 367, 378, 380
Born, R. T., 107, 121, 131, 142
Bosel, R., 229, 254
Bottini, G., 506, 525
Bouillard, J. B., 143, 157
Boulenger, J. P., 528, 544
Boulengeuz, P., 209, 215
Boulter, L. R., 246, 249

Bourbon, W. T., 240, 250
Boussaoud, D., 23, 31
Bouvier, G., 148, 160
Bowers, D., 495–496, 522–523
Bowman, E. M., 204, 207, 213, 478, 487
Boynton, G. M., 126, 140
Braak, E., 462, 480, 482
Braak, H., 462, 480, 482
Braddick, O. J., 430, 440
Bradley, C., 445, 457
Bradshaw, J. G., 496, 523
Brady, C. B., 465, 471–472, 485
Brady, T. J., 107, 121, 131, 142
Braff, D. L., 208, 213, 219, 531–532, 542, 545
Bransome, E. D., Jr., 191, 218, 237, 256, 528,
    545
Braun, J., 58, 67, 85, 91, 174–175, 177, 182–
    183, 285, 296, 309, 322, 336–337, 339–
    340, 343–345, 348–349
Braver, T. S., 538, 542
Bravo, M. J., 291–292, 296, 329, 348
Brawn, V. J., 206, 219
Brehaut, J. C., 437, 443
Breitmeyer, B., 423, 441, 478, 483, 532, 542
Brennan, C., 430, 443
Breton, F., 453, 458
Briand, K. A., 85, 91, 464, 482
Britten, K. H., 328, 348
Broadbent, D. E., 4, 13, 44, 48, 58, 67, 103,
    117, 191, 199, 213, 283, 296, 299, 313, 322,
    403, 419, 463, 482
Brodeur, D., 437, 441, 461, 486
Brody, D., 532, 542
Bronowski, J., 446, 457
Bronson, G. W., 429, 440
Brooks, D. J., 111–112, 116–117, 119, 465,
    481
Brouwer, W. H., 238, 250
Brouwers, P., 462, 485
Brown, C. M., 392, 394–396
Brown, G. M., 154, 158
Brown, J. E., 454, 456
Brown, V. J., 6, 14, 204, 206–207, 212–213,
    472, 484
Brown, W. D., 384, 389, 397
Bruce, C. J., 149, 158, 432–433, 441, 520, 522
Brugger, P., 265, 276
Bruhn, P., 454, 458
Brun, P., 45, 48
Brunn, J. L., 317, 323, 515, 521, 522
Bruno, J. P., 201, 218, 228, 247, 253
Bruyn, B., 111, 122
Bryden, M., 182

Bub, D., 384, 396, 394, 519, 521
Bucci, D. J., 209, 214
Buchsbaum, M. S., 36, 49, 228, 240, 250, 252
Buchtel, H. A., 432, 441, 469, 483
Buchwald, J. S., 150, 157
Buckle, L., 154, 161
Buckley, P., 241, 252
Buckner, R. L., 106, 115, 121, 128, 140, 154,
    157
Buda, M., 45, 48
Bullier, J., 24, 31
Bundesen, C., 168, 182, 303, 323
Bunge, M., 9, 13
Bunsey, M. D., 196, 213
Burchert, W., 84, 92, 101, 109, 119, 223, 251,
    363, 366, 379, 409, 421
Burgess, P. W., 405, 412, 422
Burkell, J., 301, 306, 324, 325
Burkhalter, A., 430, 440
Burns, R. J., 475–476, 487, 533, 546
Burt, P., 175, 182
Bush, G., 107, 117
Bushnell, I. W. R., 430, 440
Bushnell, M. C., 60, 67, 103, 117, 166, 175,
    182, 356, 365, 378
Bushnell, P. J., 200, 204, 213,
Butter, C. M., 505, 521
Butters, N., 473–476, 483, 485
Butterworth, G., 439, 440

Cabaret, M., 240, 251
Cahil, C., 99, 121
Cai, J. X., 42, 45, 47–48
Caillard, V., 528, 544
Caine, S. B., 208, 219
Callahan, M. J., 199, 213
Calvanio, R., 261, 276
Camarda, R., 206, 217, 495, 524
Cameron, S., 437, 443
Canfield, R. L., 431, 441
Canoune, H., 151, 160
Cantwell, D. P., 449, 453, 456–457, 459
Cappa, S. F., 506, 521
Caramazza, A., 144, 157, 317, 322, 390, 397,
    515, 523
Carbonnell, J., 418, 419
Cardebat, D., 387, 391, 396
Carli, M., 44, 46, 48, 191, 193, 196–197, 202,
    206–207, 214, 217
Carlson, G. A., 449, 459
Carmelli, D., 477, 486
Carmona, E., 385, 397
Carpenter, P. A., 261, 276, 317, 323, 515, 522

Carr, T. H., 387–389, 396, 398
Carson, R. E., 24, 32, 537, 543
Carter, C. S., 406–408, 419, 452, 457
Casella, V., 96, 121
Casey, B. J., 406–408, 420, 435, 443, 454, 457
Cash, T. F., 531, 542
Cassaday, H. H., 209, 215
Castro, L., 469, 487
Catena, A., 385, 397
Catsman-Berrevoets, C. E., 21, 31
Cauthen, J. C., 26, 34
Cavada, C., 28, 31
Cavallucci, C., 238, 255
Cavanagh, P., 271, 275, 281–282, 298, 471, 481
Cave, C. B., 319, 323
Cave, K. R., 6, 14, 64, 69, 85, 88, 92, 94, 112, 114, 122, 164, 170, 185, 259, 278, 464, 470, 482, 487
Caviness, V. S., Jr., 144, 159, 455, 457
Chaderjian, M., 452, 457
Chafee, M., 368–369, 378–379
Chan-Palay, V., 37, 48
Chang, L., 477, 487
Changeux, J. P., 43, 49
Chao, L. L., 148, 157
Chapin, R. I., 150, 157
Chapman, J. P., 531, 533, 544,
Chapman, L. J., 531, 533, 544
Chapman, M., 437, 441
Chase, T. N., 462, 485
Cheal, M. L., 85, 91, 170, 182
Chelazzi, L., 11, 14, 61, 63–65, 67–68, 84, 92, 113, 117, 173–174, 182, 213, 214, 273, 277, 331, 348, 350, 479, 484
Chen, P. C., 454, 457
Cherktow, H., 384, 394, 396
Cherry, S. R., 100, 122
Chesler, D. A., 124, 142
Chesney, G., 148, 160
Chiang, C., 44, 48, 199, 213, 228, 249
Chiba, A. A., 204, 209, 211, 214
Chichilnisky, E. J., 128, 141
Choate, L. S., 7, 15, 435, 443, 468, 486
Chollet, F., 387, 391, 396, 399
Christ, K., 506, 523
Christensen, B., 385, 397
Christian, D. L., 448, 459
Chugani, H. T., 434, 441
Chun, M. M., 285–286, 290, 297
Church, R. M., 202, 217
Churchland, P., 9, 14
Chwilla, D. J., 392, 396

Cizadlo, T., 154, 157, 527, 542
Claridge, G., 533, 542
Clark, C. R., 36, 42, 48, 204, 214, 533, 542
Clark, J., 99, 121, 171, 182
Clark, V. P., 77, 83–85, 91–92, 124, 128, 131–134, 140–141, 148, 158, 465, 485
Clarke, J. M., 145, 151, 158
Clayworth, C. C., 145, 159
Clements, S., 445, 457
Clevenge, W., 448, 459
Clohessy, A. B., 415, 419
Cohen, A., 11, 15, 271, 276, 430, 443, 500, 519, 522, 524
Cohen, J. D., 196, 219, 406–408, 419, 502–504, 522, 538–539, 542–543
Cohen, M. S., 124, 142
Cohen, N. J., 144, 161
Cohen, R. M., 240–242, 250
Cohen, Y., 7, 15, 26, 33, 39, 49, 171, 174, 184, 305, 324, 434, 442
Colby, C. L., 24, 28, 31, 36, 48, 59, 67, 166, 183, 257, 261, 276, 478, 482, 520, 522, 537, 543
Cole, B. J., 193–194, 196, 208, 212, 214
Colebatch, J. G., 116–117
Colebatch, J. M., 409, 419
Coleman, M., 527, 537, 546
Coles, M. G. H., 79, 91, 151, 157, 409, 420, 422
Collins, M. T., 477, 487
Collins, P., 210, 218
Colliver, J. A., 199, 215
Columbo, J., 438, 441
Conel, J. L., 434, 441
Conners, C. K., 451, 457
Connor, C. E., 58, 60, 63, 67, 69, 177, 182, 185
Connor, E., 329, 348
Constable, R. T., 388, 399
Constantinidis, C., 58, 60, 69, 177, 185, 478, 487
Contant, T. A., 45, 48, 196, 213
Cook, I. A., 481, 485
Corbetta, M., 35, 48, 103, 105–111, 114–117, 119–121, 130, 141, 212, 214, 270, 276, 362–365, 367, 378–379, 384, 396, 403, 419, 465, 482, 471, 479, 482, 529, 543
Corder, E. H., 477, 482, 487
Corkin, S., 413, 419
Corteen, R. S., 404, 419
Coryell, C., 124, 142
Coslett, H. B., 238, 255, 272–274, 276, 495–496, 522–523

Cosmides, L., 9, 15
Courchesne, E., 151, 157, 438, 440, 443
Courtney, S. M., 113–114, 117, 124, 126, 128, 130, 132–137, 140–141, 370–372, 374–375, 378
Cowan, N., 81, 94
Cowan, W. M., 21, 31, 153, 157
Cowey, 112
Cox, C., 462, 485
Cox, S. B., 97, 99–100, 117
Craig, A., 224, 250
Craik, F. I. M., 5, 15, 152, 154, 158, 161–162, 391, 396
Crayton, L., 463, 487
Creelman, C. D., 222, 252, 332, 349
Creutzfeld, O. D., 97, 117
Crick, F., 273, 277, 164, 178, 182
Crinella, F. M., 445, 457–449, 453
Crisp, J., 89, 93, 301, 310, 324
Crivello, F., 478–479, 486
Crockford, H. A., 463, 487
Crofton, K. M., 200, 213
Cromwell. R. L., 531–533, 542–543
Crooks, M., 463, 487
Crosson, B., 382, 385–386, 390, 397–399
Crovitz, H., 165, 182
Crowley, K., 448, 459
Crowne, D. P., 207, 214
Csernansky, J. G., 534, 543
Cubelli, R., 518, 523
Culhane, S. M., 59, 69
Cunningham, V. J., 409, 419
Curran, T., 148, 157, 383, 392, 396, 415, 419
Currie, J., 414, 421, 465–466, 469, 475, 485
Curry, R., 337, 349
Cutler, N. R., 465, 484

Daffner, K. R., 366, 377, 379, 469, 482, 487
Dagenbach, D., 176, 184
Dagi, T. F., 413, 419
Dale, A. M., 75, 77, 91
Daly, P. F., 144, 159
Damasio, A. R., 145, 157, 388–389, 390, 396, 412–413, 420, 527, 542
Damasio, H., 145, 157, 388, 390, 396
Daniel, R., 229, 250
Dann, O., 21, 31
D'Antono, B., 394, 396
Dark, V. J., 4, 5, 12, 14
Daves, W., 165, 182
Davidoff, D., 475, 483
Davidsen, H., 97, 101, 121
Davidson, B. J., 332, 350

Davidson, G. S., 531, 543
Davidson, J. C., 197, 203, 205, 212
Davidson, M. C., 27, 32, 40–43, 46, 48, 50, 418, 420, 528, 543
Davidson, R., 243, 251
Davies, D. R., 5, 6, 15, 222, 224–225, 229, 231, 233, 237, 246, 250, 252–254, 529–530, 545
Davies, P. W., 55, 67
Davis, B. M., 528, 543
Davis, G., 315, 318, 324
Davis, J. M., 248, 250
Davis, K. L., 528, 543
Davis, K. R., 26, 32
Davis, M., 208, 214
Davis, N., 59, 69
Davis, R. E., 199, 213
Dawson, K. A., 207, 214
Dawson, M. E., 404, 420
Dean, R. L., 45, 48, 463, 483
DeArmond, S. J., 237–238, 250
Debecker, J., 150, 157
De Bleser, R., 475, 487
De Bruyn, B., 109, 122, 365, 380
Decary, A., 148, 160
Dehaene, S., 6, 12, 15, 24, 33, 409–410, 414, 418, 420, 422
Deiber, M. P., 116–117, 409, 419
Dejerine, J., 143, 157
Delis, D. C., 473–476, 483, 485, 507–508, 522
Della Salla, S., 475, 482
DeLong, M. R., 28, 30
Del Pesce, M., 504, 523
Demadura, T. L., 474, 476, 483, 485
Dember, W. N., 7, 15, 192, 200, 217, 224, 245–246, 248, 250, 254–255, 529–530, 546
Demonet, J. F., 387, 391, 396
Dencker, S. J., 238, 250
Denckla, M. B., 454, 456–457
DePriest, D. D., 61, 63, 68
De Renzi, E., 257, 276, 361, 378
De Roo, M., 105, 107, 118
Derryberry, D., 438, 443
De Salvia, M., 210, 218
Desimone, R., 6, 8, 11, 12, 14, 22–24, 28–31, 33, 57–58, 61–65, 67–68, 84, 92–93, 96, 101–104, 109, 113, 118–119, 130, 142, 166, 172–175, 178, 182, 184, 212, 214, 257, 273, 276–277, 309, 324, 327, 329–331, 342, 346, 348–351, 357, 359, 379, 403, 420, 423, 463, 470, 479, 482, 484–485, 537, 544, 546

Desmedt, J. E., 150, 157
Despres, D., 124, 142
Des Rosiers, M. H., 96, 121
Deutsch, G., 240, 250
Devaux, B., 145, 151, 158
Dewey, M. M., 237–238, 250
DeYoe, E. A., 105, 117, 131, 257, 276
Dhawan, M., 389, 398, 404, 414, 422
Diamond, A., 433, 441
Diamond, J., 9, 14
Dias, R., 210, 214
Dickinson, A., 210, 216
Diller, L., 521–522
Dimond, S. J., 221, 242–243, 250–251
Dinner, D. S., 147, 159
Di Pellegrino, G., 355–356, 378, 508, 522
Dittmar, M. L., 246, 255
Dobmeyer, S., 104–105, 107, 114–117, 130, 141, 384, 396, 403, 419, 537, 543
Dolan, R. J., 154, 160, 406–407, 415, 419–420
Donchin, E., 79, 91, 151, 153, 157, 159, 409, 420
Donders, F. C., 99, 118
Dosher, B., 285, 292, 297
Dosher, E., 334, 336, 340, 351
Douglas, R. J., 53, 67, 167, 182
Douglas, R. M., 432, 441, 469, 483
Douglas, V. I., 445, 449, 457
Dow, B. M., 60, 66
Downing, C. J., 80, 92, 223, 251, 332, 348–349, 464, 484
Drachman, D. A., 477, 482
Drasdo, A., 37, 43, 50
Driver, J., 6, 14, 26, 33, 89, 93, 103, 109, 119, 174, 185, 261, 276, 299–311, 313–316, 318–323, 325, 463, 510–511, 513, 516, 521–522
Duara, R., 465, 477, 480–481, 484
Dudchenko, P., 199, 214, 228, 247, 253
Duerk, J. L., 241, 252
Duffy, C. J., 58, 60, 68
Duffy, E., 227, 251
Dugas, M., 453, 459
Duhamel, J. R., 166, 183, 257, 261, 276, 478, 482, 520, 522
Duncan, J., 6, 8, 11–12, 14, 24, 29–31, 58, 64–65, 67, 80, 85, 91, 102, 104–105, 109, 111–113, 118, 122, 164, 170, 172, 174, 182–183, 259, 273, 276, 287, 296, 301, 306–308, 310, 318, 322–323, 327–331, 335–337, 341–342, 346, 348, 364–365, 367, 378, 401, 403–405, 41 2, 418, 420, 463–464, 470, 482

Dunn, D., 404, 419
Dunnett, S. B., 46, 48, 207, 213
Dupont, P., 105, 107, 109, 111–112, 118, 122, 364–365, 367, 378, 380
Dykstra, L. A., 200, 213
Dziurawiec, S., 431, 438, 442

Eagger, S. A., 463, 487
Early, T. S., 414–415, 420, 422
Eason, R. G., 11, 14, 83, 91
Eeckout, H., 105, 122
Efron, R., 507–508, 522
Egeth, H. E., 64–65, 67–68, 167, 170–171, 176, 182–184, 201–202, 217, 305–306, 323, 334, 349
Eglin, M., 261, 263–265, 267–268, 276, 506, 522
Egly, R., 270, 277, 303–305, 318–319, 323
Ehlers, C. L., 150, 157
Ehrhardt, J. C., 527, 542
Eisenberg, H. M., 240, 250
Eliasson, M., 191, 216
Elkins, I. J., 532–533, 543
Ellermann, J. M., 95, 120, 124, 142
Elliott, R., 210, 215
Ellis, A. W., 383, 396
Ellis, H. D., 431, 438, 442
Emerson, J. F., 454, 457
Emerson, R. W., 5, 14
Emslie, H., 405, 412, 420
Engel, F. L., 61, 67
Engel, S. A., 126, 128, 140–141
Enns, J. T., 281, 296, 437, 440–441, 461, 486
Eriksen, B. A., 302, 323, 405, 420
Eriksen, C. W., 302, 323, 405, 420, 472, 482
Eskes, G. A., 146, 161, 361, 378
Evans, A. C., 100, 122, 369–375, 379, 388–389, 394, 396, 399
Evenden, J. L., 44, 46, 48, 191, 201, 206, 214–215
Everitt, B. J., 27, 33, 36, 44, 46, 48–49, 190–191, 194–195, 197, 201–202, 210, 214, 217–218, 227–228, 254, 462, 487
Eysenck, M. W., 44, 48

Fabiani, M., 153, 159
Fagan, J. F., 438, 441
Fan, S., 77, 83–84, 86–88, 91–92, 148, 158
Fannon, S., 131, 141
Farah, M. J., 261, 276, 301, 308–309, 317–318, 321, 323–325, 475, 483, 502–504, 515–516, 521–522
Farde, L., 528, 543

Faust, M. E., 465–466, 468, 471, 477, 483, 487

Faustman, W. O., 534, 543

Faux, S. F., 221, 253, 530, 532–533, 535, 544–545

Fedio, P., 462, 485

Feldman, M., 499, 521

Feldon, J., 209, 215

Felleman, D. J., 22, 31, 89, 91, 96, 103, 118, 257, 276, 329, 331, 348

Ferrera, V. P., 107–108, 118

Ferrier, N., 171, 182

Feskens, E. J. M., 477, 483

Fiez, J. A., 100, 105–106, 115–116, 118, 120–121, 388, 394, 396, 398, 406, 422

Filipek, P. A., 454–455, 457, 459

Filoteo, J. V., 473–476, 483, 485

Finch, D. M., 115, 122

Findlay, J., 332, 350

Fink, D. J., 97, 101, 121

Fiore, C., 453, 459

Fiori, M., 528, 543

Fische, T. D., 448, 459

Fischer, B., 60, 67, 285, 296, 301, 324, 358, 378, 432, 441, 478, 483

Fischler, I., 386, 392, 395–396, 398

Fisk, A. D., 246, 256

Fitzgerald, G. A., 454, 460

Fitzpatrick, E., 495–496, 522

Flaum, M., 527, 542

Fleming, M., 238, 255

Fletcher, J. M., 449, 459

Fletcher, P., 154, 160, 415, 420

Fletcher, W. A., 468–469, 483

Foldi, N. S., 475, 483

Folk, C. L., 170, 183

Foote, S. L., 150, 160

Ford, E., 476, 483

Ford, J. M., 534, 543

Forster, S. V., 496, 524

Forstl, H., 479, 483

Foster, J. K., 146, 161, 361, 378

Foster, N. L., 462, 485

Fowler, J., 96, 121

Fowler, S. C., 195, 197, 219

Fox, P. T., 35, 47, 49, 95, 98–100, 109, 115–116, 118, 120, 122, 124, 141, 240–241, 244, 254, 362, 378, 381, 384, 396, 398, 405, 422, 452, 458

Frackowiak, R. S. J., 99–100, 107, 110–112, 116, 118–122, 131, 134, 138, 141–142, 154, 160, 384–385, 387–389, 391, 396–399, 406–407, 409, 415, 419–420, 465, 478–479, 481, 486

Frankel, S. L., 470, 487

Franks, R. D., 531, 543

Frantik, E., 229, 251

Franzel, S. L., 64, 69, 85, 94, 112, 114, 122, 164, 170, 185, 259, 278

Frasca, R., 506, 524

Frecska, E., 528, 543

Freedman, R., 531, 543

Freeman, H., 529, 545

Freeman, R. B., 154, 158

Frey, P. W., 199, 215

Freygang, W. H. J., 98, 119

Friberg, L., 385, 397

Friederici, A., 382, 396

Friedland, R. P., 241, 252, 462, 480, 483

Friedland, R. D., 361, 380

Friedman, D. P., 24, 33, 437, 440

Friedman, H. R., 145, 158

Friedman, J. H., 502–503, 524

Friedman, L., 241, 252

Friedman-Hill, S. R., 112, 118, 269–271, 277

Friedrich, F. J., 11, 15, 204, 219, 209, 219, 314, 324, 385, 398, 465, 469, 478, 486, 499–500, 502, 515, 522, 524,

Friedrich, F. A., 267, 277, 361–362, 380

Fries, W., 28, 31

Friston, J. K., 391, 396

Friston, K. J., 99–100, 116–118, 126, 130–131, 134, 138, 141–142, 384, 387, 389, 391, 397–398, 406–407, 409, 415, 419–420

Frith, C. D., 99–100, 110, 116, 118, 120–121, 134, 138, 141, 154, 157, 388, 391, 396, 398, 401, 406–407, 415, 419–420, 478–479, 486

Frommer, D. P., 206, 215

Frost, B., 177, 184

Frostig, R. D., 97, 118

Fuentes, L. J., 385, 397

Fukushima, K., 164, 183

Fulbright, R. K., 388, 399

Fulton, J. F., 97, 118

Funahashi, S., 149, 158, 368, 378, 432–433, 441, 520, 522

Fusco, M. M., 237–238, 250

Fuster, J. M., 113, 118, 149, 158, 355, 368, 377–379

Gabrielli, J. D. E., 319, 323

Gainer, H., 97, 101, 121

Gainotti, G., 314, 323

Gal, G., 209, 215

Galambos, R., 151, 157

Gale, A., 229, 235, 251

Gall, C. M., 101, 119

Gallagher, M., 204, 209, 214

Gallant, J. L., 63, 67, 177, 182–183, 329, 348, 351

Ganz, L., 532, 542

Garbart, H., 64, 67, 170, 183

Garraghty, P. E., 24, 33

Gaskell, P. C., 477, 487

Gaymard, B., 469, 486

Gazzaniga, M. S., 9, 14, 84, 92, 101, 109, 119, 169, 184, 223, 251, 363, 366, 379, 409, 421, 516, 525

Geffen, G. M., 36, 42, 48, 204, 214, 403, 423, 475–476, 487, 533, 542, 546

Geffen, L. B., 36, 42, 48, 204, 214, 475–476, 487, 533, 542, 546

Gehring, W. J., 409, 420

Gelade, G., 80, 85, 93, 111, 121, 164, 169, 185, 258–259, 262, 278, 280, 284, 290, 298, 328–329, 351, 470–471, 487, 506, 525

Geminiani, G., 496, 521

Gendelman, P. M., 208, 214

Gennarelli, T. A., 239, 251, 253

George, M. S., 406–408, 420

Georgopoulous, A., 57, 68

Gerard, R. W., 97, 121

Gerardi, G., 417, 422

Gershberg, F. B., 154, 158, 161, 389, 397

Gerstein, G., 52, 68

Geschwind, N., 9, 14, 27, 33, 387, 397

Gettner, S. N., 321, 324

Geula, C., 28, 33, 35, 49, 235, 253

Geyer, M. A., 208–209, 213, 219–220, 531, 542

Giambra, L., 530, 545

Gianotti, G., 520, 522

Gibbs, B., 305, 323

Gibson, A. R., 21, 31

Gibson, B. S., 171, 183, 305–306, 308, 323, 334, 349

Giedd, J. N., 454, 457

Gilmore, R. O., 427, 429, 433, 441–442

Girard, P., 24, 31

Girelli, M., 89, 90–91, 300

Girgus, J. S., 437, 441

Giriunas, I. B., 413, 419

Gitelman, D. R., 110, 120, 366, 377, 379, 478–479, 486

Gjedde, A., 388–389, 399

Glazer, W., 534, 543

Glover, G. H., 126, 128, 140–141

Godefroy, O., 240, 251

Goff, W. R., 75, 91

Gold, S. M., 229, 255

Goldberg, I. E., 124, 142

Goldberg, M. E., 59–60, 67, 103, 105, 117, 122, 166, 175, 182–183, 257, 261, 276, 356, 365, 378, 478, 482, 520, 522

Goldman, R. P., 520, 522

Goldman-Rakic, P. S., 23, 27–28, 31, 34, 42, 45, 48, 100, 104, 116, 119, 145, 149, 153, 158, 368–369, 374–375, 378–379, 409, 418, 420, 423, 432–433, 441, 478–479, 483

Gomez Gonzalez, C. M., 83–84, 91, 148, 158

Gonon, F., 45, 48

Gonzalez Rothi, L. J., 385–386, 390, 397–399

Goodale, M. A., 168, 184, 257, 277

Goodman, G. S., 431, 441

Goodrich, S. J., 316, 318, 322, 325, 511, 513, 522

Gordon, B., 390, 399

Gordon, M., 450, 457

Gordon-Lickey, M. E., 204, 220

Gorman, L. K., 46, 50, 463, 487

Gös, A., 84, 92, 101, 109, 119, 365–366, 379

Gosel, A., 223, 251, 409, 421

Gottleib, D. I., 21, 31

Gottlob, L. R., 85, 91

Gould, T., 475, 483

Grabowecky, M., 146, 156, 159, 265, 269–271, 277

Grady, C. L., 24, 32, 101–102, 107–108, 112, 115, 119, 130, 132, 134–135, 138, 141–142, 149, 160, 462, 465, 471, 475, 477–481, 483–484, 486, 537, 543

Grafman, J., 146, 151, 160, 162, 241, 254

Grafton, S. T., 415, 420

Grant, P., 285, 298, 341–342, 350

Grasby, P., 154, 160

Grasby, P. M., 406–407, 415, 419–420

Gratton, G., 79, 91

Gray, C. M., 273, 277

Gray, J. A., 195, 209, 215, 218

Graybiel, A. M., 28, 32

Graziano, M. S. A., 273, 277, 495, 522

Greden, J. F., 528, 546

Green, D. M., 222, 251, 327, 332, 349

Green, M., 281, 298, 532, 543

Green, M. F., 532, 543

Greenberg, J., 96, 121

Greenberg, L. M., 450, 458

Greene, R. W., 538–539, 543

Greenwood, P. M., 461, 465, 471–472, 474–475, 477–479, 483, 486

Grier, J. B., 199, 215

Grigoryan, G. A., 209, 215

Grillon, C., 534, 543

Grindley, G. C., 61, 67
Grinvald, A., 97, 118
Grootoonk, S., 99, 121
Gross, B., 409, 420
Gross, C. G., 57, 67, 273, 277, 495, 522
Gross, M., 240–242, 250, 454, 460
Grossberg, S., 164, 183
Grossi, D., 480, 483
Grossier, D., 449, 458
Gruetter, R., 381, 391, 397
Grunze, H. C. R., 538–539, 543
Guariglia, C., 506, 520, 522, 524
Guclu, C. C., 454, 458
Guich, S., 240, 250
Guitton, D., 469, 483
Guitton, H. A., 432, 441
Gulyas, B., 8, 14, 225, 239, 241, 244, 252
Gur, R., 240, 254
Gusak, O., 209, 215
Gutman, D., 313, 324
Guze, B. H., 477, 487
Gygax, P. A., 20, 33

Habib, R., 152, 154, 162
Hadar, U., 391, 399
Haenny, P. E., 61, 63, 67, 104, 119, 331, 349
Haider, M., 230, 251
Haier, R. J., 240, 250
Haimson, J., 537, 545
Haines, J. L., 477, 482, 487
Haith, M. M., 431, 441
Hajnal, J. V., 107, 122, 131, 142
Halgren, E., 145, 151, 158, 161
Hall, F. S., 209, 220
Hall, G., 209, 215
Hall, H., 528, 543
Hall, S., 206–207, 218
Halldin, C., 528, 543
Hallen, C. C., 81, 93
Halligan, P. W., 261, 276, 315–316, 322, 324,
    493, 508, 511–512, 515, 518, 521–524
Hamburger, S. D., 454, 457
Hamel, E., 394, 396
Hammond, G. R., 208, 215
Hampson, S. A., 81, 93
Hancock, P. A., 233, 251
Hansch, E. C., 468, 486
Hansen, J. C., 81, 91, 93, 353, 355, 379
Hansma, D. I., 21, 31
Harbaugh, R. E., 199, 213
Harkness, W., 430, 440
Harley, C. W., 28, 32

Harlow, J. M., 143, 158
Harms, L., 303, 323
Harn, J., 147, 159
Harrison, A. A., 193, 195, 215
Hart, J., 390, 399
Harter, M. R., 11, 14, 83, 91, 453, 458
Hartje, W., 506, 523
Hartley, A. A., 461, 480, 483
Harvey, M., 496, 524
Hasher, L., 466, 484
Hasselmo, M. E., 538–539, 543
Haughton, V. M., 134, 139, 140
Havekes, L. M., 477, 483
Hawken, M. B., 111–112, 117, 465, 481
Hawkins, H. L., 80, 85, 92, 223, 251, 332, 349,
    464–465, 484–485
Hawley, D. K., 242, 248, 255
Haws, B., 495–496, 522
Haxby, J. V., 24, 32, 34, 46, 49, 101–102,
    107–108, 112–115, 117, 119, 124, 126,
    128, 130–138, 140–141, 149, 160, 257,
    278, 370–372, 374–375, 378, 461–463,
    465, 471, 473, 475, 477–480, 483–484,
    486, 527, 537, 542–543
Hay, D., 414, 421
Hayes, A., 418, 420
Hayhoe, M., 171, 182
Hazan, C., 431, 441
Hazelton, E., 415, 420
Hazlett, E., 240, 250
He, Z. J., 282, 287–289, 295–297, 304, 309,
    323
Head, H., 221, 232, 251
Hearne, E. F., 538–539, 543
Hedera, P., 241, 252
Heeger, D. J., 126, 140
Hegley, D. G., 533, 544
Heilman, K. M., 26, 32, 34, 145, 158, 207, 219,
    239, 251, 261, 277, 382, 399, 451, 456,
    458–459, 495–496, 507, 522–523
Heimer, L., 20–21, 31–32
Heinze, H. J., 84, 92, 101, 109, 119, 148, 158,
    223, 251, 363, 366, 379, 403, 409, 421
Heise, G. A., 189, 213
Heit, G., 145, 151, 158
Hellawell, D. J., 521, 525
Helmholtz, H., 332, 349
Hemsley, D. R., 209, 215
Hendrickson, A. E., 21, 31–32
Hendrix, J. P., 97, 121
Henik, A., 301, 323
Henriksen, L., 454, 458
Hermle, L., 533, 546

Hernandez, T. D., 207, 213
Herscovitch, P., 24, 32, 98, 120, 406–408, 420, 537, 543
Hester, D., 504, 525
Heyn, S. N., 45, 48
Hichwa, R. D., 154, 157
Hieble, J. P., 45, 49
Hier, D. B., 26, 32
Higgins, G. A., 195, 215
Hill, K., 463, 487
Hillis, A. E., 317, 322, 390, 397, 515, 523
Hillstrom, A. P., 170, 183
Hillyard, S. A., 7, 11, 14, 77, 80–81, 83–89, 91–93, 101, 109, 119, 130, 142, 145–146, 148–149, 151, 157–159, 161, 169, 184, 223, 251, 273, 277, 332, 349, 353, 355, 363, 366, 379, 382–383, 392, 394–395, 397, 403, 409, 421, 464–465, 479, 484–485, 533, 537, 544
Hink, R. F., 7, 11, 14, 81, 92
Hinke, R. M., 388, 397
Hinrichs, H., 84, 92, 101, 109, 119, 223, 251, 363, 366, 379, 409, 421
Hinshaw, S., 452, 458
Hinton, G., 177, 183
Hobson, J. A., 233, 255, 417, 421
Hockey, R., 7, 15
Hoffman, J. E., 164, 183, 308–309, 323, 533, 545
Hoffner, E., 391, 399
Hofman, E., 96, 121
Hokama, H., 527, 534, 537, 544–546
Holcomb, H. H., 240, 242, 250
Holcomb, P. J., 392, 397
Holland, P. C., 209, 214
Holley, L. A., 201, 213
Holmes, G., 269, 277
Holmes, P., 43, 50
Holmes, T. C., 150, 160
Hood, B. M., 428, 430–431, 434, 437, 440–441
Hood, P., 240, 256
Hoppel, B. E., 124, 142
Hoptman, M. J., 243, 251
Horvath, M., 229, 251
Horvath, T. B., 528, 530, 543–544
Horwitz, B., 24, 32, 101–102, 107–108, 112, 115, 119, 130, 132, 134–135, 138, 142, 149, 160, 406–408, 420, 462, 478–481, 483–484, 537, 543
Houghton, G., 35, 48
Houk, J. C., 21, 31
Houle, S., 152, 154, 158, 161–162

Howard, D., 384, 387, 389, 397, 398
Howe, S. R., 7, 15, 224, 254, 529–530, 546
Howieson, D. B., 468, 478, 486
Howland, B., 386, 396
Hoyman, L., 206, 215
Hsiao, S. S., 165, 183
Hsieh, S., 404, 419
Hu, X., 388, 397
Hubel, D. H., 89, 92, 532, 544
Huerta, M. F., 28, 32
Huguenard, J., 38, 49
Humby, T., 209, 220
Humphreys, G. W., 85, 91, 102, 111, 118, 164, 183, 259, 261–262, 276–277, 287, 296, 301, 310, 319–323, 328, 332, 341, 348, 350, 390, 399, 470, 482, 520–521, 523
Humphreys, M. S., 233, 251
Hundeshagen, H., 84, 92, 101, 109, 119, 223, 251, 363, 366, 379, 409, 421
Hung, G., 337, 349
Hunton, D. L., 111, 119
Huret, J. D., 528, 544
Hurtig, R., 154, 157
Hyde, J. S., 130, 134, 139–140
Hyder, F., 373–375, 379
Hyman, B. T., 479, 481
Hynd, G. W., 454, 458

Iadecola, C., 97, 119
Ido, T., 96, 121
Ihi, L., 175, 183
Inaccia, R., 506, 524
Incisa della Rocchetta, A., 154, 158
Inhoff, A. W., 11, 15, 385, 398, 500, 502–503, 524,
Inlow, M., 229–231, 252
Insausti, R., 153, 157
Intriligator, J. M., 144, 159
Ison, J. R., 208, 215
Ito, S., 355, 379
Ito, T., 164, 183
Iversen, S. D., 200, 218
Ivry, R., 260, 275, 41, 420, 519, 522

Jackson, G., 430, 440
Jackson, S., 35, 48
Jacobson, A., 303, 323
James, W., 4, 5, 12, 14, 170, 183, 332, 349, 446, 458, 463, 484
Jane, J. A., 239, 251
Janer, K. W., 115–116, 120, 406–407, 413–414, 421
Janowsky, J. S., 154, 158, 161

Jarrett, N., 439–440
Jasper, H. H., 38, 49
Jeffreys, D. A., 77, 92
Jenkins, I. H., 111–112, 116–117, 119, 465, 481
Jennings, C., 202, 215
Jennings, R., 240, 256
Jerabek, P., 109, 115, 122
Jerison, H. J., 221–222, 224, 245, 247, 251–252, 255
Jervey, J. P., 149, 158
Jesmanowicz, A., 130, 140
Jetter, W., 154, 158
Jewett, D. L., 77, 92
Jezzard, P., 124–126, 130, 134, 141–142
Jiang, Q., 222, 231, 253
Joanette, Y., 271, 275, 471, 481
Joel, D., 209, 215
Johannes, S., 84, 92, 101, 109, 119, 148, 158, 223, 251, 363, 366, 379, 409, 421
John, E. R., 150, 161
Johnson, D., 170, 186
Johnson, K. O., 165, 183
Johnson, M. H., 427–435, 437–439, 441–442
Johnson, R., Jr., 151, 158, 160
Johnston, J. C., 12, 14, 169–170, 183–184, 355, 380, 404, 422
Johnston, W. A., 4–5, 12, 14
Jolesz, F. A., 527, 535, 537, 545–546
Jones, D. N. C., 195, 200–201, 206, 211, 215, 218
Jones, E. G., 27, 32
Jones, T., 99, 121
Jonides, J., 6, 15, 60, 69, 85, 92, 112–114, 121, 169, 176, 183, 186, 310, 325, 353–354, 363, 369–372, 374–375, 378–380, 405, 418, 421, 423, 433, 442, 465–466, 484
Jorm, A. F., 466, 484
Joseph, J. S., 285–286, 290, 297, 310
Joseph, M. H., 209, 215
Judge, S. J., 57, 69
Julesz, B., 61, 69, 170, 176, 185, 280, 284, 293, 297, 327–329, 336–337, 340, 344–346, 348–350
Jung, T. P., 229, 252
Junque, C., 146, 162
Jurado, M. A., 146, 162
Jurica, P. J., 154, 161
Jusczyk, P. W., 439, 442
Jutagir, R., 475, 483

Kaas, J. H., 28, 32, 257, 277
Kadekard, M., 97, 122

Kahn, S., 285, 297, 299, 324, 341, 349
Kahneman, D., 283, 297, 301, 305–306, 323, 325, 385, 397
Kaiser, T., 201, 211, 216
Kalmijn, S., 477, 483
Kandel, E. R., 514–542
Kanizsa, G., 282, 287, 297
Kanter, D. R., 221, 250
Kanwisher, N. G., 6, 14, 103, 109, 119, 299, 323
Kaplan, A., 477, 487
Kapur, S., 152, 154, 158, 161–162
Karapelou, M., 534, 545
Karis, D., 153, 159
Karnath, H. O., 506, 523
Karni, A., 134, 141
Karron, D., 76, 93
Katz, D., 388, 397
Katz, S., 353, 378
Katz, W. F., 105, 118, 388, 396
Kaufman, L., 76, 93
Kawashima, R., 130, 132, 141
Kaye, J. A., 468, 478, 486
Keele, S. W., 415, 418–420
Keil, K., 113–114, 117, 124, 126, 128, 130–132, 134–137, 140–141, 370–372, 374–375, 378
Keilp, J. G., 529, 543
Kelley, K. L., 200, 213
Kemner, C., 231, 252
Kemper, T., 462, 484
Kenemans, J. L., 231, 252
Kennard, C., 111–112, 117, 131, 142, 465, 481
Kennard, M. A., 413, 421
Kennedy, D. N., 96, 107, 117, 121, 124, 142, 144, 159, 455, 457
Kershner, J. R., 456, 458
Kertzman, C., 204, 213, 478, 487
Ketter, T. A., 406–408, 420
Kety, S. S., 98, 119
Kihlstrom, J. F., 539, 544
Kikinis, R., 527, 535, 537, 545–546
Kilduff, P. T., 518, 523
Killcross, A. S., 209–210, 216, 218, 220
Kim, M. S., 88, 92
Kim, S. G., 95, 120, 124, 142, 388, 397
Kimble, M. O., 534, 537, 545
Kinchla, R. A., 332, 349
King, A. C., 240–242, 250
King, F. A., 26, 34
King, J. W., 390, 397
Kingstone, A., 435, 442, 468, 484

Kinomura, S., 8, 14, 225, 239, 241, 244, 252
Kinsbourne, M., 314, 320, 323, 504, 506, 523
Kinsella, G., 520, 523
Kinsora, J. J., 199, 213
Kirkby, D. L., 195, 215
Kirsch, N. L., 505, 521
Kishiyama, S. S., 468, 478, 486
Kleefield, J., 367, 380
Kleffener, D. A., 281, 297
Klein, G. S., 408, 421
Klein, R. M., 9, 14, 85, 91, 435, 442, 464, 468,
    482, 484
Klein, S. K., 241, 252
Klem, G., 147, 159
Klorman, R., 229, 255
Knierim, J. J., 61, 63, 68, 330–331, 349–350
Knight, R. A., 532, 544
Knight, R. T., 144–149, 151–152, 154, 156–
    157, 159–161, 261, 263–266, 268, 276,
    506–507, 522, 524
Knowlton, B., 6, 15
Koch, C., 8, 15, 53, 59, 67, 69, 164, 167, 174–
    176, 178–180, 182–185, 293, 297, 273,
    277, 329–330, 342–343, 346, 348–349,
    463–464, 471, 484
Kodaka, Y., 355–356, 379
Kodsi, M. H., 208, 216
Koek, W., 201, 216
Koelega, H. S., 44, 49, 226, 231, 252
Koenig, O., 9, 14, 319, 323
Koeppe, R. A., 112–114, 121, 353, 369–372,
    374–375, 378–380, 406–408, 418, 421,
    423, 433, 442
Koffka, K., 282, 297
Kohn, C., 519, 522
Kolb, B., 144, 159, 387, 393–394, 397
Kooistra, C. A., 507, 523
Kopriva, K., 229, 251
Kornblum, S., 406–408, 423
Kornetsky, C., 191, 216, 528–529, 544–546
Kosslyn, S. M., 9, 14, 144, 159, 233, 255, 319,
    323, 366, 377, 379
Kovelman, J. A., 527, 544
Kowler, E., 285, 292, 297
Koyama, S., 534, 544
Kraepelin, E., 528, 544
Kramer, A. F., 303, 323–324
Krantz, J., 430, 443
Kraus, N., 147, 159
Krauter, E. E., 208, 215
Krener, P., 452, 457
Kristofferson, A. B., 202, 216
Kritchevsky, M., 154, 158

Krkovic, A., 229, 250
Kroll, J. F., 394, 397
Krubitzer, L. A., 28
Krueger, G. P., 226, 252
Ksir, C., 202, 217
Kubiak, P., 44, 49, 228, 236, 249
Kubota, K., 355–356, 379
Kuhl, D. E., 96, 120–121
Kulanski, R., 131, 141
Kuljis, R. O., 480, 484
Kutas, M., 146, 148, 150, 160–161, 382–383,
    390, 392, 394–397, 533, 544
Kuypers, H. G. J. M., 21, 27, 31, 33
Kwak, H., 171, 176, 184
Kwapil, T. R., 533, 544
Kwong, K. K., 107, 121, 124, 131, 142

LaBerge, D., 6, 14, 35, 49, 228, 252, 300, 324,
    385, 397, 472, 478, 484
Lacey, 227, 252
Ladavas, E., 261, 277, 504, 508, 518, 523
Lai, Y., 59, 69
Laicona, M., 475, 482
Lalonde, F., 462, 485
Lamb, M. R., 507, 524
Landau, W. M., 98, 119
Lane, D. M., 437, 442
Lang, K., 177, 183
Lapierre, M. F., 148, 160
Larsson, J., 8, 14, 225, 239, 241, 244, 252
La Rue, A., 477, 487
Latz, E., 431, 443
Lauterborn, J. C., 101, 119
LaVail, J. H., 21, 32
LaVail, M. M., 21, 32
Lavie, N., 306, 308, 325
Law, I., 385, 397
Law, S., 534, 545
Lawrence, A. D., 463, 484
Lawson, D. S., 83, 93, 390, 398
Lazarus, J., 221, 251
LeBihan, D., 124, 142
Lecours, A. R., 519, 521
Ledoux, J. E., 516, 525
Lee, A. T., 128, 141
Lee, K., 343–344, 351
Lees, J. L., 233, 252
LeMay, M., 527, 537, 546
Lent, C., 43, 49
Leonard, C. M., 308, 322
Lerner, M., 445, 448, 459
Leser, R. P., 147, 159
Leuders, H., 147, 159

Leuschow, A., 213–214
Levander, M., 496, 524
Levere, T. E., 148, 157
Levine, D. N., 261, 276
Levy, B. S., 413, 419
Levy, J., 225, 243, 254
Levy, R., 195, 218, 463, 487
Lewin, J. S., 241, 252
Lewis, J. L., 229, 255
Lewis, T. L., 430, 442
Lhermitte, F., 146, 159
Li, C. S., 261, 275
Li, L., 101–102, 119, 172, 184, 331, 346, 349
Lickey, M. E., 41–42, 45, 50
Liddle, P. F., 99–100, 116, 118, 134, 138, 141, 391, 396
Liebenauer, L. L., 454, 460
Lieke, E. E., 97, 118
Lindsey, D. T., 80, 93
Lindsley, D. B., 227–228, 230, 251–252
Lines, C. R., 83, 93
Linnett, C. M., 285, 298, 341–342, 350
Liotti, M., 410, 423
Lippa, A. S., 463, 481
Livingstone, M. S., 89, 92, 532, 544
Lo, A., 221, 254
Lobeck, L. J., 28, 32
Loc'h, C., 528, 544
Loeb, M., 233, 252
Loewe, H., 21, 31
Lofving, B., 238, 250
Logan, G. D., 381, 394, 397
Loney, J., 450, 458
Loo, H., 528, 544
Lopez, O. L., 480, 483
Loring, D. W., 42, 49
Lorys, A. R., 454, 458
Lou, H. C., 454, 458
Lu, Z. L., 76, 93
Lubow, R. E., 209, 216
Luck, S. J., 61, 63, 68, 77, 80, 83–92, 130, 142, 148, 158, 169, 184, 223, 251, 273, 277, 300, 331–332, 349–350, 403, 421, 464–465, 479, 484–485, 537, 544
Luechter, A. F., 481, 485
Lueck, C. J., 131, 142
Lueschow, A., 113, 117, 173, 182
Luria, A. R., 269, 277, 319, 324, 445, 458
Luzzatti, C., 519, 521
Lynch, J. C., 28, 32, 57, 68, 356, 379
Lyon, D. R., 85, 91, 170, 182

MacCrimmon, D. J., 531, 542
MacDonald, B., 107, 121

Mack, A., 285, 297–299, 312–313, 324, 341–342, 349–350
Mackeben, M., 285, 297, 333, 344, 350
Mackintosh, N. J., 209, 216
Mackworth, J. F., 196, 216
Mackworth, N. H., 199, 216, 221–222, 226, 232, 236, 252
MacLeod, A. M. K., 100, 116, 120, 394, 398, 406, 422
MacLeod, C. M., 389, 395, 405, 421
Macmillan, N. A., 222, 252, 332, 349
Maddox, T., 260, 275
Magoun, H. W., 221, 227, 232, 239, 253
Maher, B. A., 533, 544, 546
Maher, L. M., 382, 398
Mahowald, M., 167, 182
Maier, S., 533, 546
Maisog, J. M., 24, 32, 101–102, 107–108, 112, 119, 124, 128, 130–132, 134, 140–141, 478, 484, 479
Makeig, S., 229–231, 252
Malach, R., 107, 121, 131, 142
Malik, J., 329, 349
Maljkovic, V., 292–295, 297
Malmo, R. R., 148, 159
Malone, M. A., 456, 458
Malone, V., 414, 421, 465–466, 469, 475, 485
Malpelli, J. G., 24, 33
Mandelkern, M. A., 477, 487
Mangels, J. A., 154, 161
Mangun, G. R., 77, 83–84, 86–87, 92, 101, 109, 119, 130, 142, 148–149, 158–159, 169, 184, 223, 251, 353, 355, 363, 366, 379, 403, 409, 421, 537, 544
Manil, J., 150, 157
Marinkovic, K., 145, 151, 158
Mark, V. W., 507, 523
Markham, J., 98, 120
Markowitsch, H. J., 152, 154, 158, 162
Marks, J., 404, 421
Marr, D. E., 99, 105, 119, 308, 316–317, 324
Marret, S., 100, 122
Marrocco, R. T., 27, 32, 40–43, 45–46, 48, 50, 197, 203–204, 205, 212, 220
Marsh, W. L., 454, 457
Marshall, J. F., 206, 215
Marshall, J. C., 316, 324, 493, 508, 511–512, 515, 518, 521–523, 524
Martin, A., 382, 398, 462, 485–486
Martin, C., 109, 115, 122
Martin, J., 527, 537, 546
Martin, K., 53, 67
Martin, K. A., 167, 182

Martin, W. R. W., 98, 120
Martinez, A. L., 480, 485
Martinot, J. L., 528, 544
Maruff, P., 414, 421, 465–466, 469, 475, 485
Marzloff, K., 479, 481
Masliah, E., 475, 487
Massman, P. J., 473–476, 483, 485
Mata, M., 97, 101, 121
Matier-Sharma, K., 451, 458
Matthews, G., 233, 252
Matthews, P. M., 124, 142
Mattingley, J. B., 315, 318, 322, 324
Matzke, M., 109, 115, 122
Mauguiere, F., 27–28, 30–31
Maunsell, J. H. R., 22–23, 32, 61, 63, 67–68,
    89, 93, 104, 107–108, 119, 213, 216, 327,
    329, 331, 349
Maurer, D., 430, 442
May, P., 171, 185, 236, 252
Mayeux, R., 465, 487
Maylor, E. A., 7, 15, 434–435, 442
Maziere, B., 528, 544
Mazoyer, B., 111–112, 120, 478–479, 486,
    528, 544
Mazziotta, J. C., 96, 100, 107, 120, 122, 131,
    142, 434, 441, 477, 487
McAndrews, M. P., 154, 159
McArthur-Jackson, C., 414, 421, 475, 485
McBurnett, K., 445, 448, 452, 459
McCann, R. S., 12, 14
McCarley, R. W., 221, 253, 527, 530, 532–
    535, 537–539, 543–546
McCarthy, G., 151, 159, 373–375, 379, 381–
    383, 388–392, 397–398, 533, 542
McCarthy, R., 240, 256
McClelland, J. E., 9, 15
McCloskey, M., 144, 161
McCormick, D. A., 38, 49
McCracken, J. T., 43, 50
McGaughy, J., 44, 49, 200, 203, 211, 216, 222,
    228, 247, 252
McGlinchey-Berroth, R., 518, 523
McGrath, S., 438, 441
McGuinness, E., 329–330, 347
McIntosh, A. R., 135, 138, 142, 159, 160
McKay, D. P. O., 404, 423
McKenna, P. J., 210, 215
McLaughlin, J. R., 58, 60, 69, 177, 185
Mclaughlin, T., 385, 397
McLeod, P., 89, 93, 301, 310, 324
McNaughton, B. L., 55, 69
McPeek, R. M., 144, 159, 165, 184, 293, 295,
    297
McWilliam, J., 533, 542

Meador, K. J., 42, 49
Mecklinger, A., 229, 254
Meissner, J., 229, 251
Melchner, J. J., 283, 298
Melchner, M. J., 333–335, 351
Meltzer, H., 241, 252
Meltzoff, A. N., 417, 421
Menon, R., 527, 542
Merkel, F., 201, 217
Messerli, P., 314, 323
Mesulam, M. M., 27–28, 31–33, 35, 49, 60,
    68, 110, 120, 152, 160, 235, 239, 253–
    354, 360–362, 366–367, 377, 379–380,
    462, 469, 477–479, 482, 485–486, 494,
    524
Metcalf, D., 527, 537, 546
Metcalfe, J., 152–153, 160
Meyer, D. E., 409, 420
Meyer, E., 388–389, 394, 396, 398
Meyer, G., 131, 141
Meyer, J., 478–479, 486
Michiels, J., 109, 112, 122
Miezin, F. M., 35, 48, 101, 104–111, 114–
    121, 130, 141, 154, 157, 161, 212, 214, 270,
    276, 329–330, 347, 362–365, 367, 378–
    379, 384, 388, 396, 403, 411, 419, 465, 479,
    482, 537, 543
Mikami, A., 355–356, 379
Milar, K. S., 189, 213
Milberg, W. P., 388, 397, 518, 523
Milewski, A., 430, 442
Milich, R., 450, 458
Miller, D. A., 214, 252
Miller, E. K., 11, 14, 64–65, 67, 101–102, 113,
    117, 119, 172–174, 182, 184, 213–214,
    331, 346, 348–349
Miller, G. A., 287, 297
Miller, J., 336–337, 339, 347, 349
Miller, J. D., 239, 254
Miller, J. G., 190, 219
Miller, M. B., 531, 544
Mills, D. L., 390, 398
Milner, A. D., 83, 93, 205, 207, 216, 257, 277,
    496, 524
Milner, B., 144, 154, 158–160, 168, 183, 362,
    378
Minoshima, S., 112–114, 121, 369–372, 374–
    375, 379, 406–408, 423, 433, 442
Mintun, M. A., 98–100, 115–116, 118, 120,
    362, 369–372, 374–375, 378–379, 385,
    398, 405–408, 419, 422, 433, 442
Mintz, J., 532, 543
Mirsky, A. F., 191, 218, 221, 236–237, 253–
    254, 260, 528–529, 544–545

Mishkin, M., 5, 14, 22, 24, 32–34, 134, 138, 141, 168, 185, 537, 543
Miyake, S., 164, 183
Miyatani, M., 534, 544
Miyazato, Y., 534, 544
Moberg, P. J., 385, 390, 397, 399
Mobley, S., 46, 50
Moe, L., 21, 32
Mohler, C. W., 60, 69, 359, 379
Mohr, J. P., 26, 32
Mohs, R. C., 528, 543
Molet, J., 146, 162
Molloy, R., 221, 238, 256
Monheit, M. A., 516, 522
Monsell, S., 403–404, 422
Moore, C. M., 65, 68
Moore, E. E., 42, 49
Moore, G., 52, 68, 179, 184
Moore, H., 228, 247, 253
Moran, J., 61–62, 68, 84, 93, 103, 109, 113, 119, 130, 142, 166, 178, 184, 257, 276, 309, 324, 330–331, 348–349, 351, 357, 359, 379, 403, 423, 479, 485, 537, 544, 546
Morant, N. J., 463, 487
Moray, N., 3–4, 14, 404, 421
Morecraft, R. J., 28, 33, 35, 49, 235, 253
Morey, M., 475, 487
Morlock, H. C., 230, 256
Morrison, J. H., 481, 485
Morrow, L. A., 516, 522
Mortelmans, L., 105, 107, 109, 111–112, 118, 122, 364–365, 367, 378, 380
Morton, J., 431, 438–439, 442
Moruzzi, G., 221, 227, 232, 239, 253
Moscovitch, M., 154, 161, 261, 276, 317–318, 322, 515, 521
Motter, B. C., 57–58, 60–61, 63–64, 66, 68, 105, 113, 119, 166, 175, 184, 300, 331, 350, 359, 379, 403, 421, 479, 485
Mouloua, M., 80, 85, 92, 223, 246, 251, 253, 332, 349, 464–465, 484–485
Mountcastle, V. B., 57–58, 60, 68–69, 105, 119, 166, 175, 184, 356, 379
Movshon, J. A., 328, 348
Mozer, M., 164, 184, 318, 322
Mueller, H. J., 332, 350
Mugnaini, E., 20, 31
Muir, J. L., 46, 49, 193, 196–198, 200, 202–203, 209–211, 217–218
Mulhall, B., 475, 485
Mulle, C., 43, 49
Muller, H. J., 164, 169–170, 183–184, 466, 485

Münte, T. F., 84, 92, 101, 109, 119, 148, 158, 363, 366, 379
Muntel, T. F., 223, 251, 409, 421
Murphy, A. Z., 246, 255
Musen, G., 6, 15
Mutter, S. A., 221, 238, 254
Myers, R., 107, 122, 131, 142

Näätänen, R., 11, 14, 234, 248, 253, 409, 421
Nadeau, S. E., 382, 385, 397, 399, 456, 458
Nageishi, Y., 534, 544
Nakagawa, A., 393, 397, 412, 421
Nakayama, K., 89, 93, 165, 170, 184, 282, 285–297, 304, 309–310, 323, 329–330, 333, 341, 344, 346, 348, 350, 470, 485
Nalcioglu, O. N., 454, 457–458
Nauta, W. J. H., 20, 33, 156, 160
Navon, D., 474, 485
Neale, J. M., 530–531, 542–544
Nealey, T. A., 61, 63, 68
Nebes, R. D., 461–462, 471–472, 465, 485
Neelin, P., 100, 122
Neisser, U., 4, 14, 164, 167, 183, 280, 298, 301, 312, 314, 324, 341, 350
Neitz, J., 105, 117
Nelson, B., 308–309, 323
Nelson, J., 177, 184
Nelson, S. B., 53, 69
Nespoulous, J. L., 387, 391, 396
Nestor, P. G., 191, 221, 252–253, 462, 486, 530, 532–535, 537, 544–545
Neville, H. J., 83, 93, 145–146, 148–150, 159–161, 390, 398
Newcorn, N., 449, 451, 457–458
Newell, A., 401–402, 421
Newsome, W. T., 22, 32, 53, 69, 328, 332, 348, 350
Newton, T. F., 481, 485
Ng, K., 520, 523
Nguyen, T., 390, 399
Nicholas, J., 331, 350
Nicholas, T., 453, 459
Nichols, M. E., 42, 49
Niebur, E., 8, 15, 170, 172–177, 179–180, 183–185, 463
Nigam, A., 533, 545
Nigg, J., 452, 458
Nimmo-Smith, I., 221, 254
Nishihara, H. K., 308, 316–317, 324
Nissen, M., 168, 171, 184
Nixon, P. D., 116–117, 119, 409, 420
Niznikiewicz, M. A., 534, 545
Nobel, B., 21, 32

Nobre, A. C., 110, 373–375, 379, 382–383, 388–390, 392, 398, 478–479, 486
Nordahl, T. T., 454, 460
Nordahl, T. E., 240–242, 250
Nordstrom, A. L., 528, 543
Norman, D. A., 7, 15, 233, 253, 283, 286, 298, 402, 409, 421
Nothcutt, C., 452, 457
Nothdurft, H. C., 329, 350
Novak, G. P., 452–453, 458
Nuechterlein, K. H., 222, 231, 240, 250, 253, 529, 532, 543, 545
Nuflo, F., 59, 69
Nunez, P. L., 75–76, 93
Nutt, D., 228, 255
Nuyts, J., 105, 107, 118

O'Craven, K. M., 128, 131, 140
O'Donnell, B. F., 534, 535, 537, 545
Ogawa, S., 95, 120, 124, 142
Ogura, C., 534, 544
O'Hanlon, J. F., 229, 253
Ohta, S., 107, 121
Ojemann, G. A., 384, 387, 398
Ojemann, J. G., 101, 121, 154, 157, 161
O'Keefe, J., 495, 524
Oken, B. S., 468, 478, 486
O'Leary, D. S., 154, 157, 527, 545
Oliver, J., 520, 523
Oliver, L. M., 202, 215, 406–408, 423
Olsen, C. R., 28, 31
Olshausen, B. A., 59, 68, 101, 120, 175, 177, 184
Olson, A., 301, 323
Olson, C. R., 155, 122, 321, 326
Oltmanns, T. F., 530, 544
Olton, D. S., 46, 50, 201–202, 204, 211, 213, 217, 219, 463, 487
Ommaya, A., 239, 253
Oram, M. W., 309, 324
Orban, G. A., 53, 69, 105, 107, 109, 111–112, 118, 122, 364–365, 367, 378, 380
O'Reilly, G., 367, 380
Oriowo, M. A., 45, 49
Orren, M. M., 237, 253
Orssaud, C., 111–112, 120, 478–479, 486
Orzack, M. H., 528–529, 545
Osborne-Shaefer, P., 367, 380
O'Scalaidhe, S. P., 23, 34
O'Shaughness, D. M., 165, 183
Oshiro, W. M., 204, 214
Osterhout, L., 382, 398
Ostry, D., 404, 421

O'Sullivan, B. T., 130, 132, 141
Ott, H., 229, 254
Ottolini, Y., 452, 458
Owen, A. M., 210, 217, 369–375, 379, 463, 481
Ozdamar, O., 147, 159
Ozonoff, S., 450, 452, 458

Pachtman, E., 531, 543
Packer, S., 520, 523
Padovani, A., 520, 522
Paladini, R., 518, 523
Paller, K. A., 150, 160
Palmer, J., 80, 93
Palumbo, C. L., 154, 161
Pandya, D. N., 23, 27–28, 33–34, 145, 160, 368, 379, 430, 443
Pang, K., 201–202, 217
Pantano, P., 520, 522
Pantev, C., 81, 93
Papanicolaou, A. C., 240, 250
Parasuraman, R., 5–7, 11, 13, 15, 44, 46, 49, 131, 141, 191–192, 200–201, 217, 221–222, 224–225, 231–233, 235, 237–238, 245–248, 250, 253–254, 382, 398, 450–451, 458, 461–463, 465–468, 471–475, 477–479, 483, 486, 529–530, 545
Pardo, J. V., 100, 115–116, 120, 240–241, 244, 254, 394, 398, 406–407, 413–414, 421–422
Pardo, P. J., 35, 47, 49, 115–116, 120, 406–407, 414, 421–422
Parekh, P. I., 406–408, 420
Parving, A., 385, 397
Pashler, H., 6, 14, 335, 350, 404, 421–422, 464, 482
Passingham, R. E., 116–117, 119, 409, 419
Pathria, M. N., 207, 214
Patlak, C. S., 96, 121
Patterson, K., 384, 387, 389, 397–398
Paul, B., 199, 214
Paulesu, E., 388, 398, 406–407, 419
Pauling, L., 124, 142
Paulsen, J., 476, 483
Pearson, D. A., 437, 442, 527, 542
Peloquin, L. J., 229, 255
Pelz, J., 171, 182
Penhune, V., 532–533, 544
Pennekamp, P., 229, 254
Pennington, B. F., 449–450, 452, 458
Perachio, N., 451, 458
Perani, D., 361, 380, 519, 521
Perenyl, A., 528, 543

Pericak-Vance, M. A., 477, 482, 487
Perkel, D. H., 52, 68, 179, 184
Perlmutter, R. A., 229, 255
Péron-Magnan, P., 528, 544
Perona, P., 329, 349
Perret, E., 407, 422
Perrett, D. I., 309, 324
Peters, S. L., 209, 215
Petersen, S. E., 7, 12, 15, 19, 26, 28, 33, 35–
  36, 43, 48–49, 95, 99–101, 104–111, 114–
  121, 128, 130, 140–141, 154, 157, 161,
  174, 185, 203, 205, 211–212, 214, 217,
  226, 236–237, 240–242, 254, 270, 276,
  330, 350, 355, 362–365, 367, 378–381,
  383–385, 388–389, 391, 394, 396, 398,
  403, 405–406, 419, 422, 434, 442, 452,
  458, 462, 465, 471, 478–479, 48 2, 486–
  487, 502–503, 524, 537, 543
Peterson, A., 530, 544
Petit, L., 111–112, 120, 478–479, 486
Petrides, M., 27, 33, 368–375, 379
Petrone, P. N., 261, 276
Petry, M. C., 385–386, 398
Pettigrew, K. D., 96, 121
Pfefferbaum, A., 534, 543
Pfittner, L., 448, 459
Phalp, R., 83, 93
Phelps, M. E., 96, 120–121, 434, 441, 477,
  487
Phillips, J. G., 496, 523
Picard, N., 115, 120
Pickett, R. M., 245, 247, 252
Picton, T. W., 7, 11, 14, 81, 92, 146, 158
Pierrot-Deseillingny, C., 469, 486
Pietrini, P., 24, 32, 101–102, 107–108, 112,
  119, 130, 132, 141, 478–479, 484
Pillon, B., 146, 159
Pineda, J. A., 150, 160
Pirozzolo, F., 468, 486
Pizzamiglio, L., 506, 520, 522, 524
Plaut, D., 308–309, 324
Plude, D. J., 461, 486
Pogue, J., 154, 161
Polansky, M., 238, 255
Poline, J. B., 109, 112, 122
Polkey, C. E., 210, 217
Pollack, S. D., 527, 537, 546
Pollak, S. D., 532–533, 535, 544
Pollatsek, A., 515, 524
Poncelet, B. P., 124, 142
Pons, T. P., 24, 33
Pontefract, A., 435, 442, 468, 484
Ponto, L. L., 154, 157

Porter, P. K., 242–243, 255
Poser, U., 154, 158
Posner, M. I., 6–7, 9, 11–12, 15, 19, 24, 26,
  28–29, 33, 35–36, 39, 43, 49, 58, 68, 85,
  93, 95, 99–101, 103–104, 109, 112, 114–
  116, 120–121, 148, 157, 171, 174, 184,
  198–199, 203, 205, 211, 223, 225–226,
  231, 235–237, 239, 241–243, 254, 259,
  267, 277, 299, 303, 309, 314, 324, 332, 350,
  355, 361–362, 380–381, 383, 385, 388–
  389, 391–392, 396, 399, 404–405, 409–
  412, 414–415, 417–418, 420, 422–423,
  428, 430, 434–435, 442–443, 446–453,
  455–456, 458–459, 462–469, 471–472,
  475, 478–479, 486, 499–500, 502–503,
  505, 515, 522, 524, 532, 545
Possamai, C. A., 336, 339, 347
Post, R. M., 406–408, 420
Potkin, S., 240, 250, 452–453, 459
Potts, G. F., 410, 423
Povlishock, J. T., 239, 254
Powell, T. P. S., 27, 32, 533, 542
Powers, R. E., 527, 542
Pratt, J., 334, 350
Preddie, D. C., 63, 67
Press, W. A., 61, 63, 68, 330–331, 350
Presti, D. E., 85, 93, 259, 277, 471, 486
Pretsell, D. O., 209, 218
Price, C. J., 384, 387, 396, 398
Price, D. L., 46, 50, 206, 219, 463, 487
Price, J. L., 21, 31
Printz, H., 196, 217
Prinzmetal, W., 85, 93, 259–260, 275, 277,
  309–310, 324, 471, 486
Provinciali, L., 504, 523
Puce, A., 151, 160, 373–375, 379
Pugh, K. R., 388, 399
Pujol, J., 146, 162
Puumala, T., 196, 217
Pylyshyn, Z., 301, 305, 324

Qiyuan, J., 529, 545
Quintana, G., 46, 50

Rabbitt, P. M. A., 169–170, 184, 466, 485
Radda, G. K., 124, 142
Rafal, R. D., 26, 33, 144, 160, 204, 217, 261,
  270–271, 274, 276–277, 301, 303–305,
  313–314, 316, 318–319, 322–324, 361–
  362, 380, 385, 398, 418, 420, 430, 435, 443,
  465, 468–469, 478–479, 486, 499, 500–
  505, 509–513, 516–517, 519, 521–522,
  524

Raichle, M. E., 9, 15, 35, 47, 49, 95–96, 98–
    101, 105–106, 108, 115–116, 118, 120–
    121, 124, 128, 140–141, 154, 157, 161,
    235, 240–241, 244, 254, 267, 277, 362,
    378, 381, 384–385, 388–389, 391, 394,
    396, 398–399, 405–407, 409–412, 414–
    415, 420–423, 446–453, 455–456, 458
Rainnie, D. G., 538, 543
Rajkowski, J., 44, 49, 228, 234, 249
Ramachandran, V. S., 281, 285, 297–298
Ramsey, S., 387, 391, 396, 398
Raney, G. E., 382, 392, 395–396, 398
Rappoport, S. I., 24, 32, 115, 119, 134–135,
    138, 141–142, 149, 160, 462, 465, 477,
    480–481, 483–484, 537, 543
Rascol, A., 387, 391, 396
Rauch, S. L., 107, 117
Rawlins, J. N. P., 209, 215
Raymer, A. M., 385, 399
Raymond, J. E., 404, 422–423
Reader, M. J., 454, 456
Reader, T. A., 38, 49
Reading, P., 202, 217
Reed, T., 477, 486
Reeder, T. M., 199, 213
Reeves, G., 505, 521
Regli, F., 504, 525
Reiman, E. M., 99, 118, 362, 378, 414–415,
    420, 422
Reinikainen, K., 171, 185
Reinitz, M. T., 80, 93
Reiss, A. L., 454, 456
Reivich, M., 96, 121, 240, 254
Remington, R. W., 12, 14, 169–170, 183–184
Renault, B., 453, 458
Rensink, R. A., 281, 296
Reppas, J. B., 107, 121, 131, 142
Reval, K., 528, 543
Revelle, W., 233, 251
Reynolds, J., 61, 63, 68, 331, 350
Rezai, K., 154, 157
Richards, J. E., 435–436, 443, 463, 487
Richards, S., 527, 542
Richardson, C. M., 207, 214
Richardson, E. P., 26, 32
Richardson, R. T., 46, 50, 204, 219, 463, 487
Richelme, C., 455, 457
Richer, F., 148, 160
Richmond, B. J., 57–58, 68–69
Richter, D. O., 242–243, 255
Riddoch, M. J., 261–262, 277, 301, 319, 321,
    323, 520–521, 523
Riley, E., 521–522

Riley, R. G., 46, 50
Ring, H., 406–408, 420
Ritter, W., 151, 160
Rivaud, S., 469, 486
Rizzolatti, G., 205, 217, 495, 518, 521, 524
Ro, T., 504, 512, 524
Robaey, P., 453, 458
RoBards, M. J., 21, 32
Robbins, T. W., 27, 33, 36, 44, 46, 48–49,
    190–191, 193–197, 200–202, 206–212,
    214–218, 220, 226–228, 254, 462, 487
Roberts, A. C., 210, 214, 218
Roberts, R. C., 496, 524
Robertson, I. H., 221, 254, 521, 524
Robertson, L. C., 112, 118, 144, 160, 204, 217,
    261, 263–271, 276–277, 300, 319, 506–
    508, 522, 524
Robinson, D. L., 60, 66–67, 103, 105, 117,
    122, 166, 174–175, 182, 185, 204, 213,
    330, 350, 356, 365, 378, 478, 487
Robinson, F. R., 21, 31
Rock, I., 285, 298, 301, 313, 324, 341–342,
    349–350
Rockland, K. S., 23, 33, 429, 443
Roediger, H. L., 5, 15
Rogers, D. C., 207, 213
Rogers, R. D., 403–404, 422
Rohrbaugh, J. W., 231–232, 235, 254
Roland, L. P., 98, 119
Roland, P. E., 8, 14, 130, 132, 141, 149, 160,
    225, 239, 241, 244, 252
Rolls, E. T., 57, 69, 308, 322
Roman, M. J., 476, 483
Romani, C., 301, 323
Romero, R. D., 502–504, 522
Ronis, V., 201, 218
Rorden, C., 318, 322
Rosen, B. R., 107, 117, 121, 128, 131, 140,
    142
Rosen, J., 465, 487
Rosen, W., 465, 487
Rosenquist, A. C., 505, 525
Roses, A. D., 477, 482, 487
Rosier, A., 111, 122
Rosicky, J., 428, 443
Rosin, C., 175, 179, 184
Rosinsky, N., 406–408, 420
Ross, W., 164, 183
Rosvold, H. E., 191, 218, 237, 240, 253–254,
    528, 545
Roth, W. T., 534, 543
Rothbart, M. K., 26, 28, 33, 417, 422, 428,
    430, 435, 438, 442–443

Rothi, L. J. G., 382, 399
Rothman, D., 381, 391, 397
Rouleau, I., 148, 160
Rousseaux, M., 240, 251
Rovainen, C. M., 97, 99–100, 117
Rowell, P., 37, 43, 50
Roy, C. S., 124, 142
Rubens, A. B., 506, 524
Rubenstein, B. S., 329, 350
Rubin, E., 301, 307–308, 310, 325
Ruchkin, D. S., 151, 160
Rudolph, K. K., 107–108, 118
Rueckert, L. M., 225, 241, 243, 254
Ruffolo, R. R. Jr., 45, 49
Rugg, M. D., 83, 93, 151, 160
Ruland, S., 201, 218
Rumelhart, D. E., 9, 15, 128, 141
Rusconi, M. L., 496, 506, 521, 525
Russell, G. S., 410, 423
Rutter, M. L., 450, 459

Saarinen, J., 170, 185, 337, 350
Sacchett, C., 390, 399
Sacuzzo, D. P., 531–532, 542, 545–546
Saffran, E., 272, 274, 276
Sagi, D., 58, 61, 67, 69, 85, 91, 174, 176, 182,
    285, 296, 309, 322, 329, 337, 339, 348, 350
Sahakian, B. J., 195, 210, 215, 217–218, 463,
    479, 483–484, 487
Sahgal, A., 199, 201, 218
Saint-Cyr, J. A., 28, 33
Saint-Hilaire, J. M., 148, 160
Sakata, H., 57, 68
Sakurada, O., 96, 121
Salamon, G., 111–112, 120
Salisbury, D. F., 534–535, 545
Salmon, D. P., 474, 476, 483, 485
Salzman, C. D., 328, 332, 350
Salzman, L. F., 229, 255
Samanin, R., 197, 214
Sandell, J. H., 24, 33
Sanders, A. F., 451, 459
Sanderson, E., 37, 43, 50
Sandon, P. A., 177, 185
Sands, S. F., 221, 253, 530, 544–545
Sandson, J., 389, 398, 404, 422
Sanghera, M. K., 57, 69
Sano, M., 465, 487
Sarason, I., 191, 218, 237, 254, 528, 545
Sarter, M., 44, 49, 199–201, 203, 211, 214,
    216, 218, 222, 226, 228, 247, 252, 254, 528,
    546
Sato, T., 57–58, 68, 346, 350

Satterfield, J. H., 453, 459
Saunders, A. M., 477, 482, 487
Savaki, L., 97, 101, 121
Savoy, R. L., 128, 131, 140
Sayer, L., 154, 161
Scabini, D., 145, 147, 151, 159
Scalaidhe, S. P. O., 418, 423
Scerbo, M. W., 246, 254
Schacter, D. L., 5, 15
Schallert, T., 206–207, 218
Schapiro, M. B., 24, 32, 134, 138, 141, 537,
    543
Schauer, C. A., 385, 398
Scheibel, A. B., 527, 544
Schein, S. G., 330, 348
Schell, A. M., 404, 420, 453, 459
Scherg, M., 79, 84, 91–92, 101, 109, 119, 223,
    251, 363, 366, 379, 409, 421
Schiepers, C., 105, 107, 118
Schiller, P. H., 24, 33, 61, 63, 67, 104, 119,
    331, 343–344, 349, 351, 429, 443
Schlageter, N. L., 465, 477, 480–481, 484
Schmechel, D. E., 477, 482
Schmidt, A., 148, 160
Schmidt, C. F., 97, 121
Schmidt, H., 259, 278
Schmidt, W., 301, 324
Schmit, P. W., 105, 117
Schmitt, M., 336, 339, 347
Schneider, W., 6, 15, 24, 30–31
Schnorr, L., 99, 121
Scholtz, M., 84, 92, 101, 109, 119, 223, 251,
    363, 366, 379, 409, 421
Schomer, D. L., 367, 380
Schroeder, M. H., 453, 458
Schubert, D. L., 532, 546
Schumacher, E. H., 112–114, 121, 353, 378
Schumsky, D. A., 242–243, 248, 255
Schwartz, M. F., 462, 487
Schwartz, M. L., 27, 34, 145, 153, 158
Schwartz, W. J., 97, 101, 121
Schwarz, U., 204, 213
Schwent, V. L., 7, 11, 14, 81, 92
Scinto, L. F. M., 366, 377, 379, 469, 482, 487
Sclar, G., 61, 63, 68
Scoville, W. B., 144, 160
Sears, C., 301, 324
Sebesteyen, G. N., 110, 120, 478–479, 486
Sedvall, G., 528, 543
See, J. E., 7, 15, 191, 224, 254, 529–530, 546
Segundo, J., 179, 184
Sejnowski, T., 9, 14
Selemon, L. D., 28, 34, 145, 153, 158

Seltzer, B., 145, 160
Semple, W. E., 240–242, 250
Semrud-Clikeman, M., 454, 457–459
Serdaru, M., 146, 159
Sereno, M. I., 75, 77, 91
Sergeant, J. A., 446, 448, 451, 459
Sergent, J., 107, 121
Serota, H. M., 97, 121
Servan-Schrieber, D., 196, 219, 502–504, 522, 538–539, 542–543
Sestokas, A. K., 57, 68, 105, 119
Seyal, M., 504, 524
Shadach, E., 209, 215
Shadlen, M. N., 53, 69, 128, 141, 328, 348
Shaffer, D., 450, 459
Shaffer, W. O., 404, 423
Shalev, U., 209, 215
Shallice, T., 7, 15, 144, 154, 160, 205, 219, 240, 256, 402, 405, 409, 412, 421–422
Shankle, W. R., 454, 457
Shapiro, K. L., 170, 183, 337, 348, 404, 422–423, 464, 482
Shapiro, M., 462, 480, 483
Sharpe, J. A., 468–469, 483
Shaw, M. L., 223, 255, 332, 351
Shaywitz, B. A., 388, 399, 449, 459
Shaywitz, S. E., 388, 399, 449, 459
Shea, C., 452, 459
Shein, S. J., 257, 276
Shenton, M. E., 221, 253, 527, 532–535, 537, 544–546
Shepherd, G. M., 528, 546
Sherman, S. M., 167, 185
Sherman, T., 531, 542
Sherrington, C. S., 124, 142
Shiffrin, R. M., 6, 15, 404, 423
Shih, S., 168, 171, 185
Shimamura, A. P., 144, 146, 154, 158, 160–161
Shimojo, S., 282, 287, 295, 297
Shimokochi, M., 534, 544
Shimp, C. P., 204, 209, 219
Shinohara, O., 96, 121
Shipp, S., 107, 122, 131, 142
Sholl, A., 394, 397
Shulman, G. L., 35, 48, 104–111, 114–117, 120–121, 130, 141, 212, 214, 270, 276, 362–365, 367, 374, 378–379, 384, 389, 396, 398, 403–404, 419, 422, 465, 482, 471, 482, 537, 543
Shulman, R. G., 381, 391, 397
Shults, C. W., 476, 485
Shuren, J. E., 382, 399

Sicotte, N., 240, 250
Sieroff, E., 515, 524
Sikkema, R., 386, 396
Silbersweig, D. A., 99, 121
Sillito, A. M., 212, 219
Silverman, G. H., 89, 93, 289, 298, 309, 323, 470, 485
Simmons, R. F., 533, 545
Simon, H. A., 401–402, 421
Simpson, G. B., 411, 423
Singer, H. S., 454, 456–457
Singer, W., 273, 277
Sinkkonen, J., 234, 252
Sirvio, J., 195–196, 217, 219
Sjouw, W., 231, 252
Skinner, J. E., 146, 161, 227, 255
Skjoldager, P., 195, 197, 219
Skudlarski, P., 388, 399
Slaghuis, W. L., 532, 546
Slamecka, N. J., 210, 219
Slangen, J. L., 201, 216
Small, G. W., 477, 482, 487
Small, S. L., 390, 399
Smith Hammond, C., 382, 399
Smith, A., 228, 255
Smith, C. B., 97, 101, 121
Smith, E. E., 112–114, 121, 353, 369–372, 374–375, 378–380, 418, 421, 433, 442
Smith, J., 430, 443
Smith, L., 534, 545
Smith, M. C., 389, 395
Smith, M. E., 151, 161
Smith, R. S., 534–535, 537, 545
Snyder, A. Z., 101, 121, 384–385, 389, 391, 398–399, 410–411, 423
Snyder, C. R., 332, 350, 414, 422
Snyder, L. H., 261, 275
Sobel, D., 81, 93
Softky, W. R., 53, 69
Sokol, S. M., 144, 161
Sokoloff, L. M., 96–98, 101, 119, 121–122
Sokolov, E. N., 151, 161
Solanto, M., 452–453, 458
Sololoff, L. M., 96, 121
Som, P., 96, 121
Somers, D. C., 53, 69
Soncrant, T. T., 134, 138, 141
Sonuga-Barke, E., 452, 459
Sorenson, L., 243, 254
Spector, A., 404, 423
Spencer, D. D., 151, 159
Sperling, G., 168, 171, 185, 283, 298, 333–336, 338, 340, 346, 351

Spieler, D. H., 471, 487
Spiers, P. A., 367, 380
Spinnler, H., 475, 482
Spitzer, H. R., 58, 69, 331, 351, 403, 423, 533, 537, 546
Spong, P., 230, 251
Sprague, J. M., 505, 524
Sprague, R. L., 242–243, 255
Sprich, S., 449, 457
Squire, L. R., 5, 15, 101, 121, 154, 157–158, 161
Squires, K. C., 151, 161
Squires, N. K., 150–151, 157, 161
Stapleton, J. M., 151, 161, 231–232, 235, 254
Stark, R., 520, 523
Starr, A., 150, 157
Starrveveld, Y., 319, 323
Stechler, G., 431, 443
Steele-Russell, I. S., 207, 214
Stein, J. F., 339, 347
Stein, L., 147, 159
Steinberg, B., 385, 397
Steingard, R. J., 454, 457
Steinmetz, M. A., 57–58, 60, 68–69, 105, 119, 177, 185, 478, 487
Stemmler, M., 177, 185
Stephens, D. N., 199, 218
Steriade, M., 227–228, 239, 255
Stern, E., 99, 121
Stern, Y., 465, 487
Sternberg, S., 99, 121, 446, 459
Steronko, R. J., 532, 546
Sterzi, R., 506, 521, 525
Steward, O., 239, 251
Stickgold, R., 233, 255
Stillman, A. E., 388, 397
Stoehr, J. D., 46, 50
Stone-Elander, S. S., 528, 543
Stookey, B., 143, 161
Storm, R. W., 305, 324
Strauss, J., 229, 255
Stricanne, B., 261, 275
Strick, P. L., 28, 30, 115, 120
Strittmatter, W. J., 477, 482
Stroop, J. R., 405, 423
Strupp, B. J., 196, 213
Sturge, C., 450, 459
Stuss, D. T., 145–146, 154, 161, 361, 378
Styles, E., 404, 419
Suarez, H., 167, 182
Suaud-Chagny, M. F., 45, 48
Sullivan, E. V., 413, 419

Sullivan, H. G., 239, 256
Sundaram, M., 462, 480, 483
Sur, M., 53, 59
Sutton, J., 107, 117
Sutton, S., 150, 161
Suzuki, S., 282, 298
Swan, G. E., 477, 486
Swanson, J. M., 445, 448, 451–453, 456, 458, 459
Swayze, V., 527, 542
Swenson, M., 476, 483
Swerdlow, N. R., 208, 219, 476, 483
Swets, J. A., 222, 251, 327, 332, 349
Swick, D., 144–146, 148, 150–151, 154, 161

Taib, C.-T., 209, 215
Talairach, J., 99, 121
Talbot, W. H., 57, 68, 356, 379
Tallal, P., 105, 118, 376, 388
Tandon, R., 528, 546
Tang, B., 285, 297, 299, 324, 341, 349
Tang, J., 319, 323
Tank, D. W., 95, 120, 124, 142
Tannock, R., 452
Tarm, L., 448, 459
Tarrasch, R., 209, 215
Taylor, J., 124, 142
Taylor, S. F., 406–408, 423
Tegner, R., 221, 256, 496, 524
Teichner, W. H., 222, 241, 255
Teitelbaum, P., 206, 215
Teleska, P., 462, 485
Ter-Pogossian, M. M., 96, 121
Thaiss, L., 475, 487
Tham, K., 221, 254, 303, 324
Tham, M. P., 643, 487
Thomas, L., 24, 30–31
Thomas-Thrapp, L., 417, 422
Thompson, L. A., 241, 252
Thompson, W., 366, 377, 379
Thulborn, K. R., 124, 142
Tiitinen, H., 171, 185, 236, 252
Tipper, S. P., 6, 15, 174, 185, 300, 304–306, 313, 317, 325, 437, 443, 514, 521
Tissot, T., 314, 323
Tobin, J. R., 46, 50206, 219, 463, 487
Tooby, J., 15
Tootell, R. B. H., 107, 121, 131, 142
Tournoux, P., 99, 121
Townsend, J., 167, 185, 438, 443
Townsend, V., 61, 67
Tranel, D., 390, 396

Treisman, A. M., 12, 15, 80, 85, 93, 111–112, 118, 121, 164, 169, 174, 185, 258–260, 262, 264, 269–271, 277–278, 280, 284, 290, 298, 301, 305–306, 309–310, 323, 325, 327–329, 340–341, 346, 351, 403, 423, 464, 470–471, 487, 506, 525
Trick, L., 301, 324
Trimble, M. R., 406–408, 420
Tsal, Y., 306, 308, 325
Tso, D. Y., 97, 118
Tsotsos, J., 167, 185
Tsotsos, J. K., 59, 69
Tucker, D. M., 148, 157, 383, 392, 396, 409–410, 414, 420, 423
Tucker, L. A., 434–435, 437, 442
Tulving, E., 5–6, 15, 152, 154, 158, 161–162, 391, 396
Tuma, R., 285, 297, 299, 324, 341, 349
Tune, L. E., 527, 542
Turchi, J., 200, 203, 213
Turner, R., 124–126, 130, 134, 141–142
Turpin, M., 202, 215
Twitchell, T. E., 413, 419
Tzourio, N., 111–112, 120, 478–479, 486

Ullman, S., 167, 172, 174, 183, 185, 329–330, 342, 346, 349, 464, 484
Ungerleider, L. G., 22–24, 28, 30–34, 96, 101–103, 107–108, 112–115, 117–119, 124, 126, 128, 130–132, 134–138, 140–142, 149, 160, 168, 185, 257, 276, 278, 330–331, 348, 351, 368, 370–372, 374–375, 377–378, 380, 478–479, 484, 537, 543
Uhourzorn, N., 448, 459
Usher, M., 170, 172–174, 177, 185

Vaituzis, A. C., 454, 457
Valenstein, E., 26, 32, 145, 158, 261, 177, 207, 219, 495, 523
Valentino, D. A., 229, 255
Vallar, G., 19, 26, 31, 361, 367, 380, 506–508, 521, 525
Van den Abell, T., 239, 251
Vanderberghe, R., 109, 111–112, 122, 364–365, 367, 378, 380
Van Der Kooy, D., 21, 31
Van der Meere, J., 451, 159
Van Essen, D. C., 22–23, 31–32, 59, 61, 63, 67–68, 89, 91, 96, 101, 103, 118, 120, 175, 177, 181–184, 257, 276, 329–331, 348–351
Van Hoesen, G. W., 27–28, 33–34, 527, 542
Van Leeuwen, T. H., 231, 252

Van Petten, C., 392, 399, 533, 542
Van Voorhis, S. T., 83, 93
Van Wolffelaar, P. C., 238, 250
Vargha-Khadem, F., 430, 440
Vaughan, H. G., 75, 91, 93
Vaughan, J., 435, 443, 468, 486
Vavrik, M., 469, 486
Vecera, S. P., 301, 308–309, 318, 323, 325
Veeraswamy, S., 109, 115, 122
Vendrell, P., 146, 162
Verbaten, M. N., 231, 252
Verfaellie, M., 518, 523
Verleger, R., 151, 162
Videen, T. O., 100–101, 116, 120–121, 154, 161, 394, 398, 406, 422
Vignal, J. P., 145, 151, 158
Villareal, M., 40–42, 48
Virzi, R. A., 64, 67, 170, 183
Voellar, K. K. S., 451, 456, 458, 459
Vogel, R., 105, 122
Vogels, R., 53, 59, 107, 118
Vogt, B. A., 28, 34, 115, 122
Volpe, B. T., 516, 525
von Restorff, H., 153, 162
Voytko, M. L., 46, 50, 204, 211, 219, 463, 487
Vuileumier, P., 504, 525

Wai, W. Y. K., 59, 69
Waldman, I., 450, 458
Waldo, M. C., 531, 342–543
Walker, E., 532, 543
Walker, J. A., 267, 277, 314, 324, 361–362, 380, 465, 469, 486, 478, 486, 499, 500–502, 515, 522, 524
Wall, T. L., 150, 157
Wallace, M. A., 276, 317–318, 323, 515, 522
Wallace, S. F., 505, 525
Walsh, 112
Walter, D. O., 481, 485
Wandell, B. A., 128, 141
Wang, Q., 281, 298
Wang, Z., 38, 49
Warburton, D. M., 43, 50, 191, 195, 199, 201, 218–219, 228, 255
Warburton, E. C., 209, 215
Ward, N. M., 206, 219
Ward, R., 109, 111–112, 122, 170, 183, 318, 325, 337, 348, 364–365, 367, 378, 413, 423, 464, 482
Warm, J. S., 7, 15, 191–192, 200, 217, 222, 226, 242, 243, 245–246, 248, 250, 254–255, 529–530, 546
Waterton, J. C., 124, 142

Watkins, G. L., 154, 157
Watson, J. D., 107, 122, 131, 142, 384, 398
Watson, J. P. G., 131, 142
Watson, R. T., 26, 34, 145, 158, 495, 523
Watt, R. J., 307, 325, 329, 351
Weaver, B., 174, 185, 304–305, 325
Weber, H., 285, 296
Weese, G. D., 206, 215
Weichselgartner, E., 338, 346, 351
Weiller, C., 348, 389, 397
Weinberger, D. R., 240, 250
Weiner, H., 209, 215
Weinstein, E. A., 361, 380
Weintraub, S. J., 367, 380, 469, 482, 487
Weisker, I., 533, 546
Weiss, I., 171, 181
Weisskoff, R. M., 124, 142
Welch, J., 521, 525
Welford, A. T., 225, 255
Weller, R. E., 24, 34
Welsh, M. C., 449, 458
Wender, P. H., 445, 459
Wenk, G. L., 46, 50, 202, 217
Wertheimer, M., 301, 325, 335, 351
Wesnes, K., 43, 50, 171, 219, 201
Wessinger, M., 24, 31–31
Westheimer, G., 165, 185
Whelan, H., 495, 523
Whishaw, I. Q., 144, 159, 207, 218, 387, 392–394
White, C., 83, 91
White, C. T., 11, 14
White, P. M., 534, 543
Whitehead, R., 225, 255
Whitteridge, D., 167, 182
Whyte, J., 238, 255
Wible, C. G., 527, 537, 546
Wiesel, F. A., 528, 543
Wigal, T., 445, 448, 459
Wilder, J., 337, 349
Wiley, C. A., 475, 487
Wilkins, A. J., 240, 256
Wilkinson, L. S., 209–210, 218, 220
Wilkinson, R. T., 191, 220, 230, 233, 256
Willait, E., 448, 459
Williams, H. L., 230, 256
Williams, L., 445, 448, 459
Williams, M. J., 202, 217
Williamson, P. D., 151, 159
Williamson, S. J., 76, 93
Wilson, A. A., 154, 158
Wilson, F. A. W., 23, 34, 418, 423
Wilson, M. A., 55, 69

Winter, M., 533, 546
Wisbord, S., 394, 396
Wise, A. L., 241, 252
Wise, R., 384, 387, 389, 391, 396–399
Wise, S. P., 355–356, 378
Witte, E. A., 27, 32, 37, 40–43, 45–46, 50, 204–205, 220
Wohlberg, G. W., 528, 546
Woldorff, M. G., 81, 85, 92–93, 109, 115, 122, 465, 485, 537, 544
Wolf, A., 96, 121
Wolfe, J. M., 64, 69, 85, 94, 112, 114, 122, 164, 170, 174, 185, 259, 278, 328, 341, 351, 470, 487
Wolfe, V., 452, 457
Wong, A. B., 261, 276, 515–516, 522
Wong, E. C., 130, 140, 317, 323
Wonnacott, S., 37, 43, 50
Woo, C., 448, 459
Wood, B., 404, 419
Wood, C. C., 151, 159, 533, 542
Wood, F. B., 453, 458
Wood, N., 81, 94
Wood, S., 202, 217
Woods, D. J., 532, 546
Woods, D. L., 145, 147–149, 151, 159
Woods, R. P., 100, 107, 122, 131, 142
Woodward, D. P., 80, 92, 223, 251, 332, 349, 464, 484
Woolsey, T. A., 21, 31, 97, 99–100, 117
Worsley, K. J., 100, 122
Wright, M. J., 475–476, 487, 533, 546
Wright, N. A., 229, 249
Wu, D., 241, 252
Wu, J., 240, 250
Wurtz, R. H., 57, 59–60, 67–69, 103, 105, 122, 175, 183, 359, 379

Yamaguchi, S., 145, 147, 151–152, 162
Yamane, S., 172, 186
Yantis, S., 6, 15, 60, 69, 169–170, 176, 183–184, 186, 305, 310, 325, 355, 363, 380, 405, 423
Yap, G. S., 495, 522
Yarowsky, P., 97, 122
Yee, B. K., 209, 215
Yeh, Y. Y., 303, 324, 472, 482
Yeo, C. H., 201, 214
Yeterian, E. H., 28, 34
Yetkin, F. Z., 134, 139–140
Yin, T. C. T., 57, 60, 68–69, 356, 379
Yingling, C. D., 146, 161, 227, 255
Yokoyama, K., 240, 256

Young, A. M. J., 209, 215
Young, A. W., 383, 396, 521, 525
Young, M. P., 22, 34, 172, 184
Youpa, 453, 459
Yuh, W. T. C., 527, 542

Zacks, R. T., 466, 484
Zametkin, A. J., 454, 460
Zamrini, E. Y., 42, 49
Zattore, R. J., 388–389, 399
Zeki, S., 107, 122, 131, 142
Zhang, Z., 77, 92
Zilles, K., 207, 220
Zisper, D., 495, 525
Zubin, J., 150, 161
Zubovic, E. A., 231–232, 235, 256

Subject Index

Acetylcholine 37, 42–43, 192–193, 197, 201, 204–205, 228, 463

Aging and attention, 461–487

Alertness. *See* Arousal

Alzheimer's disease and attention, 46, 195, 394, 461–487

Anatomy of attention, 25–30, 102–116, 405–409

Arousal, 27–28, 42, 227–229
  and attention, 189–220
  and vigilance, 44, 225–226, 229–234

Associative learning, 208–210, 538

Attention
  and alerting, 40–41, 203–205, 447–448, 455 (*see also* Arousal)
  brain imaging studies of, 95–142, 239–241, 362–377, 405–408, 453–455
  computational models of, 163–186, 538
  cognitive neuroscience and, 8–12
  covert, 164–166, 203–205, 299–301, 305, 464–472 (*see also* Orienting)
  development of, 415–416, 426–443
  in discrimination tasks, 61–63, 85, 105, 109, 115, 193–194, 202–203, 222, 231, 237, 285, 292, 335–336, 337, 344–345, 364–365, 465–470
  divided, 105–107, 190, 202–203, 306–309, 312, 327–351, 448
  executive (*see* Attention control)
  and eye movements, 59–60, 165–166, 170, 285, 358, 356, 468–469
  feature-based, 64–65, 89, 172–174, 259, 280–281, 329, 344
  feature- vs. object-based, 104–107
  in infants, 415–417, 428–438
  and language, 381–399
  location- vs. object-based, 58, 108–116, 136–137, 168–169, 302–306
  in monkeys, 35–69, 204, 234, 309, 355–359, 432–433

neurochemistry of, 35–50

neurophysiology of, 51–69, 329–332, 355–361

neurotransmitter systems, 37–38, 195–197

in rats, 46–47, 189–220

in schizophrenia, 208–209, 527–546

selective, 6, 25, 30, 56, 58–59, 64, 71–94, 105, 131–132, 136–139, 163–181, 203–205, 302, 353–380, 448–449, 461–487, 530–536

short-term memory, 113–114, 295

spatial, 109–113, 165, 191, 203–205, 353–380, 428–433 (*see also* visuospatial)

to surfaces vs. features, 286–289

sustained, 43–44, 190–192, 145–146, 149, 435–436, 448–449, 528–529 (*see also* Vigilance)

varieties of, 4–8

and visual object segmentation, 299–325

visuospatial, 39–43, 58–60, 257–278, 463–470 (*see also* Orienting)

and visual search, 64–65, 85–88, 111–113, 169–170, 470–476, 506–507

and William James, 5, 170

and working memory, 44–45, 104, 113–114, 136–137, 146, 156, 171, 172–173, 248, 353–380

Attention control, 7–8, 104, 113–116, 131, 139, 149, 154–155, 168–172, 210–211, 236, 242, 335, 367, 385, 401–423, 447–448, 450–452, 455, 537

Attention-deficit/hyperactivity disorder (ADHD), 445–460

Attentional blink, 404

Attentional resources, 44, 47, 58, 79–80, 165, 168, 190, 282–286, 385–386

Automaticity, 394–395

Balint's syndrome, 267–272, 313–314, 319–320

Brain damage, 143–162
Brain stem, 237–239

Central executive. *See* Attention control
Cingulate gyrus, 241–242, 385, 411
  anterior, 104, 114–115, 448, 455
Computational models of attention, 163–186
Cognitive neuroscience
  and attention, 8–12
  framework for, 9–10
Continuous performance task (CPT), 191–
  199, 237, 450–451, 528–530
Corpus callosum, 242–244, 454
Cortex, 22–24, 27–28, 84, 103–108, 177,
  179, 197–199, 387–388, 411–412, 429–
  431, 465, 477–478
  dorsolateral prefrontal cortex and attention,
  145–155
  parietal cortex and attention, 57–58, 111–
  112, 145–155, 356–357, 502–503
  prefrontal cortex, 172–173, 239–241, 355–
  356, 432–433
  temporal cortex and attention, 57–58, 502–
  503
Cortical lesions, 22, 112, 143–162, 197–199,
  266–267, 361–362, 412–417, 434, 499–
  502
Cytotoxic lesions, 45–47

Dopamine, 38, 42, 206–211, 418, 526–527,
  533
Dual-task performance, 285, 334–344

Early selection theory, 80–84. *See also*
  Filtering
Electroencephalogram (EEG), 72, 229–231
Event-related potentials, 11, 71–94, 145–153,
  364, 386, 391–394, 409–412, 533–535
  and eye movements, 79
  generation and localization of, 73–77
  and vigilance, 230–235
Extinction, 207, 317–318, 499–507
Eye movements, 265–266, 274, 435

Feature integration theory (FIT), 113, 169–
  170, 258–260, 310, 470
Feature-specific surround inhibition, 329–330
Filtering, 35, 63
Frontal lobe. *See* Cortex, frontal
Functional magnetic resonance imaging
  (fMRI), 78, 123–142
  and blood oxygen level dependent (BOLD)
  technique, 124–125

data analysis, 129–130
fast, 125
physical basis of, 123–124
signal changes associated with attention,
  130–139

Gestalt grouping, 287, 301–302, 335, 510–
  514

Histamine, 38

Language and resource allocation, 385–386
Late selection theory, 11

Memory, 154, 389–390, 415. *See also*
  Working memory; Short-term memory

Neglect, 19, 313–318, 489–524
  arising from subcortical lesions in animals,
  205–207
  axis-based, 316
  figure-based, 314–316
  hemispatial, 490–494
  object-based, 514–515
  perceptual and motor components of, 496–
  497
  and visual search, 260–266
Neuroanatomy
  principles of anatomical organization, 22–25
  tract tracing methods, 20–21
Neurons, 74, 109, 113
  discharge activity of, 52, 97
  integration and coding of information by,
  52–54, 177–179
Nicotine, 43, 195, 201, 205
Noradrenaline, 37–38, 41–47, 104, 194–195,
  228, 453

Orienting, 29, 39–41, 43, 59–60, 104, 203–
  205, 332–333, 428–438, 447–448, 455,
  499–508

Pop-out, 112, 279–298, 329–333, 340–345
Positron emission tomography (PET), 73, 95–
  122, 154, 241, 244, 363–364
Prepulse inhibition, 207–208
Psychopharmacology, 189–220

Regional cerebral blood flow (rCBF), 97–102

Saliency map, 177
Semantic processing, 533–534, 391–393
Sensory gating, 81, 146–148, 207–208, 531

Serotonin, 38
Schizophrenia, 414–415, 527–546
Short-term memory, 113–114. *See also*
    Working memory
Single-cell recordings, 52–57, 103, 355–361
Stroop task, 406–409, 452

Vigilance, 7, 28–29, 199–202, 221–256, 450–
    451, 529–530
  arousal and, 44, 226–234
  brain regions subserving, 104, 235–244
  brain systems of, 221–256
  decrement, 222–226
  psychophysics of, 246–248
  tasks, short- vs. long-duration, 225–226
Vision, 329
  object and spatial vision, 22–23, 102–103,
    167–168
  visual processing pathways, 25, 132, 138
Visual search, 64–65, 85–88, 257–273, 279–
    298, 470–476
  and neglect, 506–507
  segmentation and, 309–310
  serial vs. parallel, 111, 279–280
  and texture segmentation, 328–329

Working memory, 128–129, 135–137. *See*
    also Attention and working memory
  spatial, 353–380